ANTIOXIDANTS IN HUMAN HEALTH AND DISEASE

Dedicated to

Professor Dennis V. Parke
Emeritus Professor, University of Surrey, England

in recognition of his pioneering work on the interrelationships
between nutrition and chemical toxicity

ANTIOXIDANTS IN HUMAN HEALTH AND DISEASE

Edited by

TAPAN K. BASU

University of Alberta, Edmonton
Alberta, Canada

NORMAN J. TEMPLE

Athabasca University, Alberta
Canada

MANOHAR L. GARG

University of Newcastle
Callaghan, NSW, Australia

CABI *Publishing*

CABI *Publishing* is a division of CAB *International*

CABI Publishing
CAB International
Wallingford
Oxon OX10 8DE
UK

Tel: +44 (0)1491 832111
Fax: +44 (0)1491 833508
Email: cabi@cabi.org

CABI Publishing
10 E. 40th Street
Suite 3203
New York, NY 10016
USA

Tel: +1 212 481 7018
Fax: +1 212 686 7993
Email: cabi-nao@cabi.org

A catalogue record for this book is available from the British Library, London, UK

Library of Congress Cataloging-in-Publication Data
Antioxidants in human health and disease / edited by
  Tapan K. Basu, Norman J. Temple, Manohar L. Garg.
     p.   cm.
  Includes bibliographical references and index.
  ISBN 0-85199-334-6 (alk. paper)
  1. Antioxidants--Physiological effect. 2. Active oxygen in
the body. 3. Oxidation, Physiological. 4. Free radicals
(Chemistry)--Pathophysiology. I. Basu, Tapan Kumar.
II. Temple, Norman J. III. Garg, Manohar L.
  [DNLM: 1. Antioxidants--therapeutic use. 2. Antioxidants--
adverse effects. 3. Antioxidants--metabolism.
QV 800 A6325 1999]
RB170.A584   1999
616.07--dc21
DNLM/DLC
for Library of Congress   98-33114
                                                                CIP

ISBN 0 85199 334 6

Typeset in 10/12pt Garamond by Columns Design Ltd, Reading
Printed and bound in the UK by Biddles Ltd, Guildford and King's Lynn

Contents

SECTION 4 Malignant Disease

SECTION 5 Other Diseases

SECTION 6   Indicators of Oxidative Stress

SECTION 7   Consumer Issues

Contributors

Christopher R. Barnett, Cancer and Ageing Research Group, University of Ulster, Cromore Road, Coleraine, County Londonderry BT52 1SA, UK

Yvonne R. Barnett, Cancer and Ageing Research Group, University of Ulster, Cromore Road, Coleraine, County Londonderry BT52 1SA, UK

Tapan K. Basu, Department of Agricultural, Food and Nutritional Science, University of Alberta, Edmonton, Alberta T6G 2P5, Canada

Adrianne Bendich, New Product Research, SmithKline Beecham Consumer Healthcare, Parsipanny, NJ 07054-3884, USA

H.N. Bhagvan, Tishcon Corporation, Westbury, NY 11590, USA

John Belcher, Department of Medicine, Division of Hematology, University of Minnesota, Minneapolis, 516 Delaware Street SE, Box 480 UMAC, Minneapolis, MN 55455, USA

Cynthia D.K. Bottema, Department of Animal Science, Waite Agricultural Research Institute, University of Adelaide, Adelaide, SA 5000, Australia

Yuriy V. Bukin, Cancer Research Center of the Russian Academy of Medical Sciences, Kashirskoe Shosse 24, Moscow 115478, Russia

Christina Bursill, CSIRO Division of Human Nutrition, PO Box 10041 Gouger Street, Adelaide, SA 5000, Australia

Chin Wern Chan, Department of Surgery, University of Western Australia, Hollywood Private Hospital, Monash Avenue, Nedlands, WA 6009, Australia

Clare Collins, Discipline of Nutrition and Dietetics, Faculty of Medicine and Health Sciences, University of Newcastle, Callaghan, NSW 2308, Australia

Andrew R. Collins, Rowett Research Institute, Greenburn Road, Bucksburn, Aberdeen AB21 9SB, UK

Kevin D. Croft, Department of Medicine, University of Western Australia, PO Box X2213, Perth, WA 6001, Australia

A.M. Dharmarajan, Department of Anatomy and Human Biology, University of Western Australia, Nedlands, WA 6907, Australia

Vladimir A. Draudin-Krylenko, Cancer Research Center of the Russian Academy of Medical Sciences, Kashirskoe Shosse 24, Moscow 115478, Russia

Peter H. Duffy, Division of Genetic Toxicology, HFT-20, National Center for Toxicological Research, 3900 N.C.T.R. Road, Jefferson, AR 72079, USA

Mária Dušinská, Institute of Preventive and Clinical Medicine, Limbová 14, 83301 Bratislava, Slovakia

Esther Epstein, Jean Mayer USDA Human Nutrition Research Center on Aging, Tufts University, Boston, MA 02111, USA

Efi Farmakalidis, Austral Health, 17 Warwick Street, Killara, NSW 2071, Australia

Manohar Garg, Discipline of Nutrition and Dietetics, Faculty of Medicine and Health Sciences, Level 3, Medical Sciences Building, University of Newcastle, Callaghan, NSW 2308, Australia

Peter Greenwald, Division of Cancer Prevention, National Cancer Institute, Building 31, Room 10A52, National Institutes of Health, Bethesda, MD 20892, USA,

Myron Gross, Division of Epidemiology, University of Minnesota, 1300 S. 2nd Street Suite 300, Minneapolis, MN 55455, USA

Amod Gupta, Department of Ophthalmology, Postgraduate Institute of Medical Education and Research, Chandigarh 160012, India

Mary Hannon-Fletcher, Cancer and Ageing Research Group, University of Ulster, Cromore Road, Coleraine, County Londonderry BT52 1SA, UK

Ronald W. Hart, Office of the Director, HFT-20, National Center for Toxicological Research, 3900 N.C.T.R. Road, Jefferson, AR 72079, USA

Nazlin K. Howell, School of Biological Sciences, University of Surrey, Guildford, Surrey GU2 5XH, UK

Thomas A. Hughes, Department of Medicine, Division of Endocrinology, University of Tennessee-Memphis, 340M William Bowld Hospital, Memphis, TN 38105, USA

Ciara Hughes, Cancer and Ageing Research Group, University of Ulster, Cromore Road, Coleraine, County Londonderry BT52 1SA, UK

Costas Ioannides, Molecular Toxicology Group, School of Biological Sciences, University of Surrey, Guildford, Surrey GU2 5XH, UK

Paul Jacques, Jean Mayer USDA Human Nutrition Research Center on Aging, Tufts University, Boston, MA 02111, USA

Sushil K. Jain, Departments of Pediatrics, Physiology and Biochemistry and Molecular Biology, Louisiana State University Medical Center, Shreveport, LA 71130, USA

David Kritchevsky, The Wistar Institute of Anatomy and Biology, Philadelphia, PA 19104, USA

Stephen B. Kritchevsky, Department of Preventive Medicine, University of Tennessee-Memphis, 66 North Pauline Avenue, Suite 633, Memphis, TN 38105, USA

Fred A. Kummerow, University of Illinois, Burnsides Research Laboratory, 1208 W. Pennsylvania Avenue, Urbana, IL 61801, USA

Simon Laws, Department of Surgery, University of Western Australia, Hollywood Private Hospital, Monash Avenue, Nedlands, WA 6009, Australia

Ján Lietava, 2nd Department of Internal Medicine, Comenius University, Mickiewičová 13, 81369 Bratislava, Slovakia

Philippa M. Lyons Wall, Human Nutrition Unit, Department of Biochemistry, University of Sydney, Sydney, NSW 2006, Australia

Mohamedain M. Mahfouz, University of Illinois, Burnsides Research Laboratory, 1208 W. Pennsylvania Avenue, Urbana, IL 61801, USA

Ralph N. Martins, Department of Surgery, University of Western Australia, Hollywood Private Hospital, Monash Avenue, Nedlands, WA 6009, Australia

Sharon S. McDonald, The Scientific Consulting Group, Inc., 656 Quince Orchard Road, Suite 210, Gaithersburg, MD 20878, USA

Kenneth W. Moles, Altnagelvin Area Hospital, Glenshane Road, Londonderry BT47 1SB, UK

M. Moshiri, Rajai Cardiovascular Research Centre, Vali Ars Avenue, Tehran, Iran

Ravindra Nath, Department of Experimental Medicine and Biotechnology, Postgraduate Institute of Medical Education and Research, Chandigarh 160012, India

Etsuo Niki, Research Center for Advanced Science and Technology, University of Tokyo, 4-6-1 Komaba, Meguro, Tokyo 153, Japan

Kimihiro Nishino, Research Center for Advanced Science and Technology, University of Tokyo, 4-6-1 Komaba, Meguro, Tokyo 153, Japan

Noriko Noguchi, Research Center for Advanced Science and Technology, University of Tokyo, 4-6-1 Komaba, Meguro, Tokyo 153, Japan

Maurice J. O'Kane, Altnagelvin Area Hospital, Glenshane Road, Londonderry BT47 1SB, UK

Begoña Olmedilla, Servicio de Nutrición, Clínica Puerta de Hierro, San Martin de Porres 4, 28035 Madrid, Spain

Sebely Pal, CSIRO Division of Human Nutrition, PO Box 10041 Gouger Street, Adelaide, SA 5000, Australia

Surinder S. Pandav, Department of Ophthalmology, Postgraduate Institute of Medical Education and Research, Chandigarh 160012, India

Dennis V. Parke, Division of Molecular Toxicology, School of Biological Sciences, University of Surrey, Guildford, Surrey GU2 5XH, UK

Walter J. Perrig, Institute of Psychology, University of Bern, Muesmattstrasse 45, CH-3000 Bern 9, Switzerland

Pasqualina Perrig, Institute of Psychology, University of Bern, Muesmattstrasse 45, CH-3000 Bern 9, Switzerland

Rajendra Prasad, Department of Biochemistry, Postgraduate Institute of Medical Education and Research, Chandigarh 160012, India

P. Quaggiotto, Discipline of Nutrition and Dietetics, Faculty of Medicine and Health Sciences, Level 3, Medical Sciences Building, University of Newcastle, Callaghan, NSW 2308, Australia

Katarína Rašlová, Institute of Preventive and Clinical Medicine, Limbová 14, 83301 Bratislava, Slovakia

S.S. Rastogi, Centre for Diabetes and Clinical Nutrition, 112 Saini Enclave, Vikas Marg, Delhi 110092, India

Ravinder Reddy, University of Pittsburgh Medical Center, Western Psychiatric Institute and Clinic, 3811 O'Hara Street, Pittsburgh, PA 15213, USA

Paul D. Roach, CSIRO Division of Human Nutrition, PO Box 10041 Gouger Street, Adelaide, SA 5000, Australia

Suhur Saeed, School of Biological Sciences, University of Surrey, Guildford, Surrey GU2 5XH, UK

Samir Samman, Human Nutrition Unit, Department of Biochemistry, University of Sydney, Sydney, NSW 2006, Australia

Honglian Shi, Research Center for Advanced Science and Technology, University of Tokyo, 4-6-1 Komaba, Meguro, Tokyo 153, Japan

R.B. Singh, Medical Hospital and Research Centre, Civil Lines, Moradabad-10, (U.P.) 244 001, India

Susan Southon, Institute of Food Research, Norwich Research Park, Colney, Norwich NR4 7UA, UK

Hannes B. Stähelin, Institute of Psychology, University of Bern, Muesmattstrasse 45, CH-3000 Bern 9, Switzerland

Allen Taylor, Jean Mayer USDA Human Nutrition Research Center on Aging, Tufts University, Boston, MA 02111, USA

Rajinder Thakur, Department of Biochemistry, Postgraduate Institute of Medical Education and Research, Chandigarh 160012, India

Angelo Turturro, Division of Biometry and Risk Assessment, HFT-20, National Center for Toxicological Research, 3900 N.C.T.R. Road, Jefferson, AR 72079, USA

Gerlad Veurink, Department of Surgery, University of Western Australia, Hollywood Private Hospital, Monash Avenue, Nedlands, WA 6009, Australia

Emma Waddington, Department of Surgery, University of Western Australia, Hollywood Private Hospital, Monash Avenue, Nedlands, WA 6009, Australia

Eiichi Washio, Research Center for Advanced Science and Technology, University of Tokyo, 4-6-1 Komaba, Meguro, Tokyo 153, Japan

Ted Wilson, La Crosse Exercise and Health Program and Department of Biology, University of Wisconsin–La Crosse, La Crosse, WI 54601, USA

Lisa Wood, Discipline of Nutrition and Dietetics, Faculty of Medicine and Health Sciences, University of Newcastle, Callaghan, NSW 2308, Australia

Jayne V. Woodside, Department of Surgery, University College London Medical School, 67–73 Riding House Street, London W1P 7LD, UK

Jeffrey K. Yao, University of Pittsburgh Medical Center, Western Psychiatric Institute and Clinic, 3811 O'Hara Street, Pittsburgh, PA 15213, USA

John W.G. Yarnell, Department of Epidemiology and Public Health, Institute of Clinical Science, Grosvenor Road, Belfast BT12 6BJ, UK

Ian S. Young, Department of Clinical Biochemistry, Institute of Clinical Science, Grosvenor Road, Belfast BT12 6BJ, UK

Gaoli Zheng, Department of Pharmacology, Zhejiang Academy of Medical Sciences, 60 Tianmushan Road, Hangzhou, Zhejiang 310013, People's Republic of China

Qi Zhou, University of Illinois, Burnsides Research Laboratory, 1208 W. Pennsylvania Avenue, Urbana, IL 61801, USA

Shoumin Zhu, Zhejiang Medical University, Research Centre of Nutrition and Food, 353 Yana Road, Hangzhou, Zhejiang 310006, People's Republic of China

Preface

The realization that reactive oxygen species and oxidative stress play an important role in the aetiology and progression of major human degenerative diseases has triggered enormous and worldwide interest in endogenous and exogenous antioxidants. The 1990s have seen the explosion of interest in antioxidants. There is now abundant evidence that substances in fruit and vegetables are potent preventives of various diseases, especially cancer, heart disease, diabetes and cataracts. With these recent developments in scientific knowledge which firmly establish the links between food factors and the prevention of disease, it appeared opportune and constructive to bring together some of the experts on these matters, to gain a better insight into the key food factors that are responsible for these health-giving benefits and how they work.

All of the experts approached were enthusiastically supportive of arranging the 6th World Congress on Clinical Nutrition (WCCN) on 'Antioxidants and Disease'. This scientific meeting was sponsored by the International College of Nutrition and held in Banff, Canada, on 23–26 July 1997.

Essentially, this volume emanated from the presentations made at the WCCN. However, some authors in this text were later invited for their contributions; this was to add any aspects that were felt to be pertinent for the scope of the book but were not covered in the meeting. As a scientific meeting, the congress was an outstanding success, as the chapters in this volume will amply testify.

This book is a timely publication, dealing with up-to-date information by scientists actively researching in the area of antioxidants and disease. The principal attraction of this book, however, is its breadth of scope. There are 31 chapters in seven sections, comprising: (i) Antioxidants and Their Mechanisms of Action, (ii) Food Factors as Antioxidants, (iii) Coronary Heart Disease, (iv) Malignant Disease, (v) Other Diseases, (vi) Indicators of Oxidative Stress, and (vii) Consumer Issues.

We wish to express thanks to Dr Ram B. Singh, the president of the International College of Nutrition, for sponsoring the 6th World Congress on

Clinical Nutrition, to Linda Callan, Judy Carss and other members for their unstinting help in the organization of the meeting, to the speakers and chairpersons for their excellent and stimulating presentations, to sponsors for their most generous financial support, and to Linda Callan for her invaluable service toward the preparation of this volume. Last, but not least, we would like to thank each of the authors for their contribution and for their cooperation and patience in revising and updating their papers. This volume is the result of special team effort.

Tapan K. Basu
Norman J. Temple
Manohar L. Garg

Acknowledgements

We gratefully acknowledge the following organizations who generously donated funds to support the 6th World Congress on Clinical Nutrition, held in Banff, Alberta, Canada, 23–26 July 1997:

University of Alberta (U of A)
Faculty of Agriculture, Forestry and Home Economics (U of A)
Alberta Heritage for Medical Research (U of A)
Hoffman-LaRoche Vitamin Information Centre, Canada

Hoffman-LaRoche Inc. USA
Dairy Farmers of Canada
Monsanto Canada Inc.
Matol Botanic International
Natural Factors
New Era Nutrition
American Journal of Clinical Nutrition
Carfax Publishing Company
Queen and Company Health Communications
Whitehall Robins

Foreword

The whole issue of the beneficial effect of antioxidants on cellular function and the maintenance of health in man has become a subject that has engrossed many scientific groups across the world over the last decade. Following the Second World War there was a complete change in nutrition and food policy in the West based on the recognition that animal protein, derived from either meat or milk, was particularly valuable in promoting the growth of relatively stunted children. The emphasis was on providing enough energy and high-quality food to sustain optimum growth in children. Fruit and vegetables were seen as a useful addition to the diet but these foods were required simply to avoid the development of such unusual problems as scurvy. It is little wonder, therefore, that in many societies there was a steady decline in vegetable consumption. Since the 1950s we have seen an emerging epidemic of chronic adult diseases, such as cardiovascular disease and cancer. Then slowly, with the development of biological insight into the pathophysiological processes, it became apparent that there were much more complex homeostatic mechanisms which were involved in preserving the integrity of cellular systems and tissue responsiveness into old age.

Over the last 10 years we have seen a plethora of studies looking at the importance of vitamin E and other antioxidant nutrients in cardiovascular disease, and there are now emerging very carefully controlled double-blind trials with nutrient supplements which attempt to discern the specific effects of the classic vitamins as well as the more newly recognized antioxidants, such as β-carotene, on the morbidity and, indeed, mortality of different population groups.

This book reviews and often presents new evidence on the whole gamut of effects which different bio-active components of the diet, derived particularly from fruit and vegetables, might have on different cellular processes, and on the health of population groups in many parts of the world. A reader who is not familiar with this field will therefore find a wealth of information and often, as is appropriate in a multi-authored volume, a variety of views on the relative importance of the antioxidant role of particular dietary compounds and the priority assigned to particular antioxidants. I very much hope that, as a result of the types of interactions embodied in this book, we can move forward to the point where we will have a much more coherent understanding of what is appropriate in establishing a new wave of nutrition and food policies which can indeed promote healthy ageing.

Professor W.P.T. James
CBE, MD, DSc, FRSE
Rowett Research Institute, Aberdeen, UK

Nutritional Antioxidants and Disease Prevention: Mechanisms of Action

DENNIS V. PARKE

Division of Molecular Toxicology, School of Biological Sciences, University of Surrey, Guildford, UK

Introduction

It has been known for 50 years or longer that much disease is caused by reactive oxygen species (ROS). At an international meeting of the World Health Organization in the mid-1960s, the distinguished Russian toxicologist, Professor Sanojki, presented a major treatise on the 'rusting diseases', a phrase not understood by many American and European delegates, but intended to mean diseases attributed to oxygen toxicity, such as rheumatoid arthritis. Since that time it has been increasingly realized that because of the ubiquitous biological toxicity of ROS, the similarity of ROS-induced pathology to that of many spontaneous diseases, and the relative ease with which ROS are produced, particularly by bacteria and other invasive organisms, much disease, from malignancy to cardiovascular disease and dementia, is associated with ROS. Indeeed, ROS are also responsible for ageing and death, and were it not for the existence of a highly effective biological system for antioxidant defence, life as we know it could not exist.

Sources of Reactive Oxygen

ROS, comprising the superoxide anion radical ($O_2^-\cdot$), the peroxide anion (O_2^{2-}), and singlet oxygen ($^1O_2$), are highly reactive entities, produced from molecular oxygen (O_2) by the gain of electrons, or the realignment of the electron spins. The hydroxyl radical ($\cdot OH$), the most highly reactive species of ROS, is formed by dismutation of peroxide catalysed by Fe^{2+}. The hypochlorite ion (OCl^-) is yet another highly reactive oxygen species which, together with the former ROS, is produced by leukocytes to kill invading microorganisms.

© CAB *International* 1999. *Antioxidants in Human Health*
(eds T.K. Basu, N.J. Temple and M.L. Garg)

The free radical, nitric oxide (NO), identical with endothelium-derived relaxing factor (EDRF), is an important cytotoxic molecule, active in defence against malignant cells, fungi and protozoa; it results in vasodilation and inflammation (Valance and Moncada 1994). It is generated from L-arginine, and contributes to the endogenous nitrosation of secondary amines; its formation is decreased in old age, hence the increase in fungal infections and malignancies at that time.

ROS are formed spontaneously by many biological processes, and may be considered as a measure of biological inefficiency, since they are formed by electron leakage from membranes and inadequately coupled reactions (Table 1.1); the released electrons reduce molecular oxygen stepwise to superoxide anion, then peroxide. Electron leakage occurs continuously from the mitochondrial membranes and the endoplasmic reticulum; also from the futile cycling of the various cytochromes P450 in the catalysis of microsomal oxygenations, especially with CYP2E1 which acts primarily as a ROS generator to oxidize resistant chemicals such as benzene and ethanol. ROS are also produced by activated leukocytes and protect the organism against bacteria and viruses, and initiate the mechanism of the inflammation (Parke and Parke, 1995). Other ROS-generating systems include the reduction of tissue oxygen by iron and other redox metal systems, the redox cycling of quinones, and as a side-reaction in the conversion of PGG_2 to PGH_2 in prostaglandin biosynthesis (Parke and Parke, 1995).

Table 1.1. Origins of reactive oxygen species.

Origins	References
Homolytic scission of water by ionizing radiation	Halliwell and Gutteridge (1989)
Leaking of electrons from membranes and reduction of O_2	Sohal *et al.* (1990)
Futile cycling of CYPs	Ekström and Ingelman-Sundgerg (1989)
Activation of CYP2E1	Ekström and Ingelman-Sundgerg (1989)
Reduction of tissue O_2 by Fe^{2+}/Fe^{3+} and other metal redox systems	Minotti and Aust (1989)
Activation of leukocytes in inflammation	Biemond *et al.* (1986)
Redox cycling of quinones	Powis *et al.* (1981)
Prostaglandin biosynthesis	Eling and Kraus (1985)

Mechanisms of ROS Toxicity

ROS are the mediators of inflammation, and through this their interaction with platelets, neutrophils, macrophages and other cells can involve the synthesis of eicosanoids and the activation and release of various cytokines, propagating the inflammatory process from one organ system (liver) to another (kidney, lungs, etc.). This results in tissue oxidative stress and multiple-system organ failure (Parke and Parke, 1995). Generation of ROS in experimental animals by induction of CYP2E1 by fasting, or by exposure to ether anaesthesia, results in tissue oxidative stress by depletion of tissue glutathione (GSH), and restoration of the GSH can prevent the oxidative stress and tissue injury (Lui *et al.*, 1993).

ROS-mediated inflammation is involved in the pathogenesis of infectious disease, including tuberculosis and septic shock (Welbourn and Young, 1992), and in immune and autoimmune diseases such as rheumatoid arthritis and inflammatory bowel disease (Parke *et al.*, 1991). More recent studies have also implicated the involvement of ROS in cancer (Witz, 1991; Ames *et al.*, 1993), atherosclerosis (Halliwell, 1994), hepatitis (Elliot and Strunin, 1993), AIDS (Baruchel and Wainberg, 1992), Alzheimer's dementia (Evans, 1993), multiple-system organ failure (Fry, 1992; Parke and Parke, 1995) and respiratory distress syndrome (ARDS) (McLean and Byrick, 1993). Molecular mechanisms of ROS toxicity and ROS-mediated disease, include: (i) oxidation of vital thiol compounds to disulphides, (ii) loss of tissue GSH, (iii) impairment of energy generation (ATP, NADH, NADPH), (iv) inhibition of Ca^{2+} transport and electrolyte homeostasis, (v) oxidation of cytochromes, (vi) DNA strand cleavage, and (vii) the initiation and promotion of mutations and carcinogenesis (Parke, 1994a).

Biological Defence Against ROS Injury

Biological defence against ROS comprises a complex array of endogenous antioxidant enzymes, numerous endogenous antioxidant factors including GSH and other tissue thiols, haem proteins, coenzyme Q, bilirubin and urates, and a variety of nutritional factors, primarily the antioxidant vitamins (Table 1.2).

Tissue GSH and other tissue thiols are the ultimate bastion against oxidative stress and tissue injury (Liu *et al.*, 1993), although these are maintained in the reduced state by the concerted action of tissue ascorbate, tocopherols and other reducing factors such as bilirubin and urates.

The cascade of endogenous antioxidant enzymes requires energy to maintain the living system in the reduced state. GSH reductase maintains tissue glutathione in the reduced state (GSH) at the expense of reduced NADP and FAD (Fig. 1.1). The GSH peroxidases reduce soluble peroxides (GSH peroxidase; GPX), and membrane-bound peroxides (phospholipid

Table 1.2. Antioxidant defence.

Endogenous factors	Endogenous enzymes	Nutritional factors
Glutathione and other thiols	GSH reductase	Ascorbic acid (vitamin C)
Haem proteins	GSH transferases	Tocopherols (vitamin E)
Coenzymes Q	GSH peroxidases (GPX and PHGPX)	β-Carotene and retinoids
Bilirubin	Superoxide dismutase	Selenium – essential dietary component of peroxidase
Urates	Catalase	Methionine or lipotropes for choline biosynthesis

hydroperoxide GSH peroxidase; PHGPX) to the corresponding alcohols, at the expense of GSH which is oxidized to GSSG (Fig. 1.2). The enzyme, superoxide dismutase, catalyses the conversion of superoxide anion radical to peroxide and oxygen, and catalase converts the peroxide to water.

These endogenous antioxidant enzymes and other factors operate a number of repair systems which: (i) reduce toxic disulphides and quinones; (ii) scavenge ROS; and (iii) reduce soluble and membrane-bound peroxides, etc. (Box 1.1). The vital repair systems require constant replenishment of energy (NADH and NADPH) and antioxidant vitamins to function efficiently. Ascorbic acid, α-tocopherol and GSH, interact as a complex system to reduce ROS and other oxidants (Fig. 1.1).

Mechanisms of Nutritional Antioxidant Defence

Among the various mechanisms for nutritional defence and disease prevention are: (i) ROS scavenging; (ii) reduction of peroxides and repair of peroxidized biological membranes; (iii) sequestration of iron to decrease ROS formation; (iv) utilization of dietary lipids (rapid energy production and ROS scavenging by short-chain fatty acids, ROS scavenging by cholesteryl esters); and (v) alternative biological pathways as occur in stomach cancer, multiple-system organ failure and diabetes.

ROS Scavenging

Dietary vitamin C, vitamin E and retinoids provide an integrated antioxidant system, with tissue GSH scavenging ROS and protecting tissues from ROS-induced oxidative damage, characteristic of acute inflammation and chronic inflammatory diseases. This ascorbate–tocopherol–GSH antioxidant system

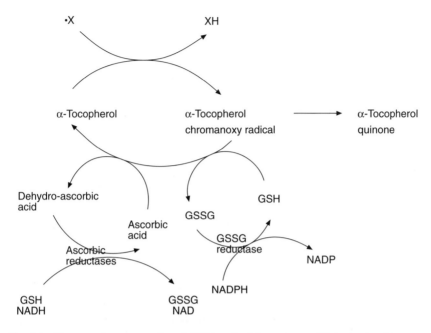

Fig. 1.1. The ascorbate–tocopherol–GSH antioxidant system. Biological oxidants and ROS (represented by ·X) are reduced directly by the tocopherols. The oxidized tocopheryl chromanoxy radical is cyclically reduced back to the tocopherols by ascorbic acid or GSH. The dehydro-ascorbic acid is cyclically reduced back to ascorbic acid at the expense of GSH or NADH, and oxidized glutathione (GSSG) is reduced back to GSH by NADPH in the presence of glutathione reductase.

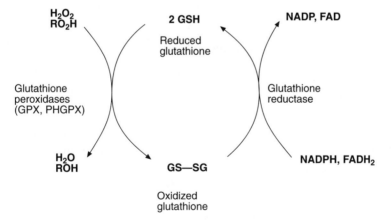

Fig. 1.2. Reduction of disulphides and peroxides by GSH reductase and GSH peroxidase. The GSH peroxidases are selenium-containing enzymes which reduce soluble peroxides by GPX, and reduce phospholipid membrane peroxides by PHGPX.

Box 1.1. Antioxidant nutrient repair systems.

Reduction of disulphides, peroxides, quinones, etc., by GSH, with GSH
   reductase and GSH peroxidase
Radical scavenging by the GSH/ascorbate/tocopherol system
Reduction of soluble peroxides by GSH peroxidase (GPX)
Reduction of phospholipid membrane peroxides by GSH phospholipid
   peroxidase (PHGPX)
Phospholipid membrane integrity, methylation of ethanolamine to choline, to
   prevent electron loss
Defence against NO nitrosation in stomach by ascorbate

is self-regenerating, at the expense of energy (NADH, NADPH) (Fig. 1.1), so
that as long as the subject is well-nourished, the integrated antioxidant system protects the individual against oxidative stress. Patients with systemic
sclerosis had lower than normal concentrations of ascorbic acid, tocopherols, retinoids, folate and vitamin B_{12}, and enjoyed lower dietary intakes
of fruit and vegetables (Lundberg *et al.*, 1992). Similarly, rheumatoid arthritis patients had lower than normal levels of blood and joint ascorbate
(Panush, 1991; Parke *et al.*, 1996).

Retinoids scavenge ROS and act directly on polymorphonuclear leukocytes to prevent their generation of hydroxyl radicals (Yoshioka *et al.*, 1986).
In addition to ROS scavenging by the natural integrated antioxidant system,
synthetic antioxidants, such as BHT (butylated hydroxytoluene), BHA (butylated hydroxyanisole) have long been used for this purpose as food additives, especially to prevent the peroxidation of lipids (Parke and Lewis,
1992).

Reduction of peroxides

Reversal of oxidative damage is also affected by the antioxidant defence system, thereby arresting progression into oxidative stress and tissue damage.
The dietary mineral element selenium is essential for this aspect of antioxidant protection and disease prevention, as it is a vital component of the two
peroxidase enzymes, GPX, which reduces soluble peroxides and PHGPX,
which removes lipid peroxides from biological membranes (Fig. 1.2).
Dietary selenium, as selenomethionine, protects against ethanol-induced
lipid peroxidation (Parke, 1994b), cirrhosis, cancer and cardiovascular disease. Selenium deficiency, through lower GPX and PHGPX activities, results
in increased formation of thromboxanes (TXB_2) at the expense of
prostaglandin (PGI_2) formation, leading to thrombotic and inflammatory
episodes and vascular injury (Schoene *et al.*, 1986).

Selenium deficiency has also been associated with Kashin-Beck and
Keschin disease (Diplock, 1993). Dietary supplementation of rheumatoid

arthritis patients with L-selenomethionine restored levels of serum and erythrocyte selenium and GPX to normal after prolonged treatment, but had no effect on leukocyte GPX (Tarp *et al.*, 1992).

Sequestration of iron

Among some of the most toxic substances known are the transitional metals, especially iron (Fe^{2+}/Fe^{3+}), as these are potent generators of ROS from molecular O_2. Since iron catalyses ROS generation, it is also highly effective as a biological catalyst of oxidation reactions, and consequently is found in haemoglobin, the mitochondrial cytochromes responsible for energy production, and the microsomal cytochromes which catalyse the insertion of oxygen into biological compounds to form cholesterol, the steroid hormones, bile acids and many other essential molecules.

Therefore, iron, from the time of its absorption from the gut to its incorporation into haem and other stable organic iron complexes (transferrin, ferritin) has to be sequestered in biological systems to prevent toxicity through ROS generation. Inorganic iron, or simple complexes such as iron nitriloacetate, are highly toxic and carcinogenic (Preece *et al.*, 1989), and intraperitoneal injection of iron nitriloacetate into rodents results in hepatic and renal necrosis, malignancy and death. Intramuscular injection preparations of iron have been extensively prescribed for use in Africa and other developing countries for the treatment of hookworm anaemia; their prescription in more advanced countries would not have been countenanced because of the high incidence of tumours at the site of injection.

Silicic acid, a ubiquitously distributed component of cereals and other foods, forms complexes with inorganic iron, which enable the safe sequestration of iron in tissues, decreasing its ability to generate ROS, initiate membrane lipid peroxidation, and to mobilize leukocytes (Birchall, 1993). Iron, *per se*, as oxygen-bridged ferrous–ferric complexes may initiate lipid peroxidation (Minotti and Aust, 1989). Dietary supplementation of iron-enhanced dimethylhydrazine-induced colorectal cancer in rats, but this was reversed by phytic acid, a component of dietary fibre, probably due to the chelation of the iron by phytic acid, with the consequent decreased ability of the iron to generage ROS (Nelson *et al.*, 1989).

Dietary lipids

The most common targets for autoxidative stress and oxidative tissue injury and disease are the biological membranes. These comprise a variety of lipids, including many different phospholipids and cerebrosides, short-chain and long-chain saturated, unsaturated and polyunsaturated fatty acids. This diversity reflects the multiplicity of membrane functions. The short-chain fatty acid, butyrate, is known to protect against ROS damage, inflammation and cancer (Hill, 1995), possibly by ROS scavenging, or rapid production of

energy. However, the most fundamental membrane function is electron conductance, which appears to depend to a large extent on the presence of
choline, a charged molecule, and a zwitterion [OCH$_2$CH$_2$N(CH$_3$)$_3$]; which
may facilitate membrane electron transport by Grotthüs conduction.
Deficiency of dietary choline or dietary lipotropes (vitamin B$_{12}$, folate, pyri-
doxal, glycine, PO$_4^{3-}$, etc.) (Fig. 1.3) leads to ROS production, lipid peroxidation, tissue injury, malignancy and death (Vance, 1990; Lombardi *et al.*,
1991; Schrager and Newberne, 1993).

Although much attention has been focused on the causation of coronary heart disease (CHD), namely by dietary fats and cholesterol, it would
appear that the mechanisms generally assumed by physicians are somewhat
incorrect. Firstly, dietary cholesterol has little affect on blood cholesterol
levels, and in any event probably leads to the decrease of cholesterol by

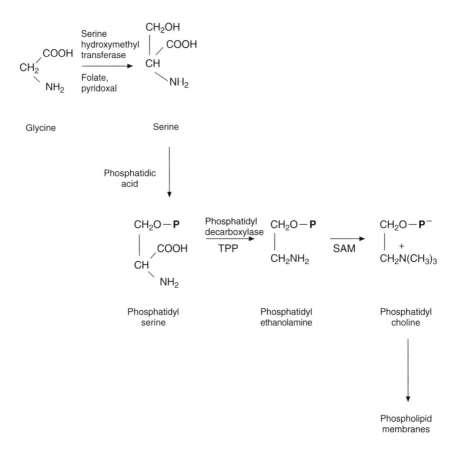

Fig. 1.3. Choline biosynthesis for membranes: choline occurs in the lecithins of
membrane phospholipids. SAM, *S*-adenosylmethionine (folate + vitamin B$_{12}$);
TPP, thiamin pyrophosphate; P, phosphatidic acid.

enhancing cholesterol 7α-hydroxylase activity and promoting bile acid production (Björkhem *et al.*, 1991). High dietary fibre keeps the bile acid in the
stool and hence removes the negative feedback of cholic acid on cholesterol
7α-hydroxylase. So for lower blood cholesterol dietary restriction is value-
less, but a high fibre diet is highly efficacious (Anderson and Tietyen-Clark,
1986). Most cholesterol is synthesized in the body where it is needed, from
fatty acids which may be derived from dietary carbohydrate (Lewis and
Watts, 1997). However, reduction of low-density lipoprotein (LDL) cholesterol by 35% led to a 40% decrease in adverse CHD events (Shepherd *et al.*,
1995). Cholesterol is relatively inert, but some of its polyunsaturated fatty
acid esters are highly peroxidisable, and form peroxyl radicals capable of
converting cholesterol to toxic oxidation products. Nutritional prophylaxis
in CHD should focus on prevention of lipid peroxidation, by the use of
antioxidants, instead of concentrating on cholesterol removal. Oestrogens
also act as antioxidant cardioprotectants; and oxidative damage of LDL,
which is implicated in atherogenesis, is inhibited by 17β-oestradiol
(Wiseman and O'Reilly, 1997).

Alternative pathways

Much disease is due to a sequential series of interactive phenomena, and
disease prevention can best be achieved by studying the mechanisms
involved and arresting one or more of the critical stages. For example, in
multiple system organ failure, a disease syndrome seen in critical infections
and accident trauma (Fry, 1992; Parke and Parke, 1995), systemic inflammation progresses from one organ to another, due primarily to the linking
of these different systems by the actions of the cytokines, eicosanoids and
ROS. A simple gut infection, or road traffic accident, or even elective minor
surgery, may lead to liver involvement progressing to hepatic failure. When
this is corrected by modern sophisticated medical procedures, inflammation
may not be totally arrested but may progress to the kidneys, then the lungs,
and even return again to the liver. The phenomena linking these organ fail-
ures are inflammation and the cytokines, and in addition to aggressive res-
cue and resuscitation by perfusion, nutrition and appropriate medication,
the use of antioxidants to arrest ROS production is indicated.

A further example is gastric cancer, now attributed to *Helicobacter
pylorii* infections, but known to result also from surgical vagotomy, and
from stress and trauma mediated by the cytokines (Fig. 1.4). A sequence of
pathological events has been elucidated, progressing from stress to inflammation of the gastric mucosa, to achlorhydria, bacterial invasion of the gastric mucosal barrier, depletion of antioxidant protectants, formation of
nitrosamines in the gastric lumen, mutations and malignancy (Parke, 1997).
Although the *H. pylorii* infection appears to be a most critical factor, this
microorganism is highly resistant to antibiotic treatment. A more successful
approach appears to be to administer ascorbic acid to inhibit nitrosation,

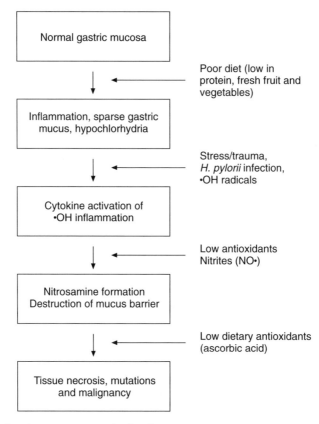

Fig. 1.4. Gastric cancer, stages in development.

and subsequently, with the aid of antibiotics, to eliminate the microbial overgrowth and restore the normal gastric equilibrium.

References

Ames, B.N., Shinenaga, M.K. and Hagen, T.M. (1993) Oxidants, antioxidants and the degenerative diseases of aging. *Proceedings of the National Academy of Sciences, USA* 90, 7915–7922.

Anderson, J.W. and Tietyen-Clark, J. (1986) Dietary fibre: hyperlipidemia, hypertension and coronary heart disease. *American Journal of Gastroenterology* 81, 907–919.

Baruchel, S. and Wainberg, M.A. (1992) The role of oxidative stress in disease progression in individuals infected by the human immunodeficiency virus. *Journal of Leukocyte Biology* 52, 111–114.

Biemond, P., Swaak, A.J.G., Penders, J.M.A., Beindorff, C.M. and Koster, J.F. (1986) Superoxide production by polymorphonuclear leucocytes in rheumatoid arthritis and osteoarthritis: *in vivo* inhibition by the anti-rheumatic drug, piroxicam, due to interference with the activation of the NADPH-oxidase. *Annals of Rheumatic Disease* 45, 249–255.

Birchall, J.D. (1993) Silicon and the bioavailability of aluminum – nutritional aspects. In: Parke, D.V., Ioannides, C. and Walker, R. (eds) *Food, Nutrition and Chemical Toxicity.* Smith-Gordon, London, pp. 215–226.

Björkhem, I., Eggertsen, G., and Andersson, U. (1991) On the mechanism of stimulation of cholesterol 7α-hydroxylase by dietary cholesterol. *Biochemica et Biophysica Acta* 1085, 329–335.

Diplock, A.T. (1993) Low dietary selenium and its relationship to human disease. In: Parke, D.V., Ioannides, C. and Walker, R. (eds) *Food, Nutrition and Chemical Toxicity.* Smith-Gordon, London, pp. 395–402.

Ekström, G. and Ingelman-Sundberg, M. (1989) Rat liver microsomal NADPH-supported oxidase activity and lipid peroxidation dependent on ethanol-inducible cytochrome P450 (P450IIE1). *Biochemical Pharmacology* 38, 1313–1319.

Eling, T.E. and Krause, R.S. (1985) Arachidonic acid-dependent metabolism of chemical carcinogens and toxicants. In: Marnett, L. (ed.) *Arachidonic Acid and Tumour Initiation.* Martinus Nijhoff, Boston, Massachusetts, pp. 83–124.

Elliot, R.H. and Strunin, L. (1993) Hepatotoxicity of volatile anaesthetics. *British Journal of Anaesthaesia,* 70, 339–349.

Evans, P.H. (1993) Free radicals in brain metabolism and pathology. *British Medical Bulletin* 49, 577–587.

Fry, D.E. (1992) Multiple system organ failure. In: Fry, D.E. (ed.) *Multiple System Organ Failure.* Mosby Year Book, St Louis, Missouri, pp. 3–14.

Halliwell, B. (1994) Free radicals and antioxidants: a personal view. *Nutrition Review* 52, 253–265.

Halliwell, B. and Guttteridge, J.M.C. (1989) *Free Radicals in Biology and Medicine.* Clarendon Press, Oxford.

Hill, M.J. (1995) Introduction: dietary fibre, butyrate and colerectal cancer. *European Journal of Cancer Prevention* 4, 341–344.

Lewis, B. and Watts, G.F. (1997) Paradise regained: insight into coronary heart disease prevention from recent clinical trials and basic research. *Journal of the Royal College of Physicians, London* 31, 263–275.

Liu, P.T., Ioannides, C., Symons, A.M. and Parke, D.V. (1993) Role of tissue glutathione in prevention of surgical trauma. *Xenobiotica* 23, 899–911.

Lombardi, B., Chandard, N. and Locker, J. (1991) Nutritional model of hepatocarcinogenesis. Rat fed choline-devoid diet. *Digestive Disease Sciences* 36, 979–984.

Lundberg, A.C., Åkesson, A. and Åkesson, B. (1992) Dietary intake and nutritional status in patients with systemic sclerosis. *Annals of Rheumatic Disease* 51, 1143–1148.

McLean, J.S. and Byrick, R.J. (1993) ARDS and sepsis – definitions and new therapy. *Canadian Journal of Anaesthaesia* 40, 585–590.

Minotti, G. and Aust, S.D. (1989) The role of iron in oxygen radical-mediated lipid peroxidation. *Chemico-Biological Interactions* 71, 1–19.

Nelson, R.L., Yoo, S.J., Tanure, J.C., Adrianopoulos, G. and Misumi, A. (1989) The effect of iron on experimental colorectal carcinogenesis. *Anticancer Research* 9, 1477–1482.

Panush, R.S. (1991) Does food cause or cure arthritis. *Rheumatic Disease Clinics* 17, 259–272.

Parke, A. and Parke, D.V. (1995) The pathogenesis of inflammatory disease: surgical shock and multiple system organ failure. *Inflammopharmacology* 3, 149–168.

Parke, A.L., Ioannides, C., Lewis, D.F.V. and Parke, D.V. (1991) Molecular pathology of drugs – disease interaction in chronic autoimmune inflammatory diseases. *Inflammopharmacology* 1, 3–36.

Parke, A.L., Parke, D.V. and Avery Jones, F. (1996) Diet and nutrition in rheumatoid arthritis and other chronic inflammatory diseases. *Journal of Clinical Biochemistry and Nutrition* 20, 1–26.

Parke, D.V. (1994a) The cytochromes P450 and mechanisms of chemical carcinogenesis. *Environmental Health Perspectives*, 102, 852–853.

Parke, D.V. (1994b) The role of nutrition in the prevention and treatment of degenerative disease. *Saudi Medical Journal* 15, 17–25.

Parke, D.V. (1997) Sixty years of research into gastric cancer. *Toxicology Ecotoxicology News* 4, 132–137.

Parke, D.V. and Lewis, D.F.V. (1992) Safety aspects of food preservatives. *Food Additives and Contaminants* 9, 562–577.

Parke, D.V. and Sapota, A. (1996) Chemical toxicity and reactive oxygen species. *International Journal of Occupational Medicine and Environmental Health* 9, 331–340.

Powis, G., Svingen, P.A. and Appel, P. (1981) Quinone stimulated superoxide formation by subcellular fractions, isolated hepatocytes and other cells. *Molecular Pharmacology* 20, 387–394.

Preece, N.E., Evans, P.F., Howarth, J.A., King, L.J. and Parke, D.V. (1989) Effects of acute and sub-chronic administration of iron nitrilotriacetate in the rat. *Toxicology* 59, 37–58.

Schoene, N.W., Morris, V.C. and Levander, O.A. (1986) Altered arachidonic acid metabolism in platelets and aortas from selenium-deficient rat. *Nutrition Research* 6, 75–83.

Schrager, T.F. and Newberne, P.M. (1993) Lipids, lipotropes and malignancy: a review and introduction of new data. In: Parke, D.V., Ioannides, C. and Walker, R. (eds) *Food, Nutrition and Chemical Toxicity.* Smith-Gordon, London, pp. 227–247.

Shepherd, J., Cobbe, S.M., Ford, I. and Isles, C.G. (1995) Prevention of coronary heart disease with pravastatin in men with hypercholesterolemia. *New England Journal of Medicine* 333, 1301–1307.

Sohal, R.S., Svensson, I. and Brunk, U.T. (1990) Hydrogen peroxide production by liver mitochondria in different species. *Mechanisms of Aging and Development* 53, 209–215.

Tarp, V., Stengaard-Pedersen, K., Hansen, J.C. and Thorling, E.B. (1992) Glutathione redox cycle enzymes and selenium in severe rheumatoid arthritis: lack of antioxidative response to selenium supplementation in polymorphonuclear leucocytes. *Annals of Rheumatic Disease* 51, 1044–1049.

Valance, P. and Moncada, S. (1994) Nitric oxide – from mediator to medicines. *Journal of the Royal College of Physicians, London* 28, 209–219.

Vance, D.E. (1990) Phosphatidylcholine metabolism: masochistic enzymology, metabolic regulation and lipoprotein assembly. *Biochemical Cell Biology* 68, 1151–1165.

Welbourn, C.R.B. and Young, Y. (1992) Endotoxin, septic shock and acute lung injury: neutrophils, macrophages and inflammatory mediators. *British Journal of Surgery* 79, 998–1003.

Wiseman, H. and O'Reilly, J.O. (1997) Oestrogens as antioxidant cardioprotectants. *Biochemical Society Transactions* 25, 54–58.

Witz, G. (1991) Active oxygen species as factors in multistage carcinogenesis. *Proceedings of the Society of Experimental Biology and Medicine* 198, 675–682.

Yoshioka, A., Miyachi, Y., Imamura, S. and Niwa, Y. (1986) Anti-oxidant effects of retinoids on inflammatory skin diseases. *Archives of Dermatology Research* 278, 177–183.

Potential Role of Antioxidant Vitamins 2

TAPAN K. BASU

*Department of Agricultural, Food and Nutritional Science,
University of Alberta, Edmonton, Canada*

Introduction

Oxygen-derived free radicals are the by-products of aerobic metabolism. A free radical is an atom or molecule with one or more unpaired electron(s). This electron imbalance causes high reactivity, creating other free radicals by chain reactions. These reactive compounds and their products (reactive oxygen species, ROS) are created through various physiological and biochemical processes such as mitochondrial respiration, the activation of phagocytes, the biosynthesis of endoperoxides by cyclooxygenase and lipooxygenase, the oxidation of various compounds by enzymes such as xanthine oxidase, and the presence of transition state metals such as Fe^{2+} and Cu^{2+} (Halliwell, 1994, 1996; Yucan and Kitts, 1997). Oxygen-derived free radicals and other pro-oxidants are important mediators in signal transduction and play a vital role in the production of biologically active and essential compounds. At the same time, however, they are toxic and known to inflict damage upon cells by promoting the oxidation of lipids, proteins and DNA to induce peroxidation, modification and strand break. In addition to the reactive agents derived from biological processes, humans are also exposed to environmental sources of pro-oxidants such as cigarette smoke, ultraviolet (UV) radiation and oxidizing agents (Schefller *et al.*, 1992; Gutteridge, 1994). There are, however, many naturally occurring substances, which function to protect against the potentially harmful effects of pro-oxidants. These substances, termed antioxidants, can be defined simply as chemical compounds or substances that inhibit oxidation. Antioxidant compounds must be present in biological systems in sufficient concentrations to prevent an accumulation of pro-oxidant molecules, a state known as oxidative stress. In recent years, oxidative stress is increasingly being implicated in the pathogenesis of many degenerative diseases, including coronary heart disease (CHD), cancer, diabetes, cataracts, and rheumatoid arthritis (Gey *et al.*, 1987; Jacob, 1995; Thompson and Godin, 1995).

© CAB *International* 1999. *Antioxidants in Human Health*
(eds T.K. Basu, N.J. Temple and M.L. Garg)

A variety of proteins and enzymes synthesized in the body may function as antioxidants. Such substances include catalase, selenium-dependent glutathione peroxidase, copper and zinc-dependent superoxide dismutase, uric acid and the transition metal-binding proteins, such as transferrin and ceruloplasmin (Halliwell and Chirico, 1993; Halliwell, 1996). Being derived from protein, the levels of these antioxidants are determined by their rate of synthesis, and therefore cannot be manipulated easily. In addition to these endogenous antioxidants, one can obtain oxygen scavengers from dietary sources. The common dietary antioxidants are tocopherols (vitamin E), ascorbic acid (vitamin C), carotenoids and flavonoids. Since these dietary antioxidants are exogenous in nature, their levels can be manipulated by supplements and dietary modifications. There also appear to be a variety of synthetic compounds such as probucol and butylated hydroxytoluene (BHT), with an antioxidant activity. The use of these compounds, however, is limited by their possible unwanted side-effects (Thompson and Moldeus, 1988).

The potential of dietary antioxidants to reduce the risk of coronary vascular disease (CVD), is gaining a great deal of interest in the medical and scientific communities. In this chapter the evidence supporting the use of naturally occurring antioxidants, with particular references to vitamins C and E, and the carotenoids in the prevention of atherosclerosis, will be discussed.

Oxidative Stress

The development of atherosclerotic lesions in the coronary arteries of the heart, if left untreated may lead to CHD, the leading cause of death in affluent communities (Simon, 1992). Atherogenesis is proving to be a very complex process to resolve. One theory is that this process is initiated by oxidative injury to the endothelial lining of the arteries (Fig. 2.1). It is postulated that oxidative stress leading to peroxidation of endothelial membrane lipids, may be cytotoxic to endothelial cells, thus compromising the integrity of the arterial wall (Esterbauer *et al.*, 1991). As part of the inflammatory response, monocytes migrate to the site of injury and begin to infiltrate the area beneath the endothelial lining. Due to some unknown stimulus, these monocytes differentiate into macrophages and begin to imbibe impressive amounts of lipid, whereupon they become foam cells (Steinberg, 1987; Esterbauer *et al.*, 1991; Naito *et al.*, 1994). This process leads to the formation of a fatty streak underneath the endothelium. Macrophages also secrete a number of cytokines that promote their own growth and differentiation, and cause the migration of smooth muscle cells into the intimal area. In addition, smooth muscles are believed to differentiate into a macrophage-like state, where they start to accumulate lipid and become foam cells. Furthermore, they secrete a number of cell matrix com-

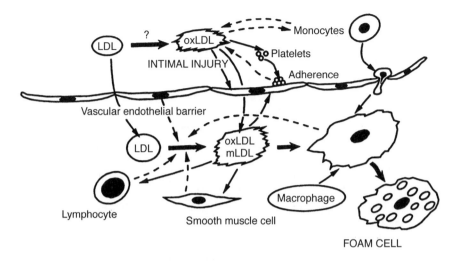

Fig. 2.1. A hypothetical model for low-density lipoprotein-mediated atherogenesis. (Reproduced from Shireman, 1996, with permission.)

ponents, such as proteoglycans, which contribute to the hardening of the lesion. At this stage, the lesion becomes a plaque, composed of cells, cell debris and lipid, laying underneath the endothelial lining. Continuous growth of the plaque leads to necrosis of the tissue, which may eventually block the circulation of blood, thus causing a heart attack (Gorog, 1992).

Oxidized LDL

Epidemiological evidence suggests that high concentrations of cholesterol in the plasma, especially in the form of low-density lipoprotein (LDL), is a high predictor of atherosclerotic risk (Kritchevsky *et al.*, 1995; Jailal and Devaraj, 1996). Why is LDL atherogenic? An emerging theory is that under certain conditions, LDL is susceptible to modification particularly by oxidation, and it is this oxidatively modified LDL that triggers foam cell formation. Oxidation of LDL has been shown to occur *in vitro* upon treatment with metal ions such as Cu^{2+} and Fe^{2+}, with cigarette smoke, and even with arterial cells, including endothelial, macrophage and smooth muscle cells. In fact, cigarette smoking, and high serum concentrations of Cu^{2+} and Fe^{2+}, are believed to correlate positively with incidence of atherosclerosis (Lynch and Frei, 1996). Iron is a major generator of free radicals (Herbert *et al.*, 1996). At physiological levels, the free radicals generated by iron are essential for cell regeneration, while an excess amount of iron could be potentially detrimental to the cell through generating large quantities of free radicals. There are, however, two circulating iron-binding proteins: transferrin and ferritin which, to some extent, counteract the toxicity of moderately excessive quantities of iron in the body.

In addition to endothelial cells, other arterial cells are also believed to be affected by oxidative processes, and the changes induced in these cells may contribute to the progression of atherosclerosis. Oxidative stress has been shown to stimulate chemotactic responses in macrophages and promote smooth muscle cell proliferation and differentiation (Steinberg, 1992; McMurray *et al.*, 1993).

The likely candidate responsible for the oxidative modification of LDL and arterial cells, is the oxygen-derived free radical. It is believed to interact with the lipid component of LDL particles and cause this lipid to become peroxidatively modified. Polyunsaturated fatty acids contained within the LDL particle are especially susceptible to attack by free-radical species (Yla-Herttuala *et al.*, 1989). These reactive compounds are capable of abstracting one of the double allylic hydrogen atoms on the carbon atom between the double bonds of the fatty acid. The reaction then proceeds as depicted below:

$$LH + R\cdot \rightarrow L\cdot \tag{2.1}$$
$$L\cdot + O_2 \rightarrow LOO\cdot \tag{2.2}$$
$$LOO\cdot + LH \rightarrow LOOH + L \tag{2.3}$$
$$LOOH + Fe^{3+} \rightarrow LOO\cdot + H^+ + Fe^{2+} \tag{2.4}$$
$$LOOH + 2GSH \rightarrow LOH + GSSG + H_2O \tag{2.5}$$

The product of a reaction between a free radical $(R\cdot)$ and a polyunsaturated fatty acid, LH (Equation 2.1), is the pentadienyl radical $(L\cdot)$, which can immediately react with oxygen to form the peroxyl radical, $LOO\cdot$ (Equation 2.2). This process may be propagated if peroxyl radical reacts with another polyunsaturated fatty acid molecule to form another lipid free-radical and a lipid peroxide, LOOH (Equation 2.3). Lipid peroxides may re-initiate this chain reaction if converted to a free radical (Equation 2.4). Instead, they may be converted to an alcohol (LOH) by enzymes such as selenium-dependent glutathione peroxidase (GSH), and thus become inactivated (Equation 2.5).

The pathological consequences of lipid free-radical and peroxide productions have been well documented, and they have been implicated for their role in atherogenesis (Steinberg, 1987). It has been suggested that the concentrations of lipid peroxides in the plasma correlate well with the severity of atherosclerotic lesions. It is believed that these reactive substances eventually react with apolipoprotein B (apo-B), the sole protein component of LDL, and promote its oxidation.

Oxidatively modified forms of LDL have been produced *in vitro* by treating the native lipoprotein with endothelial cells or copper (Steinberg *et al.*, 1989). The physico-chemical properties of this form of LDL (oxidized

LDL) have been shown to be different from that of native LDL (Esterbauer *et al.*, 1991). It has, thus, a greater density and increased negative changes compared to native LDL. The oxidation of lipids in LDL is characterized by the conversion of polyunsaturated fatty acids into lipid hydroxyperoxides with conjugated double bonds, called conjugated dienes. Further oxidation of LDL causes the conjugation of lysine residues of apo-B with lipid peroxide products such as malondialdehyde, and ultimately the fragmentation of the protein (Esterbauer *et al.*, 1991).

What is the physiological significance of this *in vitro*-modified LDL? It may be that LDL is similarly modified *in vivo* under oxidative conditions, and that this modified LDL is atherogenic. To test this hypothesis, Yla-Herttuala *et al.* (1989) extracted LDL from the atherosclerotic lesions of human subjects. This LDL showed physical, chemical and immunological characteristics of *in vitro*-oxidized LDL. The finding of this peroxidatively modified lipoprotein predominantly in the atherosclerotic lesions but not in normal human intima, suggests its atherogenic nature. Additional evidence for the occurrence of LDL oxidation *in vivo*, and its accumulation in atherosclerotic lesions was provided by others, who identified auto-antibodies to malondialdehyde-modified LDL in human serum and in the atherosclerotic lesions of humans and rabbits (Jailal and Devaraj, 1996). Furthermore, an epidemiological study reported that the titre of auto-antibodies recovered from the serum of a group of Finnish men was able to effectively predict the progression of atherosclerosis in these individuals (Salonen *et al.*, 1992).

Since the aetiology of atherosclerosis seems to involve lipid peroxidation, it is conceivable that processes limiting lipid peroxidation may retard or prevent the progression of atherosclerosis. In general, antioxidants function by impairing oxidative chain reactions involved in lipid peroxidation, converting reactive radical species to relatively inert compounds. Examples of antioxidants are the lipid-soluble group such as vitamin E and the carotenoids, and plasma-soluble vitamin, ascorbic acid.

Ascorbic Acid (Vitamin C)

As a water-soluble compound, ascorbic acid may be the front-line of defence against free radicals created by metabolism. Ascorbic acid has been found to react with hydrogen peroxide (H_2O_2), the hydroxyl radical ($\cdot OH$), peroxyl radical ($ROO\cdot$) and singlet oxygen ($O_2^{-}\cdot$), to form the semidehydroascorbate radical (A^-) and dehydroascorbate (A) as shown in Equations 2.6–2.9 (Thompson and Goldin, 1995; Duell, 1996; Kitts, 1997).

$$AH^- + \cdot OH \rightarrow H_2O + A\cdot^- \tag{2.6}$$
$$AH^- + O_2^{-}\cdot + H^+ \rightarrow H_2O_2 + A\cdot^- \tag{2.7}$$
$$AH^- + ROO\cdot \rightarrow RH + A\cdot^- \tag{2.8}$$
$$AH^- + H_2O_2 + H^+ \rightarrow 2H_2O + A \tag{2.9}$$

Ascorbic acid acts in the plasma to scavenge free radicals, dissipating these reactive species before they can react with biological membranes and lipoproteins. This was demonstrated by a study in which human blood plasma exposed to a water-soluble radical initiator, or to the oxidants generated by polymorphonuclear leukocytes, did not show any signs of lipid peroxidation as long as ascorbate was present (Frei *et al.*, 1989). In addition, plasma devoid of ascorbate but no other endogenous antioxidants, such as α-tocopherol, was found to be extremely susceptible to lipid peroxidative damage. Animal studies have reported that marginal ascorbate deficiency induced by diet leads to myocardial injury as evidenced by lipid peroxidation; this damage was prevented by ascorbic acid supplementation. Such observations have also been made in human studies. Thus, elderly subjects receiving 400 mg of ascorbic acid daily for 1 year, experienced a 13% decrease in serum peroxide levels. Similarly, ascorbic acid supplementation of 1.5 g day^{-1} for 4 weeks was shown to protect against the cigarette smoking-associated rise of lipid peroxidation by-products, thiobarbituric acid-reactive substances (TBARS) in plasma as well as in LDL. Ascorbic acid also has the ability to regenerate the activity of lipid-soluble antioxidants, such as γ-tocopherol and β-carotene, by interacting with biological membranes at the aqueous–lipid interphase (Steinberg *et al.*, 1989; Stadtman, 1991; Jailal and Grundy, 1991). The sparing effect of ascorbate on lipid-soluble antioxidants has been demonstrated essentially *in vitro*. Consistent with this finding, studies have reported α-tocopherol to be ineffective in cardiac tissue that contained relatively low levels of ascorbic acid (Jailal and Grundy, 1991; Sies *et al.*, 1992; Simon, 1992). Taken together, this evidence suggests that ascorbate may have a dual antioxidant function in biological systems: to inactivate damaging radicals in the plasma and to preserve the activity of lipophilic antioxidants.

According to many epidemiological studies, there appears to be an inverse relationship between ascorbic acid intake and mortality from CHD (Simon, 1992). However, the mechanisms responsible for this effect appear to be complex. In addition to preventing lipid peroxidation, ascorbate has been shown to affect other potential risk factors associated with the disease. There is some evidence that ascorbic acid lowers plasma total cholesterol by promoting its conversion to bile acids (Ginter, 1975). In addition, the atherosclerotic lesions seen in animals and humans with chronic ascorbic acid deficiency may result from increased vascular fragility secondary to a deficiency in collagen synthesis. Ascorbic acid supplementation has also been shown to lower blood pressure, possibly by influencing prostaglandin synthesis (Jacques, 1992). Ascorbic acid may thus have additional anti-atherosclerotic effects that are unrelated to its antioxidant activity.

Tocopherols (Vitamin E)

The most commonly found members of the vitamin E family in humans are the group of tocopherols, α-tocopherol being the most abundant and the most active isomer in this group. The other group, the tocotrienols are more highly unsaturated, and possibly more potent antioxidants, however, they are present in much smaller quantities. Once absorbed from the gut, vitamin E is transported to target tissues and cells via the lipoproteins. It is estimated that LDL carries about 50% of circulating vitamin E (Esterbauer *et al.*, 1991). Normally, an average of six molecules of α-tocopherol are present in each LDL particle. Other lipid-soluble antioxidants, including γ-tocopherol, β-carotene, and α-carotene are found in LDL in much lower quantities, one-12th, one-20th, and one-50th of the α-tocopherol concentration, respectively. The proximity of vitamin E to lipids in LDL explains its unique ability to directly prevent lipid peroxidation within the LDL particle.

Vitamin E functions by donating hydrogen to fatty peroxyl radicals, thereby halting lipid peroxidation. This antioxidant can potentially react with two peroxyl radicals, as shown below:

$$\alpha\text{-tocopherol} \rightarrow \alpha\text{-tocopherol} \cdot + \text{LOOH} \tag{2.10}$$
$$\alpha\text{-tocopherol} \cdot + \text{LOO} \cdot \rightarrow \text{LOO}-\alpha\text{-tocopherol} \tag{2.11}$$

The α-tocopherol radical produced in Equation 2.10 assumes a resonance-stabilized conformation, enabling the molecule to react with another peroxyl radical to form a stable adduct, LOO–α-tocopherol (Equation 2.11).

Vitamin E has been touted to be the most effective antioxidant for reducing lipid peroxidation (Jailal and Grundy, 1992). An abundance of evidence exists to support this claim. Epidemiological studies have shown that vitamin E is the strongest contributor to the inverse relationship between serum antioxidant concentrations and ischaemic heart disease (Gey *et al.*, 1991). An 8-year follow-up study involving over 87,000 female nurses has also found that women with the highest intake of vitamin E had a relative risk of CHD 0.66 of that of the group which consumed the least amount of the vitamin, after adjustment for age and smoking (Stampfer *et al.*, 1993). Experimentally, it has been shown that dietary vitamin E can ameliorate the development of spontaneous atherosclerosis in nutritional models of cardiovascular disease (Verlangieri and Bush, 1992). Atherosclerotic lesions in the carotic arteries were induced in a primate model over a period of time by feeding the animals a high cholesterol diet. α-Tocopherol supplementation was shown to decrease the severity of atherosclerosis and promote the regression of diet-induced atherosclerotic lesions. Studies involving rabbits have also shown that supplementation with vitamin E inhibits oxidative LDL modification, however, it failed to prevent dietary cholesterol-induced atherosclerosis (Morel *et al.*, 1994).

Inadequate dietary intake of vitamin E and its low plasma level have been shown to result in heart failure and death in a primate model (Verlangieri and Bush, 1992). Examination of the cardiac tissue revealed fatty streaks in the myocardium of all animals examined. Increased vitamin E intake of deficient animals restored serum values to normal levels and prevented subsequent death from cardiac disease. In humans, levels of vitamin E in the plasma have been shown to correlate inversely with the serum levels of lipid peroxides. Indeed, dietary vitamin E administration was found to decrease the susceptibility of LDL isolated from hypercholesterolaemic men to oxidative modification. Vitamin E supplementation of 600 mg day^{-1} had a protective effect against smoking-induced LDL oxidation (Harats *et al.*, 1989). Following 90 min of acute smoking, the plasma and LDL contents of TBARS were significantly reduced in subjects receiving α-tocopherol. Treatment of LDL with vitamin E, either *in vivo* by supplementing a diet with the vitamin, or *in vitro* by incubation of the lipoprotein with vitamin E has been shown to reduce the rate of TBARS formation in LDL samples incubated with Cu^{2+} (Esterbauer *et al.*, 1991). In fact the onset of lipid peroxidation, demonstrated by TBARS formation, occurs only after LDL is depleted of vitamin E.

As previously mentioned, the antioxidant activity of vitamin E relies, to some extent, on the availability of ascorbic acid. α-Tocopherol radical is thus reduced by ascorbic acid, resulting in the regeneration of the metabolically active form of vitamin E. Selenium is another antioxidant which is involved in vitamin E function. This trace element is a necessary component of the enzyme glutathione peroxidase (GSH). Like vitamin E, selenium-dependent glutathione peroxidase functions to inactivate lipid peroxides (Equation 2.5). The anti-atherogenic property of selenium has been evident in many studies. High incidence of atherosclerosis and CHD has thus been reported in populations with low serum selenium concentrations compared with those with adequate selenium (Salonen *et al.*, 1988).

Carotenoids

Like vitamin E, the carotenoids including β-carotene, γ-carotene and lycopene, are lipid soluble, and are therefore carried within lipoprotein particles. Normally, 1 mol of LDL contains only about 0.29 mol of β-carotene, 0.12 mol of α-carotene and 0.16 mol of lycopene (Esterbauer *et al.*, 1991). Carotenoids are thought to be highly efficient quenchers of singlet oxygen, $^1O_2$. At a low oxygen pressure (15–160 torr O_2), normally present in the physiological situation, carotenoids are also an excellent substrate for free radical attack (Sies *et al.*, 1992; Krinsky, 1993). β-Carotene has an added advantage of being able to trap more lipid free-radicals than α-tocopherol, the latter being able to trap a maximum of two. This is because of β-carotene's ability to form multiple resonance stabilized molecules as subsequent binding of free radicals occurs. The reaction of β-carotene (CAR) with lipid peroxyl radicals (LOO·), to form multiple carbon-centred radicals (LOO-CAR·, LOO-CAR-OOL, $(LOO)_2$-CAR-OOL·, and $(LOO)_2$-CAR-$(OOL)_2$) is depicted in Equations 2.12–2.15. Another unique action of the carotenoids is that as they trap singlet oxygen the energy is released in the form of heat, and thus a regeneration system, such as that required for α-tocopherol, is not needed (Sies *et al.*, 1992).

$$CAR + LOO· \rightarrow LOO\text{-}CAR· \qquad (2.12)$$
$$LOO\text{-}CAR· + LOO \rightarrow LOO\text{-}CAR\text{-}OOL \qquad (2.13)$$
$$LOO\text{-}CAR\text{-}OOL + LOO·- \rightarrow (LOO)_2\text{-}CAR\text{-}OOL· \qquad (2.14)$$
$$(LOO)_2\text{-}CAR\text{-}OOL· + LOO· \rightarrow (LOO)_2\text{-}CAR\text{-}(OOL)_2 \qquad (2.15)$$

A single β-carotene molecule is believed to eliminate up to 1000 singlet oxygens by physical mechanisms involving energy transfer, before it is oxidized and loses its antioxidant properties. The rate of oxidation of β-carotene is dependent on the oxygen partial pressure. The carbon-centred radicals are resonance-stabilized when the oxygen pressure is lowered. The equilibrium reactions (Equations 2.12–2.15) shift sufficiently to the left to effectively lower the concentrations of peroxyl radicals (LOO·); the rate of autooxidation of β-carotene is thus reduced. The reactivity of β-carotene towards peroxyl radicals and the stability of the resulting carbon-centred radicals are two important features that give the carotene molecule antioxidant capabilities (Burton, 1989).

In vitro studies have shown that 2 μM of β-carotene is more potent than 40 μM of α-tocopherol in inhibiting the oxidative modification of LDL (Jailal and Grundy, 1991; Woodall *et al.*, 1996). Further, populations who consume high levels of fruit and vegetables have been found to be associated with a lower risk of cardiovascular disease. However, a major problem in interpreting epidemiological studies is that there is uncertainty if the apparent benefits are due to carotenoids, or are related to other dietary or life-style characteristics. A randomized double-blind, placebo-controlled trial involving over 22,000 subjects taking 50 mg β-carotene on alternate days for 12 years, revealed no beneficial outcomes of β-carotene supplementations in relations to chronic disease (Hennekens *et al.*, 1996). The lack of a beneficial effect of β-carotene has also been reported in another study involving smokers and non-smokers taking 30 mg of β-carotene per day for 4 years (Omenn *et al.*, 1996).

Conclusions

Foam cells are thought to be the major constituents of the fatty streak, an early lesion associated with developing atherosclerosis. It is believed that oxidized LDL is responsible for the lipid loading of macrophages in arterial walls resulting in the formation of foam cells. Ascorbic acid, tocopherols and carotenoids are notable non-enzymatic dietary antioxidants, which could potentially reduce the rate of initiation or prevent the propagation of free radicals, and thereby inhibit the oxidation of LDL. Evidence to date suggests that the tocopherols play the most effective role in this respect; but their activities depend upon the presence of other factors, such as their reactivity and concentrations as well as the availability of their regenerating systems, including ascorbic acid and selenium. Ascorbic acid, on the other hand, requires cellular thiols such as glutathione in order to be regenerated from its radical form (see Chapter 1, Fig. 1.1).

The potential role of antioxidants in atherosclerosis prevention requires further study. It is possible that a cocktail of antioxidants is more effective than one individual antioxidant in isolation. More basic research including the unequivocal demonstration of oxidized LDL in the arterial wall, is important. The therapeutic use of antioxidant vitamins requires validation through prospective, randomized, double-blind clinical studies. All antioxidants can potentially become pro-oxidants subject to their concentrations. It is, therefore, critical that a guideline for an effective dose level for each antioxidant is formulated. Only then can antioxidant vitamins be recommended as a therapeutic tool for general use in the prevention of atherosclerosis.

References

Burton, G.W. (1989) Antioxidant action of carotenoids. *Journal of Nutrition* 119, 109–111.

Duell, P.B. (1996) Prevention of atherosclerosis with dietary and antioxidants: fact or fiction. *Journal of Nutrition* 126, 1067S–1071S.

Esterbauer, H., Dieber-Rotheneder, M., Striegl, G. and Waeg, G. (1991) Role of vitamin E in preventing the oxidation of low-density lipoproteins. *American Journal of Clinical Nutrition* 53, 312S–321S.

Frei, B., England, L. and Ames, B.N. (1989) Ascorbate is an outstanding antioxidant in human blood plasma. *Proceedings of the National Academy of Sciences, USA* 86, 6377–6381.

Gey, K.F., Brubacher, G.B. and Stahelin, H.B (1987) Plasma levels of antioxidant vitamins in relation to ichemic heart disease and cancer. *American Journal of Clinical Nutrition* 45, 1368–1377.

Gey, K.F., Puska, P., Jordan, P. and Moser, U.K. (1991) Inverse correlation between plasma vitamin E and mortality from ischemic heart disease in cross-cultural epidemiology. *American Journal of Clinical Nutrition* 53, 326S–334S.

Ginter, E. (1975) Ascorbic acid in cholesterol and bile acid metabolism. *Annals of the New York Academy of Science* 258, 410–421.

Gorog, P. (1992) Neutrophil-oxidized low density lipoprotein: generation in and clearance from the plasma. *International Journal of Experimental Pathology* 73, 485–490.

Gutteridge, J.M. (1994) Biological origin of free radicals, and mechanisms of antioxidant protection. *Chemico-Biological Interactions* 91, 133–140.

Halliwell, B. (1994) Free radicals and antioxidants: a personal review. *Nutrition Review* 52, 253–265.

Halliwell, B. (1996) Mechanisms involved in the generation of free radicals. *Pathologie and Biology* 44, 6–13.

Halliwell, B. and Chirico, S. (1993) Lipid peroxidation: its mechanism, measurement and significance. *American Journal of Clinical Nutrition* 57, 715–725.

Harats, D., Ben-Naim, M., Dabach, Y., Hollander, G., Stein, O. and Stein, Y. (1989) Cigarette smoking renders the LDL susceptible to peroxidative modification and enhances metabolism by macrophages. *Atherosclerosis* 79, 245–252.

Hennekens, C.H., Buring, J.E., Manson, J.E. and Stampfer, M. (1996) Lack of effect of long-term supplementation with beta-carotene on the incidence of malignant neoplasms and cardiovascular disease. *New England Journal of Medicine* 334, 1145–1149.

Herbert, V., Shaw, S. and Jayatilleke, E. (1996) Vitamin C-driven free radical generation from iron. *Journal of Nutrition* 126, 1213S–1220S.

Jacob, R.A. (1995) The integrated antioxidant system. *Nutrition Research* 15, 755–766.

Jacques, P.F. (1992) Effects of vitamin C on high-density lipoprotein cholesterol and blood pressure. *Journal of the American College of Nutrition* 11, 139–144.

Jailal, I. and Devaraj, S. (1996) The role of oxidized low-density lipoprotein in atherogenesis. *Journal of Nutrition* 126, 1053S–1057S.

Jailal, I. and Grundy, S.M. (1991) Preservation of the endogenous antioxidants in low density lipoprotein by ascorbate but not probucol during oxidative modification. *Journal of Clinical Investigation* 87, 597–601.

Jailal, I. and Grundy, S.M. (1992) Effect of dietary supplementation with alpha-tocopherol on the oxidative modification of low-density lipoproteins. *Journal of Lipid Research* 33, 899–906.

Kitts, D.D. (1997) An evaluation of the multiple effects of the antioxidant vitamins. *Trends in Food Science and Technology* 8, 198–203.

Krinsky, N.I. (1993) Actions of carotenoids in biological systems. *Annual Review of Nutrition* 13, 561–587.

Kritchevsky, S.B., Shimakawa, T., Grethe, S.T., Dennis, B., Carpenter, M., Eckfeldt, J.H., Peacher-Ryan, H. and Heiss, G. (1995) Dietary antioxidants and carotid artery wall thickness: the ARIC study. *Circulation* 92, 2142–2150.

Lynch, S.M. and Frei, B. (1996) Mechanisms of metal ion-dependent oxidation of human low-density lipoprotein. *Journal of Nutrition* 126, 1063S–1066S.

McMurray, H.F., Parthasarathy, S. and Steinberg, D. (1993) Oxidatively modified low-density lipoprotein is a chemoattractant for human T lymphocytes. *Journal of Clinical Investigation* 92, 1004–1008.

Morel, D.W., dela Llera-Moyaa, M. and Friday, K.E. (1994) Treatment of cholesterol-fed rabbits with vitamins E and C inhibit lipoprotein oxidation but not development of atherosclerosis. *Journal of Nutrition* 124, 2123–2130.

Naito, M., Yamada, K., Hayashi, T., Asai, K., Yoshimine, N. and Iguchi, A. (1994) Comparative toxicity of oxidatively modified low-density lipoprotein and lysophosphatidylcholine in cultured vascular endothelial cells. *Heart and Vessels* 9, 183–187.

Omenn, G.S., Goodman, G.E., Thornquist, M.D. and Balms, J. (1996) Effects of a combination of beta-carotene and vitamin A on lung cancer and cardiovascular disease. *New England Journal of Medicine* 334, 1150–1155.

Salonen, J.L., Salonen, R. and Seppanen, K. (1988) Relationship of serum selenium and antioxidants to plasma proteins and platelet disease in Eastern Finnish men. *Atherosclerosis* 70, 155–160.

Scheffler, E., Wiest, E and Woehrle, J. (1992) Smoking influences the atherogenic potential of low-density lipoprotein. *Journal of Clinical Investigation* 70, 263–268.

Shireman, R. (1996) Formation, metabolism and physiologic effects of oxidatively modified low-density lipoproteins: overview. *Journal of Nutrition* 126, 1049S–1052S.

Sies, H., Stahl, W. and Sundquist, A.R. (1992) Antioxidant functions of vitamins: vitamins E and C, beta-carotene and other carotenoids. *Annals of the New York Academy of Science* 669, 7–20.

Simon, J.A. (1992) Vitamin C and cardiovascular disease: a review. *Journal of the American College of Nutrition* 11, 107–125.

Stadtman, E.R. (1991) Prooxidant activity of ascorbic acid. *American Journal of Clinical Nutrition* 54, 1125S–1127S.

Stampfer, M.F., Hennekins, C.H., Manson, J.E., Colditz, G.A., Rosner, B. and Willet, W.C. (1993) Vitamin E consumption and the risk of coronary heart disease in women. *New England Journal of Medicine* 328, 1444–1449.

Steinberg, D. (1987) Lipoproteins and pathogenesis of atherosclerosis. *Circulation* 76, 508–514.

Steinberg, D. (1992) Antioxidants in the prevention of human atherosclerosis. *Circulation* 85, 2338–2344.

Steinberg, D., Parthasarathy, S. and Carew, T.E. (1989) Modifications of low-density lipoprotein that increase its atherogicity. *New England Journal of Medicine* 320, 915–924.

Thompson, K.H. and Goldin, D.V. (1995) Micronutrients and antioxidants in the progression of diabetes. *Nutrition Research* 15, 1377–1410.

Thompson, M. and Moldeus, P. (1988) Cytotoxicity of butylated hydroxyanisole and butylated hydroxytoluene in isolated rat hepatocytes. *Biochemical Pharmacology* 37, 2201–2207.

Verlangieri, A.J. and Bush, M.J. (1992) Effects of alpha-tocopherol supplementation on experimentally induced primate atherosclerosis. *Journal of the American College of Nutrition* 11, 131–138.

Woodall, A.A., Britton, G. and Jackson, M.J. (1996) Dietary supplementation with carotenoids: Effects on alpha-tocopherol levels and susceptibility of tissues to oxidative stress. *British Journal of Nutrition* 76, 307–317.

Yla-Herttuala, S., Palinsky, W., Rosenfeld, M.E., Parthasarathy, S., Carew, T.E., Butler, S., Witztum, J.L. and Steinberg, D. (1989) Evidence for the presence of oxidatively modified low-density lipoproteins in arteriosclerotic lesions of rabbit and man. *Journal of the Clinical Investigation* 84, 1086–1095.

Yucan, Y.V. and Kitts, D.D. (1997) Endogenous antioxidants: role of antioxidant enzymes in biological system. In: Shaihids, F. (ed.) *Natural Antioxidants: Chemistry, Health Effects and Applications*. AOCS Press, Champaign, Illinois, pp. 258–270.

Immunological Role of Antioxidant Vitamins

3

ADRIANNE BENDICH
New Product Research, SmithKline Beecham Consumer Healthcare, Parsippany, New Jersey, USA

Introduction

Free radicals, which are highly reactive molecules with one or more unpaired electrons, can cause damage to cell structures and consequently may adversely affect immune functions (Machlin and Bendich, 1987; Halliwell, 1995; Bendich, 1996).

Antioxidants interfere with the production of free radicals and/or inactivate them once they are formed. Three essential micronutrients are antioxidants and can act by either interfering with the propagation stage of free radical generation or act directly as free radical scavengers. Vitamin E (α-tocopherol), the major lipid-soluble antioxidant in cellular membranes, protects against lipid peroxidation and prevents the loss of membrane fluidity. Vitamin E has been characterized as the most critical antioxidant in blood (Burton *et al.*, 1983). Vitamin C (ascorbic acid) is water soluble and, along with vitamin E, can quench free radicals as well as singlet oxygen (Frei, 1991). Ascorbate can also regenerate the reduced, antioxidant form of vitamin E (Bendich *et al.*, 1986).

β-Carotene, a pigment found in all photosynthetic plants, is an efficient quencher of singlet oxygen and can function as an antioxidant (Krinsky, 1989; Bendich, 1993). Carotenoid-rich diets are consistently associated with reduced risk of many cancers (Ziegler and Subar, 1991); β-carotene supplementation has been shown to enhance natural killer (NK)-immune cell functions such as the killing of tumour cells (Garewal and Shamdas, 1991) and also increases the secretion of tumour necrosis factor from human monocytes (Hughes *et al.*, 1997). β-Carotene is the major dietary carotenoid precursor of vitamin A. Vitamin A cannot quench singlet oxygen and has less antioxidant activity than the other nutrients discussed, however its importance in clinical medicine (Bendich, 1994a) and for the immune system is well recognized (Bendich, 1993; Semba, 1997).

© CAB *International* 1999. *Antioxidants in Human Health*
(eds T.K. Basu, N.J. Temple and M.L. Garg)

The objective of this review is to examine the data from clinical studies on antioxidants and immune functions. As a number of these studies involved subjects over the age of 60, the effects of ageing on immune responses are reviewed as well.

Immune System Functions

The primary functions of the immune system are to protect against invasion by pathogens, to remove damaged or aged cells, and to seek out and destroy altered cells with the potential to cause cancer (Chandra and Kumari, 1994). The immune system can also become imbalanced and result in the development of autoimmune disease; there can also be the loss of immune responses (Bendich and Cohen, 1996).

Measuring Immune Responses

Non-invasive measures of immune function include documentation of infection rates, number of days of fever, days of use of antibiotics and consequent days of hospitalization. Invasive measures are defined as those which require either the non-oral administration of agents to the subject or the removal of blood or other internal body fluids. Invasive measures of immune function include delayed-type hypersensitivity (DTH) skin test responses discussed in detail below; blood sample analyses for number and types of white blood cells, antibody titres to vaccines, serum concentrations of acute phase proteins and virus concentrations. Determination of white blood cell classes has improved considerably with the advent of the fluorescence-activated cell sorter which provides an accurate and rapid means for determining subsets of immune cells, their receptors and their state of activation. Functional assays of immune cells, such as NK cell function, macrophage and neutrophil phagocyte functions, T and B lymphocyte proliferation as well as measurement of interleukins and cytokines (such as interferons) have also improved during the last decade (Bendich, 1996).

The major classes of lymphocytes are T cells and B cells. T cells are further characterized as helper, cytotoxic or suppressor cells, and T helper cells have been recently divided into T-helper 1 and 2 subclasses. T-helper 1 (Th1) cells are primarily responsible for cell-mediated immune responses, enhancement of interleukin 2 (IL-2) and γ-interferon production and cytotoxic T-cell activities. T-helper 2 (Th2) cells modulate antibody responses of B cells, and increase inflammatory responses via release of interleukins 4, 5, 6 and 10. B cells are responsible for secretion of all classes of antibodies as immunoglobulins (Male, 1996; Roitt et al., 1996).

DTH responses are mainly a reflection of Th1's cell-mediated immune functions. The DTH response is invoked by re-exposure to an antigen;

usually seven antigens are tested at the same time. The magnitude of the immune response is reflected by the summation of the number of responses and the diameter of the elevated area of the skin surrounding each site of antigen placement (induration), usually under the skin of the forearm, as assessed 24–48 h after exposure. In addition to Th1 responses, DTH is also dependent upon the interaction of antigen-presenting cells such as macrophages, cytokine and interleukin production, and inflammatory responses at the site of antigen exposure. A vigorous DTH response (increased induration) reflects the effective interactions of all cells and factors necessary to mount a similar immune response should an adult individual be exposed to most pathogens in the environment. The DTH response is also similar to the response seen post-vaccination with a common pathogen. Thus DTH is an indirect measure of an individual's capacity to mount an immune response to infection or immune-related disease. Clinically, DTH is equally important as an index of immune compromise; lack of DTH to all seven antigens is defined as anergy and is reflective of increased risk of morbidity and mortality, especially in the elderly (Marrie *et al.*, 1988; Christou, 1990; Wayne *et al.*, 1990).

Responses to vaccines are determined by the vigour of the antibody response to the viral or bacterial antigen challenge as determined by measuring the antibody titre in the blood. Th2-cell responses are required for proper formation and secretion of antibodies. The elderly may have an imbalance in Th2 responses which is seen in an overproduction of autoantibodies at the same time as reduced antibody titres are produced to flu and other vaccines (Chandra, 1992; Bogden and Louria, 1997).

Free Radicals and Immune Cell Function

There are numerous links between free-radical reactions and immune cell functions. White blood cell membranes, as with all cellular membranes, are composed of lipids containing saturated and unsaturated fatty acids. Unsaturated bonds in fatty acids are highly susceptible to free-radical attack, one consequence of which is to adversely affect the integrity of the cell's membranes. For instance, oxygen-containing radicals and the products of their reactions have been shown to decrease the fluidity of white blood cell membranes (reviewed in Baker and Meydani, 1994) and synovial fluids, consequently reducing their function (Merry *et al.*, 1989). Loss of membrane fluidity has been directly related to the decreased ability of lymphocytes to respond to challenges to the immune system (Bendich, 1990, 1994b). Free radicals can also damage DNA and result in mutations, altered capacity of cells to produce critical factors and derangement of the capacity to proliferate. Systemic free-radical damage is often measured by examining oxidative damage to DNA in lymphocytes. Duthie *et al.* (1996) have shown that supplementation with vitamins C, E and β-carotene significantly reduces endogenous DNA damage to lymphocytes and increases lymphocyte resistance to exogenous oxidative challenge.

Effects of Antioxidant Deficiency on Immune Function

One of the most obvious factors that could reduce antioxidant status is a dietary deficiency. Jacob *et al.* (1991) examined the effects of marginal vitamin C deficiency on immune and other parameters in healthy males. Serum, white blood cell and sperm vitamin C levels were significantly reduced when the daily diet contained 5, 10 or 20 mg of vitamin C for 2 months. DTH responses to seven antigens were also significantly depressed during the period of low vitamin C intake. In fact, when subjects initially consumed 250 mg day^{-1} of vitamin C, they responded to 3.3 out of seven antigens, which were reduced to less than one antigen after only 1 month at 5 mg day^{-1} of vitamin C. Even when intakes were increased back to 250 mg day^{-1} for 1 month, the average number of DTH responses did not increase above one out of seven antigens. The robustness of the responses (i.e. the diameter of the induration) was 35 mm at baseline, dropped to 11 mm when vitamin C intakes were 5, 10 or 20 mg for 2 months and increased to half of the initial level (17 mm) when either 60 mg (the current recommended daily allowance (RDA)) or 250 mg of vitamin C was consumed daily for 1 month. It is important to note that immune function did not return to baseline levels even though the serum and white blood cell vitamin C concentrations did return to baseline levels when vitamin C intake was increased to 250 mg day^{-1}. This carefully controlled study clearly demonstrates the importance of the balance between antioxidant status, oxidant levels and immune response. This study is especially noteworthy since all other dietary antioxidants, such as vitamin E and β-carotene were provided throughout the study at RDA levels and only one antioxidant, vitamin C, was reduced.

Several recent reports have noted that low serum vitamin E levels are associated with impaired immune responses. Von Herbay *et al.* (1996) reported that serum vitamin E levels were significantly lower in patients with severe viral hepatitis compared with controls and returned to control levels when the hepatitis subsided. These data suggest that hepatitis involves oxidative reactions which consume vitamin E and may consequently decrease potential immune responses to the disease. Comstock *et al.* (1997) found that lower than average serum vitamin E levels preceded the diagnosis of two autoimmune diseases, rheumatoid arthritis and systemic lupus erythematosus. Low vitamin E status has been associated with the conversion of an avirulent viral strain to a virulent one in an animal model (Beck, 1997).

Effects of Ageing and Antioxidant Status on Immune Functions

The cumulative effects of free radical damage throughout the life span are graphically seen in the pigmented age spots of the elderly which are a consequence of lipid oxidation. Oxidative damage to the lens of the eye is associated with cataract formation and increased concentrations of free radical-mediated peroxides are seen in several other tissues in the aged. Cumulative oxidative damage visible in the skin and cataracts of the elderly can also be seen in deposits of oxidized lipids in blood vessels (atherosclerosis) and organs. The overall increased oxidative stress associated with ageing is thought to also adversely affect many aspects of immune responses (Bendich, 1995, 1996).

Immune function impacts on the health and well being of all individuals, but is especially critical in the elderly because immune responses generally decline with age (Miller, 1994; Chandra, 1995). The consequences of suboptimal immune responses are particularly detrimental in the elderly, who have an increased risk of infections as well as immune-mediated cancers, adverse hospital outcomes and increased risk of autoimmune diseases (Meydani and Blumberg, 1993; Bogden and Louria, 1997).

The cell-mediated immune responses involving Th1-lymphocyte functions (cytotoxicity, IL-2 production, proliferation) are the most sensitive to the age-related decline in immune responses (Ernst, 1995). As a consequence of an imbalance between Th1 and Th2 responses, DTH responses to skin test antigens are significantly diminished in the elderly, and can often result in complete loss of response to antigen challenge (anergy) in the most immunosuppressed (Marrie *et al.*, 1988; Christou, 1990). Marrie *et al.* (1988) have documented the progressive decline in both number and diameter of skin test responses to seven test antigens in individuals aged 66–82 compared with those aged 25–40. They observed that 35% of those aged 25–40 had positive responses to five of seven antigens whereas none of the matched group aged 66–82 had five responses. Likewise, only 1.5% of the younger group were anergic (no responses to the seven antigens) whereas 18% of the older group had no responses. In addition to responding to fewer antigens, the older group also had approximately half the induration response of that seen in the younger group.

Clinical studies have shown that DTH can be used as a predictor of morbidity and mortality in the elderly (i.e. elderly with anergy had twice the risk of death from all causes as elderly that responded to the antigens) (Wayne *et al.*, 1990). Moreover, in hospitalized elderly who had undergone surgery for any reason, anergy was associated with a more than tenfold increased risk of mortality and a fivefold increased risk of sepsis (Christou, 1990). DTH responses are also indicative of morbidity within an age-matched elderly population as documented in a study by Marrie *et al.* (1988). They showed that those who lived at home and were self-sufficient averaged positive responses to two antigens and indurations of about 8 mm compared with those in nursing homes who were self-sufficient (1.1 responses and 4 mm induration) and nursing home residents that were not self-sufficient (0.5 responses and 1.7 mm induration). Thus, if micronutrient supplements could improve DTH responses in the elderly, the health effects could be substantial (Goodwin, 1995).

Clinical studies in the elderly: multivitamins

Multivitamins usually contain 100% of the daily value (100% DV – the new term which has replaced US RDA on product labels) of vitamins C and E (60 mg and 30 IU, respectively). Beginning in the 1990s, most multivitamins began to contain some portion of vitamin A activity as β-carotene (about 1–2 mg dose^{-1}). Average daily adult dietary intake of vitamin C is about 100 mg; vitamin E, 8 IU, and β-carotene, 3 mg. Thus the level of vitamin E in the multivitamin represents about three times the usual intake levels whereas vitamin C and β-carotene levels approximate usual intake levels (Alaimo *et al.*, 1994).

Intake of a one-a-day type multivitamin/mineral supplement for 12 months significantly enhanced DTH in healthy elderly compared with the placebo group (Bogden *et al.*, 1994). There was a less than 10% increase in both the number of responses and level of induration over the 12 months compared with baseline values in the placebo group but a more than 60% increase in the supplemented group. Because the multivitamin included β-carotene (approximately 1 mg), vitamin E (30 IU), vitamin C (60 mg) and all other vitamins as well as several minerals, it is not possible to determine whether the antioxidants or the other components in the multivitamin supplement were responsible for the improved DTH responses. However, it should be noted that the only significant changes in serum micronutrient levels were for vitamins C, E, B$_6$, β-carotene and folic acid.

Pike and Chandra (1995) have shown an increase in the number of NK cells in 35 healthy elderly (69 years average age) who participated in a 1 year, placebo-controlled, double-blind study involving a multivitamin/mineral supplement that contained 45 IU of vitamin E and 90 mg of vitamin C. There was a significant decrease in T-helper cells in the placebo group which resulted in a significant decline in the helper/suppressor ratio; this was not seen in the supplemented group.

In another placebo-controlled intervention trial, elderly subjects with marginal intakes of several vitamins were given a multivitamin daily for 1 year which contained approximately eight times the standard level of intake of β-carotene (16 mg). The supplemented group had significantly fewer infections than the placebo group. Responses to influenza vaccine, as measured by increased antibody titres, were also improved in the supplemented group (Chandra, 1992).

The ability to survive pneumonia and influenza is significantly reduced in the elderly (MMWR, 1995). Of the 20,000 pneumonia- and influenza-associated deaths reported in 1991 in the USA, more than 90% were in persons aged 65 and older. For bacterial pneumonia, there is a vaccine, which, however, is only 56% effective in preventing pneumococcal pneumonia, the most common cause of bacterial pneumonia. Currently, only 28% of the elderly receive pneumococcal vaccination; 52% receive influenza vaccination. Thus, it is especially important to improve immune responses in this at-risk population because another major consequence of reduced immune responses in the elderly is decreased effectiveness of vaccination (which can be predicted by reduced antibody titre following inoculation). Poor immune responses to vaccines, such as the pneumococcal, hepatitis and flu vaccines, can increase the risk of morbidity and mortality, especially in the frail elderly.

Clinical studies: antioxidants in the elderly

There is evidence that a supplement containing only antioxidants can improve the immune cell profile of aged hospitalized patients. Elderly, who were hospitalized for at least 2 months following a stroke, were given a supplement of 8000 IU of vitamin A, 50 IU of vitamin E and 100 mg of vitamin C for 28 days. Supplementation resulted in an increase in total T lymphocyte numbers and T-helper cell markers as well as enhanced lymphocyte proliferation. It is not possible in this study to differentiate either the direct immunoenhancing effects of vitamin A or its weak antioxidant effects, from the stronger antioxidant effects of vitamins C and E. Improvement in the immunosuppressed state of long-term, hospitalized elderly may decrease the prolonged morbidity often associated with respiratory infections seen in this population (Penn *et al.*, 1991).

Vitamin E studies in the elderly

One of the first studies to associate vitamin E status with immune function in the elderly was published in 1984. Chavance *et al.* (1984), in a retrospective epidemiological study, found a significant association between high plasma vitamin E levels and a lower number of infections in healthy adults over the age of 60.

Two placebo-controlled, double-blind studies conducted in the elderly have found that vitamin E supplementation alone can significantly enhance DTH responses, antibody titres to certain vaccines, and proliferative responses as well as IL-2 activities. In a carefully controlled study conducted in a metabolic ward where the daily diet contained approximately RDA levels of all nutrients, vitamin E supplementation (800 IU day^{-1}) for 1 month resulted in significantly increased DTH responses of healthy elderly subjects (Meydani *et al.*, 1990). Lymphocyte vitamin E levels increased over threefold with supplementation and were correlated with enhanced immune responses such as enhanced IL-2 production. The vitamin E-supplemented group showed no adverse effects (Meydani *et al.*, 1994a); in fact, the beneficial effects included enhanced lymphocyte proliferation, decreased production of immunosuppressive prostaglandin E2 as well as decreased levels of serum lipid peroxides. The subjects in this study all consumed meals containing the recommended levels of all nutrients including vitamin E while they were residents of a metabolic ward. Thus, the diets and environments of the placebo and vitamin E groups were very similar. The authors concluded that '... it is encouraging to note that a single nutrient supplement can enhance immune responsiveness in healthy elderly subjects consuming the recommended amounts of all other nutrients'.

Meydani *et al.* (1997) extended their earlier findings and examined the effects of 6 months of supplementation with 60, 200, or 800 IU day^{-1} of vitamin E in a placebo-controlled, double-blind study in healthy, free-living elderly subjects. In addition to DTH responses, they determined *in vitro* proliferation and *ex vivo* antibody titres to clinically relevant vaccines. DTH responses were significantly increased above placebo levels in all three supplemented groups; the greatest responses were seen in the 200 IU group. *In vitro* proliferative responses were highest in the 800 IU group. Antibody titres to tetanus were unaffected by vitamin E supplementation, but titres to hepatitis B vaccine were highest in the 200 IU group.

There is also growing interest in the potential for vitamin E to reduce cardiovascular disease (CVD) risk; CVD is the leading cause of death. There are data indicating that vitamin E's beneficial effects on monocyte function may be one mechanism by which vitamin E prevents CVD (Devaraj *et al.*, 1996; Lander, 1997; Martin *et al.*, 1997).

Vitamin C and E studies

In contrast to the extensive studies of the effects of vitamin E on immune function in the elderly, there have been neither many nor recent studies of the effects of vitamin C, a critical water-soluble antioxidant which functions to regenerate the antioxidant form of vitamin E (Niki *et al.*, 1995). In one study, DTH was enhanced in an elderly population following injections of 500 mg day^{-1} of vitamin C (Kennes *et al.*, 1983). In another study, oral supplementation with vitamin C (2 g day^{-1}) in an elderly population enhanced *in vitro* lymphocyte proliferative responses but did not affect DTH (Delafuente *et al.*, 1986). Jeng *et al.* (1996) examined the interactions of vitamins C and E on cytokine production in healthy adults. Vitamin C (1 g day^{-1}) did not increase either IL1-β or tumour necrosis factor production following 14 days of supplementation whereas vitamin E (400 IU day^{-1}) significantly enhanced both; the combination of both supplements resulted in a further, significant enhancement in production of these cytokines, suggesting a synergistic action on immune functions which had been reported previously in an animal model (Bendich *et al.*, 1984).

β-Carotene in the elderly

β-Carotene has traditionally been seen solely as a source of vitamin A activity. However, several studies have shown that carotenoids can enhance immune functions independently of any provitamin A activity (Bendich, 1994a). The mechanisms of immunoenhancement may include the antioxidant and singlet oxygen-quenching capacities. In animal studies, comparisons between β-carotene and canthaxanthin, a non-pro-vitamin A carotenoid, have shown that both carotenoids enhance T and B lymphocyte proliferative responses to mitogens, increase cytotoxic T-cell and macrophage tumour killing activity, and stimulate the secretion of tumour necrosis factor-α, and, at the same time, lower the tumour burden (reviewed in Bendich, 1991).

In a clinical study, vegetarians were found to have similar serum levels of all of the vitamins measured (including vitamin A) compared with a matched non-vegetarian population. However, serum β-carotene levels were twice as high in the vegetarian group. NK from the vegetarian group lysed double the number of tumour cells as compared to NK from the non-vegetarian group. It may be that β-carotene or other carotenoids enhance NK functions independent of provitamin A activity (Malter *et al.*, 1989). Kramer *et al.* (1995), in a preliminary report, found that carotenoid-rich vegetable consumption enhanced NK cell number as well as lymphocyte proliferation.

Carotenoids containing nine or more conjugated double bonds can quench the high energy from ultraviolet (UV) light and block the subsequent formation of singlet oxygen. Herraiz *et al.* (1999) have examined the effect of β-carotene in healthy elderly subjects who were exposed to a controlled level of UV light. In a placebo-controlled, double-blind trial, 32 males about 65 years of age had baseline DTH responses determined and then were placed on a low-carotene diet and all were given 1.5 mg day^{-1} of β-carotene (the USA average daily intake) for the duration of the study. The supplement, 30 mg β-carotene, or the placebo was taken for 28 days prior to UV exposure and a pre-UV DTH response was determined. The third and final DTH response was determined following 12 exposures over 16 days to a relatively low level of UV for 2–6 min day^{-1} for a total of 15 J cm^{-2} of UV light; the supplement or placebo was taken during this time. The placebo group showed a 50% decline in serum β-carotene between baseline and pre-UV whereas the supplemented group had a tenfold increase in serum β-carotene. There were no changes seen in the β-carotene-supplemented group's serum levels of the other carotenoids or vitamin E during the study.

Following UV exposure there were decreases in DTH responses. However, β-carotene supplementation at 30 mg day^{-1} protected against the UV-induced immunosuppression significantly better than 1.5 mg day^{-1}. It should be noted, however, that the 1.5 mg day^{-1} of β-carotene apparently did render some benefit because in an earlier, similar protocol, young men fed a β-carotene-depleted diet had significantly greater declines in DTH following UV exposure than was seen in the placebo group in this study (Fuller *et al.*, 1992).

Meydani *et al.* (1995) reported preliminary results from a short-term, placebo-controlled, double-blind intervention study in which elderly women (average age 70) were given 90 mg day^{-1} of β-carotene for 3 weeks and were not exposed to UV. Serum β-carotene levels increased tenfold in the supplemented group; there was also a significant 35% increase in DTH response ($P < 0.05$). There were no effects on mitogen responses, IL-2 production or total lymphocyte count and lymphocyte subsets; there was no report of effects on NK cell number or activity. Concomitantly, there was an increase in the antioxidant capacity of the plasma of the β-carotene-supplemented group (Meydani *et al.*, 1994b).

There have been several other studies to determine the effect of β-carotene supplementation on NK function in adults over 50. In the first published report, healthy middle-aged individuals (average age 56) were supplemented for 2 months with either 0, 15, 30, 45 or 60 mg day^{-1} of β-carotene. The groups given 45 or 60 mg day^{-1} had increases in the percent of T helper and NK cells, and a concomitant increase in immune cells expressing the IL-2 receptor (Watson *et al.*, 1991). IL-2, a cytokine secreted by activated T cells, is thought to bind to the IL-2 receptor on NK cells and result in proliferation. In this short-term study, however, there was no determination of either IL-2 production or the capacity of the NK cells to kill tumour cells.

Recently, Santos *et al.* (1997) examined the effect of long-term β-carotene supplementation on NK cell number and function as well as production of the NK cell stimulatory cytokine, IL-2. The study population was a cohort from the Physicians Health Study, a placebo-controlled, double-blind intervention trial to determine the effects of aspirin and/or β-carotene (50 mg every other day for more than 10 years) on cancer and cardiovascular outcomes. The subjects were divided into two groups based on age. The middle-aged (MA) group's average age was 57 and the elderly (E) were about 73 years old. These two groups were further divided into β-carotene (BC)-supplemented and matched placebo groups (P); both groups took aspirin every other day for at least 5 years. There was a threefold increase in serum β-carotene levels in the supplemented groups, regardless of age (Fotouhi *et al.*, 1995). Compared with the respective P groups, white blood cell β-carotene levels were increased sixfold in the MA-BC group but only 3.5-fold in the E-BC group. NK killing of tumour cells was significantly diminished in the E-P compared with MA-P group. However, the E-BC group had a significantly increased NK activity compared with E-P, which was increased to the level seen in the MA-BC group. No increase in IL-2 production was found although there was a non-significant decrease in prostaglandin E2 production in the β-carotene supplemented group.

Conclusions

The data reviewed suggest that critical aspects of immune function can be enhanced by improving the micronutrient intakes of certain population groups, especially the elderly (Kelley and Bendich, 1996; Bogden and Louria, 1997; Chandra, 1997). Well controlled clinical trials indicate that micronutrients with antioxidant capacity consistently improve delayed hypersensitivity responses in the elderly. This is particularly important as DTH responses decline with age and the decline is associated with increased morbidity and mortality.

The research into the immunomodulating effects of antioxidants, especially vitamin E, has also led investigators to examine the role of antioxidants in modulating immune cells involved in atherosclerosis and CVD. These data and the new research on alteration of the virulence of pathogens based upon the antioxidant state of the host provide many opportunities for further research into the role of antioxidants in the immune system.

Acknowledgements

The author thanks Dr B. Daggy for his valuable comments and Ms J. Miller for her assistance in manuscript preparation.

References

Alaimo, K. *et al.* (1994) Dietary intake of vitamins, minerals, and fiber of persons ages 2 months and over in the United States: Third National Health and Nutrition Examination Survey, Phase 1, 1988–91. In: *Advance Data from Vital and Health Statistics*, No. 258. National Center for Health Statistics, Hyattsville, Maryland, pp. 1–26.

Baker, K.R. and Meydani, M. (1994) Beta-carotene in immunity and cancer. *J. Opt. Nutr.* 3, 39–50.

Beck, M.A. (1997) Increased virulence of coxsackievirus B3 in mice due to vitamin E or selenium deficiency. *Journal of Nutrition* 127, 966S–970S.

Bendich, A. (1990) Antioxidant micronutrients and immune responses. In: Bendich, A. and Chandra, R.K. (eds) *Micronutrients and Immune Functions*, Vol. 587. New York Academy of Sciences, New York, pp. 168–180.

Bendich, A. (1991) Carotenoids and immunity. *Clinics in Applied Nutrition: Nutrition in Immune Function* 1, 45–51.

Bendich, A. (1993a) Clinical importance of beta carotene. *Perspectives in Applied Nutrition* 1, 14–22.

Bendich, A. (1993b) Biological functions of dietary carotenoids. In: Canfield, L.M., Krinsky, N.I. and Olson, J.A. (eds) *Carotenoids in Human Health*, Vol. 691. New York Academy of Sciences, New York, pp. 61–67.

Bendich, A. (1994a) Recent advances in clinical research involving carotenoids. *Pure and Applied Chemistry* 66, 1017–1024.

Bendich, A. (1994b) Role of antioxidants in the maintenance of immune functions. In: Frei, B. (ed.) *Natural Antioxidants in Human Health and Disease.* Academic Press, New York, pp. 447–467.

Bendich, A. (1995) Criteria for determining recommended dietary allowances for healthy older adults. *Nutrition Review* 53, S105–S110.

Bendich, A. (1996) Antioxidant vitamins and the immune response. *Vitamins and Hormones* 52, 35–62.

Bendich, A. and Cohen M. (1996) Vitamin E, rheumatoid arthritis and other arthritic disorders. *Journal of Nutrition Immunology* 4, 47–65.

Bendich, A., D'Apolito, P., Gabriel, E. and Machlin, L.J. (1984) Interaction of dietary vitamin C and vitamin E on guinea pig immune responses to mitogens. *Journal of Nutrition* 114, 1588–1593.

Bendich, A. *et al.* (1986) The antioxidant role of vitamin C. *Advances in Free Radical Biology and Medicne* 2, 419–444.

Bogden, J.D. and Louria, D.B. (1997) Micronutrients and immunity in older people. In: Bendich, A. and Deckelbaum, R. (eds) *Preventive Nutrition: the Comprehensive Guide for Health Professionals.* Humana Press, Totowa, New Jersey, pp. 317–336.

Bogden, J.D., Bendich, A., Kemp, F.W., Bruening, K.S., Skurnick, J.H., Denny, T., Baker, H. and Louria, D.B. (1994) Daily micronutrient supplements enhance delayed-hypersensitivity skin test responses in older people. *American Journal of Clinical Nutrition* 60, 437–447.

Burton, G.W. *et al.* (1983) Is vitamin E the only lipid-soluble, chain-breaking antioxidant in human blood plasma and erythrocyte membranes? *Archives of Biochemistry and Biophyics* 221, 281–290.

Chandra, R.K. (1992) Effect of vitamin and trace-element supplementation on immune responses and infection in elderly subjects. *Lancet* 340, 1124–1127.

Chandra, R.K. (1995) Nutrition and immunity in the elderly: clinical significance. *Nutrition Review* 53, S80–S83.

Chandra, R.K. (1997) Graying of the immune system. *Journal of the American Medical Association* 277, 1398–1399.

Chandra, R.K. and Kumari, S. (1994) Effects of nutrition on the immune system. *Nutrition* 10, 207–210.

Chavance, M. *et al.* (1984) Immunological and nutritional status among the elderly. *Topics in Aging Research in Europe* 1, 231–237.

Christou, N. (1990) Perioperative nutrition support: immunologic defects. *Journal of Enteral and Parenteral Nutrition* 14, 186S.

Comstock, G.W. *et al.* (1997) Serum concentrations of α tocopherol, β-carotene, and retinol preceding the diagnosis of rheumatoid arthritis and systemic lupus erythematosus. *Annals of the Rheumatic Diseases* 56, 323–325.

Delafuente, J.C. *et al.* (1986) Immunologic modulation by vitamin C in the elderly. *International Journal of Immunopharmacology* 8, 205–211.

Devaraj, S. *et al.* (1996) The effects of alpha tocopherol supplementation on monocyte function. *Journal of Clinical Investigation* 98, 756–763.

Duthie, S.J. *et al.* (1996) Antioxidant supplementation decreases oxidative DNA damage in human lymphocytes. *Cancer Research* 56, 1291–1295.

Ernst, D.N. (1995) Aging and lymphokine gene expression by T cell subsets. *Nutrition Review* 53, S18–S26.

Fotouhi, N. *et al.* (1995) The effect of long term β-carotene (B-C) supplementation on carotenoids and tocopherol concentration in plasma, RBC, and peripheral blood mononuclear cells (PBMC). *Federation of the American Society of Experimental and Biological Journal* A170.

Frei, B. (1991) Ascorbic acid protects lipids in human plasma and low-density lipoprotein against oxidative damage. *American Journal of Clinical Nutrition* 54, 1113S–1118S.

Fuller, C.J. *et al.* (1992) Effect of beta-carotene supplementation on photosuppression of delayed-type hypersensitivity in normal young men. *American Journal of Clinical Nutrition* 56, 684–690.

Garewal, H.S. and Shamdas, G.J. (1991) Intervention trials with beta-carotene in precancerous conditions of the upper aerodigestive tract. In: Bendich, A. and Butterworth, C.E. (eds) *Micronutrients in Health and in Disease Prevention.* Marcel Dekker, New York, pp.127–140.

Goodwin, J.S. (1995) Decreased immunity and increased morbidity in the elderly. *Nutrition Review* 53, S41–46.

Halliwell, B. (1995) Oxygen radicals, nitric oxide and human inflammatory joint disease. *Annuals of the Rheumatic Diseases* 54, 505–510.

Herraiz, L.A. *et al.* (1998) Effect of β-carotene supplementation on photosuppression of delayed-type hypersensitivity in healthy older men. *Journal of the American College of Nutrition* 17, 617–624.

Hughes, D.A. *et al.* (1997) The effect of β-carotene supplementation on the immune function of blood monocytes from healthy male nonsmokers. *Journal of Laboratory Clinical Medicine* 129, 309–317.

Jacob, R.A. *et al.* (1991) Immunocompetence and oxidant defense during ascorbate depletion of healthy men. *American Journal of Clinical Nutrition* 54, 1302S–1309S.

Jeng, K.G. *et al.* (1996) Supplementation with vitamins C and E enhances cytokine production by peripheral blood mononuclear cells in healthy adults. *American Journal of Clinical Nutrition* 64, 960–965.

Kelley, D.S. and Bendich, A. (1996) Essential nutrients and immunologic functions. *American Journal of Clinical Nutrition* 63, 994S–996S.

Kennes, B. *et al.* (1983) Effect of vitamin C supplements on cell-mediated immunity in old people. *Gerontology* 29, 305–310.

Kramer, T.R. *et al.* (1995) Carotenoid–flavonoid modulated immune responses in women. *Federation of the American Society of Experimental and Biological Journal* A170.

Krinsky, N.I. (1989) Carotenoids in medicine. In: Krinsky, N.I., Mathews-Roth, M.M. and Taylor, R.F. (eds) *Chemistry and Biology.* Plenum Press, New York, pp. 279–291.

Lander, H.M. (1997) An essential role for free radicals and derived species in signal transduction. *Federation of the American Society of Experimental and Biological Journal* 11, 118–124.

Machlin, L.J. and Bendich, A. (1987) Free radical damage: antioxidant defenses. *Federation of the American Society of Experimental and Biological Journal* 1, 441–445.

Male, D. *et al.* (1996) Initiation of the immune response. *Advanced Immunology.* Mosby, London, pp. 8.40–8.15.

Malter, M. *et al.* (1989) Natural killer cells, vitamins, and other blood components of vegetarian and omnivorous men. *Nutr. Can.* 12, 271–280.

Marrie, T.J. *et al.*(1988) Cell-mediated immunity of healthy adult Nova Scotians in various age groups compared with nursing home and hospitalized senior citizens. *Journal of Allergy and Clinical Immunology* 81, 836–844.

Martin, A. *et al.* (1997) Vitamin E inhibits low-density lipoprotein-induced adhesion of monocytes to human aortic endothelial cells *in vitro*. *Arteriosclerosis, Thrombosis and Vascular Biology* 17, 429–436.

Merry, P. *et al.* (1989) Oxygen free radicals, inflammation, and synovitis: the current status. *Annals of Rheumatic Disease* 48, 864–870.

Meydani, S.N. and Blumberg, J.B. (1993) Vitamin E and the immune response. In: Cunningham-Rundles, J. (ed.) *Nutrient Modulation of the Immune Response.* Marcel Dekker, New York, pp. 223–238.

Meydani, S.N. *et al.* (1990) Vitamin E supplementation enhances cell-mediated immunity in healthy elderly subjects. *American Journal of Clinical Nutrition* 52, 557–563.

Meydani, S.N. *et al.* (1994a) Assessment of the safety of high-dose, short-term supplementation with vitamin E in healthy older adults. *American Journal of Clinical Nutrition* 60, 704–709.

Meydani, M. *et al.* (1994b) β-carotene supplementation increases antioxidant capacity of plasma in older women. *Journal of Nutrition* 124, 2397–2403.

Meydani, S.N. *et al.* (1995) Effect of β-carotene (B-C) on the immune response of elderly women. *Federation of the American Society of Experimental and Biological Journal* A170.

Meydani, S.N. *et al.* (1997) Vitamin E supplementation and *in vivo* immune response in healthy elderly subjects. *Journal of the American Medical Association* 277, 1380–1386.

Miller, R.A. (1994) Aging and immune function: cellular and biochemical analyses. *Experimental Gerontology* 29, 21–35.

MMWR. (1995) Increasing influenza vaccination rates for Medicare beneficiaries – Montana and Wyoming, 1994. *MMWR* 44, 744–746.

Niki, E. *et al.* (1995) Interaction among vitamin C, vitamin E, and β-carotene. *American Journal of Clinical Nutrition* 62, 1322S–1326S.

Penn, N.D. *et al.* (1991) The effect of dietary vitamin supplementation with vitamins A, C and E on cell-mediated immune function in elderly long-stay patients: a randomized controlled trial. *Age and Aging* 20, 169–174.

Pike, J. and Chandra, R.K. (1995) Effect of vitamin and trace element supplementation on immune indices in healthy elderly. *International Journal of Vitamin Nutrition Research* 65, 117–120.

Roitt, I. *et al.* (1996) Cell-mediated immune reactions. In: *Immunology*, 4th edn. Mosby, London, pp. 9.2–9.4.

Santos, M.S. *et al.* (1997) Natural killer cell activity in elderly men is enhanced by beta-carotene supplementation. *American Journal of Clinical Nutrition* 64(5), 772–777.

Semba, R.D. (1997) Impact of vitamin A on immunity and infection in developing countries. In: Bendich, A. and Deckelbaum, R.J. (eds) *Preventive Nutrition: the Comprehensive Guide for Health Professionals.* Humana Press, Totowa, New Jersey, pp. 337–350.

Von Herbay, A. *et al.* (1996) Diminished plasma levels of vitamin E in patients with severe viral hepatitis. *Free Radical Research* 25, 461–466.

Watson, R.R. *et al.* (1991) Effect of beta-carotene on lymphocyte subpopulations in elderly humans: evidence for a dose response relationship. *American Journal of Clinical Nutrition* 53, 90–94.

Wayne, S.J. *et al.* (1990) Cell-mediated immunity as a predictor of morbidity and mortality in subjects over 60. *Journal of Gerontology and Medical Science* 45, M45–M48.

Ziegler, R.G. and Subar, A.F. (1991) Vegetables, fruits and carotenoids and the risk of cancer. In: Bendich, A. and Butterworth, C.E. (eds) *Micronutrients in Health and in Disease Prevention.* Marcel Dekker, New York, pp. 97–126.

The Effect of Antioxidants on the Production of Lipid Oxidation Products and Transfer of Free Radicals in Oxidized Lipid–Protein Systems 4

NAZLIN K. HOWELL AND SUHUR SAEED

School of Biological Sciences, University of Surrey, Guildford, UK

Introduction

Epidemiological studies suggest that a high fat intake is associated with atherosclerosis, and with colon and breast cancer (Doll and Peto, 1981; Kinlen, 1983; Harris, 1989). In contrast, fatty fish and fish oils are reported to be beneficial and their consumption has increased in recent years. However, if the oils are not stabilized, their degradation by oxidation can produce toxic compounds (Blankenhorn *et al.*, 1990). In this chapter, methods for assessing lipid oxidation and lipid oxidation mechanisms are reviewed, as well as the effect of lipids and lipid oxidation products on proteins. In addition, we discuss how antioxidants might prevent the degradation of proteins.

Lipids in Fatty Fish

Fatty fish typically contain a fat content of about 7 g per 100 g (range 3–20 g 100 g^{-1}). The lipid comprises mainly triglycerides (75%) and phospholipids (25%). Most fish oils are composed mainly of 8–10 fatty acids including saturated acids: myristic, palmitic and stearic; monounsaturated acids: palmitoleic, oleic, 11-eicosenoic and 11-docosenoic; and polyunsaturated fatty acids (PUFA): docosapentaenoic acid (DHA) and eicosapentaenoic acid (EPA). Fatty fish generally contain a high proportion of the unsaturated fatty

© CAB *International* 1999. *Antioxidants in Human Health*
(eds T.K. Basu, N.J. Temple and M.L. Garg)

acids with four to six double bonds. For example, lipids from Atlantic mackerel (*Scomber scombrus*) contain about 70% unsaturated fatty acids of which 30% are PUFA (Ackman and Eaton, 1971; Ackman, 1990).

Unsaturated fatty acids and cholesterol in fat are easily oxidized during cooking and storage. In particular, fish oils are rich in the polyunsaturated DHA (20:5w3) and EPA (22:6w3). Although these ω-3 fatty acids are implicated in reducing atherosclerosis and lowering blood cholesterol (Harris, 1989), their presence in fatty fish or fish oils can result in oxidation and rancidity which greatly shortens the product shelf-life (Shenouda, 1980). The lipid oxidation chain reaction leads to rancidity, which yields different groups of chemicals including: various mutagens (Halliwell and Gutteridge, 1995); promoters and carcinogens such as fatty acid hydroxides; cholesterol hydroxides (Bischoff, 1969), endoperoxides, cholesterol and fatty acid epoxides (Bischoff, 1969; Imai *et al.*, 1980; Petrakis *et al.*, 1981); enals and other aldehydes and alkoxy and hydroperoxide radicals. Therefore, the stabilization of PUFA with the aid of antioxidants as well as processing, encapsulation and packaging is essential.

Lipid Oxidation Mechanisms

Lipid peroxidation is a complex process which occurs in the presence of oxygen and transition metal ions or enzymes. There are usually three stages in the oxidation process, as described in the following sections.

Initiation stage

A hydrogen atom is abstracted from a methylene group (-CH$_2$-) in the PUFA by a reactive species such as a hydroxyl radical (·OH) leaving behind an unpaired electron on the carbon (-CH- or lipid radical). The carbon radical is stabilized by a molecular rearrangement to form a conjugated diene which can combine with oxygen to form a peroxy radical ROO· or RO$_2$·.

$$RH \quad \rightarrow \quad R\cdot + H\cdot \tag{4.1}$$

Propagation stage

The peroxy radical can abstract another H from another lipid molecule and this leads to an autocatalytic chain reaction by which lipid oxidation proceeds. The peroxy radicals can combine with the H which they abstract to form lipid hydroperoxides and cyclic peroxides. Since H abstraction can occur at different points on the carbon chain, the peroxidation of arachidonic acid, for example, is reported to give six lipid hydroperoxides.

$$R\cdot + O_2 \rightarrow RO_2\cdot \tag{4.2}$$
$$RO_2\cdot + RH \rightarrow ROOH + R\cdot \tag{4.3}$$

Secondary products

Hydroperoxides are the primary molecular products which are unstable and degrade to various secondary products including hydroxy-fatty acids, epoxides and scission products such as aldehydes (including malondialdehyde), ketones and lactones many of which are toxic (Halliwell and Gutteridge, 1995).

The degradation of lipid hydroperoxides can be initiated by the presence of transition metal ions including traces of iron and copper salts. The metal ions can cause fission of an O–O bond to form an alkoxy radical $RO\cdot$ as well as peroxy radicals $RO_2\cdot$. In the presence of thiols or other reducing agents such as ascorbic acid, O_2 is reduced to superoxide anion ($O_2^-\cdot$), which then dismutates to H_2O_2 or reduces Fe^{3+} to Fe^{2+}. The hydroxy radical ($OH\cdot$) is produced via the Fenton reaction between the Fe^{2+} and H_2O_2 and can initiate further chain reactions. The reaction of iron, which is present in the fish myoglobin, with lipid peroxides can generate a wide range of products; for example pentane gas can be produced from linoleic acid and arachidonic acid, and ethane and ethylene gases are produced by a similar β-scission reaction from linolenic acid in the presence of Fe^{2+}.

Termination stage

The free radicals produced can combine with each other, or more likely with protein molecules, and end the chain reaction. The latter reaction, which causes cross-linking and severe damage to the protein, is depicted below.

$$R\cdot + R\cdot \rightarrow R - R \tag{4.4}$$
$$nRO_2\cdot \rightarrow (RO_2)n \tag{4.5}$$
$$RO_2\cdot + R\cdot \rightarrow RO_2R \tag{4.6}$$

Enzymic Peroxidation

In contrast with the non-enzymic lipid peroxidation described above for oxygen and metal ions, the enzymes lipoxygenase, cycloxygenase and peroxidase promote the controlled peroxidation of fatty acids to give hydroperoxides and endoperoxides that are stereospecific. Lipoxygenase (EC 1.13.11.12) is commonly found in foods and catalyses peroxidation of PUFA to primary and secondary oxidation products (Hildebrand, 1989; German and Crevelling, 1990).

Lipoxygenase contains one iron atom per molecule and will abstract a hydrogen atom from an unsaturated fatty acid following which bonds rearrange and oxygen is added to form hydroperoxides. The reactions are more complex than those found for non-enzymic hydroperoxides described above, and the hydroperoxide products may interact further with the enzyme. The action of lipoxygenase may produce co-oxidation of other materials, for example carotenoid pigments or proteins. We have recently undertaken the isolation of the crude enzyme and studied its action on the oxidation of fish lipids from Atlantic mackerel, *S. scombrus* (Saeed, 1998).

Effect of Antioxidants

Antioxidants can retard lipid oxidation through competitive binding of oxygen, retardation of the initiation step, blocking the propagation step by destroying or binding free radicals, inhibition of catalysts, or stabilization of hydroperoxides (Halliwell, 1994). Antioxidants can scavenge the active forms of oxygen involved in the initiation step of oxidation, or can break the oxidative chain reaction by reacting with the fatty acid peroxy radicals to form stable antioxidant radicals which are either too unreactive for further reactions or form non-radical products.

Synthetic Antioxidants

Synthetic antioxidants which contain phenolic groups, such as gallic acid esters, butylated hydroxyanisole (BHA), butylated hydroxytoluene (BHT) and tertiary butyl hydroxyquinone (BHQ), are the most widely used food synthetic antioxidants (Fig. 4.1). The effectiveness of phenolic antioxidants depends on the resonance stabilization of the phenoxy radicals determined by the substitution at the ortho and para positions on the aromatic ring and by the size of the substituting group (Shahidi *et al.*, 1992). The presence of carbonylic and carboxylic groups in numerous phenolic compounds can also result in the inhibition of oxidative rancidity by metal chelation (Hudson and Lewis, 1983).

In spite of the widespread use of phenolic antioxidants, there is increasing concern over their safety. The potential toxicity of some phenolic antioxidants in biological models has been described (Thompson and Moldeus, 1988). Thus the replacement of synthetic antioxidants by 'safe, natural' antioxidants such as vitamins E and C, flavonoids and other plant phenolics has been increasingly advocated (see Chapter 2).

Analysis of Lipid Oxidation Products

Since lipid oxidation products are so varied, it is necessary to use several sophisticated techniques to analyse them reliably. Most studies, undertaken

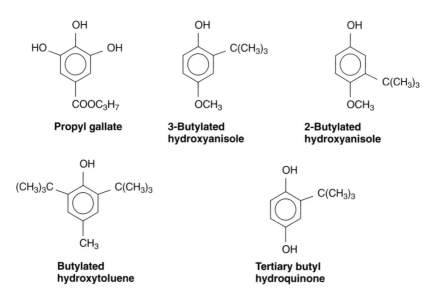

Fig. 4.1. The chemical structure of synthetic antioxidants.

over 20 years ago, examined final lipid oxidation products such as malondialdehyde and peroxides using traditional methods which lack sensitivity and specificity.

The formation of hydroperoxides from PUFA generates a conjugated diene as the double bonds rearrange. Previously reported methods for fatty acid hydroperoxide quantitation include the measurement of absorbance at 234 nm (Corongiu and Banni, 1994), iodometric titration (Jessup *et al.*, 1994), xylenol orange reactivity and glutathione oxidation (O'Gara *et al.*, 1989); however, these methods are not sensitive.

High pressure liquid chromatography (HPLC) and spectroscopy

An HPLC method, developed by the authors for identifying breakdown products of hydroperoxides (Saeed and Howell, 1999), provides a simple and very useful method for investigating the initiation, propagation and termination stages of lipid oxidation in detail. Lipids are transesterified according to Schmarr *et al.* (1996) and the hydroperoxides are purified by liquid chromatography fractionation on amino-phase SPE cartridges. Since the hydroperoxides are very unstable, they spontaneously give rise to oxidation products which are separated on a reverse-phase HPLC Hichrom Kromasil 100 5C18 column using acetic acid–methanol–water (0.1–65–35) solvent. Figure 4.2 shows the development of hydroperoxide alcohol derivatives from methyl linoleate, oxidized under ultraviolet (UV) radiation for 6 and 24 h. The oxidation products were 9-, 10-, 12- and 13-hydroxylinoleate, with the 9-hydroxylinoleate (*trans–cis*) being the most abundant.

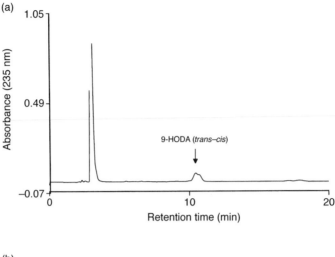

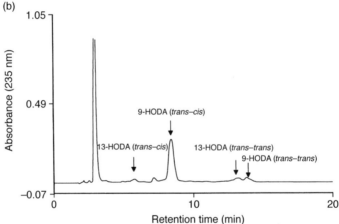

Fig. 4.2. HPLC chromatograms of methyl linoleate oxidized under UV radiation for (a) 6 h and (b) 24 h. HODA, hydroxyoctadecadienoic acid.

Gas chromatography–mass spectroscopy (GC-MS) of oxidized methyl linoleate revealed three GC peaks which represent isomers of molecular weight 382 and are consistent with the molecular formula $C_{22}H_{42}O_3Si$, which is the alcohol derivative of the hydroperoxide. Ion fragmentation spectra of these three peaks indicated that the major high-mass fragment had a mass to charge ratio (m/e) value of 225 (Saeed and Howell, 1999).

The presence of the alcohol derivative of methyl linoleate oxidized by UV radiation was also confirmed by ^{13}C nuclear magnetic resonance (NMR) spectroscopy. However, in this case, a peak at 87 ppm, corresponding to a carbon atom carrying the alcohol derivative of hydroperoxides, was observed only for samples oxidized for longer periods (24 h and 48 h). Although ^{13}C NMR is less sensitive than HPLC for measurements of products generated in the initial stages of oxidation, it is a useful technique for measuring the high concentrations in the later stages (Saeed and Howell, 1999).

In addition to the simple lipid methyl linoleate, the HPLC method also works well for complex lipids extracted from mackerel. One major peak, assigned as 13-HODA, was observed in chromatograms of oil obtained from fish stored at both −20°C and −30°C (Fig. 4.3a). However, for mackerel stored at −20°C the peak was bigger and two extra minor peaks were evident; these were absent from the spectra obtained from control fish fillets stored at −30°C. When α-tocopherol, vitamin C, BHT and BHA were added to the mince fish prior to storage at −20°C (Fig. 4.3b and c), fewer peaks, which were also smaller, were observed compared to the mixture of peaks evident in the chromatograms of the control fish.

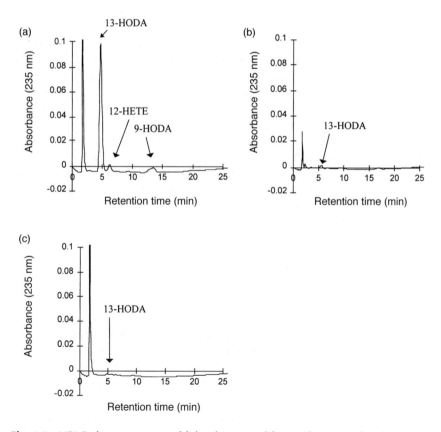

Fig. 4.3. HPLC chromatograms of fish oil extracted from Atlantic mackerel stored (a) at −20°C for 6 months, (b) with BHT, and (c) with vitamin C.
HETE, hydroxyeicosatetraenoic acid; HODA, hydroxyoctadecadienoic acid.

Protein–Lipid Interactions

Oxidized lipids are known to interact with proteins, causing undesirable changes in the nutritional and functional properties of proteins. The interactions can form covalent bonds which may involve hydroperoxides, saturated and unsaturated aldehydes, ketones, ketols, diketones and epoxides in the oxidized lipid. These can react with amines, thiols, disulphides and phenolic groups in the protein (Schaich and Karel, 1975; Schaich, 1980). Non-covalent hydrogen bonds involving hydroxyls and carboxyl groups in proteins and lipids may also be formed (Pokorny, 1987).

In addition, there is a loss of specific amino acids such as cysteine, lysine, histidine and methionine; cross-linking; and damage to DNA as well as to other pigmented proteins such as cytochrome C and haemoglobin (Roubal and Tappel, 1966). An increase in fluorescence has been reported which is attributed to the formation of certain oxidized lipid–protein complexes; for example, fluorescent compounds containing phosphorus and C=N functional groups have been isolated from the oxidation reaction of linoleate and myosin in frozen Coho salmon (Braddock and Dugan, 1973). It has also been reported that aldehydes can react with -SH groups, and dialdehydes such as malondialdehyde can attack amino groups to form intramolecular cross-links as well as cross-links between different proteins. The aldehyde–amine Schiff bases can result in non-enzymic browning pigments (Gardner, 1979, 1983). Malondialdehyde is also reported to form interaction compounds related to lipofucsin-like substances in ageing human cells (Aubourg, 1993).

In addition, it is believed that interaction of free radicals with specific groups on amino acids may be involved (Varma, 1967); for example, alkoxy radicals can attack tryptophan and cysteine residues (Halliwell and Gutteridge, 1995).

Electron Spin Resonance (ESR) Spectroscopy

Radicals involved in lipid oxidation are short-lived species and are measured by ESR spectroscopy, or electron paramagnetic resonance spectroscopy (EPR), which is the only method available for directly detecting free radicals in biological systems. Only one ESR study of free-radical transfer in fish lipid–protein systems has been reported to date; this was done on freeze-dried fish as well as proteins and amino acids in the presence of various lipids such as DHA and an antioxidant hydroquinone (Roubal, 1970). We have recently observed direct evidence using ESR spectroscopy of the presence of short-lived radicals produced during lipid oxidation of either methyl linoleate or fish oil *and the subsequent transfer of the free radicals* to the carbon and sulphydryl groups of amino acids and proteins (Saeed, 1998).

Proteins, including egg lysozyme, egg ovalbumin, fish myosin and the amino acids arginine, lysine and histidine, were exposed to oxidized lipids, namely methyl linoleate and oil extracted from Atlantic mackerel (*S. scombrus*). A strong central singlet signal was induced in the proteins and amino acids which was detected by ESR spectroscopy and assigned to the carbon radical (Fig. 4.4). With the amino acids, ovalbumin and fish myosin, downfield shoulders were also observed which were due to the radical residing on sulphydryl groups. With the addition of antioxidants a reduction in free radicals was observed (Fig. 4.4).

The above changes in the proteins were accompanied by an increase in fluorescence (Fig. 4.5) indicating the formation of cross-links between the individual amino acids as well as conformational changes in the proteins. Synthetic antioxidants, such as BHT and BHA as well as vitamins C and E, inhibited the development of both the free radical peak and fluorescence when added to the proteins prior to incubation with oxidized lipids.

Conclusions

Lipid oxidation products can be monitored successfully and specifically using HPLC combined with NMR and GC-MS techniques. In addition, the

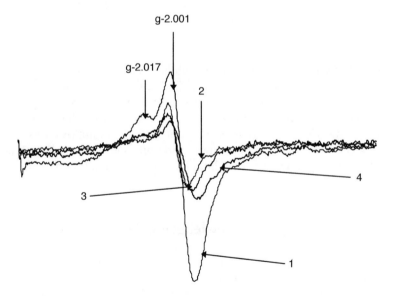

Fig. 4.4. ESR spectra of Atlantic mackerel myosin. Myosin incubated with oxidized mackerel oil (1); control – myosin incubated without oxidized fish oil (2); myosin incubated with BHT and oxidized fish oil (3); and myosin incubated with vitamin C and oxidized fish oil (4). Settings: power 5 mW, central field 328 mT, sweep width 10 mT, modulation 0.5 mT and receiver gain 200.

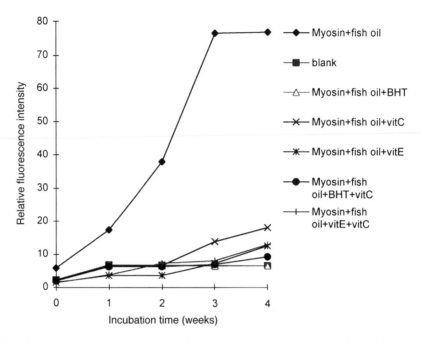

Fig. 4.5. Fluorescence formation in fish myosin: molar fluorescence intensities relative to quinine sulphate in 0.1 mol l^{-1} H_2SO_4 solution. Emission wavelength 420 nm and excitation wavelength 360 nm.

transfer of free radicals from oxidized lipids to proteins in protein–lipid systems has been shown to result in cross-linking of proteins and can be monitored by ESR spectroscopy and fluorescence spectroscopy, respectively. The damage caused by lipid oxidation products in model systems and whole fish muscle can be minimized by the addition of antioxidants, in particular a combination of water-soluble ascorbic acid with the lipophilic α-tocopherol. These advances may help to enhance the nutritional and safety aspects of food.

Acknowledgements

This research project was financed by The Commission of the European Communities within the STD Framework Contract No. TS3*-CT94–0340 awarded to and coordinated by Dr Nazlin K. Howell.

References

Ackman, R.G. (1990) Seafood lipids and fatty acids. *Food Reviews International* 6, 617–646.

Ackman, R.G. and Eaton, C.A. (1971) Mackerel lipids and fatty acids. *Canadian Institute of Food Science and Technology Journal* 4, 169–172.

Aubourg, S.O. (1993) Review: interaction of malondialdehyde with biological molecules – new trends about reactivity and significance. *International Journal of Food Science and Technology* 28, 323–335.

Bischoff, F. (1969) Carcinogenic effects of steroids. *Advances in Lipid Research* 7, 165–244.

Blankenhorn, D.H., Johnson, R.L., Mack, W.J., El Zain, H.A. and Vailas, L.I. (1990) The influence of diet on the appearance of new lesions in human coronary arteries. *Journal of the American Medical Association* 263, 1646–1652.

Braddock, R.J. and Dugan, L.R. (1973) Reaction of autoxidizing linoleate with Coho salmon myosin. *Journal of the American Oil Chemists' Society* 50, 343–346.

Corongiu, F.P. and Banni, S. (1994) A sensitive electrochemical method for quantitative hydroperoxide determination. *Methods in Enzymology* 233, 303–310.

Doll, R. and Peto, J. (1981) The causes of cancer – quantitative estimates of avoidable risks of cancer in the United States today. *Journal of the National Cancer Institute* 66, 1191–1308.

Gardner, H.W. (1979) Lipid hydroperoxide reaction with proteins and amino acids. A review. *Journal of Agricultural and Food Chemistry* 27, 220–229.

Gardner, H.W. (1983) Effects of lipid hydroperoxides on food components. In: Finley, J.W. and Schwass, D.E. (eds) *Xenobiotics in Food and Feeds.* American Chemical Society, Washington, DC, pp. 63–84.

German, J.B. and Crevelling, R.K. (1990) Identification and characterization of a 15-lipoxygenase from fish gills. *Journal of Agricultural and Food Chemistry* 38, 2144–2147.

Halliwell, B. (1994) Free radicals and antioxidants: a personal view. *Nutrition Reviews* 52, 253–265.

Halliwell, B and Gutteridge, J.M.C. (1995) *Free Radicals in Biology and Medicine,* 2nd edn. Clarendon Press, Oxford.

Harris, W.S. (1989) Fish oils and plasma lipid and lipoprotein metabolism in humans. A critical review. *Journal of Lipid Research* 30, 785–807.

Hildebrand, D.F. (1989) Lipoxygenases. *Physiologia Plantarum* 76, 249–253.

Hudson, B.J. and Lewis, J.I. (1983) Polyhydroxy flavonoid antioxidants for edible oils: structural criteria for activity. *Food Chemistry* 10, 47–51.

Imai, H., Weithesser, N.T., Subramosyam, V., Lequesne, P., Suoway, W.A.H. and Kanisawa, M. (1980) Angiotoxicity of oxygenated sterols and possible precursors. *Science* 207, 651.

Jessup, W., Dean, R.T. and Gebicki, J.M. (1994) Iodometric determination of hydroperoxides in lipids and proteins. *Methods in Enzymology* 233, 289–303.

Kinlen, L.J. (1983) Fat and cancer. *British Medical Journal* 286, 1081–1082.

Nagaoka, S., Sawada, K., Fukumoto, Y., Nagashima, U., Katsumata, S. and Mukai, K. (1992) Mechanism of antioxidant reaction of vitamin E: Kinetics, spectroscopic and an *in vivo* study of proton-transfer reactions. *Journal of Physical Chemistry* 96, 6663–6668.

O'Gara, C.Y., Rao, K.M. and Marnett, L.J. (1989) A sensitive electrochemical method for quantitative hydroperoxide determination. *Chemical Research in Toxicology* 2, 295–300.

Patterson, L.K. (1981) Studies of radiation-induced peroxidation in fatty acid micellers. In: Rodgers, M.A.J. and Powers, E.L. (eds*)* *Oxygen and Oxy-radicals in Chemistry and Biology.* Academic Press, New York, pp. 89–95.

Petrakis, N.L., Gruenke, L.D. and Craig, J.C. (1981) Cholesterol and cholesterol epoxides in nipple aspirates of human breast fluid. *Cancer Research* 41, 2563–2566.

Pokorny, J. (1987) Major factors affecting the autoxidation of lipids. In: Chan, H.W.S. (ed.) *Autoxidation of Unsaturated Lipids.* Academic Press, London, pp 141–206.

Pryor, W.A. (1976) *Free Radicals in Biology.* Academic Press, New York.

Roubal, W.T. (1970) Trapped radicals in dry lipid–protein systems undergoing oxidation. *Journal of the American Oil Chemists' Society* 47, 141–144.

Roubal, W.T. and Tappel, A.L. (1966) Damage to proteins, enzymes and amino acids by peroxidizing lipids. *Archives of Biochemistry and Biophysics* 5, 113–117.

Saeed, S. (1998) Lipid oxidation mechanisms and lipid–protein interactions in frozen mackerel (*Scomber scombrus*). PhD thesis, University of Surrey, Guildford, UK.

Saeed, S. and Howell, N.K. (1998) High performance liquid chromatography (HPLC) and NMR studies on oxidation products extracted from Atlantic mackerel. *Journal of the American Oil Chemists' Society* 76, 1–7.

Schaich, K.M. (1980) Free radical initiation in proteins and amino acids by ionizing and ultraviolet radiation and lipid oxidation. *CRC Critical Reviews in Food Science and Nutrition* 13, 131–159.

Schaich, K.M. and Karel, M. (1975) Free radical reactions of peroxidizing lipids with amino acids and proteins: an ESR study. *Lipids* 11, 392–400.

Schmarr, H.G., Gross, H.B. and Shabamoto, T. (1996) Analysis of polar cholesterol oxidation products, evaluation of a new method involving transesterification. Solid-phase extraction and gas chromatography. *Journal of Agricultural and Food Chemistry* 44, 512–517.

Shahidi, F., Janitha, P.K. and Wanasundara, P.D. (1992) Phenolic antioxidants. *CRC Critical Reviews in Food Science and Nutrition* 32, 67–103.

Shenouda, S.Y.K. (1980) Theories of protein denaturation during frozen storage of fish flesh. *Advances in Food Research* 26, 273–311.

Thompson, M. and Moldeus, P. (1988) Cytotoxicity of butylated hydroxyanisole and butylated hydroxytoluene in isolated rat hepatocytes. *Biochemical Pharmacology* 37, 2201–2207.

Varma, T.M.R. (1967) Protein–lipid interaction affecting the quality of protein foods. *Journal of Food Science and Technology* 4, 12–13.

Regulation of the Low-density Lipoprotein Receptor by Antioxidants

5

SEBELY PAL[1,2,4], CHRISTINA BURSILL[1,3], CYNTHIA D.K. BOTTEMA[2] AND PAUL D. ROACH[1]

[1]*CSIRO Division of Human Nutrition, Adelaide;* [2]*Department of Animal Science, Waite Agricultural Research Institute, University of Adelaide, Adelaide, Australia;* [3]*Department of Physiology, University of Adelaide, Adelaide, Australia;* [4]*Department of Medicine, University of Western Australia, Perth, Australia*

Introduction

Low-density lipoproteins (LDL) carry the majority of the cholesterol in the blood and the LDL cholesterol concentration is strongly correlated with the risk of developing heart disease. The clearance of the lipoproteins from the circulation is mediated by a specific cell-surface receptor called the LDL receptor (Brown and Goldstein, 1986); the LDL receptor pathway is therefore one of the mechanisms by which the blood concentration of cholesterol is controlled (Brown and Goldstein, 1981). This is most evident in familial hypercholesterolaemic (FH) subjects who are deficient in LDL receptors; they can have untreated cholesterol concentrations up to eight times higher than normal and often suffer from heart disease in their first decade of life. The level of LDL receptors expressed by cells can be regulated by a number of factors. The most well known is feedback downregulation by sterols which occurs at the level of gene transcription (Wang *et al.*, 1994; Sanchez *et al.*, 1995).

Since the advent of the oxidation hypothesis of atherosclerosis there has been much interest in the role of antioxidants in protecting against the oxidation of LDL (Witztum and Steinberg, 1991). However, the present studies stem more from reports that antioxidants such as vitamin C, vitamin E and catechins can lower blood cholesterol in various animal models of hypercholesterolaemia (Westrope *et al.*, 1982; Muramatsu *et al.*, 1986; Phonpanichrasamee *et al.*, 1990; Hemila, 1992). The aim was to determine whether this effect of antioxidants on blood cholesterol could be related to upregulation of the LDL receptor. Nutrient antioxidants (vitamin A, C, E and β-carotene) and non-nutrient antioxidants found in green tea and red wine (catechins) were studied for their effects on the LDL receptor of the human liver HepG2 hepatoma cell line in culture.

Methods

Cell cultures

The HepG2 cells were grown under 5% CO_2 at 37°C in Dulbecco's Modified Eagles Medium (DMEM) supplemented with 12 mg ml^{-1} penicillin, 16 mg ml^{-1} gentamicin, 20 mM HEPES buffer, 10 mM NaOH, 2 mM L-glutamine and 10% (v/v) fetal calf serum (Kambouris *et al.*, 1990). For experiments, cells were grown to near-confluency (usually 80–90%), incubated for 24 h in the presence of the desired compounds and then extensively washed in phosphate-buffered saline (PBS: 10 mM phosphate, 154 mM NaCl, pH 7), scraped from the flasks and suspended in PBS.

LDL receptor binding assay

Harvested HepG2 cells were assayed for LDL receptor binding activity as described for mononuclear cells (Roach *et al.*, 1993a). Human LDL, $1.025 > d > 1.050$ g ml^{-1}, was isolated from 2–4 day old blood (Red Cross, Adelaide, Australia) and conjugated to colloidal gold (LDL–gold) as previously described (Roach *et al.*, 1987, 1993a). The cells, 100 μg of protein (Lowry *et al.*, 1951), were incubated for 1 h at room temperature with LDL–gold (20 μg protein ml^{-1}) and buffer (60 mM Tris-HCl, pH 8.0, and 20 mg ml^{-1} bovine serum albumin) in a total volume of 300 μl either in the presence of 2 mM $Ca(NO_3)_2$ to measure total binding or 20 mM ethylene diamine tetraacetic acid (EDTA) to measure calcium-independent binding. The cells were then centrifuged at $400 \times g$ for 10 min, resuspended and washed in 300 ml of 2 mM $Ca(NO_3)_2$ for total binding or 300 ml of 20 mM EDTA (pH 8.0) for calcium-independent binding and centrifuged at $400 \times g$ for 10 min. The HepG2 cells were finally resuspended in 120 μl of 4% (w/v) gum arabic and the cell-bound LDL–gold was quantified using a silver enhancement solution (IntenSE BL kit, Amersham, Sydney, Australia) and a Cobas Bio autoanalyser (Roche Diagnostica, Nutley, New Jersey). The binding of LDL to its receptor (calcium-dependent binding) was calculated as the total binding minus the calcium-independent binding and this was taken to be the LDL receptor-binding activity of the cells and expressed as ng LDL mg^{-1} cell protein.

LDL receptor protein assay

The LDL receptor protein in the HepG2 cells was measured as described for rat liver (Roach *et al.*, 1993b; Balasubramaniam *et al.*, 1994). The cells were solubilized by incubation for 12 h in a solution of 1.5% (w/v) Triton X-100 containing 50 mM Tris-maleate (pH 6), 2 mM $CaCl_2$, 1 mM phenylmethyl-sulphonyl fluoride (PMSF) and 10 mM n-ethylmaleamide. Solubilized cell protein (100 mg) (37) and rainbow molecular weight markers (Pharmacia LKB, Uppsala, Sweden) were separated by electrophoresis on 2–15% SDS–polyacrylamide gradient gels at 30 mA for 5 h. Separated proteins were electrotransferred at 45 V for 12 h on to 0.45 μm nitrocellulose membranes (Schleicher and Schuell, Dassel, Germany) and the membranes were blocked for 1 h at room temperature in 10 mM Tris-HCl buffer, pH 7.4, containing 154 mM NaCl and 10% (w/v) skim milk powder. After washing in 10 mM Tris-HCl buffer, pH 7.4, containing 154 mM NaCl and 1% (w/v) skim milk powder, the membranes were incubated with a polyclonal anti-LDL receptor antibody (3.7 mg protein ml^{-1} in 10 mM Tris-HCl buffer, pH 7.4, containing 154 mM NaCl and 1% (w/v) skim milk powder). The membranes were then incubated with anti-rabbit IgG linked to horseradish peroxidase (Amersham, North Ryde, Australia), diluted 1:5000 in 10 mM Tris-HCl buffer, pH 7.4, containing 154 mM NaCl and 1% (w/v) skim milk powder and washed twice with 10 mM Tris-HCl buffer, pH 7.4, containing 154 mM NaCl and 2 mM $CaCl_2$. The membranes were then soaked in enhanced chemiluminescence substrate solution for horseradish peroxidase (ECL detection kit, Amersham, North Ryde, Australia) and exposed to hyper-film ECL (Amersham, North Ryde, Australia) for 1–5 min. The films were then scanned to determine the intensity of the LDL receptor protein bands using an LKB Ultrascan XL laser densitometer (Pharmacia LKB Biotechnology, North Ryde, Australia) and the absorbance was taken as the measure of the LDL receptor protein.

LDL receptor mRNA assay

Cellular RNA was isolated using the procedure of Chomczynski and Sacchi (1987). The LDL receptor mRNA was then measured using reverse transcription and the polymerase chain reaction (PCR) to incorporate a nucleotide conjugated with digoxygenin into an amplified LDL receptor sequence (Powell and Kroon, 1992).

The isolated HepG2 cell total RNA was reversed transcribed into cDNA along with a synthetic piece of cRNA, AW109 (Perkin-Elmer Cetus Instruments, Norwalk, Connecticut) which contains primer site sequences unique to the LDL receptor. The reverse transcription reaction mixture (11.94 ml) contained 1 ml of cell total RNA (120 ng ml^{-1}), 1 ml of AW109 cRNA (4×10^4 copies ml^{-1}), 1 ml of PCR buffer (100 mM Tris-HCl, pH 8.3, 500 mM KCl), 2 ml of 25 mM $MgCl_2$, 0.5 ml of RNasin (20 U ml^{-1}; Perkin-Elmer

Cetus Instruments, Norwalk, Connecticut), 0.5 ml of random hexanucleotide primers (50 mM; Perkin-Elmer Cetus Instruments, Norwalk, Connecticut), 1.5 ml each of 10 mM dGTP, 10 mM dATP and 10 mM dCTP, 0.94 ml of 10 mM dTTP (Perkin-Elmer Cetus Instruments, Norwalk, Connecticut) and 0.5 ml of Moloney murine leukaemia virus reverse transcriptase (50 U ml^{-1}; Perkin-Elmer Cetus Instruments, Norwalk, Connecticut). It was then sequentially incubated at 23°C for 10 min, 45°C for 15 min, 95°C for 5 min in a thermal cycler (Perkin-Elmer Cetus Instruments, Norwalk, Connecticut) and finally chilled on ice.

The LDL receptor sequences were then amplified using PCR and the modified nucleotide, dUTP conjugated to digoxygenin (DIG), was incorporated. The PCR mixture (20 ml) contained 5 ml of the reverse transcription reaction mixture, 0.5 ml of 1 mM digoxygenin-11-dUTP, 2 ml of PCR buffer (100 mM Tris-HCl, pH 8.3, 500 mM KCl), 0.25 ml of AmpliTaq DNA polymerase (5 U ml^{-1}, Perkin-Elmer Cetus Instruments, Norwalk, Connecticut), 0.60 ml of the LDL receptor dowstream primer AW125 (25 mM, Perkin-Elmer Cetus, Norwalk, Connecticut), 0.60 ml of the LDL receptor upstream primer AW126 (25 mM, Perkin-Elmer Cetus, Norwalk, Connecticut) and 11.05 ml deionized H$_2$O. The mixture was overlaid with mineral oil and the amplification was done with a DNA thermal cycler (Perkin Elmer Cetus, Norwalk, Connecticut) for 27 cycles of denaturation at 95°C for 1 min, primer annealing at 55°C for 1 min and extension at 72°C for 1 min. After 27 cycles a further extension period of 10 min at 72°C was done. Each PCR reaction mixture (10 ml) was size fractionated by electrophoresis for 90 min at 90 V in 3% (w/v) agarose gels with 0.8 mM Tris-acetate, pH 8.5, and 0.04 mM EDTA as running buffer and the DNA transferred on to positively charged nylon membranes (Boehringer Mannheim, Rose Park, Australia) by blotting for 4 h in 0.15 M Na$_3$citrate, pH 7.6 and 1.5 M NaCl. The nylon membranes were baked for 1 h at 100°C and rinsed in 30 mM Na$_3$citrate, pH 7.6, and 0.3 M NaCl, incubated in 0.1 mM Tris-HCl, pH 7.5, and 0.1 M NaCl for 5 min at room temperature and blocked for 30 min at room temperature in 0.1 mM Tris-HCl, pH 7.5, 0.1 M NaCl and 10% (w/v) skim milk powder. The membranes were then incubated for 30 min with an anti-digoxygenin–IgG antibody conjugated to alkaline phosphatase (Boehringer Mannheim, Rose Park, Australia) diluted 1:1000 in 0.1 mM Tris-HCl, pH 7.5, 0.1 M NaCl and 1% (w/v) skim milk powder, washed three times for 20 min in 0.1 mM Tris-HCl, pH 7.5, 0.1 M NaCl, incubated in 0.1 M Tris-HCl, pH 9.5, 0.1 M NaCl and 50 mM MgCl$_2$ for 5 min and soaked for 5 min in ECL alkaline phosphatase substrate solution consisting of 100 mg ml^{-1} AMPPD (disodium 3-(4-methoxyspiro{1,2-dioxetane-3,2-(5-chloro) tricyclo[3.3.1.1]decan}-4-y)phenylphosphate) (Boehringer Mannheim, Rose Park, Australia) in 0.1 M Tris-HCl, pH 9.5, 0.1 M NaCl and 50 mM MgCl$_2$. They were then blotted dry, sealed in plastic, incubated at 37°C for 20 min and exposed to hyper-film ECL (Amersham, North Ryde, Australia) for 5–30 min. The films were then scanned using the LKB

Ultrascan XL enhanced laser densitometer (Pharmacia LKB Biotechnology, North Ryde, Australia) to determine the intensity of the two bands corresponding to: (i) cellular LDL receptor mRNA at 258 bp, and (ii) synthetic AW109 internal standard RNA at 301 bp. The amount of LDL receptor mRNA in the HepG2 cells was calculated relative to the intensity of the band for the known amount of AW109 RNA added as internal standard and was expressed as copies per mg of cellular RNA.

Green tea preparations

Green tea was prepared by brewing 10 g of green tea leaves for 10 min in 100 ml of just-boiled hot water. Organic solvent extracts were prepared as described by Huang *et al.* (1992). Green tea leaves (2.5 kg) were extracted with 15 l of methanol at 50°C for 3 h (methanol extract). The methanol was removed using a rotary evaporator. The residue was dissolved in 5 l of 50°C water and extracted three times with hexane (hexane wash), once with chloroform (chloroform wash) and once with ethyl acetate (ethyl acetate extract). The solvents were removed from the extracts using a rotary evaporator and the residues were redissolved in 50°C water and freeze dried.

Measurement of tocopherols in cells

Cellular tocopherols were measured as described by Yang and Lee (1987). A 200 µl sample containing 0.1 mg of cell protein in PBS and 12.5 µg of α-tocopherol acetate as internal standard was extracted with 175 µl of ethanol and 400 µl hexane. The sample was vortexed and centrifuged for 10 min at 10,000 × g at 4°C. The hexane phase (300 µl) was transferred into another tube, dried under nitrogen, and the residue was redissolved in 200 µl of the mobile phase (methanol:acetonitrile:dichloromethane:hexane, 22:55:11.5:11.5). The sample was analysed using a Supelcosil LC-18-DB column (Sigma-Aldrich, Castle Hill, Australia) and a ICI modular HPLC system (ICI, Dingley, Australia).

Results

Nutrient antioxidants

When HepG2 cells were incubated for 24 h in the presence of the antioxidant vitamins A, C, E (α-tocopherol) and β-carotene at 50 or 100 µM, the LDL receptor binding activity was increased two- to threefold in all cases except in the presence of 100 µM vitamin E (Fig. 5.1). Increases in LDL receptor protein (data not shown) or mRNA (Fig. 5.2) were also observed except for vitamin E at 100 µM. As seen in Fig. 5.2, vitamin E increased the LDL receptor mRNA tenfold at the 50 µM concentration but it had no effect at 100 µM. Vitamin A and C and β-carotene increased the LDL receptor

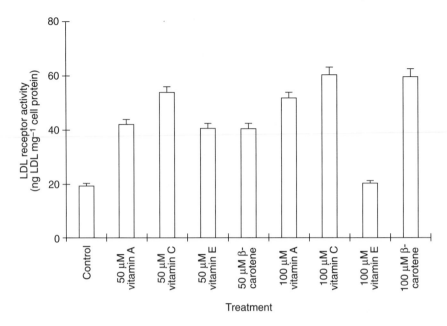

Fig. 5.1. The effect of nutrient antioxidants on LDL receptor activity. HepG2 cells were incubated for 24 h with either 50 or 100 μM vitamin A, C, E or β-carotene as indicated. Control cells were not exposed to any nutrient antioxidants. The LDL receptor activity was measured in duplicate using the LDL colloidal gold method as described in the 'Methods' section. The results represent the calcium-dependent LDL binding activity of the cells, expressed as ng LDL bound mg^{-1} cell protein, and are means ± SEM of three experiments.

mRNA two- to fourfold at the 50 μM concentration and eight- to tenfold at 100 μM.

Further dose–response experiments confirmed the biphasic 'up-then-down' nature of the effect of vitamin E; the LDL receptor activity was progressively increased by α-tocopherol at concentrations up to 50 μM but it was decreased from this peak at higher vitamin concentrations (Fig. 5.3). The same biphasic effect was observed when LDL receptor protein (Fig. 5.4) or mRNA (Fig. 5.5) was measured. The effect was specific for α-tocopherol in that δ- and γ-tocopherol downregulated the receptor at all concentrations tested (Fig. 5.5) despite all three analogues being similarly taken up by the HepG2 cells (Fig. 5.6).

Non-nutrient antioxidants

Green tea and red wine were also found to upregulate the LDL receptor at least twofold when incubated with HepG2 cells (Fig. 5.7). The upregulating

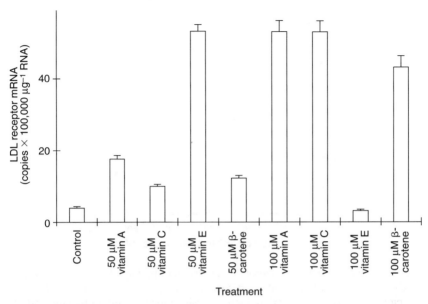

Fig. 5.2. The effect of nutrient antioxidants on LDL receptor mRNA. HepG2 cells were incubated for 24 h with either 50 or 100 μM vitamin A, C, E or β-carotene as indicated. Control cells were not exposed to any nutrient antioxidants. The LDL receptor mRNA was measured in duplicate using the ECL–digoxygenin method as described in the 'Methods' section. The results were expressed as copies of LDL receptor mRNA μg^{-1} cellular RNA and are means ± SEM of three experiments.

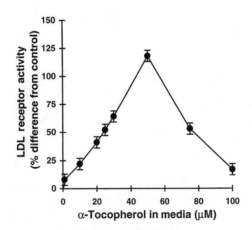

Fig. 5.3. The effect of α-tocopherol on LDL receptor activity. HepG2 cells were incubated for 24 h with the indicated concentration of α-tocopherol. The LDL receptor activity was measured in duplicate using the LDL–colloidal gold method as described in the 'Methods' section. The results represent the calcium-dependent LDL binding activity of the cells, expressed as the percent difference from the binding obtained in control cells and are means ± SEM of three experiments. Control cells were not exposed to any α-tocopherol and the activity in these cells was 30±4 ng LDL mg^{-1} cell protein.

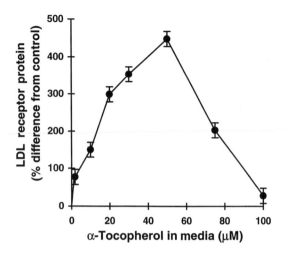

Fig. 5.4. The effect of α-tocopherol on LDL receptor protein. HepG2 cells were incubated for 24 h with the indicated concentration of α-tocopherol. The LDL receptor protein was measured in duplicate using the ECL Western blot method as described in the 'Methods'. The results represent the percentage difference from the amount of protein measured in control cells and are means ± SEM of three experiments. Control cells were not exposed to any α-tocopherol and the amount of LDL receptor protein measured in these cells was 0.2±0.09 densitometer absorbance units.

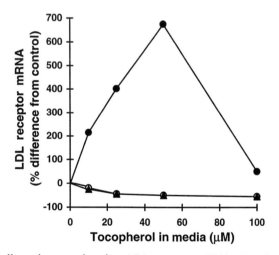

Fig. 5.5. The effect of α-tocopherol on LDL receptor mRNA. HepG2 cells were incubated for 24 h with the indicated concentration of α-(●), δ- (○) or γ-tocopherol (▲). The LDL receptor mRNA was measured in duplicate using the ECL dioxygenin method as described in the 'Methods' section. The results represent the percentage difference from the amount of mRNA measured in control cells and are means ± SEM of three experiments. Control cells were not exposed to any α-tocopherol and the amount of LDL receptor mRNA measured in these cells was 4.2±0.8 × 10^5 copies μg^{-1} RNA.

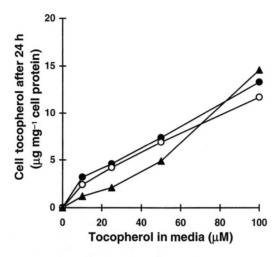

Fig. 5.6. The enrichment of HepG2 cells with the different tocopherols. Cells were incubated for 24 h with the indicated concentration of α-(●), δ- (○) or γ-tocopherol (▲). The tocopherols were measured by HPLC as described in the 'Methods' section and are means of duplicate determinations.

activity was extracted from green tea with methanol and retained in the polyphenol-enriched ethyl acetate extract (Fig. 5.8). The upregulating activity was not extracted by hexane or chloroform.

Of the polyphenolic compounds which are abundant in green tea (epicatechin, epicatechin gallate, epigallocatechin and epigallocatechin gallate) epigallocatechin gallate was the most potent at upregulating the HepG2 cell LDL receptor (Fig. 5.9). Propyl gallate, a preservative often added to food, had little upregulating activity. Upregulation of the LDL receptor by epigallocatechin gallate followed saturation kinetics with no evidence of a biphasic 'up-then-down' regulation as found for α-tocopherol.

Discussion

We present here the novel observation that antioxidants can modulate the expression of the LDL receptor in the human liver HepG2 hepatoma cell line. The effect appeared to be a 'general antioxidant effect' as the effectors, whether they were nutrients (vitamins) or non-nutrients (catechins), had the common property of being antioxidants. The regulation appeared to be at the level of gene transcription as similar effects were found whether LDL receptor-binding activity, protein or mRNA was measured.

All the nutrient antioxidants tested, vitamins A, C and E as well as β-carotene, were able to upregulate the receptor. However, in contrast to the other antioxidants, vitamin E (α-tocopherol) was observed to have a

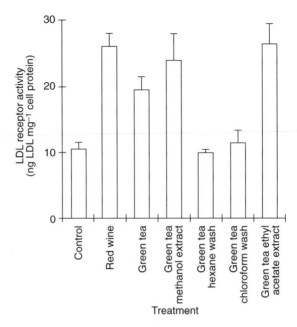

Fig. 5.7. The effect of non-nutrient antioxidant preparations on LDL receptor activity. HepG2 cells were incubated for 24 h with the indicated preparations of green tea, red wine or different extracts of green tea prepared as described in the 'Methods' section. The amount of green tea extracts and red wine used were based on containing the equivalent of 100 μM epigallocatechin gallate and 100 μM quercetin respectively. Control cells were not exposed to any preparation. The LDL receptor activity was measured in duplicate using the LDL–colloidal gold method as described in the 'Methods' section. The results represent the calcium-dependent LDL binding activity of the cells, expressed as ng LDL bound mg^{-1} cell protein, and are means ± SEM of triplicate incubations.

biphasic 'up-then-down' effect. Up to 50 μM, it progressively upregulated the receptor but then it downregulated it at higher concentrations. The biphasic effect was specific for α-tocopherol in that the δ and γ analogues downregulated the LDL receptor at all the concentrations tested. Green tea and red wine also upregulated the receptor. The upregulating activity was retained in a polyphenol-enriched ethyl acetate extract of green tea leaves and, of the polyphenolic compounds found in green tea, epigallocatechin gallate was the most potent at upregulating the receptor. Interestingly, epigallocatechin gallate is the most abundant of the catechins in green tea (Huang *et al.*, 1992) and also the strongest antioxidant (Jovanovic *et al.*, 1995).

Upregulation of the LDL receptor by vitamin C, vitamin E and green tea catechins is consistent with previous reports that these antioxidants can

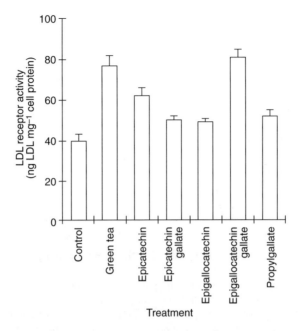

Fig. 5.8. The effect of catechins on LDL receptor activity. HepG2 cells were incubated for 24 h with 100 μM of the indicated catechins, green tea or propyl gallate as described in the 'Methods' section. Control cells were not exposed to any preparation. The LDL receptor activity was measured in duplicate using the LDL–colloidal gold method as described in the 'Methods'. The results represent the calcium-dependent LDL binding activity of the cells, expressed as ng LDL bound mg^{-1} cell protein, and are means ± SEM of triplicate incubations.

lower blood cholesterol in various animal models of hypercholesterolaemia (Westrope *et al.*, 1982; Muramatsu *et al.*, 1986; Phonpanichrasamee *et al.*, 1990; Hemila, 1992). It may therefore also be that the LDL receptor is down-regulated in animal models of vitamin C and vitamin E deficiency where plasma cholesterol is increased (Yasuda *et al.*, 1979; Holloway *et al.*, 1981; Chupukcharoen *et al.*, 1985). At least, the effect of deficiency could be relevant to the present vitamin E experiments because there was no measurable vitamin E in the HepG2 cells incubated in the absence of added vitamin. Upregulation of the LDL receptor of HepG2 cells by vitamin A and β-carotene also suggests that the effect may be a general antioxidant phenomenon, but there is no evidence that these two nutrients can lower blood cholesterol. The lack of upregulation with the weaker antioxidants such as δ- and γ-tocopherol and some of the catechins also suggests a general antioxidant effect.

The biphasic effect observed with vitamin E is difficult to explain but it is consistent with the 'up-then-down' biphasic effect of increasing amounts

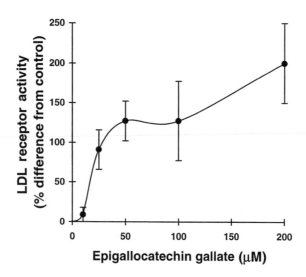

Fig. 5.9. The effect of epigallocatechin gallate on LDL receptor activity. HepG2 cells were incubated for 24 h with the indicated concentrations of epigallocatechin gallate. The LDL receptor activity was measured in duplicate using the LDL–colloidal gold method as described in the 'Methods'. The results represent the calcium-dependent LDL-binding activity of the cells, expressed as ng LDL bound mg^{-1} cell protein, and are means ± SEM of triplicate incubations.

of α-tocopherol on the activity of phospholipase A$_2$ *in vitro* (Tran *et al.*, 1996). In keeping with the 'general antioxidant effect' the biphasic regulation may be related to the recent observation that α-tocopherol can become a strong oxidant if it is oxidized into a tocopheroxy radical and there are no other antioxidants such as vitamin C or ubiquinol 10 to regenerate the radical to its tocopherol form (Thomas *et al.*, 1995), as was the case in the present experiments. It may be that enough tocopheroxy radicals are produced as the vitamin E concentration increases to counterbalance the antioxidant effect.

The mechanism of action by which antioxidants upregulate the LDL receptor is currently under investigation using the HepG2 cell line. Our preliminary studies indicate that green tea and epigallocatechin gallate decrease the amount of cholesterol in the cell (unpublished data). This could upregulate the LDL receptor by decreasing the sterol feedback downregulation of the gene's transcription (Brown and Goldstein, 1986; Wang *et al.*, 1994; Sanchez *et al.*, 1995). The conversion of cholesterol to bile acids will also be studied because studies in animal models have found that vitamin C (Holloway, 1981) and vitamin E (Chupukcharoen, 1985) increase the activity of the hepatic cholesterol 7α-hydroxylase, the rate-limiting enzyme in bile acid synthesis.

Upregulation of the LDL receptor by antioxidants, if it occurs in humans, may or may not decrease blood cholesterol, as it is only one of the factors which modulates its concentration. The steady-state balance between the entry of cholesterol into and its clearance from the circulation ultimately determines its concentration (Dietschy *et al.*, 1993). Accordingly, there is some evidence that antioxidants may affect plasma cholesterol in humans (Kono *et al.*, 1992; Gatto *et al.*, 1996), but intervention studies with antioxidants have found little effect on plasma cholesterol. However, upregulation of the LDL receptor may still be beneficial if it occurs without a decrease in blood or LDL cholesterol; upregulation of the receptor could still increase the LDL turnover rate, thereby reducing its circulatory half-life and its exposure to oxidative modification, an initiating factor in atherogenesis (Witztum and Steinberg, 1991).

In conclusion, antioxidants have been found to upregulate the LDL receptor in culture experiments with the human liver HepG2 hepatoma cell line. The effect may be relevant to the lowering of blood cholesterol in animal models of hypercholesterolaemia. However, its relevance to hypercholesterolaemia and atherosclerosis in humans remains to be determined.

Acknowledgements

We would like to thank Dr Paul Kroon and Dr Elizabeth Powell (Dept of Biochemistry, University of Queensland, Brisbane, Australia), for teaching us how to measure mRNA by quantitative PCR with a non-radioactive label. Special thanks are also due to our colleagues Calliope Triantifilidis (CSIRO) for all her technical help and to Dr Mavis Abbey (CSIRO), Dr Paul Nestel (CSIRO) and Dr Andrew Thomson (Adelaide University) for their support and advice.

References

Balasubramniam, S., Szanto, A. and Roach P.D. (1994) Circadian rhythm in hepatic low-density-lipoprotein (LDL)-receptor expression and plasma LDL levels. *Biochemical Journal* 298, 39–43.

Brown, M.S. and Goldstein, J.L. (1981) Lowering plasma cholesterol by raising LDL receptors. *New England Journal of Medicine* 305, 515–517.

Brown, M.S. and Goldstein, J.L. (1986) A receptor-mediated pathway for cholesterol homeostasis. *Science* 232, 34–47.

Chomczynski, P. and Sacchi, N. (1987) Single-step method of RNA isolation by acid guanidium thiocyanate-phenol–chlorophorm extraction. *Annals of Biochemistry* 162, 156–159.

Chupukcharoen, N., Komaratat, P. and Wilairat, P. (1985) Effects of vitamin E deficiency on the distribution of cholesterol in plasma lipoproteins and the activity of cholesterol 7a-hydroxylase in the rabbit liver. *Journal of Nutrition* 115, 468–472.

Dietschy, J.M., Turley, S.D. and Spady, D.K. (1993) Role of liver in the maintenance of cholesterol and low density lipoprotein homeostasis in different animal species, including humans. *Journal of Lipid Research* 34, 1637–1659.

Gatto, L.M., Hallen, G.K., Brown, A.J. and Samman, S. (1996) Ascorbic acid induces a favourable lipoprotein profile in women. *Journal of the American College of Nutrition* 15, 154–158.

Hemila, H. (1992) Vitamin C and plasma cholesterol. *Critical Research in Food Science and Nutrition* 32, 33–57.

Holloway, D.E., Peterson, F.J., Prigge, W.F. and Gedhard, R.L. (1981) Influence of dietary ascorbic acid upon enzymes of sterol biosynthesis in guinea pigs. *Biochemistry and Biophysics Research Communications* 102, 1283–1289.

Huang, M.T., Ho, C.T., Wang, Z.Y., Ferraro, T., Finnegan-Olive, T., Lou, Y.R., Mitchell, J.M., Laskin, J.D., Newmark, H., Yang, C.S. and Conney, A.H. (1992) Inhibitory effect of topical application of a polyphenol fraction on tumour initiation and promotion in mouse skin. *Carcinogenesis* 13, 947–954.

Jovanovic, S., Hara, Y., Steenken, S. and Simic, M.G. (1995) Antioxidant potential of gallocatechins. A pulse radiolysis and laser photolysis study. *Journal of the American Chemistry Society* 117, 9881–9888.

Kambouris, A.M., Roach, P.D., Calvert, G.D. and Nestel, P.J. (1990) Retroendocytosis of high density lipoproteins by the human hepatoma cell line, HepG2. *Arteriosclerosis* 10, 582–590.

Kono, S., Shinchi, K., Ikeda, N., Yanai, F. and Imanishi, K. (1992) Green tea consumption and serum lipid profiles: a cross-sectional study in Northern Kyushi, Japan. *Preventive Medicine* 21, 526–531.

Lowry, O.H., Rosebrough, N.J., Farr, A.L. and Randall R.J. (1951) Protein measurement with the Folin phenol reagent. *Journal of Biological Chemistry* 193, 265–275.

Muramatsu, K., Fukuyo, M. and Hara, Y. (1986) Effect of green tea catechins on plasma cholesterol level in cholesterol-fed rats. *Journal of Nutritional Science and Vitaminology* 32, 613–622.

Phonpanichrasamee, C., Komaratat, P. and Wilairat, P. (1990) Hypocholesterolemic effect of vitamin E on cholesterol-fed rabbit. *International Journal of Vitamins and Nutrition Research* 60, 240–245.

Powell, E.E. and Kroon, P.A. (1992) Measurement of mRNA by quantitative PCR with a nonradioactive label. *Journal of Lipid Research* 33, 609–614.

Roach, P.D., Zollinger, M. and Noël, S.-P. (1987) Detection of the low density lipoprotein (LDL) receptor on nitrocellulose paper with colloidal gold–LDL conjugates. *Journal of Lipid Research* 28, 1515–1521.

Roach, P.D., Hosking, J., Clifton, P.M., Bais, R., Kusenic, B., Coyle, P., Wight, M.B., Thomas, D.W. and Nestel, P.J. (1993a) The effects of hypercholesterolemia, simvastatin and dietary fat on the low density lipoprotein receptor of unstimulated mononuclear cells. *Atherosclerosis* 103, 245–254.

Roach, P.D., Balasubramaniam, S., Hirata, F., Abbey, M., Szanto, A., Simons, L.A. and Nestel, P.J. (1993b) The low density lipoprotein receptor and cholesterol synthesis are affected differently by dietary cholesterol in the rat. *Biochimica et Biophysica Acta* 1170, 165–172.

Sanchez, H.B., Yieh, L. and Osborne, T.F. (1995) Cooperation by sterol regulatory element-binding protein and Sp1 in sterol regulation of low density lipoprotein receptor gene. *Journal of Biological Chemistry* 270, 1161–1169.

Thomas, S.R., Neuzil, J., Mohr, D. and Stocker, R. (1995) Coantioxidants make α-tocopherol an efficient antioxidant for low-density lipoprotein. *American Journal of Clinical Nutrition* 62, 1357S–1364S.

Tran, K., Wong, J.T., Lee, E., Chan, A.C. and Choy, P.C. (1996) Vitamin E potentiates arachidonate release and phospholipase A_2 activity in rat heart myoblastic cells. *Biochemical Journal* 319, 385–391.

Wang, X., Sato, R., Brown, M.S., Hua, X. and Goldstein, J.L. (1994) SREBP-1, a membrane-bound transcription factor released by sterol-regulated proteolysis. *Cell* 77, 53–62.

Westrope, K.L., Miller, R.A. and Wilson, R.B. (1982) Vitamin E in a rabbit model of endogenous hypercholesterolemia and atherosclerosis. *Nutrition Reports International* 25, 83–88.

Witztum, J.L. and Steinberg, D. (1991) Role of oxidized low density lipoprotein in atherogenesis. *Journal of Clinical Investigation* 88, 1785–1792.

Yang, C.S. and Lee, M.J. (1987) Methodology of plasma retinol, tocopherol and carotenoid assays in cancer prevention studies. *Journal of Nutrients and Growth of Cancer* 4, 19–27.

Yasuda, M., Fujita, T. and Mizunoya, Y. (1979) Liver and plasma lipids in vitamin E-deficient rats. *Chemical and Pharmacological Bulletin* 27, 447–451.

Carotenoid and Lipid/Lipoprotein Correlates of the Susceptibility of Low-density Lipoprotein to Oxidation in Humans

6

STEPHEN B. KRITCHEVSKY[1], THOMAS A. HUGHES[2], JOHN BELCHER[3] AND MYRON GROSS[4]

[1]*Department of Preventive Medicine, University of Tennessee-Memphis, Memphis, Tennessee;* [2]*Department of Medicine, Division of Endocrinology, University of Tennessee-Memphis, Memphis, Tennessee;* [3]*Department of Medicine, Division of Hematology, University of Minnesota, Minneapolis, Minnesota;* [4]*Division of Epidemiology, University of Minnesota, Minneapolis, Minnesota, USA*

Introduction

Recently, four clinical trials have reported results on the effect of β-carotene on the occurrence of cardiovascular disease (CVD). The Alpha-Tocopherol Beta-Carotene Trial was designed to assess the effect of those two anti-oxidants on lung cancer among Finnish male smokers (The Alpha-Tocopherol Beta-Carotene Prevention Study Group, 1994). Contrary to expectation, there was a small but statistically significant increase in the risk of coronary heart disease (CHD) death among those receiving β-carotene. In the CARET trial, Omenn *et al.* studied the effect of both β-carotene and vitamin A in a population at high risk of lung cancer, including both long-term heavy smokers and people with documented asbestos exposure (Omenn *et al.*, 1996). They found a 26% increase in the risk of CVD death among those receiving the supplement. The Physicians Health Trial evaluated the effect of 50 mg of β-carotene taken every other day in primarily non-smoking physicians, and no effect on either incident myocardial infarction

© CAB *International* 1999. *Antioxidants in Human Health*
(eds T.K. Basu, N.J. Temple and M.L. Garg)

or CVD death was found (Hennekens *et al.*, 1996). Finally, Greenberg and colleagues (1996), in a study to evaluate the effect of β-carotene on the occurrence of skin cancer among adults who had had a prior pathologically confirmed basal or squamous cell carcinoma, also found a slight elevation in the risk of CVD death (Greenberg *et al.*, 1996).

The findings in the above trials are in contrast to several promising, albeit inconsistent, epidemiologic results relating both increased dietary and increased plasma β-carotene to lower rates of CHD and CVD reported by several authors (Riemersma *et al.*, 1991; Bolton-Smith *et al.*, 1992; Gey *et al.*, 1993; Kardinaal *et al.*, 1993; Rimm *et al.*, 1993; Morris *et al.*, 1994; Street *et al.*, 1994; Gaziano *et al.*, 1995b; Pandey *et al.*, 1995; Kushi *et al.*, 1996; Evans *et al.*, 1998). The discrepancy between the epidemiological and the clinical trial results is exemplified by data from the Skin Cancer Prevention Trial (Greenberg *et al.*, 1996). While the trial showed that those taking β-carotene had a 15% excess rate of CVD death, the relative risk of CVD death was significantly lower in those with an increased level of prerandomization plasma β-carotene levels. Those with β-carotene levels above the median (greater than 0.33 µmol l^{-1}) had nearly a 50% lower rate of CVD death compared to those with levels in the lowest quartile (less than or equal to 0.21 µmol l^{-1}).

What can explain the discrepancy between the encouraging epidemiologic findings and the discouraging clinical trial results? The dose could be wrong. It is unlikely that the dose was too low. The blood levels achieved in the Finnish trial among the supplemented group should have protected them if the epidemiological evidence is to be used as a guide (The Alpha-Tocopherol Beta-Carotene Prevention Study Group, 1994). If anything, the dose might be too high. Perhaps the β-carotene was given at the wrong stage in the natural history of the disease. This may well be an issue in explaining the null findings with respect to cancer occurrence. As far as CHD is concerned, trials of effective interventions, such as HMG-CoA inhibitors, find a protective effect beginning no later than 2 years following the initiation of treatment (Shah, 1996). All of the β-carotene trials were of sufficient duration to show an effect on CHD given this time frame. Perhaps β-carotene is not the correct substance to test: people eat foods not micronutrients. Those consuming foods rich in β-carotene are also consuming any number of other plant-derived substances, as well as other carotenoids. Data from the Lipids Research Clinics study underscore that point (Morris *et al.*, 1994). In this population of type II hyperlipidaemics, total serum carotenoids levels were strongly and inversely associated with the risk of incident CHD. Since β-carotene constitutes only about one-quarter of the serum carotenoids, it is certainly plausible that the reduced risk of disease is due to the action of other carotenoids.

One conclusion that can be reached from the discrepancy between the trial results and the epidemiological data is that carotenoids other than β-carotene should be investigated with respect to their role in CHD. One possible mechanism by which carotenoids might exert a protective influence is through their antioxidant properties. The potential for antioxidants to prevent heart disease has become apparent with the growing appreciation of the atherogenic nature of oxidized LDL (Steinberg, 1995). Thus, it is worthwhile to ask whether carotenoids other than β-carotene are associated with the susceptibility of LDL to oxidation.

Study Population

The associations between the susceptibility of LDL to oxidation and plasma carotenoids, α-tocopherol, lipids and lipoproteins were examined in 22 men participating in a pilot study of carotid artery wall lesions determined by B-mode ultrasound. On the basis of self-reports, the participants were in good general health. The group was older (average age: 64 years (range 49–71)) and generally overweight (average body mass index: 27.7 kg m^{-2} (range 22.3–38.8)). Nine participants (41%) reported taking multivitamin supplements and two participants (9%) were current smokers. Following an overnight fast, blood was collected in ethylene diamine tetraacetic acid (EDTA) tubes. Samples were spun at approximately 1500 × g for 20 min and plasma transferred to storage tubes shortly after phlebotomy. Aliquots of plasma were stored at −70°C until analysis. The carotenoids are stable to these handling conditions (Gross *et al.*, 1995).

Laboratory Methods

Plasma carotenoids, α- and β-carotene, β-cryptoxanthin, lycopene, and the combination of zeaxanthin/lutein as well as α-tocopherol were estimated by high performance liquid chromatography (HPLC; Bieri *et al.*, 1979, 1985). Zeaxanthin and lutein are presented together because they could not be analysed individually due to limitations of the HPLC method. Instrument calibration utilized a crystalline standard for each carotenoid and an internal standard to account for variation in recoveries. Quality control procedures included the routine analysis of plasma control pools containing high and low concentrations of each analyte. In addition, the laboratory routinely analyses National Institutes of Standards and Technology reference sera and is a participant in the National Institutes of Standards and Technology Fat-soluble Vitamin Quality Assurance Group. Typical coefficients of variation for all analytes were less than 8%, recoveries of the internal standard were greater than 90% and values from analysis of the reference sera were within 10% of certified values.

Plasma lipoproteins (very-low-density lipoprotein (VLDL), low-density lipoprotein (LDL), and high-density lipoprotein (HDL) subfractions) were isolated by gradient ultracentrifugation as previously described (Hughes *et al.*, 1988) except for minor modifications of the salt gradient which short-ened the necessary spin time (Hughes *et al.*, 1991). Apolipoproteins were measured by reverse-phase HPLC (Hughes *et al.*, 1988). The total and free cholesterol (Boehringer Mannheim Diagnostics) and triglyceride (Sigma) concentrations of each lipoprotein subfraction were determined with com-mercially available enzymatic assays. The apolipoprotein B (apoB) content of LDL was determined by the Lowry assay in 50 mM sodium dodecyl sul-phate (SDS) and 0.1 M NaOH using bovine serum albumin (BSA) as a stan-dard. The apolipoprotein (apoB) concentrations in VLDL were determined in a similar manner after precipitating the apoB and resolubilizing in SDS (Hughes *et al.*, 1988).

LDL susceptibility to oxidation was measured by the following method (Belcher *et al.*, 1993). LDL was isolated by rate zonal density gradient ultra-centrifugation. LDL was oxidized with hemin and H_2O_2 in 96-well microtitre plates. The oxidation of LDL was monitored by measuring the decreasing absorbance of hemin at 405 nm. This parallels the increase in thiobarbituric acid-reactive substances and conjugated dienes. The final assay concentra-tions for the microtitre assay were 100 mg l^{-1} LDL cholesterol, 2.5 µmol l^{-1} hemin and 50 µmol l^{-1} H_2O_2 in HEPE/NaCl (10/150 µmol l^{-1}) buffer, pH 7.4, in a final assay volume of 0.15 ml. The susceptibility of LDL to oxida-tion was measured as the time required for the reaction to reach maximum velocity (i.e. time to V_{max}). V_{max}, as measured by the change in hemin absorbance, was reached near the midpoint of the propagation phase. The time to V_{max} was computed by software linked to the plate reader (Molecular Devices, Menlo Park, California). The greater the time to V_{max}, the greater the resistance of the LDL to oxidation. Other researchers have used the time until the beginning of the propagation phase to index oxida-tive resistance. The correlation between this lag time and the time to V_{max} in 56 samples was 0.992; however, time to V_{max} was approximately 10 min longer than lag time.

Results

Table 6.1 shows the cholesterol and triglyceride levels of the study partici-pants. The levels are not remarkable except for one participant with a triglyceride level of 15.4 µmol l^{-1}. In the table, the results for the plasma lipids are given, both including and excluding this subject. Given this extreme level it is likely that he has type V dyslipoproteinaemia. In many subsequent analyses this individual was a statistical outlier. In those cases, the results are shown both including and excluding his data.

The average lag time was 81.6 min (SD = 20 min, range 54–133 min). As shown in Fig. 6.1, the lag time for men using vitamin supplements aver-aged 11.6 min longer than the non-users but the difference was not statisti-cally significant (P = 0.18, *t*-test). In subsequent analyses, the relationships

Table 6.1. Plasma lipid levels (mmol l^{-1}) of subjects.

Lipid	Level (SD)	Range
Total cholesterol	5.82 (0.88)	4.16–7.52
	5.73 (0.81)[a]	4.16–7.21
LDL-C	3.26 (0.85)	0.98–4.57
	3.38 (0.68)[a]	2.02–4.57
HDL-C	1.34 (0.34)	0.82–1.94
	1.35 (0.32)[a]	0.82–1.94
VLDL-C	0.76 (0.99)	0.13–4.69
	0.58 (0.47)[a]	0.13–1.84
Triglyceride	2.30 (3.06)	0.61–15.35
	1.68 (0.97)[a]	0.61–3.92

[a] Values with one type V hyperlipidaemic removed.

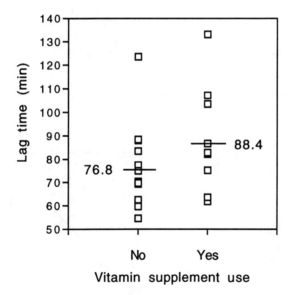

Fig. 6.1. Lag time before maximal LDL oxidation comparing vitamin supplement users with non-users.

between lag time and the carotenoids and α-tocopherol did not differ by supplement use (data not shown). Supplement users tended to have higher levels of the plasma antioxidants. Compared with non-users, supplement users had 15% higher lutein+zeaxanthin levels (P = 0.28, t-test), 34% higher cryptoxanthin levels (P = 0.38, t-test), 123% higher α-carotene levels (P = 0.08, t-test), 182% higher β-carotene levels (P = 0.04, t-test), 39% higher levels of α-tocopherol (*P* = 0.02, Wilcoxon rank sum test) but 9.6% lower lycopene levels (*P* = 0.52, *t*-test).

The mean levels and range of plasma carotenoids and α-tocopherol are shown in Table 6.2. They are listed in descending order of the Pearson product moment correlation with lag time. Among the carotenoids, lycopene was present at the highest concentration followed by β-carotene and lutein+zeaxanthin. Lutein+zeaxanthin levels were highly correlated with the lag time (*r* = 0.81; Fig. 6.2), as were α-tocopherol levels (*r* = 0.76). β-

Table 6.2. Plasma α-tocopherol and carotenoid levels and correlations with time until maximum LDL oxidation.

Substance	Mean (SD) (μmol I^{-1})	Range	Correlation with lag time
Lutein+ zeaxanthin	0.31 (0.09)	0.18–0.48	0.81*
α-Tocopherol	36.2 (16.0)	33.8–85.9	0.76*
β-Carotene	0.48 (0.47)	0.11–1.77	0.36
β-Cryptoxanthin	0.13 (0.10)	0.02–0.46	0.04
α-Carotene	0.10 (0.10)	0.03–0.46	0.02
Lycopene	0.73 (0.25)	0.16–1.07	−0.54*

*$P<0.05$.

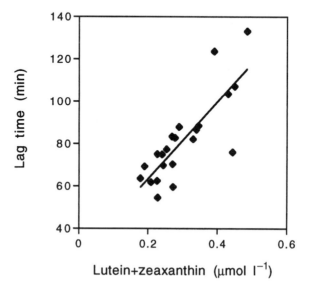

Fig. 6.2. The relationship between plasma lutein+zeaxanthin levels and lag time before maximal LDL oxidation.

Carotene was less strongly correlated with lag time, and there was no relationship between either β-cryptoxanthin or α-carotene and lag time. Surprisingly, lycopene was inversely correlated with lag time ($r = -0.54$). When the relationships were examined expressing the antioxidant levels per apoB molecule in LDL, there was little change in the relationship between lutein+zeaxanthin or α-tocopherol and lag time ($r = 0.83$ and 0.73, respectively). The correlation between β-carotene and lag time increased to 0.48 ($P = 0.02$) and the correlation with lycopene became -0.29 ($P = 0.19$).

Correlations between the lipid content of the major lipoprotein fractions and lag time are shown in Table 6.3. Overall, there was no relationship between total serum cholesterol and lag time. VLDL cholesterol was associated with increased lag time and both HDL and LDL cholesterol with reduced lag time. The triglyceride levels in each of the fractions was associated with increased lag time. However, all of these associations were greatly diminished when the type V hyperlipidaemic was removed from consideration.

Table 6.4 shows the associations between lag time and apoproteins. ApoB levels were associated with modestly shorter lag times, and each of the three C apolipoproteins with increased lag times. The relationships between C-II and C-III were statistically significant. However, these associations diminished after the removal of the type V hyperlipidaemic.

Discussion

In this study, the triglyceride content of the lipoprotein fractions were associated with reduced oxidative susceptibility. VLDL cholesterol was associated with reduced oxidative susceptibility but HDL and LDL cholesterol

Table 6.3. Correlations between lipid subfractions and time until maximum LDL oxidation.

Fraction	Cholesterol	Triglyceride
Total	0.07	0.51*
		[0.24]
VLDL	0.53*	0.52*
	[0.30]	[0.28]
HDL	−0.27	0.47*
	[−0.17]	[0.08]
LDL	−0.51*	0.36
	[−0.32]	[−0.16]

Values in brackets are after one type V hyperlipidaemic was removed from the analysis.
*$P<0.05$.

Table 6.4. Plasma apolipoproteins levels and correlations with time until maximum LDL oxidation.

Apoprotein	Level (SD) (μmol l⁻¹)	Range	Correlation with lag time
B	1.78 (0.36)	1.20–2.55	−0.20 [−0.03]
A-I	55.83 (9.19)	37.45–75.26	0.07
C-I	14.39 (4.24)	7.73–25.45	0.32 [0.07]
C-II	6.70 (2.73)	3.87–13.75	0.46* [0.27]
C-III	19.47 (11.16)	9.58–63.05	0.52*
	[17.37 (5.68)]	[9.58–30.74]	[0.27]

Values in brackets are after one type V hyperlipidaemic was removed from the analysis.
*$P < 0.05$.

were associated with increased oxidative susceptibility. The relationships involving the lipoproteins were strongly influenced by one subject with profoundly elevated triglycerides. When this participant was omitted from the analysis, there were no significant correlations between either lipoprotein cholesterol or triglycerides and oxidative susceptibility. All three of the C apolipoproteins were associated with low oxidative susceptibility. Again, after the omission of the one participant with extremely high triglycerides, these correlations were attenuated, though there was still a modest correlation ($r = 0.27$) between lag time and apoproteins C-II and C-III.

In this investigation, plasma lutein+zeaxanthin and α-tocopherol levels had statistically significant associations with reduced susceptibility of LDL to *in vitro* oxidation. Surprisingly, lycopene levels were associated with higher oxidative susceptibility. As calculated by Esterbauer *et al.* (1992), individual carotenoids are probably not present in high enough concentrations in the LDL particle to affect LDL's properties. Our findings suggest, therefore, a common factor associated with both lutein+zeaxanthin levels and LDL's susceptibility to oxidation. This common factor might involve absorption of these carotenoids or their subsequent metabolism. Goulinet and Chapman (1997) recently showed that the concentration of both α-tocopherol and the oxygenated carotenoids (lutein+zeaxanthin and canthaxanthin) are related to LDL particle size. Denser LDL carries less oxy-carotenoids. LDL's susceptibility to oxidation has been shown to increase with increasing density (Esterbauer *et al.*, 1992). It is possible that in our population lutein+zeaxanthin and α-tocopherol levels are a proxy for LDL density. Along these lines, the apolipoproteins C-II and C-III are not found in LDL. But, because of their apparent role in the transfer of triglycerides and cholesterol between lipoprotein fractions, they may have a role in determining the density of the LDL molecule.

Two important caveats should be observed concerning the present study. The subjects were selected for a pilot study of carotid ultrasound abnormalities and antioxidants. They had been screened previously and those who had either very low or very high levels of carotid disease were invited to participate. It is possible that the results derived from a small study involving a selected population may not be substantiated by other studies. Indeed, the correlations between α-tocopherol and the oxidative susceptibility of LDL are considerably larger than that reported by others (Esterbauer *et al.*, 1992; Iribarren *et al.*, 1997).

Our findings do not imply that supplementation will have an effect on either the susceptibility of LDL to oxidation or CHD incidence. In our study, β-carotene was modestly associated with increased lag time but supplementation with β-carotene does not affect LDL susceptibility to oxidation (Gaziano *et al.*, 1995a).

Epidemiologists look for explanations of the distribution and determinants of disease. From an epidemiological perspective, LDL oxidation theory has been both exciting and frustrating. On the one hand, it has opened an important new avenue in the epidemiology of heart disease. On the other, the data have been inconsistent, and there is still much to be learned regarding the role of antioxidants and their interplay with established CVD determinants.

A number of studies of various rigour have evaluated the role of the carotenoids other than β-carotene on CVD. In addition to the data presented in this report, two other studies support a protective role for lutein. Fig. 6.3 is redrawn from an ecological study by Howard *et al.* (1996). It compares the average plasma levels of various carotenoids between two of the MONICA populations in Europe, namely Belfast, an area with a high rate of heart disease, and Toulouse, an area with a low rate. While there are many possible explanations for the differences in carotenoid levels between the two populations, it is interesting that the carotenoid showing the largest difference was lutein, and that there was no difference in the levels of either β-carotene or lycopene. In the ARIC study, Iribarren *et al.* (1997) compared serum levels of various carotenoids between two groups. One group had severe but asymptomatic carotid artery disease, the other was a matched control group with little carotid disease. Since the carotid arteries can be imaged non-invasively, they provide an opportunity to observe early presymptomatic atherosclerotic changes. After adjusting for potential confounders, neither serum β-carotene nor α-tocopherol were associated with carotid artery disease. Of the carotenoids examined (the same ones included in the present report) only lutein+zeaxanthin was associated with lower levels of carotid artery disease. Contrary to these findings, Kohlmeier *et al.* (1997) recently reported adipose lycopene levels to be inversely associated with the risk of non-fatal myocardial infarction. The carotenoid story is still unfolding, and despite the disappointing results of the β-carotene trials, the epidemiologic data are intriguing enough to motivate the further evaluation of other carotenoids and their role in the prevention of CVD.

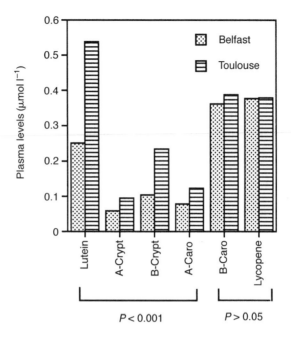

Fig. 6.3. Comparison of mean carotenoid levels between a high CHD area (Belfast) and a low CHD area (Toulouse). Redrawn from Howard *et al.* (1996).

Acknowledgements

Thanks to Dr Susan Carlson for performing the α-tocopherol measurement and to Dr William B. Applegate for facilitating recruitment for this study.

References

The Alpha-Tocopherol Beta-Carotene Cancer Prevention Study Group (1994) The effect of vitamin E and beta carotene on the incidence of lung cancer and other cancers in male smokers. *New England Journal of Medicine* 330, 1039–1035.

Belcher, J.D., Balla, J., Balla, G., Jacobs, D.R. Jr, Gross, M., Jacob, H.S. and Vercellotti, G.M. (1993) Vitamin E, LDL, and endothelium: brief oral vitamin supplementation prevents oxidized LDL-mediated vascular injury *in vitro*. *Arteriosclerosis and Thrombosis* 13, 1779–1789.

Bieri, J.G., Tolliver, T.J. and Catignani, G.L. (1979) Simultaneous determination of alpha-tocopherol and retinol in plasma or red cells by high pressure liquid chromatography. *American Journal of Clinical Nutrition* 32, 2143–2149.

Bieri, J.G., Brown, E.O. and Smith, J. (1985) Determination of individual carotenoids in human plasma by high performance chromatography. *Journal of Liquid Chromatography* 8, 473–484.

Bolton-Smith, C., Woodward, M. and Tunstall-Pedoe, H. (1992) The Scottish Heart Health Study. Dietary intake by food frequency questionnaire and odds ratios for coronary heart disease risk. II. The antioxidant vitamins and fibre. *European Journal of Clinical Nutrition* 46, 85–93.

Esterbauer, H., Gebicki, J., Puhl, H. and Jürgens, G. (1992) Role of lipid peroxidation and antioxidants in oxidative modification of LDL. *Free Radical Biology and Medicine* 13, 341–390.

Evans, R.W., Shaten, B.J., Day, B.W. and Kuller, L.H. (1998) Prospective association between lipid soluble antioxidants and coronary heart disease in men: The Multiple Risk Factor Intervention Trial. *American Journal of Epidemiology* 147, 180–186.

Gaziano, J.M., Hatta, A., Flynn, M., Johnson, E.J., Krinsky, N.I., Ridker, P.M., Hennekens, C.H. and Frei, B. (1995a) Supplementation with beta-carotene *in vivo* and *in vitro* does not inhibit low density lipoprotein oxidation. *Atherosclerosis* 112, 187–195.

Gaziano, J.M., Manson, J.E., Branch, L., Colditz, G., Willett, W. and Buring, J. (1995b) A prospective study of consumption of carotenoids in fruits and vegetables and decreased cardiovascular mortality in the elderly. *Annals of Epidemiology* 5, 255–260.

Gey, K.F., Stähelin, H.B. and Eicholzer, M. (1993) Poor plasma status of carotene and vitamin C is associated with higher mortality from ischemic heart disease and stroke. *Basel Prospective Study. Clinical Investigator* 71, 3–6.

Goulinet, S. and Chapman, M.J. (1997) Plasma LDL and HDL Subspecies are heterogeneous in particle content of tocopherols and oxygenated and hydrocarbon carotenoids: relevance to oxidative resistance and atherogenesis. *Arteriosclerosis, Thrombosis and Vascular Biology* 17, 786–796.

Greenberg, E.R., Baron, J.A., Karagas, M.R., Stukel, T.A., Nierenberg, D.W., Stevens, M.M., Mandel, J.S. and Haile, R.W. (1996) Mortality associated with low plasma concentration of beta carotene and the effect of oral supplementation. *Journal of the American Medical Association* 275, 699–703.

Gross, M.D., Prouty, C.B. and Jacobs, D.R. Jr (1995) Stability of carotenoids and α-tocopherol during blood collection and processing procedures. *Clinical Chemistry* 41, 943–944.

Hennekens, C.H., Buring, J.E., Manson, J.E., Stampfer, M., Rosner, B., Cook, N.R., Belanger, C., LaMotte, F., Gaziano, J.M., Ridker, P.M., Willett, W. and Peto, R. (1996) Lack of effect of long-term supplementation with beta carotene on the incidence of malignant neoplasms and cardiovascular disease. *New England Journal of Medicine* 334, 1145–1149.

Howard, A.N., Williams, N.R., Palmer, C.R., Cambou, J.P., Evans, A.E., Foote, J.W., Marques-Vidal, P., McCrum, E.E., Ruidavets, J.B., Nigdikar, S.V., Rajput-Williams, J. and Thurnham, D.I. (1996) Do hydroxy-carotenoids prevent coronary heart disease? A comparison between Belfast and Toulouse. *International Journal of Vitamins and Nutritional Research* 66, 113–118.

Hughes, T.A., Moore, M.A., Neame, P., Medley, M.F. and Chung, B.H. (1988) Rapid quantitative apolipoprotein analysis by gradient ultracentrifugation and reversed-phase HPLC. *Journal of Lipid Research* 29, 363–376.

Hughes, T.A., Gaber, A.O. and Montgomery, C.E. (1991) Plasma distribution of cyclosporin within lipoproteins and 'in vitro' transfer between very-low density lipoproteins, low density lipoproteins, and high density lipoproteins. *Therapeutic Drug Monitoring* 13, 289–295.

Iribarren, C., Folsom, A.R., Jacobs, D.R. Jr, Gross, M.D., Belcher, J.D. and Eckfeldt, J.H. (1997) Association of serum vitamin levels, LDL susceptibility to oxidation, and autoantibodies against MDA-LDL with carotid atherosclerosis: a case–control study. *Arteriosclerosis, Thrombosis and Vascular Biology* 17, 1171–1177.

Kardinaal, A.F., Kok, F.J., Ringstad, J., Gomez-Aracena, J., Mazaev, V.P., Kohlmeier, L., Martin, B.C., Aro, A., Kark, J.D., Delgado-Rodriguez, M., Riemersma, R.A., van 't Veer, P., Huttunen, J.K. and Martin-Moreno, J.M. (1993) Antioxidants in adipose tissue and risk of myocardial infarction: the EURAMIC study. *Lancet* 342, 1379–1384.

Kohlmeier, L., Kark, J.D., Gomez-Garcia, E., Martin, B.C., Steck, S.E., Kardinaal, A.F.M., Ringstad, J., Thamm, M., Masaev, V., Riemersma, R., Martin-Moreno, J.M., Huttunen, J.K. and Kok, F.J. (1997) Lycopene and myocardial infarction risk in the EURAMIC Study. *American Journal of Epidemiology* 146, 618–626.

Kushi, L.H., Folsom, A.R., Prineas, R.J., Mink, P.J., Wu, Y. and Bostick, R.M. (1996) Dietary antioxidant vitamins and death from coronary heart disease in postmenopausal women. *New England Journal of Medicine* 334, 1156–1162.

Morris, D.L., Kritchevsky, S.B. and Davis, C.E. (1994) Serum carotenoids and coronary heart disease: the Lipid Research Clinics Coronary Primary Prevention Trial and Follow-up Study. *Journal of the American Medical Association* 272, 1439–1441.

Omenn, G.S., Goodman, G.E., Thornquist, M.D., Balmes, J., Cullen, M.R., Glass, A., Keogh, J.P., Meyskens, F.L., Valanis, B., Williams, J.H. Jr, Barnhart, S. and Hammar, S. (1996) Effects of a combination of beta carotene and vitamin A on lung cancer and cardiovascular disease. *New England Journal of Medicine* 334, 1150–1155.

Pandey, D.K., Shekelle, R., Selwyn, B.J., Tangney, C. and Stamler, J. (1995) Dietary vitamin C and B-carotene and risk of death in middle-aged men: the Western Electric Study. *American Journal of Epidemiology* 142, 1269–1278.

Riemersma, R.A., Wood, D.A., Macintyre, C.C., Elton, R.A., Gey, K.F. and Oliver, M.F. (1991) Risk of angina pectoris and plasma concentrations of vitamins A, C, and E and carotene. *Lancet* 337, 1–5.

Rimm, E.B., Stampfer, M.J., Ascherio, A., Giovannucci, E., Colditz, G.A. and Willett, W.C. (1993) Vitamin E consumption and the risk of coronary heart disease in men. *New England Journal of Medicine* 328, 1450–1456.

Shah, P. (1996) Pathophysiology of plaque rupture and the concept of plaque stabilization. *Cardiology Clinics* 14, 17–29.

Steinberg, D. (1995) Role of oxidized LDL and antioxidants in atherosclerosis. In: Longnecker, J.B., Kritchevsky, D. and Drezner, M. (eds) *Nutrition and Biotechnology in Heart Disease and Cancer*. Plenum Press, New York, pp. 39–48.

Street, D.A., Comstock, G.W., Salkeld, R.M., Schüep, W. and Klag, M.J. (1994) Serum antioxidants and myocardial infarction: are low levels of carotenoids and alpha-tocopherol risk factors for myocardial infarction? *Circulation* 90, 1154–1161.

Antioxidation and Evolution: Dietary Restriction and Alterations in Molecular Processes

7

ANGELO TURTURRO[1], PETER H. DUFFY[2]
AND RONALD W. HART[3]

[1]Division of Biometry and Risk Assessment, [2]Division of Genetic Toxicology, [3]Office of the Director, National Center for Toxicological Research, Jefferson, Arkansas, USA

Introduction

The administration of compounds with an antioxidant activity has been reported to have both beneficial (Kushi *et al.*, 1996) and detrimental (Omenn *et al.*, 1996) effects. Factors such as timing of dosing, duration, levels, etc., can potentially affect the result, and comparative analyses of antioxidation across species have been conflicting. Recent studies have shown an inverse relationship of antioxidation potential and species longevity (Perez-Campo *et al.*, 1998). In order to understand better the consequences of exogenous exposure to these agents, it is useful to consider the endogenous role that antioxidants play in the development and survival of an organism in a broad evolutionary context. A tool to explore this role, especially from an evolutionary perspective, is dietary restriction (DR), which has been found to alter the oxidation patterns of macromolecules (Hart *et al.*, 1992).

Antioxidation appears to be part of an integrated set of responses to DR by an organism which helps to stabilize the genomic integrity of cells in the face of exogenous and endogenous stress (Hart *et al.*, 1993). These responses lead to a decrease in the cancer rates with lowered dietary intake at a number of sites (Turturro *et al.*, 1993, 1994, 1995, 1996, 1997, 1998). DR also inhibits other chronic diseases (Berg and Simms, 1960; Turturro and Allaben, 1995; Sheldon *et al.*, 1995a) and, consequently, extends longevity. Since antioxidation may play a role in inhibiting these diseases, antioxidation may thus appear to be a longevity-related process (LRP) (Turturro and Hart, 1991). Besides consequences for longevity, DR also affects reproduction, as discussed earlier in the adaptive-longevity-related process theory of restriction (Turturro and Hart, 1991) and its elaboration (Hart and Turturro, 1998). These efforts partly explored the role of DR in an evolutionary context.

The evolutionary context for DR is further expanded in this report. The importance of the alteration of molecular processes as a result of these LRP (such as antioxidation) for evolution is discussed, along with the mechanisms for potential alterations in the rate of the molecular clocks used in dating evolutionary events.

Alteration of Molecular Processes by DR

One of the most important discoveries of the action of DR made in the last decade is that this environmental alteration can alter molecular processes previously thought to be fixed by the genetic background of organisms. The best example of this was the ability of DR to stimulate DNA excision repair. Until the late 1980s (Licastro *et al.*, 1988; Lipman *et al.*, 1989; Weraarchakul *et al.*, 1989), DNA excision repair was considered a characteristic of the species genome (e.g. see Hart and Setlow, 1974). Recent work involving humans, in our laboratory, has shown that this is truly a stimulation of DNA excision repair with a decreased dietary intake, not simply a slowed rate of its decline with age (data not shown).

The production of oxidative damage and the components of the systems that protect from this damage were also once thought to be a fixed genomic characteristic, but are, instead, likewise mutable by DR. With DR, the production of oxygen free radicals appears to decrease (Weindruch and Walford, 1988). A number of defence mechanisms have evolved to inactivate free radicals prior to their interactions with macromolecules, including the inducible enzymes: superoxide dismutase, glutathione peroxidase, catalase and haem oxygenase. The efficiency of these enzymes appears to increase with DR (Feuers *et al.*, 1995). For example, the time to maximum substrate inhibition by catalase increases with DR, thus increasing the enzyme's effectiveness. Cells from DR animals exposed to hydrogen peroxide resisted oxidative damage much better than cells from *ad libitum* (AL)-fed animals (Li *et al.*, 1998).

While free radical formation may have a beneficial role to play in recruitment of polymorphonuclear leukocytes and other phagocytes important in the inactivation of pathogens, they have also been implicated in the development of many diseases including ischaemia–reperfusion injury in heart attacks, stroke, cancer, emphysema, immune and neurodegenerative disorders, and ageing (McCord, 1995; Spitzer, 1995). With DR in the absence of malnutrition, the times to occurrence or the severities of many of these diseases are decreased (Hart and Turturro, 1995). Using direct measurements, DR significantly decreases 5-hydroxymethyluracil levels in the DNA of both liver and mammary gland tissue (Djuric *et al.*, 1992, 1995), and decreases oxidative damage in ageing mice (Sohal *et al.*, 1994).

In addition to elevating both DNA excision repair and antioxidation, DR also increases the fidelity of the polymerases responsible for DNA replication (Srivastra *et al.*, 1993), and suppresses the expression of oncogenes associated with cancer (Nakamura *et al.*, 1989; Lyn-Cook *et al.*, 1995). Thus, DR has the effect of preserving genomic fidelity through a series of LRP, including antioxidation.

Adaptive-longevity-related Process Theory of DR

In order to understand the evolutionary consequences of the protection of genomic fidelity by DR, it is important to know the characteristics of the adaptive-longevity-related process theory of DR, as outlined below:

1. DR mimics a situation very common in the wild, i.e. food scarcity at different times of the year, or for years on end.

2. A successful species preserves itself during these difficult times by either forming some metabolically quiescent stage (e.g. sporification) or adapting the organism through some method, such as hibernation, to a phase so that it will live long enough to reproduce when times become better again. Reproduction is often suspended, with reproductive capacity being preserved. One aspect of this adaptation phase is that energy-intensive non-food-gathering activities are curtailed. One of the first activities to be curtailed with DR is the maintenance of body temperature. Average body temperature falls by approximately 1.5°C for mice (Duffy *et al.*, 1990) and 0.75°C for rats (Duffy *et al.*, 1989) and primates (Lane *et al.*, 1996). Cellular proliferation, another energy-intensive process, is significantly decreased throughout the organism (Lu *et al.*, 1993; Wolf and Pendergrass, 1995). Reproduction itself is severely decreased (Merry *et al.*, 1985) or, in some species such as mice, stopped (Nelson *et al.*, 1985). In these same mice, however, reproduction can be re-initiated by refeeding, even at very advanced ages, past the average lifespan of the AL-fed animals. In these aspects, DR is similar to hibernation.

3. The ability to extract energy from foods is increased, with systems becoming more efficient. This is, in part, accomplished by the enzymatic changes discussed above, presumably enabling an organism to optimize the food that is available. For instance, the efficiencies of a number of key enzymes in intermediary metabolism such as glucose 6-phosphate dehydrogenase and pyruvate kinase are increased with DR (Feuers *et al.*, 1991). These enzymes then function at full efficiency instead of being inhibited by the usual regulatory processes involving the addition of phosphates. Metabolism rises following feeding, with the respiratory quotient indicating direct utilization of foodstuffs, with little storage or diversion of food energy for any process except its direct utilization (Duffy *et al.*, 1989, 1990, 1994, 1995).

4. In addition to the 'hibernation-like' slowdown of non-essential functions, animals with DR appear to increase those activities important to food acquisition and competition. Thus, they become very active around feeding time. They also become more prone to escape encagement than AL-fed animals. DR animals become more aggressive, presumably permitting them to be better able to forage and compete for food in times of scarcity. Consistent with this increased aggressiveness in behaviour is the observation that levels of the glucocorticoids, which indicate activation of fight-or-flight stimuli, are elevated in DR animals (Leakey *et al.*, 1995), especially during the early stages of DR (Leakey *et al.*, 1994). In addition, adrenal glands are larger (per gram body weight) in DR animals than in AL-fed ones (Merry and Holehan, 1985). It appears that this increase in food acquisition activity requires so much energy that even the hungry animal is able to maintain it for only part of the day. Presumably, increasing this activity around the animal's usual feeding time maximizes its chances for obtaining food. It is not clear whether this increased food acquisition activity is an LRP or a negative process that limits the positive influence that DR has on lifespan. Increased activity induced by lowering environmental temperature has a detrimental effect on lifespan in mammals (Kibler and Johnson, 1961), suggesting that the increase in activity seen in DR animals may be an antagonistic, pleiotropic effect (Williams, 1957), which sacrifices long-term benefits for short-term survival ones.

5. The mechanisms used to increase lifespan are the specific LRPs that the species normally uses, and emerge in long-lived members of the species. The best candidates for these LRPs are those directly related to reproduction or tied to the processes that directly regulate reproduction. However, other, more distal phenomena, such as alteration of hormone levels and physical activity, also seem to be important.

6. The organism not only delays reproduction, it also increases the protection of the cells involved in reproduction (e.g. by increasing their ability to withstand oxidative damage) by an increase in the activity of the processes discussed above which are believed to protect genomic integrity. This presumably occurs so that the delay in reproduction will not simply result in damaged or dead offspring as a result of the longer time that the organism and its gametes are exposed to damage-inducing agents such as oxidative stress.

Consequences of DR for Evolution

One of the consequences of the improvement in the processes of genomic integrity is that DR decreases variability in a number of parameters. This is shown most clearly for body weight (which has a direct influence on tumorigenesis at a number of sites (Turturro *et al.*, 1995, 1996, 1998)) and is illustrated in Fig. 7.1 for B6C3F1 male mice. This decrease in variability indicates that the factors important to tumorigenesis are maintained at a uniform low level. The factors include mutation, fixation of mutation by cell proliferation and survival. These factors are also important in speciation, both in the generation of new combinations of nucleotides and in their fixation and selection. Conversely, the increase in variability as a result of AL feeding after a period of DR indicates poorer regulation of such factors and greater chance of individual variation.

This analysis helps to explain what has been observed after some mass extinctions, like the one that occurred at the end of the Cretaceous era. If some celestial boloid caused a prolonged winter-like period (Kerr, 1997), the animals who survived would have gone through a period of dietary restriction, preserving both reproductive capacity and genomic integrity. After the effects of the extinction event subsided, there would have been a wide variety of ecological niches available that were basically unpopulated. With little or no competition, the animals would have been similar to AL-fed

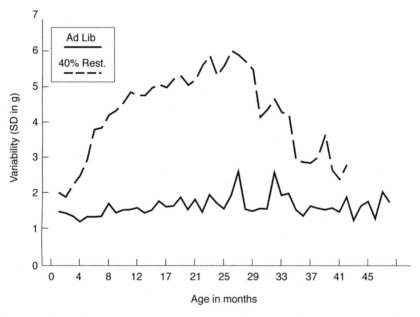

Fig. 7.1. Variability of body weight by age and diet. Standard deviations of similar cohorts (*n* = 54) of B6C3F1 male mice in grams with either *ad libitum* (Ad Lib) or dietary restricted to 40% of *ad libitum* consumption (40% Rest.) as a function of age in months. The Ad Lib cohort suffers the onset of significant mortality after 24 months, while the 40% Rest. group starts this mortality after 30 months of age (see Sheldon *et al.*, 1995b, for mortality and body weight curves).

animals, with little protection from genomic alterations. Under these circumstances, it is likely that speciation would have occurred at a relatively rapid rate after the catastrophe. This is consistent with recent findings about the Tertiary radiation (Normile, 1998).

As the niches were filled, the normal competition for food would have resulted in a level of DR (probably less than that observed during the extinction event) which would have re-established some genetic stability as the genomic integrity processes were again activated. This normal competition could be a stabilizing factor for species, and would result in a long period of relatively little speciation while competition remained high. This is consistent with evidence from bird speciation in the Pleistocene, which indicates longer times for successive speciation events as the present is approached (Zink and Slowinski, 1995) and from evidence in man (Ninio, 1997).

The LRP approach emphasizes that environmental alterations and catastrophes directly affect the molecular processes contributing to evolution, not only selection factors. It leads to predictions that the molecular clocks, i.e. the mutation rates in genes which are used to predict the time of species divergence, besides being different for different members of a gene family (Gibb *et al.*, 1998), should overall speed up under conditions leading to AL feeding and slow down during periods of DR. The normal food-competitive condition should result in a clock rate that is a function of the intensity of the competition. The molecular clocks can be thought of as a quartz clock in which the resonant frequency is a function of temperature, which is controlled by the amount of fuel (food) available. The LRP approach is also consistent with the observation of punctuated equilibrium, adding molecular stability to species segregation leading to new species (Gould, 1998). Interestingly, since most mutations are deleterious, and would probably contribute to decreased capacity for food gathering, there appears to be an actual 'restorative force' for the equilibrium, which is a dampening of the molecular processes that lead to speciation under normal conditions of food competition. Finding a new niche would disturb this equilibrium, but increasing numbers and the competition for food would stabilize it again. The LRP approach also is consistent with different speciation rates in groups of related species (Vrba, 1985), which in this analysis would depend on the history of food availability and intra- and inter-species competition.

The LRP approach predicts that extinction events that make habitats unavailable should result in fewer species being generated than those events that simply depopulate niches, despite strong selection pressure. This prediction is consistent with the loss of species that is presently occurring despite the creation of man-made habitats, since man already occupies many of these new habitats. An interesting prediction also generated by this approach is that man, and his parasites, should now, after a long period of relatively low mutation rates, be found to be mutating fairly rapidly in the developed countries as the food supply becomes unlimited. This would result in an elevated rate of genetic polymorphisms in the well-fed industrialized countries compared with countries with limited food supplies. Also, the generation of new forms of viruses, bacterial diseases, etc., would be expected as these 'parasites' are released from their energy-restricted controls as they migrated to industrialized countries from poorer ones.

Conclusions

DR, and the LRPs it induces such as antioxidation, seem to play a role in the rate of development of new species, as well as preserving the integrity of members in an existing one. DR initially protects an animal and its reproductive potential through a period of extreme want, and then the increased variability of the AL condition can thus result in the better exploitation of various niches when conditions are favourable. These factors complicate comparative analyses of factors important in intraspecies survival, such as the LRPs. Thus an LRP such as antioxidation may be well correlated to survival within a species, and might be poorly correlated to survival times between species (e.g. Perez-Campo *et al.*, 1998). Between species, the time since initial formation of the species and the length of the period of genetic stability may be factors. In addition, the impact of an environmental factor such as DR on rates of genetic change should point to other factors, such as hormonal changes and regulatory gene changes, which will also be altered by the environment, as potential modifiers of the rate of molecular evolution.

Finally, the ability to manipulate genetic expression with environmental changes adds another tool for experimenters to better fine-tune the alterations they make to genomes and their consequences.

References

Allaben, W., Chou, M., Pegram, R., Leakey, J., Feuers, R., Duffy, P., Turturro A. and Hart, R. (1990) Modulation of toxicity and carcinogenicity by caloric restriction. *Korean Journal of Toxicology* 6, 167–182.

Berg, B.N. and Simms, H.S. (1960) Nutrition and longevity in the rat: II. Longevity and onset of disease with different levels of food intake. *Journal of Nutrition* 71, 255–263.

Djuric, Z., Lu, M.H., Lewis, S.M., Luongo, D.A., Chen, X.W., Heilbrun, L.K., Reading, B.A., Duffy, P.H. and Hart, R.W. (1992) Oxidative DNA damage levels in rats fed low-fat, high-fat, or caloric-restricted diets. *Toxicology and Applied Pharmacology* 115, 156–160.

Djuric, Z., Lu, M.H., Lewis, S.M., Luongo, D.A., Chen, X.W., Heilbrun, L.K., Reading, B.A., Duffy, P.H. and Hart, R.W. (1995) Effects of dietary calories and fat on levels of oxidative DNA damage. In: Hart, R.W., Neuman, D. and Robertson, R. (eds) *Dietary Restriction: Implications for the Design and Interpretation of Toxicity and Carcinogenicity Studies.* ILSI Press, Washington, DC, pp. 197–212.

Duffy, P.H., Feuers, R., Leakey, J., Nakamura, K., Turturro, A. and Hart, R.W. (1989) Effect of chronic caloric restriction on physiological variables that modulate energy metabolism in the male Fischer-344 rat. *Mechanisms of Ageing and Development* 48, 117–133.

Duffy, P.H., Feuers, R., Leakey, J. and Hart, R.W. (1990) Sex-related differences in adaption to caloric restriction in old B6C3F1 mice: implications for chronopharmacology and chronotherapy. *Annual Review of Chronopharmacology* 7, 95–98.

Duffy, P.H., Feuers, R., Pipkin, J. and Hart, R.W. (1994) Effect of chronic caloric restriction: physiological and behavioral response to alternate day feeding in old female B6C3F1 mice. *Age* 17, 13–21.

Duffy, P.H., Feuers, R., Pipkin, J., Berg, T., Leakey, J., Turturro, A. and Hart, R.W. (1995) The effect of dietary restriction and aging on the physiological response of rodents to drugs. In: Hart, R.W., Neuman, D. and Robertson, R. (eds) *Dietary Restriction: Implications for the Design and Interpretation of Toxicity and Carcinogenicity Studies*. ILSI Press, Washington, DC, pp. 127–140.

Feuers, R., Hunter, J.D., Casciano, D.A., Shaddock, J.G., Leakey, J., Duffy, P.H., Scheving, L.E. and Hart, R.W. (1991) Modifications in regulation of intermediary metabolism by caloric restriction in rodents. In: Fishbein, L. (ed.) *Biological Effects of Dietary Restriction*. Springer-Verlag, New York, pp. 198–206.

Feuers, R., Duffy, P.H., Chen, F., Desai, V., Oriaku, E., Shaddock, J.G., Pipkin, J.L., Weindruch, R. and Hart, R.W. (1995) Intermediary metabolism and antioxidant systems. In: Hart, R.W., Neuman, D. and Robertson, R. (eds) *Dietary Restriction: Implications for the Design and Interpretation of Toxicity and Carcinogenicity Studies*. ILSI Press, Washington, DC, pp. 181–195.

Hart, R.W. and Setlow, R.B. (1974) Correlation between deoxyribonucleic acid excision-repair and life-span in a number of mammalian species. *Proceedings of the National Academy of Sciences, USA* 71, 2169–2173.

Hart, R.W. and Turturro, A. (1995) Dietary restriction: an update. In: Hart, R.W., Neuman, D. and Robertson, R. (eds) *Dietary Restriction: Implications for the Design and Interpretation of Toxicity and Carcinogenicity Studies*. ILSI Press, Washington, DC, pp. 1–13.

Hart, R.W. and Turturro, A. (1998) Evolution and dietary restriction. *Experimental Gerontology* 33, 53–60.

Hart, R.W., Chou, M., Feuers, R., Leakey, J., Duffy, P.H., Lyn-Cook, B., Turturro, A. and Allaben, W. (1992) Caloric restriction and chemical toxicity/carcinogenesis. *Quality Assurance: Good Practice, Regulation, and Law* 1, 120–131.

Hart, R.W., Leakey, J., Allaben, W., Chou, M., Duffy, P.H., Feuers, R. and Turturro, A. (1993) Role of nutrition and diet in degenerative processes. *International Journal of Toxicology, Occupational and Environmental Health* 1, 26–32.

Gibb, P.E., Witke, W.F. and Dugaiczyk, A. (1998) The molecular clock runs at different rates among closely related members of a gene family. *Journal of Molecular Evolution* 46, 552–561.

Gould, S.J. (1998) Gulliver's further travels: the necessity and difficulty of a hierarchical theory of selection. *Philosophical Transactions of the Royal Society of London, Series B: Biological Sciences* 353, 307–314.

Kerr, R. (1997) Cores document ancient catastrophe. *Science* 275, 1265.

Kibler, H. and Johnson, H. (1961) Metabolic rate and aging in rats during exposure to cold. *Journal of Gerontology* 16, 13–16.

Kushi, L., Folsom, A., Prinas, R., Mink, P., Wu, Y. and Bostick, R. (1996) Antioxidant vitamins and coronary heart disease. *New England Journal of Medicine* 334, 1156–1162.

Lane, M., Baer, D., Rumpler, W., Weindruch, R., Ingram, D., Tilmont, E., Cutler, R. and Roth, G. (1996) Calorie restriction lowers body temperature in rhesus monkeys, consistent with a postulated anti-aging mechanism in rodents. *Proceedings of the National Academy of Science, USA* 93, 4159–4164.

Leakey, J., Chen, S., Manjgaladze, M., Turturro, A., Duffy, P.H., Pipkin, J. and Hart, R.W. (1994) Role of glucocorticoids and 'caloric stress' in modulating the effects of caloric restriction in rodents. *Annals of the New York Academy of Sciences* 719, 171–194.

Leakey, J., Seng, J., Manjgaladze, M., Kozlovskaya, N., Xia, S., Lee, M., Frame, L., Chen, S., Rhodes, C., Duffy, P.H. and Hart, R.W. (1995) Influence of caloric intake on drug metabolizing enzyme expression: relevance to tumorigenesis and toxicity testing. In: Hart, R.W., Neuman, D. and Robertson, R. (eds) *Dietary Restriction: Implications for the Design and Interpretation of Toxicity and Carcinogenicity Studies*. ILSI Press, Washington, DC, pp. 167–180.

Li, Y., Yan, Q., Pendergrass, W.R. and Wolf, N.S. (1998) Response of lens epithelial cells to hydrogen peroxide stress and the protective effect of caloric restriction. *Experimental Cell Research* 239, 254–263.

Licastro, F., Weindruch, R., Davis, L.I. and Walford, R.L. (1988) Effect of dietary restriction upon the age-associated decline of lymphocyte DNA repair activity in mice. *Age* 11, 48–52.

Lipman, J., Turturro, A. and Hart, R.W. (1989) The influence of dietary restriction on DNA repair in rodents: a preliminary study. *Mechanisms of Ageing and Development* 48, 135–143.

Lu, M., Hinson, W., Turturro, A., Sheldon, W. and Hart, R.W. (1993) Cell proliferation by cell cycle analysis in young and old dietary restricted mice. *Mechanisms of Ageing and Development* 68, 151–162.

Lyn-Cook, B., Blann, E., Hass, B. and Hart, R.W. (1995) Oncogene expression and cellular transformation: The effects of dietary restriction. In: Hart, R.W., Neuman, D. and Robertson, R. (eds) *Dietary Restriction: Implications for the Design and Interpretation of Toxicity and Carcinogenicity Studies*. ILSI Press, Washington, DC, pp. 271–278.

McCord, J.M. (1995) Superoxide radical: controversies, contradictions, and paradoxes. *Proceedings of the Society for Experimental Biology and Medicine* 109, 112–117.

Merry, B. and Holehan, A. (1985) The endocrine response to dietary restriction in the rat. In: Woodhead, A., Blackett, A. and Holleander, A. (eds) *Molecular Biology of Aging*. Plenum Press, New York, pp. 117–141.

Merry, B., Holehan, A. and Philips, J. (1985) Modification of reproductive decline and life span by dietary manipulation in CFY Sprague-Dawley rats. In: Lofts, B. and Holmes, W. (eds) *Current Trends in Comparative Endocrinology*. Hong Kong University Press, Hong Kong, pp. 621–624.

Nakamura, K., Duffy, P., Lu, M., Turturro, A. and Hart R. (1989) The effect of dietary restriction on myc protooncogene expression in mice: a preliminary study. *Mechanisms of Ageing and Development* 48, 199–205.

Nelson, J., Gosden, R. and Felicio, L. (1985) Effect of dietary restriction on estrous cyclicity and follicular reserves in aging C57Bl/6J mice. *Biology and Reproduction* 32, 515–522.

Ninio, J. (1997) The evolutionary design of error-rates, and the fast fixation enigma. *Origins of Life and Biosphere* 27, 609–621.

Normile, D. (1998) New views of the origins of mammals. *Science* 281, 774–775.

Omenn, G.S., Goodman, G.E., Thornquist, M.D., Balmes, J., Cullen, M.R., Glass, A., Keogh, J.P., Meyskens, F.L., Jr, Valanis, B., Williams, J.H., Jr, Barnhart, S., Cherniack, M.G., Brodkin, C.A. and Hammar, S. (1996) Risk factors for lung cancer and for intervention effects in CARET, the Beta-Carotene and Retinol Efficacy Trial. *Journal of the National Cancer Institute* 88, 1550–1559.

Perez-Campo, R., Lopez-Torres, M., Cadenas, S., Rojas, C. and Barja, G. (1998) The rate of free radical production as a determinant of the rate of aging: evidence from the comparative approach. *Journal of Comparative Physiology – B Biochemistry, Systematics, and Environmental Physiology* 168, 149–158.

Sheldon, W., Warbritton, A., Bucci, T. and Turturro, A. (1995a) Primary glaucoma in food restricted and *ad libitum* fed DBA/2NNia mice. *American Association of Laboratory Animal Science* 45, 508–518.

Sheldon, W., Bucci, T., Hart, R.W. and Turturro, A. (1995b) Age-related neoplasia in a lifetime study of *ad libitum*-fed and food restricted B6C3F1 mice. *Toxicology Pathology* 23, 458–476.

Sohal, R.S., Agarwal, S., Candas, M., Forster, M. and Lal, H. (1994) Effect of age and caloric restriction on DNA oxidative damage in different tissues of C57BL/6 mice. *Mechanisms of Ageing and Development* 76, 215–224.

Spitzer, J.A. (1995) Active oxygen intermediates – beneficial or deleterious? An introduction. *Proceedings of the Society for Experimental Biology and Medicine* 209, 102–123.

Srivastava, V.K., Miller, S., Schroeder, M.D., Hart, R.W. and Busbee, D. (1993) Age-related changes in expression and activity of DNA polymerase α: some effects of dietary restriction. *Mutation Research* 295, 265–280.

Turturro, A. and Allaben, W. (1995) Rodent survival, body weight and degenerative diseases. In: *Proceedings of the Special Symposium on Rodent Survival and Interpretation of Toxicological Evaluations in Chronic Studies.* Toxicology Forum, Washington, DC, pp. 11–30.

Turturro A. and Hart R.W. (1991) Longevity-assurance mechanisms and caloric restriction. *Annals of the New York Academy of Sciences* 621, 363–372.

Turturro, A., Duffy, P.H. and Hart, R.W. (1993) Modulation of toxicity by diet and dietary macronutrient restriction. *Mutation Research* 295, 151–164.

Turturro, A., Blank K., Murasko, D. and Hart, R.W. (1994) Mechanisms of caloric restriction effecting aging and disease. *Annals of the New York Academy of Sciences* 719, 159–170.

Turturro, A., Duffy, P.H. and Hart, R.W. (1995) The effect of caloric modulation on toxicity studies. In: Hart, R.W., Neuman, D. and Robertson, R. (eds) *Dietary Restriction: Implications for the Design and Interpretation of Toxicity and Carcinogenicity Studies.* ILSI Press, Washington, DC, pp. 79–98.

Turturro, A., Duffy, P.H., Hart, R.W. and Allaben, W. (1996) Rationale for the use of dietary control in toxicity studies – B6C3F1 mouse. *Toxicologic Pathology* 24, 769–775.

Turturro, A., Leakey, J., Allaben, W. and Hart, R.W. (1997) Letter to the Editor, Response to Michael Festing's "Fat Rats". *Nature* 389, 326.

Turturro, A., Duffy, P.H., Hart, R.W. and Allaben, W. (1998) Body weight impact on spontaneous and agent-induced diseases in chronic bioassays. *International Journal of Toxicology* 17, 79–100.

Vrba, E. (1985) Environment and evolution: alternative causes of the temporal distribution of evolutionary events. *South African Journal of Science* 81, 229–236.

Weindruch, R. and Walford, R.L. (1988) *The Retardation of Ageing and Disease by Dietary Restriction*. Charles C. Thomas, Springfield, Illinois.

Weraarchakul, N., Strong, R., Wood, W.G. and Richardson, A. (1989) The effect of aging and dietary restriction on DNA repair. *Experimental Cell Research* 181, 197–204.

Williams, G. (1957) Pleiotrophy, natural selection and the evolution of senescence. *Evolution* 11, 398–411.

Wolf, N. and Pendergrass, W. (1995) *In vivo* cell replication rates and *in vitro* replication capacity are modulated by caloric intake. In: Hart, R.W., Neuman, D. and Robertson, R. (eds) *Dietary Restriction: Implications for the Design and Interpretation of Toxicity and Carcinogenicity Studies*. ILSI Press, Washington, DC, pp. 299–310.

Zink, R.M. and Slowinski, J.B. (1995) Evidence from molecular systematics for decreased avian diversification in the Pleistocene epoch. *Proceedings of the National Academy of Sciences, USA* 92, 5832–5835.

Evaluation of the Contribution of Flavanols and Caffeine to the Anticarcinogenic Potential of Tea

8

COSTAS IOANNIDES

Molecular Toxicology Group, School of Biological Sciences, University of Surrey, Guildford, UK

Introduction

The identification and isolation of the components of food of plant origin that may afford protection against major chronic diseases, such as cancer and cardiovascular disease, is currently the subject of worldwide research activity. One of the extensively studied dietary components is tea (*Camellia sinensis*), the most widely consumed beverage after water worldwide.

In the East, green tea is by far the most popular beverage but in the Western hemisphere black tea and, increasingly, decaffeinated black tea are the favourite types. Black tea is produced by the controlled fermentation of green tea, during which the flavanols present in tea are oxidized by polyphenol oxidase to yield the reddish-brown dimeric theaflavins and polymeric thearubigins that are responsible for the characteristic colour of black tea. Consequently, the level of flavanols in black tea is much lower than in green tea (Lunder, 1992; Wang *et al.*, 1994; Harbowy and Balentine, 1997). Semi-fermented teas, such as oolong and pouchong, are also available.

Anticarcinogenic Potential of Tea

A large number of laboratory studies have documented the chemo-preventive effect of tea, particularly green tea, against structurally diverse classes of chemical carcinogens as well as radiation-induced tumours (Table 8.1). Tea can suppress the carcinogenic response in many tissues. Moreover,

© CAB *International* 1999. *Antioxidants in Human Health*
(eds T.K. Basu, N.J. Temple and M.L. Garg)

Table 8.1. Anticarcinogenic potential of tea.

Initiator of carcinogenesis	Cancer site	Type of tea
UVB light	Mouse skin	GT, BT
7,12-Dimethylbenz[a]anthracene	Mouse skin	GT, BT, DGT, DBT
N-Nitrosodiethylamine	Mouse lung and forestomach	GT
Benzo[a]pyrene	Mouse lung and forestomach	GT
NNK	Mouse lung	GT, BT
Aflatoxin B_1	Rat liver	GT
N-Nitrosomethylbenzylamine	Rat oesophagus	GT, BT
7,12-Dimethylbenz[a]anthracene	Rat mammary gland	BT
IQ	Rat mammary gland	BT

NNK, 4-(methylnitrosamino)-1-(3-pyridyl)1-butanone; IQ, 2-amino-3-methylimidazo [4,5-f]quinoline; GT, green tea; BT, black tea; DGT, decaffeinated green tea; DBT, decaffeinated black tea.

the anticarcinogenic effect of green tea is manifested at very low concentrations; when the model carcinogen was N-methyl-N-nitrosourea, green tea extracts at the low concentration of 0.002% (w/v) effectively decreased colon carcinogenesis induced by the nitrosamine (Narisawa and Fukaura, 1993). The strength of brews consumed by humans is about 2–3%.

It appears that tea exerts its anticarcinogenic effect by modulating all stages of chemical carcinogenesis. In chemical systems, aqueous extracts of green and black tea prevented the formation of heterocyclic amines and the nitrosation of methylurea (Weisburger *et al.*, 1994; Constable *et al.*, 1996). Numerous studies have demonstrated the ability of tea aqueous extracts to impair the initiation stage of carcinogenesis, as exemplified by the marked suppression of the mutagenicity of chemical carcinogens, both direct- and indirect-acting, in *in vitro* studies (Bu-Abbas *et al.*, 1994; Apostolides *et al.*, 1996; Stavric *et al.*, 1996; Yen and Chen, 1996). Furthermore, in *in vivo* human studies, the excretion of mutagens in the urine of women consuming cooked beef was suppressed by the intake of Tochu tea (*Eucommia ulmoides*) (Sasaki *et al.*, 1996), a type of tea taken in Japan. Green tea, administered orally or topically, reduced the epidermis DNA binding of the two polycyclic aromatic hydrocarbons 3-methylcholanthrene and 7,12-dimethylbenz[a]anthracene (Wang *et al.*, 1989). The *in vivo* binding of 2-amino-3-imidazo[4,5-f]quinoline (IQ) to hepatic DNA in rats was inhibited by infusions of green and black tea (Xu *et al.*, 1996).

The anticarcinogenic effect of tea, however, is not exclusively due to inhibition of the initiation stage of carcinogenesis. Extracts of green and black decaffeinated tea inhibited DNA synthesis and cell proliferation in a rat hepatoma and a murine erythroleukaemia cell line (Lea *et al.*, 1993). In the mouse skin model, aqueous extracts of green tea inhibited the promotion stage of carcinogenesis initiated by 7,12-dimethylbenz[*a*]anthracene and promoted by 12-*O*-tetradecanoylphorbol-13-acetate (TPA) in SENCAR mice (Katiyar *et al.*, 1993a). Similarly, aqueous extracts of green tea, administered to mice at the post-initiation stage, afforded protection against forestomach and lung tumours induced by benzo[*a*]pyrene and diethylnitrosamine in A/J mice (Katiyar *et al.*, 1993b). The same workers demonstrated that green tea can also influence the progression stage of carcinogenesis, as exemplified by the ability of a tea polyphenolic fraction to inhibit the transformation of benign skin papillomas to squamous cell carcinomas induced by benzoyl peroxide and 4-nitroquinoline-*N*-oxide in SENCAR mice (Katiyar *et al.*, 1993c, 1997). Clearly, green tea has the potential to suppress all the stages of chemical carcinogenesis.

Despite the numerous epidemiological studies which have examined the chemopreventive effects of tea, no convincing and consistent relationship between cancer incidence and tea consumption could be established (IARC, 1991; Kohlmeier *et al.*, 1997; Yang *et al.*, 1997; Ahmad *et al.*, 1998). However, in most of these studies no adjustment was made for confounding factors such as consumption of fruit and vegetables. Moreover, no attempt was made to adjust for the method of preparation of the tea (e.g. the strength of the infusion, temperature of the water, the addition of milk, lemon, etc.). Such factors are likely to affect the composition of the tea brew. For example, it has been reported that the flavonoid content of tea prepared using tea bags is higher than that prepared using loose leaves (Hertog *et al.*, 1993). It is noteworthy that in a recent population-based case–control study conducted in Shanghai, after adjusting for smoking, consumption of fruit and vegetables, and other factors, green tea consumption was inversely correlated with pancreatic and colorectal tumours (Ji *et al.*, 1997).

Contribution of Flavanols to the Anticarcinogenic Activity of Green Tea

Flavanols (catechins, flavan-3-ols), a major group of tea polyphenolics, a large part of which exist as gallate esters, are considered by many to be responsible for the anticarcinogenic effects of green tea. However, this view is based largely on speculation, with little experimental evidence to support it.

Tea flavanols have received enormous attention, primarily for two reasons. Firstly, they are present in green tea at high concentrations, comprising more than a quarter of all solids in tea infusions (Wang *et al.*, 1994; Constable *et al.*, 1996; Yen and Chen, 1996) and nearly a third of the total dry weight (Lunder, 1992). The major flavanols present in green tea are (−)-epigallocatechin and its gallate ester, and to a lesser extent (−)-epicatechin and its gallate ester and (−)-catechin (Fig. 8.1). Secondly, tea flavanols have been shown to possess potent antioxidant properties in

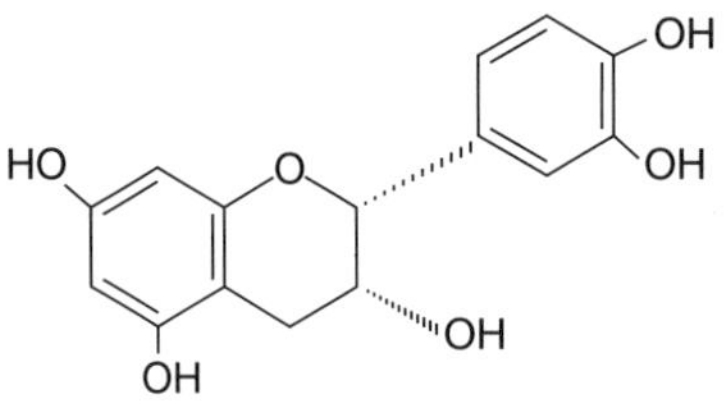

(—)-Epicatechin (EC)

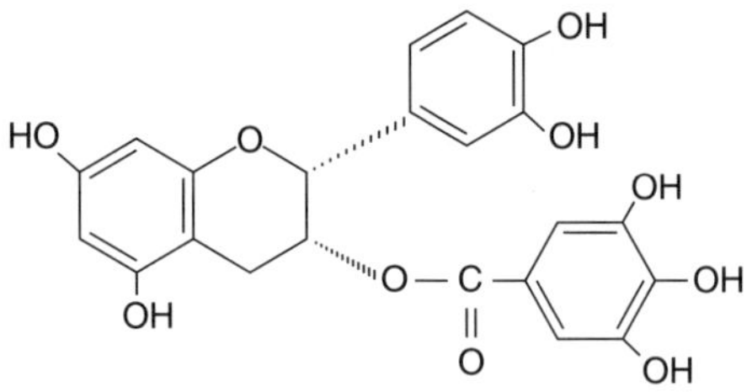

(—)-Epicatechin-3-gallate (ECG)

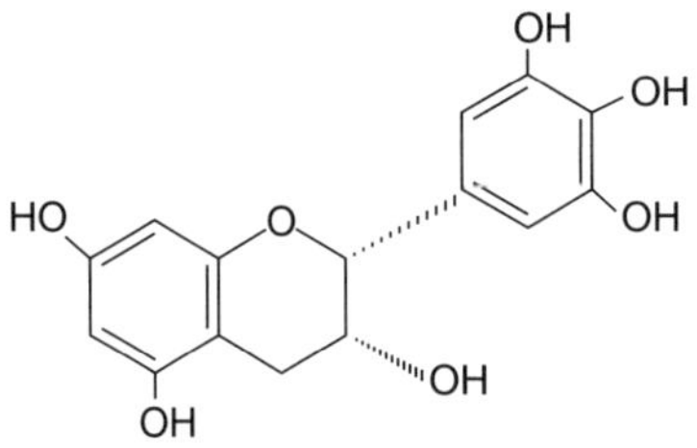

(—)-Epigallocatechin (EGC)

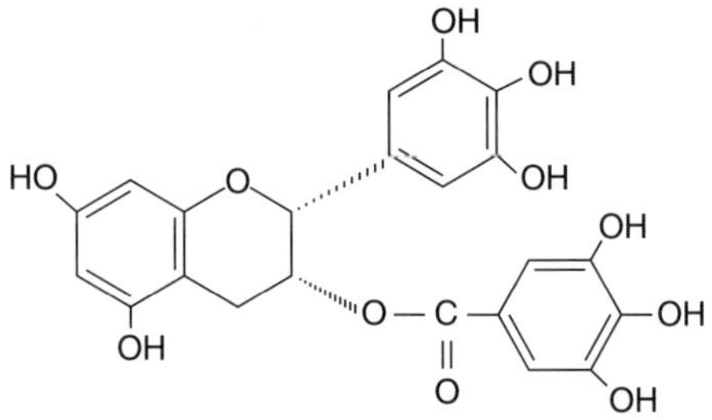

(—)-Epigallocatechin-3-gallate (EGCG)

Fig. 8.1. Chemical structure of tea flavanols.

a number of experimental systems. Green tea extracts inhibited lipid peroxidation and oxidative DNA damage induced by the carcinogen 1,2-dimethylhydrazine in rats (Inagake *et al.*, 1995; Matsumoto *et al.*, 1996). Individual tea flavanols markedly inhibited the *in vitro* oxidation of human lipoproteins by cupric ions, being the most effective among many groups of naturally occurring polyphenolic compounds (Vinson *et al.*, 1995). Similarly, in phospholipid bilayers, (−)-epicatechin and its gallate ester were potent inhibitors of oxygen radical-induced lipid peroxidation (Terao *et al.*, 1994). Finally, aqueous extracts of both green and black tea suppressed the IQ-generated production of oxygen free radicals in the presence of NADPH–cytochrome P450 reductase (Hasaniya *et al.*, 1997). However, in certain *in vitro* model systems tea extracts can display pro-oxidant activity (Yen *et al.*, 1997). It must be emphasized that all the above studies have been conducted *in vitro* and their relevance to the *in vivo* situation remains to be critically assessed.

Anticarcinogenic potential of tea flavanols

Only one of the green tea flavanols, namely (−)-epigallocatechin gallate, has been studied for possible anticarcinogenic activity (Fujiki *et al.*, 1992). At high doses (approximately 100 mg kg^{-1} day^{-1}, given 5 days per week by stomach perfusion) it antagonized the intestinal carcinogenicity of 1,2-dimethylhydrazine in mice (Pingzhang *et al.*, 1994). The same flavanol afforded protection against N-methyl-N'-nitro-N-nitrosoguanidine-induced tumours in the stomach of rats (Yamane *et al.*, 1995) and N-ethyl-N'-nitro-N-nitrosoguanidine-induced tumours in the mouse duodenum (Fujita *et al.*, 1989). In the mouse skin carcinogenesis system, topical application of (−)-epigallocatechin gallate inhibited skin tumorigenicity initiated by 7,12-dimethylbenz[*a*]anthracene and promoted by TPA in SENCAR mice (Katiyar *et al.*, 1992). Finally, (−)-epigallocatechin gallate, administered to mice in the drinking water, prevented the appearance of spontaneous hepatomas (Nishida *et al.*, 1994). The possible anticarcinogenic effects of the other tea flavanols have not been investigated.

Antimutagenic activity of tea flavanols

The antimutagenic effect of green as well as black tea appears to involve at least two distinct mechanisms: (i) inhibition of the cytochrome P450-dependent metabolic activation of chemical carcinogens, and (ii) scavenging of the generated reactive intermediates (Bu-Abbas *et al.*, 1994, 1996). It is not yet clear whether the same component(s) of tea mediates both mechanisms.

The antimutagenic activity of green tea against a number of model food mutagens in the Ames test was found to be very similar to that exhibited by black tea, despite the lower flavanol content of the latter, indicating that flavanols are unlikely to be the constituents of green tea responsible for its antimutagenic activity (Bu-Abbas *et al.*, 1996). This view is supported by the studies of Yen and Chen (1994) who showed that semifermented teas were more potent antimutagens than green and black tea against a number of model food mutagens. The same authors in subsequent studies failed to obtain clear correlations between, on the one hand, the antimutagenic activity of four teas, including fermented, semifermented and non-fermented teas, against a number of carcinogens and, on the other hand, the levels of individual flavanols, although a significant positive correlation was noted in the case of IQ (Yen and Chen, 1996). In their studies, Apostolides *et al.* (1996) reported that black tea polyphenolics were more potent anti-mutagens against 2-amino-1-methyl-6-phenylimidazo[4,5-*b*]pyridine (PhIP) than those derived from green tea. Moreover, instant teas, which are prepared from black teas and contain very low levels of flavanols as a result of their further oxidation during manufacture, exhibited the same anti-mutagenic potency as green and black tea against a number of heterocyclic amines in the Ames test (Constable *et al.*, 1996).

Antimutagenic studies employing the isolated tea flavanols have also been conducted. In these studies the heterocyclic amine PhIP (10 μmol l^{-1}) served as the model mutagen (Apostolides *et al.*, 1997). (−)-Epicatechin and (−)-epigallocatechin failed to suppress the mutagenicity of PhIP even at concentrations as high as 1 mmol l^{-1}; their gallate esters, however, inhibited the PhIP-induced mutagenic response with IC_{50} values of 0.5 and 0.7 mmol l^{-1}, respectively. Bearing in mind that the mutagenicity of the related heterocyclic amine IQ was inhibited by 80% in the presence of only 100 μl of a 2.5% infusion of green tea (Bu-Abbas *et al.*, 1994), the antimutagenic effect of green tea cannot be attributed to the flavanoids.

In a recent study aimed at establishing the role of individual flavanols in the antimutagenic activity of green tea (Bu-Abbas *et al.*, 1997), green tea aqueous extracts were decaffeinated and then fractionated into four distinct fractions, each of which had a different flavanol composition that was fully defined. The antimutagenic activity of these fractions against four carcinogens was determined; no correlation was evident between antimutagenic potency and the levels of (−)-epicatechin, (−)-epigallocatechin and of their gallate esters. Clearly, there is overwhelming experimental evidence that tea flavanols are not responsible for the *in vitro* antimutagenic activity and are therefore unlikely to play a major role in the ability of green tea to impair the initiation stage of chemical carcinogenesis.

An alternative mechanism through which tea can influence the initiation of chemical carcinogenesis is by modulating the phase II enzyme systems involved in the metabolism of xenobiotics. Treatment of rats and mice with aqueous extracts or polyphenolic fractions of green tea enhanced hepatic glucuronosyl transferase activity, facilitating the deactivation of chemical carcinogens, and glutathione S-transferase activity leading to the detoxication of the electrophilic reactive intermediates of chemical carcinogens (Khan *et al.*, 1992; Bu-Abbas *et al.*, 1995, 1999; Sohn *et al.*, 1994). The constituent(s) of green tea mediating its effects on the phase II activities has not yet been identified, but any contribution of flavanols is likely to be minimal. This is indicated by the fact that black tea, despite having a much lower content of flavanols than green tea, was a more effective inducer of the glucuronosyl transferase and glutathione S-transferase activities in rat liver (Bu-Abbas *et al.*, 1999).

Effect of tea flavanols on the promotion and progression stages of carcinogenesis

Reactive oxygen species are believed to act as tumour promoters (Oberley and Oberley, 1995), so that flavanols, by virtue of their potent antioxidant activity (*vide supra*), could contribute to the documented ability of green tea to impair this stage of chemical carcinogenesis. (−)-Epigallocatechin gallate, following topical application, inhibited the promoting effect of teleocidin and okadaic acid (Yoshizawa *et al.*, 1987; Huang *et al.*, 1992). In recent studies, (−)-epigallocatechin gallate was shown to suppress the radiation-induced oncogenic transformation of C3H10T1/2 mouse embryo fibroblast cells (Komatsu *et al.*, 1997). Whether flavanols can bring about such effects at the concentrations present in tea, remains to be established.

Pharmacokinetic characteristics of tea flavonoids

Despite the important contribution to the anticarcinogenic activity of tea ascribed to flavanols, their pharmacokinetic behaviour, and especially their absorption and distribution, are only now being investigated. These compounds are not very lipophilic and, in addition, the presence of phenolic groups that can readily conjugate sulphate and glucuronide, and thus facilitate their elimination, make it difficult to envisage sufficiently high tissue concentrations to exert a biological effect. However, the concentration of these compounds in tea, particularly green tea, is high (Wang *et al.*, 1994) and the daily intake of these compounds from tea, one of the major sources, is substantial.

When a single 50 mg dose of (−)-epigallocatechin gallate was administered to fasted 150 g body weight rats, absorption was rapid, reaching a maximum of about 0.2 μg ml^{-1} of plasma within an hour (Unno and Takeo, 1995). The levels, however, declined rapidly, being barely detectable 2 h after administration. In more recent studies, the levels of flavanols in the plasma of rats were monitored following a single intragastric administration of decaffeinated green tea (200 mg kg^{-1}); maximum plasma levels of (−)-epigallocatechin gallate, (−)-epicatechin and (−)-epigallocatechin were attained within an hour (Chen *et al.*, 1997). (−)-Epicatechin and (−)-epigallocatechin had a much higher bioavailability than (−)-epigallocatechin gallate. The same authors studied the pharmacokinetic behaviour of pure (−)-epigallocatechin gallate, the major tea flavonoid with the strongest antioxidant activity, following an intragastric dose of 75 mg kg^{-1} and showed that the bioavailability was only 1.5%, compared to the intravenous administration of the compound. However, in contrast to the studies of Unno and Takeo (1995), the plasma disappearance was slow. It is noteworthy that when (−)-epigallocatechin gallate was given in tea rather than in pure form it was more readily absorbed but less readily eliminated. In both the urine and plasma the flavanols are present largely as conjugates with sulphate and glucuronide (Lee *et al.*, 1995).

The poor bioavailability of flavanols may be partly attributed to biotransformation by intestinal microorganisms. Rat faecal preparations extensively metabolized (−)-epicatechin and (−)-epigallocatechin but their gallate esters were resistant (Meselhy *et al.*, 1997). Interestingly, when human faecal preparations were used, the free compounds as well as the gallate esters were metabolized.

Contribution of caffeine to the anticarcinogenic activity of green tea

Caffeine (1,3,7-trimethylxanthine) is a major component of tea that may contribute to its anticarcinogenic activity. It is present in green and black tea, comprising 5% of all solids and in 1.25% (w/v) brew is present at a concentration of about 220 μg ml^{-1} (Wang et al., 1994). The ability of caffeine to modulate the tumorigenicity of chemicals is well documented. However, caffeine has been demonstrated to both inhibit and potentiate chemically induced cancers in rats and mice (Nomura, 1976; Hiroshino and Tanooka, 1979; Denda et al., 1983; Welsch et al., 1988a). Similarly, some epidemiological studies established correlations between coffee consumption and certain cancers (MacMahon et al., 1981; Boyle et al., 1984) whereas others failed to detect an association (Rosenberg et al., 1985; Wynder et al., 1986). A comparison of the anticarcinogenic potential of green and black teas with that of their decaffeinated derivatives against ultraviolet B (UVB) light-induced skin carcinogenesis in mice showed that the decaffeinated teas were markedly less effective and at a high dose even exacerbated the carcinogenic response (Huang et al., 1997). Adding caffeine back to the decaffeinated teas restored their higher anticarcinogenic activity thus establishing, at least in this case, a role for caffeine. The decaffeinated teas, however, displayed a similar anticarcinogenic activity against UVB-induced skin cancer in mice initiated with 7,12-dimethylbenz[a]anthracene (Wang et al., 1994). The fact that decaffeinated teas also displayed anticarcinogenic activity in this animal model indicates that other components in green and black tea also possess anticarcinogenic properties. Whether the presence of caffeine in the tea affords protection against chemically induced cancers remains to be established.

Antimutagenic activity of caffeine

Caffeine is a selective substrate of CYP1A2, an isoform of cytochrome P450 that is closely associated with the activation of many planar chemical carcinogens (Ioannides and Parke, 1990), including heterocyclic amines (Kleman and Övervik, 1995). It would be anticipated, therefore, that caffeine would inhibit the bioactivation of carcinogens that rely on this cytochrome P450 for their activation. Indeed, caffeine, at a final concentration of about 100 μmol l^{-1}, inhibited the bioactivation of mutagens in the Ames test in a concentration-dependent fashion (Alldrick and Rowland, 1988). In studies where the antimutagenic properties of black tea and decaffeinated black tea were compared, no difference could be discerned when the model carcinogens were polycyclic aromatic hydrocarbons, heterocyclic amines or nitrosamines (Bu-Abbas et al., 1996). Thus it appears that caffeine, at the concentrations encountered in tea, does not play a major role in the anti-mutagenic activity of tea against indirect-acting mutagens. Moreover, both caffeinated and decaffeinated black tea suppressed the mutagenicity of direct-acting mutagens that do not require bioactivation in order to express their mutagenicity (Bu-Abbas *et al.,* 1996). In contrast, caffeine has been reported to have no influence on the mutagenic response of direct-acting mutagens (Yamaguchi and Nakawa, 1983). It can be inferred from these observations that the antimutagenic activity of tea cannot be attributed to the presence of caffeine. This is further supported by recent observations that fractions of green tea retained their antimutagenic activity even after caffeine had been extracted (Bu-Abbas *et al.,* 1997).

Effect of caffeine on the promotion stage of carcinogenesis

In studies conducted in female rats using the mammary carcinogen 7,12-dimethylbenz[*a*]anthracene, caffeine suppressed the carcinogenic response when administered during the initiation phase. However, it failed to attenuate the carcinogenic response when administered during the promotion stage (Welsch *et al.,* 1988b; Welsch and DeHoog, 1988) and even stimulated the carcinogenic activity in female mice (Welsch *et al.,* 1988a). Clearly, caffeine is unable to influence the promotion stage of carcinogenesis and is even less likely to have such an effect when consumed as tea, where the level is relatively low.

Conclusions

An increasing number of naturally occurring chemicals, including many polyphenolics, have been shown to afford effective protection against cancer and cardiovascular disease. Many of these have been shown to possess antioxidant activity, largely in *in vitro* systems, and could conceivably exert their cancer chemopreventive activity by lowering the levels of reactive oxygen species, which can not only induce DNA damage, but also plays an important role in the promotion stage of carcinogenesis. However, experimental evidence to link anticarcinogenic activity with antioxidant potency is lacking.

Similarly, in the case of green tea, flavanols have been implicated in the anticarcinogenic response as these compounds are abundant in tea. Overall, experimental evidence indicates that these compounds do not possess significant antimutagenic activity and thus if these compounds make a contribution to the chemopreventive activity of green tea, they are likely to exert their effects on a subsequent stage of carcinogenesis, namely promotion or progression. Whether this is related to their antioxidant activity remains to be established.

In most experimental studies, oral administration of decaffeinated tea was as effective as caffeinated tea in antagonizing the carcinogenic response elicited by chemicals, but in a recent study caffeine, through an as yet undefined mechanism, was important in the suppression by tea of the UVB-induced skin carcinogenesis in mice (Huang *et al.,* 1997). Clearly, the role of caffeine, if any, in the tea-mediated suppression of chemically induced cancers still remains to be established.

Tea is a very complex mixture (Harbowy and Balentine, 1997) which contains, in addition to flavanols and caffeine, many other chemicals, including other polyphenolics such as flavonols, flavones and their glycosides, albeit at lower concentrations, one or more of which may contribute substantially to the anticarcinogenic activity of tea. It is likely that different tea constituents influence the various stages of carcinogenesis and, furthermore, this depends on the nature of the carcinogenic agent. As already described, caffeine does not appear to be significantly involved in the antitumorigenic activity of tea against chemical carcinogens, but plays a dominant role when cancer is induced by UVB radiation.

References

Ahmad, N., Katiyar, S.K. and Mukhtar, H. (1998) Cancer chemoprevention by tea polyphenols. In: Ioannides, C. (ed.) *Nutrition and Chemical Toxicity.* John Wiley & Sons, Chichester, pp. 301–343.

Alldrick, A.J. and Rowland, I.R. (1988) Caffeine inhibits hepatic-microsomal activation of some dietary genotoxins. *Mutagenesis* 3, 423–427.

Apostolides, Z., Balentine, D.A., Harbowy, M.E. and Weisburger, J.H. (1996) Inhibition of 2-amino-1-methyl-6-phenylimidazo[4,5-b]pyridine (PhIP) mutagenicity by black and green tea extracts and polyphenols. *Mutation Research* 359, 159–163.

Apostolides, Z., Balentine, D.A., Harbowy, M.E., Hara, Y. and Weisburger, J.H. (1997) Inhibition of PhIP mutagenicity by catechins, and by theaflavins and gallate esters. *Mutation Research* 389, 167–172.

Boyle, C.A., Berkowitz, G.S., Li Volsi, V.A., Ort, S., Merino, M.J., White, C. and Kelsey, J.S. (1984) Caffeine consumption and fibrocystic breast disease: case–control epidemiology study. *Journal of the National Cancer Institute* 72, 1015–1019.

Bu-Abbas, A., Clifford, M.N., Walker, R. and Ioannides, C. (1994) Marked antimutagenic potential of aqueous green tea extracts: mechanism of action. *Mutagenesis* 9, 325–331.

Bu-Abbas, A., Clifford, M.N., Walker, R. and Ioannides, C. (1995) Stimulation of rat hepatic UDP-glucuronosyl transferase activity following treatment with green tea. *Food and Chemical Toxicology* 33, 27–30.

Bu-Abbas, A., Nunez, X., Clifford, M.N., Walker, R. and Ioannides, C. (1996) A comparison of the antimutagenic potential of green, black and decaffeinated teas: contribution of flavanols to the antimutagenic effect. *Mutagenesis* 11, 597–603.

Bu-Abbas, A., Clifford, M.N., Walker, R. and Ioannides, C. (1997) Fractionation of green tea extracts: correlation of antimutagenic effect with flavanol content. *Journal of the Science of Food and Agriculture* 75, 453–462.

Bu-Abbas, A., Clifford, M.N., Walker, R. and Ioannides, C. (1999) Contribution of caffeine and flavanols in the induction of hepatic phase II activities by green tea. *Environmental Pharmacology and Toxicology* (in press).

Chen, L., Lee, M.-J., Li, H. and Yang, C.S. (1997) Absorption, distribution, and elimination of tea polyphenols in rats. *Drug Metabolism and Disposition* 25, 1045–1050.

Constable, A., Varga, N., Richoz, J. and Stadler, R.H. (1996) Antimutagenicity and catechin content of soluble instant teas. *Mutagenesis* 11, 189–194.

Denda, A., Yokose, Y., Emi, Y., Murata, Y., Ohara, T., Sunagawa, M., Mikami, S., Takahoshi, S. and Konishi, Y. (1983) Effects of caffeine on pancreatic carcinogenesis by 4-hydroxyamino-quinoline 1-oxide in partially pancreatectomized rats. *Carcinogenesis* 4, 17–22.

Fujiki, H., Yoshizawa, S., Horiuchi, T., Suganuma, M., Yatsunami, S., Nishiwaki, S., Okabe, S., Nishiwaki, M.R., Okuda, T. and Sugimura, T. (1992) Anticarcinogenic effect (−)-epigallocatechin gallate. *Preventive Medicine* 21, 503–509.

Fujita, M., Yamane, T., Tanaka, M., Kuwata, K., Okuzumi, J., Takahashi, T, Fujiki, H. and Okuda, K. (1989) Inhibitory effect of (−)-epigallocatechin gallate on carcinogenesis with *N*-ethyl-*N'*-nitro-*N*-nitrosoguanidine in mouse duodenum. *Japanese Journal of Cancer Research* 80, 503–505.

Harbowy, M.E. and Balentine, D.A. (1997) Tea chemistry. *Critical Reviews in Plant Sciences* 16, 415–480.

Hasaniya, N., Youn, K., Xu, M., Hernaez, J. and Dashwood, R. (1997) Inhibitory activity of green and black tea in a free radical-generating system using 2-amino-3-methylimidazo[4,5-*f*]quinoline as substrate. *Japanese Journal of Cancer Research* 88, 553–558.

Hertog, M.G.L., Hollman, P.C.H. and van de Putte, B. (1993) Content of potentially anticarcinogenic flavonoids of tea infusions, wines, and fruit juices. *Journal of Agricultural and Food Chemistry* 41, 1242–1246.

Hiroshino, H. and Tanooka, H. (1979) Caffeine enhances skin tumour induction in mice. *Toxicology Letters* 4, 83–85.

Huang, M.-T., Ho, C.-T., Wang, Z.Y., Ferraro, T., Finnegan-Olive T., Lou, Y.-R., Mitchell, J.M., Laskin, J.D., Newmark, H., Yang, C.S. and Conney, A.H. (1992) Inhibitory effect of topical application of a green tea polyphenol fraction on tumour initiation and promotion in mouse skin. *Carcinogenesis* 13, 947–954.

Huang, M.-T., Xie, J.-G., Wang, Z.Y., Ho, C.-T., Lou, Y.-R., Wang, C.-X, Hard, G.C. and Conney, A.H. (1997) Effects of tea, decaffeinated tea, and caffeine on UVB light-induced complete carcinogenesis in SKH-1 mice: demonstration of caffeine as a biologically important constituent of tea. *Cancer Research* 52, 2623–2629.

IARC (1991) Coffee, tea, mate, methylxanthines and methylglyoxal. In: *Monographs on the Evaluation of Carcinogenic Risks to Humans,* Vol. 51. International Agency for Research on Cancer, Lyon, pp. 207–271.

Inagake, M., Yamane, T., Kitano, Y., Oya, K., Matsumoto, M., Kiluoka, N., Nakatani, H., Takahashi, T., Nishimura, H. and Iwashima, A. (1995) Inhibition of 1,2-dimethylhydrazine-induced oxidative DNA damage by green tea extract in rat. *Japanese Journal of Cancer Research* 86, 1106–1111.

Ioannides, C. and Parke, D.V. (1990) The cytochrome P450I gene family of microsomal haemoproteins and their role in the metabolic activation of chemicals. *Drug Metabolism Reviews* 22, 1–85.

Ji, B.-T., Chow, W.-H., Hsing, A.W., McLaughlin, J.K., Gao, Y.-T., Blot, W.J. and Faumeni, J.F. Jr (1997) Green tea consumption and the risk of pancreatic and colorectal cancers. *International Journal of Cancer* 70, 255–258.

Katiyar, S.K., Agarwal, R., Wang, Z.Y., Bhatia, A.K. and Mukhtar, H. (1992) (−)-Epigallocatechin-3-gallate in *Camellia sinensis* leaves from Himalayan region of Sikkim: inhibitory effects against biochemical events and tumour initiation in SENCAR mouse skin. *Nutrition and Cancer* 18, 73–83.

Katiyar, S.K., Agarwal, R. and Mukhtar, H. (1993a) Inhibition of both stage I and stage II skin tumor promotion in SENCAR mice by a polyphenolic fraction isolated from green tea: inhibition depends on the duration of polyphenol treatment. *Carcinogenesis* 14, 2641–2643.

Katiyar, S.K., Agarwal, R., Zaim, M.T. and Mukhtar, H. (1993b) Protection against *N*-nitrosodiethylamine and benzo[α]pyrene-induced forestomach and lung tumorigenesis in A/J mice by green tea. *Carcinogenesis* 14, 849–855.

Katiyar, S.K., Agarwal, R. and Mukhtar, H. (1993c) Protection against malignant conversion of chemically induced benign skin papillomas to squamous cell carcinomas in SENCAR mice by a polyphenolic fraction isolated from green tea. *Cancer Research* 53, 5409–5412.

Katiyar, S.K., Agarwal, R. and Mukhtar, H. (1997) Protection against induction of mouse skin papillomas with low and high risk of coversion to malignancy by green tea polyphenols. *Carcinogenesis* 18, 497–502.

Khan, S.G., Katiyar, S.K., Agarwal, R. and Mukhtar, H. (1992) Enhancement of antioxidant and phase II enzymes by oral feeding of green tea polyphenols in drinking water to SKH-1 hairless mice: possible role in cancer chemoprevention. *Cancer Research* 52, 4050–4052.

Kleman, M.I. and Övervik, E. (1995) Carcinogens formed during cooking. In: Ioannides, C. and Lewis, D.F.V. (eds) *Drugs, Diet and Disease*, Vol. 1, *Mechanistic Approaches to Cancer*. Ellis Horwood, Hemel Hempstead, pp. 66–93.

Kohlmeier, L., Weterings, K.G.C., Steck, S. and Kok, F.J. (1997) Tea and cancer prevention: an evaluation of the epidemiologic literature. *Nutrition and Cancer* 27, 1–13.

Komatsu, K., Tauchi, H., Yano, N., Endo, S., Matsuura, S. and Shoji, S. (1997) Inhibitory action of (−)-epigallocatechin gallate on radiation-induced mouse oncogenic transformation. *Cancer Letters* 112, 135–139.

Lea, M.A., Xiao, Q., Sadhukhan, A.K., Cottle, S., Wang, Z.-Y. and Yang, C.S. (1993) Inhibitory effects of tea extracts and (−)-epigallocatechin gallate on DNA synthesis and proliferation of hepatoma and erythroleukemia cells. *Cancer Letters* 68, 231–236.

Lee, M.J., Wang, Z.Y., Li, H., Chen, L., Sun, Y., Gabbo, S., Balentine, D.A. and Yang, C.S. (1995) Analysis of plasma and urinary tea polyphenols in human subjects. *Cancer Epidemiology, Biomarkers and Preventors* 4, 393–399.

Lunder, T.E. (1992) Catechins of green tea: antioxidant activity. In: Huang, M.-T., Ho, C.-T. and Lee, C.Y. (eds) *Phenolic Compounds in Food and Their Effects on Health II*. ACS Symposium series 507, Washington DC, pp. 114–120.

MacMahon, B., Yen, S., Trichopoulos, D., Warren, K. and Nardi, G. (1981) Coffee and cancer of the pancreas. *New England Journal of Medicine* 304, 630–633.

Matsumoto, H., Yamane, T., Inagake, M., Nakatani, H., Iwata, Y., Takahashi, T., Nishimura, H., Nishino, H., Nagawa, K. and Miyazawa, T. (1996) Inhibition of mucosal lipid hyperoxidation by green extract in 1,2-dimethylhydrazine-induced rat colonic carcinogenesis. *Cancer Letters* 104, 205–209.

Meselhy, M.R., Nakamura, M. and Hattori, M. (1997) Biotransformation of (−)-epicatechin 3-O-gallate by human intestinal bacteria. *Chemical and Pharmacological Bulletin* 45, 888–893.

Narisawa, T. and Fukaura, T. (1993) A very low dose of green tea polyphenols in drinking water prevents *N*-methyl-*N*-nitrosurea-induced colon carcinogenesis in F344 rats. *Japanese Journal of Cancer Research* 84, 1007–1009.

Nishida, H., Omori, M., Fukutomi, Y., Ninomiya, M., Nishiwaki, S., Suganuma, S., Moriwaki, H. and Muto, Y. (1994) Inhibitory effects of (−)-epigallocatechin gallate on spontaneous hepatoma-derived PLC/PRF/5 cells. *Japanese Journal of Cancer Research* 85, 221–225.

Nomura, T. (1976) Diminution of tumorigenesis initiated by nitroquinoline-1-oxide by post-treatment with caffeine in mice. *Nature* 260, 547–549.

Oberley, L.W. and Oberley, T.D. (1995) Reactive oxygen species in the aetiology of cancer. In: Ioannides, C. and Lewis, D.F.V. (eds) *Drugs, Diet and Disease*, Vol. 1, *Mechanistic Approaches to Cancer*. Ellis Horwood, Hemel Hempstead, pp. 47–63.

Rosenberg, L., Miller, D.R., Helmrick, S.P., Kaufman, D.W., Schottenfeld, D., Stolley, P.D. and Shapiro, S. (1985) Breast cancer and the consumption of coffee. *American Journal of Epidemiology* 122, 391–399.

Sasaki, Y.F., Chiba, A., Murakami, M., Sekihashi, K., Tanaka, M., Takahoko, M., Moribayashi, M., Kudou, C., Hara, Y., Nakazawa, Y., Nakamura, T and Onizuka, S. (1996) Antimutagenicity of Tochu tea (an aqueous extract of *Eucommia ulmoides* leaves): 2. Suppressing effect of Tochu tea on the urine mutagenicity after ingestion of raw fish and cooked beef. *Mutation Research* 371, 203–214.

Sohn, O.S., Surace, A., Fiala, E.S., Richie, J.P., Jr, Colosimo, S., Zang, E. and Weisburger, J.H. (1994) Effects of green and black tea on hepatic xenobiotic metabolizing systems in the male F344 rat. *Xenobiotica* 24, 119–127.

Stavric, B., Matula, T.I., Klassen, R. and Downie, R.H. (1996) The effect of teas on the *in vitro* mutagenic potential of heterocyclic aromatic amines. *Food and Chemical Toxicology* 34, 515–523.

Terao, J., Piskula, M. and Yao, K. (1994) Protective effects of epicatechin, epicatechin gallate, and quercetin on lipid peroxidation in phospholipid layers. *Archives of Biochemistry and Biophysics* 308, 278–284.

Unno, T. and Takeo, T. (1995) Absorption of (−)-epigallocatechin gallate into the circulation system of rats. *Bioscience, Biotechnology and Biochemistry* 59, 1558–1559.

Vinson, J.A., Dabbagh, Y.A., Serry M.M. and Jang, J. (1995) Plant flavonoids, especially tea flavonols, are powerful antioxidants using an *in vitro* oxidation model for heart disease. *Journal of Agricultural and Food Chemistry* 43, 2800–2802.

Wang, Z.Y., Khan, W.A., Bickers, D.R. and Mukhtar, H. (1989) Protection against polycyclic aromatic hydrocarbon-induced skin tumor initiation in mice by green tea polyphenols. *Carcinogenesis* 10, 411–415.

Wang, Z.Y., Huang, M.-T., Lou, Y.-R., Xie, J.-G., Reuhl, K.R., Newmark, H.L., Ho, C.-T., Yang, C.S. and Conney, A.H. (1994) Inhibitory effects of black tea, green tea, decaffeinated black tea, and decaffeinated green tea on ultraviolet B light-induced skin tumorigenesis in 7,12-dimethylbenz(*a*)anthracene-initiated SKH-1 mice. *Cancer Research* 54, 3428–3435.

Weisburger, J.H., Nagao, M., Wakabyashi, K. and Oguri, A. (1994) Prevention of heterocyclic amine formation by tea and tea polyphenols. *Cancer Letters* 83, 143–147.

Welsch, C.W. and DeHoog, J.V. (1988) Influence of caffeine consumption on 7,12-dimethylbenz(α)anthracene-induced rat mammary gland tumorigenesis in female rats fed a chemically defined diet containing standard and high levels of unsaturated fat. *Cancer Research* 48, 2074–2077.

Welsch, C.W., DeHoog, J.V. and O'Connor, D.H. (1988a) Influence of caffeine consumption on carcinomatous and normal mammary gland development in mice. *Cancer Research* 48, 2078–2082.

Welsch, C.W., DeHoog, J.V. and O'Connor, D.H. (1988b) Influence of caffeine and/or coffee consumption on the initiation and promotion phases of 7,12-dimethyl-benz(α)anthracene-induced rat mammary gland tumorigenesis. *Cancer Research* 48, 2068–2073.

Wynder, E.L., Hall, N.E.L. and Polansky, M. (1986) Epidemiology of coffee and pancreatic cancer. *Cancer Research* 43, 3900–3906.

Xu, M., Bailey, A.C., Hernaez, J.F., Taoka, C.R., Schut, H.A.J. and Dashwood, R.H. (1996) Protection by green tea, black tea, and indole-3-carbinol against colonic aberrant crypts induced by rat 2-amino-3-methylimidazo[4,5-*f*]quinoline. *Carcinogenesis* 17, 1429–1434.

Yamaguchi, T. and Nagaawa, K. (1983) Reduction of induced mutability with xanthine- and imidazole-derivatives through inhibition of metabolic activation. *Agricultural and Biological Chemistry* 47, 1673–1677.

Yamane, T., Takahashi, T., Kuwata, K., Oya, K., Inagake, M., Kitao, Y., Suganuma, M. and Fujiki, H. (1995) Inhibition of N-methyl-N'-nitro-N-nitrosoguanidine-induced carcinogenesis by (−)-epigallocatechin gallate in the rat glandular stomach. *Cancer Research* 55, 2080–2084.

Yang, C.S., Lee, M.-J., Chen, L. and Yang, G.-Y. (1997) Polyphenols as inhibitors of carcinogenesis. *Environmental Health Perspectives* 105, 971–976.

Yen, G.-C. and Chen, H.-Y. (1994) Comparison of the antimutagenic effect of various tea extracts (green, oolong, pouchong, and black tea). *Journal of Food Protection* 57, 54–58.

Yen, G.-C. and Chen, H.-Y. (1996) Relationship between antimutagenic activity and major components of various teas. *Mutagenesis* 11, 37–41.

Yen, G.-C., Chen, H.-Y. and Peng, H.H. (1997) Antioxidant and pro-oxidant effects of various tea extracts. *Journal of Agricultural and Food Chemistry* 45, 30–34.

Yin, P., Zhao, J., Cheng, S., Hara, Y., Zhu, Q. and Zhengguo, L. (1994) Experimental studies of the inhibitory effects of green tea catechin on mice large intestinal cancers induced by 1,2-dimethylhydrazine. *Cancer Letters* 79, 33–38.

Yoshizawa, S., Horiuchi, T., Fujiki, H., Yoshida, T., Okuda, T. and Sugimura, T. (1987) Antitumor promoting activity of (−)-epigallocatechin gallate, the main constituent of 'tannin' in green tea. *Phytotherapy Research* 1, 44–47.

Antioxidant Effects of Plant Phenolic Compounds 9

KEVIN D. CROFT

Department of Medicine,
University of Western Australia, Perth, Australia

Introduction

Phenolic compounds are widely distributed in plants. One of the major groups of phenolic compounds is the flavonoids, which are important in contributing to the flavour and colour of many fruits and vegetables and products derived from them such as wine, tea and chocolate. The biological role of some of the other simple phenolic compounds is not well understood; they may play a role as building blocks for other compounds or in plant defence mechanisms. Dietary phenolic compounds have generally been considered as non-nutrients and their possible benefit to human health has only recently been considered. There is now much interest in the biological effects of phenolic compounds since evidence was found that diets rich in fruit and vegetables appear to protect against cardiovascular disease and some forms of cancer (Block, 1992; Hertog *et al.*, 1993; Block and Langseth, 1994). Since oxygen free radicals and lipid peroxidation are thought to be involved in several conditions such as atherosclerosis, cancer and chronic inflammation the antioxidant activity of phenolic compounds has been of primary interest (Halliwell, 1994). There have been several excellent recent reviews on the antioxidant activity of the flavonoids (Bors *et al.*, 1990; Rice-Evans *et al.*, 1996; Cook and Saman, 1996), while less information is available on other phenolic species.

Despite major advances in understanding the *in vitro* antioxidant activity of phenolic compounds and a number of studies on absorption in animals, there are few data available on either the absorption or antioxidant effects of these compounds *in vivo* in man. This chapter will outline our current understanding of the antioxidant activity of flavonoids and phenolic acids, their bioavailability and the most appropriate methods for assessing antioxidant effects *in vivo*.

© CAB *International* 1999. *Antioxidants in Human Health*
(eds T.K. Basu, N.J. Temple and M.L. Garg)

Chemistry and Biosynthesis

The term 'phenolic compound' embraces a wide range of plant substances which possess an aromatic ring bearing one or more hydroxyl substituents. They frequently occur attached to sugars (glycosides) and as such tend to be water soluble. The flavonoids are the largest single group of phenolic compounds. Flavonoids are C15 compounds composed of two phenolic rings connected by a three-carbon unit. The flavonoids are biosynthetically derived from acetate and shikimate (Mann, 1978) such that the A ring has a characteristic hydroxylation pattern at the 5 and 7 position. The B ring is usually 4', 3'4' or 3'4'5' hydroxylated. Figure 9.1 shows these major structural features with examples of the chalcone, flavonol and flavone groups. The isoflavonoids are derived by cyclization of the chalcones such that the B ring is located at the 3 position (Fig. 9.1). Other major groups of flavonoids include the catechins (often found as esters with gallic acid in tea) and the anthocyanidins, which are highly coloured pigments (Fig. 9.2).

Of the simple phenolic acids, cinnamic acid and its derivatives are widespread in plants. They are derived primarily from the shikimate

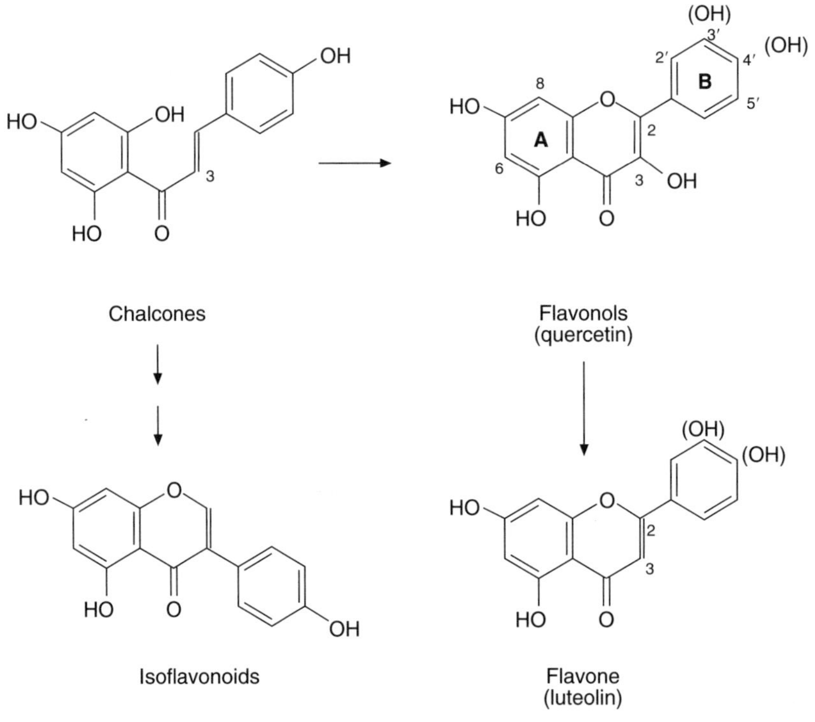

Fig. 9.1. Structural features of chalcones and their products.

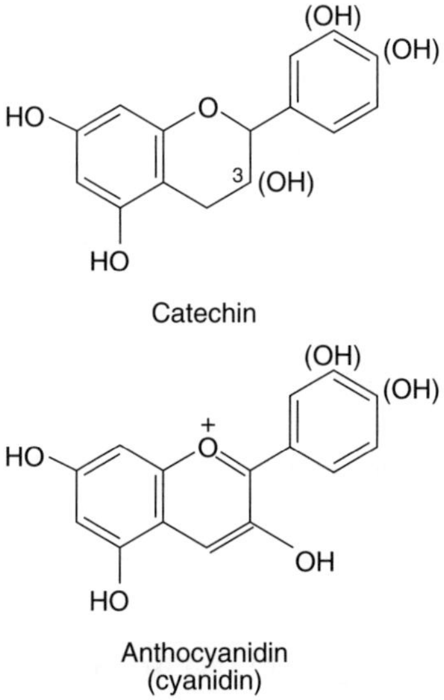

Fig. 9.2. Structural features of catechin and anthocyanidin.

pathway via phenylalanine or tyrosine (Mann, 1978) and major examples are coumaric acid (single hydroxyl group) and caffeic acid (Fig. 9.3). Oxidation of the side chain can produce derivatives of benzoic acid such as protocatechuic acid and gentisic acid. These compounds are usually found in nature as glucose ethers or in ester combination with quinic acid. Other phenolic compounds of interest include resveratrol, a hydroxy stilbene found in red wine (Pace-Asciak *et al.*, 1995), oleuropein, a bitter principle of olives (Visioli and Galli, 1994), and complex compounds which may be derived by oxidative coupling of more simple phenolics, e.g. salvianolic acid isolated from *Salvia miltiorrhiza*, a plant used in traditional Chinese medicine (Lin *et al.*, 1996).

Some major dietary sources of phenolic compounds are outlined in Table 9.1. The daily intake of flavonoids has been estimated at between 20 mg and 1 g (Hertog *et al.*, 1993). The flavanols, particularly catechin and catechin–gallate esters and the flavonol quercetin, are found in beverages such as green and black tea (Stagg and Millin, 1975) and red wine (Frankel *et al.*, 1995). Quercetin is also a predominant component of onions, apples and berries. The flavanones, such as naringin, are mainly found in citrus fruits. The phenolic acids are widespread but are also found in red wine. Patterns of polyphenolic compounds in wines are being studied as a means of 'fingerprinting' wine (Soleas *et al.*, 1997).

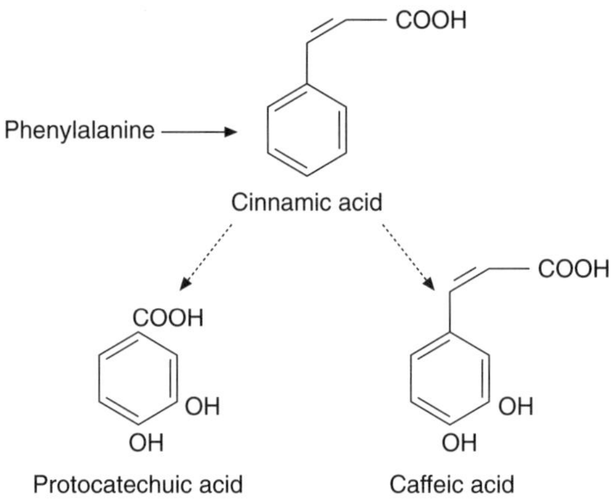

Fig. 9.3. Cinnamic acid and its derivatives.

Antioxidant Activity of Flavonoids and Phenolic Acids

Free radicals are produced in the body as part of normal metabolism, for example superoxide, $O_2^-\cdot$ and nitric oxide, $NO\cdot$ which have important physiological functions. In general, free radicals are highly reactive and can attack membrane lipids for example, generating a carbon radical which in turn reacts with oxygen to produce a peroxyl radical which may attack adjacent fatty acids to generate new carbon radicals. This process leads to a chain reaction producing lipid peroxidation products (Halliwell, 1994). By this means a single radical may damage many molecules by initiating lipid peroxidation chain reactions. Because of the potential damaging nature of free radicals, the body has a number of antioxidant defence mechanisms which include enzymes such as superoxide dismutase, catalase, copper and iron transport and storage proteins, and both water-soluble and lipid-soluble molecular antioxidants. Oxidative stress may result when antioxidant

Table 9.1. Some dietary sources of flavonoids and phenolic acids.

Flavonoid	Source
Catechins	Tea, red wine
Flavanones	Citrus fruits
Flavonols (e.g. Quercetin)	Onions, olives, tea, wine, apples
Anthocyanidins	Cherries, strawberries, grapes, coloured fruits
Caffeic acid	Grapes, wine, olives, coffee, apples, tomatoes, plums, cherries

defences are unable to cope with the production of free radicals, and may result from the action of certain toxins or by physiological stress (Halliwell, 1994).

Flavonoids and phenolic acids can act as antioxidants by a number of potential pathways. The most important is likely to be by free radical scavenging in which the polyphenol can break the free radical chain reaction. For a compound to be defined as an antioxidant it must fulfil two conditions: (i) when present at low concentrations compared with the oxidizable substrate it can significantly delay or prevent oxidation of the substrate; (ii) the resulting radical formed on the polyphenol must be stable so as to prevent it acting as a chain propagating radical (Halliwell *et al.*, 1995). This stabilization is usually through delocalization, intramolecular hydrogen bonding or by further oxidation by reaction with another lipid radical (Shahidi and Wanasundara, 1992). A number of studies have been carried out on the structure–antioxidant activity relationships of the flavonoids (Bors *et al.*, 1990; Chen *et al.*, 1996; Rice-Evans *et al.*, 1996; Van Acker *et al.*, 1996; Cao *et al.*, 1997). The main structural features of flavonoids required for efficient radical scavenging could be summarized as follows:

1. An ortho-dihydroxy (catechol) structure in the B ring, for electron delocalization;
2. A 2,3 double bond in conjugation with a 4-keto function, provides electron delocalization from the B ring;
3. Hydroxyl groups at positions 3 and 5, provide hydrogen bonding to the keto group.

These structural features are illustrated in Fig. 9.4.

The phenolic acids may also be good antioxidants, particularly those possessing the catechol-type structure such as caffeic acid (Laranjinha *et al.*, 1994; Nardini *et al.*, 1995; Abu-Amsha *et al.*, 1996). Recent studies have indicated that simple cell-derived phenolic acids such as 3-hydroxyanthranilic acid may also be efficient co-antioxidants for α-tocopherol, able to inhibit lipoprotein and plasma lipid peroxidation in humans (Thomas *et al.*, 1996). The possible interaction between flavonoids and phenolic acids with other physiological antioxidants such as ascorbate or tocopherol is another possible antioxidant pathway for these compounds. The synergistic inter-action of these antioxidants may be exemplified by the enhancement of the antiproliferative effect of quercetin by ascorbic acid, possibly due to its ability to protect the polyphenol from oxidative degradation (Kandaswami *et al.*, 1993). In a similar manner, coincubation of low-density lipoprotein (LDL) with ascorbate and caffeic or coumaric acid resulted in a synergistic protection from oxidation promoted by ferrylmyoglobin (Vieira *et al.*, 1998a).

Another pathway of apparent antioxidant action of the flavonoids, particularly in oxidation systems using transition metal ions such as copper or iron, is chelation of the metal ions. Chelations of catalytic metal ions may

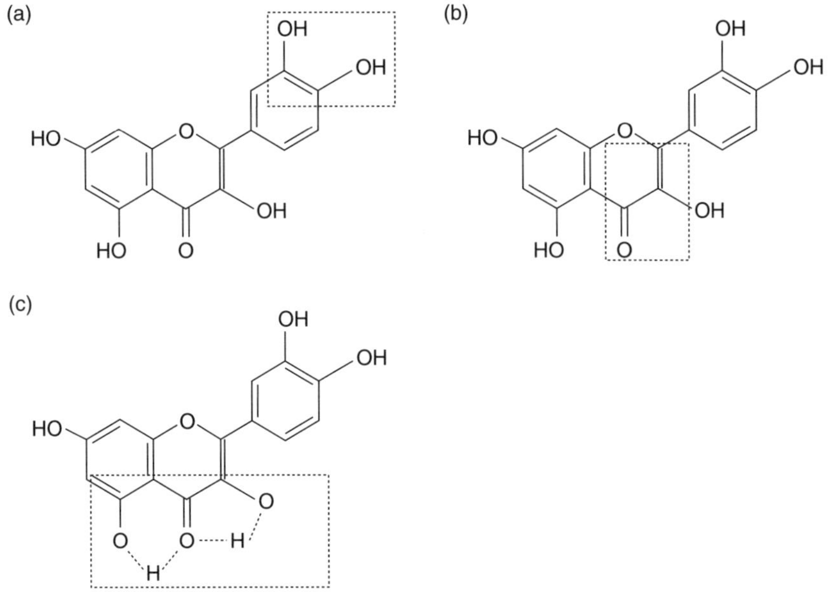

(a)

(b)

(c)

Fig. 9.4. Structural groups for radical scavenging.

prevent their involvement in Fenton-type reactions which can generate highly reactive hydroxyl radicals (reactions 9.1 and 9.2) (Halliwell *et al.*, 1995).

$$H_2O_2 + Cu^+ \rightarrow \cdot OH + OH^- + Cu^{2+} \qquad (9.1)$$
$$Cu^{2+} + O_2^- \cdot \rightarrow Cu^+ + O_2 \qquad (9.2)$$

The ability of polyphenolics to react with metal ions may also render them pro-oxidant. For example, in a recent study by Cao *et al.* (1997) using three diffferent oxidation systems, flavonoids had potent antioxidant activity against peroxyl radicals generated from AAPH and against hydroxyl radicals but were pro-oxidant with Cu^{2+}. Presumably flavonoids can reduce Cu^{2+} to Cu^+ and hence allow the formation of initiating radicals. Caffeic acid has also been shown to have pro-oxidant activity on Cu^{2+}-induced oxidation of LDL (Yamanaka *et al.*, 1997). It should be noted that this pro-oxidant activity was seen only in the propagation phase of the oxidation, not in the initiation phase in which caffeic acid inhibited lipoprotein oxidation, in agreement with previous findings (Laranjinha *et al.*, 1994; Nardini *et al.*, 1995; Abu-Amsha *et al.*, 1996).

The possible pro-oxidant effects of flavonoids may be important *in vivo* if free transition metal ions are involved in oxidation processes. In the healthy human body, metal ions appear largely sequestered in forms that are unable to catalyse free radical reactions (Halliwell and Gutteridge, 1990).

However, injury to tissues may release iron or copper (Halliwell *et al.*, 1992) and catalytic metal ions have been measured in atherosclerotic lesions (Smith *et al.*, 1992). In these cases the potential for flavonoids to act as pro-oxidants cannot be ignored.

Other biological actions of phenolic compounds have been noted which may be relevant to their effects on human health. For example, caffeic acid may have cytoprotective effects on endothelial cells related not only to its antioxidant action but also to its ability to block the rise in intracellular calcium in response to oxidized lipoproteins (Vieira *et al.*, 1998b). Some phenolic compounds may also inhibit platelet aggregation (Pace-Asciak *et al.*, 1996), while others may act as inhibitors of nuclear transcription factor NF-κB (Natarajan *et al.*, 1996). The ability of phenolic compounds to trap mutagenic electrophiles such as reactive nitrogen species may also protect biological molecules from damage (Kato *et al.*, 1997).

Absorption and Bioavailability

An understanding of the absorption and bioavailability of phenolic compounds, as well as appropriate measures or markers of their effects on steady-state oxidative damage *in vivo*, are necessary to evaluate optimal dietary intake of these substances. While data on the bioavailability of phenolic compounds in humans are scarce, there is enough evidence to suggest that flavonoids are absorbed in significant quantities (Hollman, 1997). Flavonoids such as quercetin can be absorbed both as the free aglycone and glycoside, and have been detected in blood and urine (Cova *et al.*, 1992; Hollman *et al.*, 1995). There is some evidence that peak absorption may be 2–3 h after ingestion (Hackett, 1983). Flavonoids that are absorbed may form conjugates such as glucuronides or sulphates in the liver. The metabolism of flavonoids is determined by the hydroxylation pattern, with compounds having 5,7 and 3′,4′ hydroxylation being susceptible to hydrolysis and heterocyclic ring cleavage by microbiological degradation in the colon (Griffiths, 1982). Whether hydrolysis of the flavonoid glycosides is necessary for absorption is uncertain, although recent methods have detected flavonoids as glycosides in human plasma (Paganga and Rice-Evans, 1997). Catechins are another major group of flavonoids which have been shown to be absorbed; they are present in plasma after 1 hour and also detected in a 24 h urine sample after a single oral dose (Lee *et al.*, 1995).

Further evidence for the absorption of flavonoids comes from a number of studies with isoflavonoids. Plasma concentrations of daidzein and genistein were found to be 15–40 times higher in Japanese men compared with men eating a European diet (Adlercreutz *et al.*, 1993). This reflects the high soybean (which is rich in isoflavonoids) content of the Japanese diet.

Humans supplemented with a single soybean drink containing 2 mg of isoflavone showed plasma concentrations of 2 μM after 6.5 h (Xu *et al.*, 1994).

While many aspects of flavonoid metabolism and bioavailability are still not known, there is enough evidence to suggest that some flavonoids are found in the plasma in concentrations high enough to have biological effects. Improvements in methodologies for measuring flavonoids in plasma will continue to provide valuable information in this area.

Information about the absorption of phenolic acids in humans is very limited. Our own recent research data suggest that plasma levels of caffeic acid are significantly increased within 1–4 h of drinking a glass of red wine (Abu-Amsha-Caccetta, unpublished results). The increase in plasma caffeic acid occurred using red wine with or without the alcohol removed (Fig. 9.5).

Methods for Assessment of Oxidative Damage *in Vivo*

The development of suitable methods and biomarkers for determining oxidative damage in humans is critical to the assessment of nutritional antioxidants (Halliwell, 1996). For example, methods for the assessment of total lipid peroxidation in humans have been limited to measurements of MDA excretion or hydrocarbon gases in exhaled air. These methods can be non-specific and influenced by components in the diet or environment (Halliwell, 1996). The F_2 isoprostanes formed by free-radical damage to

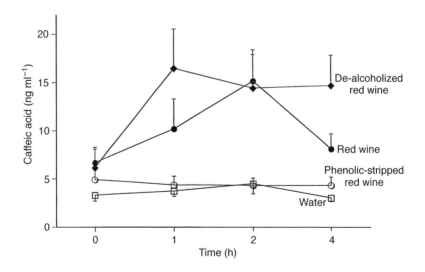

Fig. 9.5. Plasma caffeic acid concentration measured by gas chromatography–mass spectrometry in subjects who consumed 200 ml of either red wine, de-alcoholized red wine, phenolic-stripped red wine or water (*n*=12).

arachidonic acid in the body can be measured in plasma or urine and may be a good measure of steady-state lipid peroxidation (Morrow and Roberts, 1996). While the ideal method of analysis requires negative chemical ionization gas chromatography–mass spectrometry (GC-MS), a commercial enzyme immunoassay kit has become available, and measurements in agreement with the GC-MS method have been reported (Wang *et al.*, 1995). For measurement of oxidative DNA damage, the urinary excretion of 8-hydroxydeoxyguanine has been used but may suffer from several technical problems as well as a contribution from dietary intake (Halliwell, 1996). Assessment of oxidative damage to proteins can involve measurement of specific amino acid adducts with MDA or derived by attack of reactive oxygen or nitrogen species (e.g. hydroxytyrosine or nitrotyrosine) (Halliwell, 1996).

Assessment of the *in vivo* effect of dietary phenolic compounds can be very difficult. Recently, we have studied the effects of antioxidant polyphenolics in beverages such as red wine on LDL oxidation (Abu-Amsha *et al.*, 1996). Since oxidative damage to low-density lipoproteins has been linked to the development of atherosclerosis and heart disease, the rich flavonoid content of red wine has led to its appeal as possibly being beneficial against heart disease. While a number of *in vitro* studies clearly show strong antioxidant effects of red wine phenolics against LDL oxidation (Frankel *et al.*, 1993; Abu-Amsha *et al.*, 1996; Puddey and Croft, 1997), several human intervention trials have given conflicting results (Fuhrman *et al.*, 1995; Sharpe *et al.*, 1995; De Rijke *et al.*, 1996). This may arise from the fact that alcohol itself is a pro-oxidant and the overall effects of a beverage may be due to a balance between its pro-oxidative and antioxidant components (Puddey and Croft, 1997). In addition, most studies use oxidative susceptibility of isolated LDL which may not necessarily relate to oxidative damage occuring *in vivo*. Furthermore, it may be important to consider the possible location of phenolic compounds *in vivo*. In a recent interesting study, Carbonneau *et al.* (1997) fed red wine phenolic compounds to 20 volunteers, which increased the antioxidant capacity of their plasma but had no effect on the oxidizability of isolated LDL. It is presumed that phenolic compounds may act in the aqueous phase or at the surface of lipoprotein particles, and that these may be stripped from the particles during the dialysis step of lipoprotein isolation.

Conclusion

There is good evidence that many flavonoids and phenolic acids are potent antioxidants *in vitro*. The possible pro-oxidative effects of flavonoids due to interaction with metal ions may be important in some conditions where there are available or releasable transition metals. While there is still much to be learnt about the absorption and bioavailability of these compounds there is evidence that they may occur in plasma at concentrations high enough to have biological effects. On the basis of our current scientific knowledge it is not yet possible to determine the optimal level of dietary antioxidants to prevent disease. The application of state-of-the-art 'biomarkers' of oxidative damage and sensitive methods for the analysis of phenolic compounds or their metabolites in plasma and urine are needed to fully evaluate their role in human health.

Acknowledgements

The author would like to thank his colleagues, Ian Puddey, Lawrie Beilin and Trevor Mori for many helpful discussions, and PhD student Rima Abu-Amsha Caccetta for her work on antioxidants in red wine. The financial support of the National Heart Foundation of Australia and the Medical Research Foundation of Royal Perth Hospital are gratefully acknowledged.

References

Abu-Amsha, R., Croft, K.D., Puddey, I.B., Proudfoot, J.M. and Beilin, L.J. (1996) Phenolic content of various beverages determines the extent of inhibition of human serum and low density lipoprotein oxidation *in vitro*: identification and mechanism of action of some cinnamic acid derivatives from red wine. *Clinical Science* 91, 449–458.

Adlercreutz, H., Markkanen, H. and Watenabe, S. (1993) Plasma concentrations of phytoestrogens in Japanese men and women consuming a traditional Japanese diet. *Lancet* 342, 1209–1210.

Block, G. (1992) A role for antioxidants in reducing cancer risk. *Nutrition Review* 50, 207–213.

Block, G and Langseth, L. (1994) Antioxidant vitamins and disease prevention. *Food Technology* July, 80–84.

Bors, W., Heller, W., Michel, C. and Saran, M. (1990) Flavonoids as antioxidants: Determination of radical-scavenging efficiencies. *Methods in Enzymology* 186, 343–355.

Cao, G., Sofic, E. and Prior, R.L. (1997) Antioxidant and pro-oxidant behaviour of flavonoids: structure–activity relationships. *Free Radical Biology and Medicine* 22, 749–760.

Carbonneau, M.-A., Leger, C.L., Monnier, L., Bonnet, C., Michel, F., Fouret, G., Deieu, F. and Descomps, B. (1997) Supplementation with wine phenolic compounds increases the antioxidant capacity of plasma and vitamin E of low-density lipoprotein without changing the lipoprotein Cu^{2+} oxidizability: possible explanation by phenolic location. *European Journal of Clinical Nutrition* 51, 682–690.

Chen, Z.Y., Chan, P.T., Ho, K.Y., Fung, K.P. and Wang, J. (1996) Antioxidant activity of natural flavonoids is governed by number and location of their aromatic hydroxyl groups. *Chemistry and Physics of Lipids* 76, 157–163.

Cook, N.C. and Samman, S. (1996) Flavonoids, chemistry, metabolism, cardio-protective effects and dietary sources. *Journal of Nutritional Biochemistry* 7, 66–76.

Cova, D., De Angelis, L., Giavarini, F., Palladini, G. and Parego, R. (1992) Pharmacokinetics and metabolism of oral diosmin in healthy volunteers. *International Journal of Clinical Pharmacology Therapeutics and Toxicology* 30, 279–286.

De Rijke, X.B., Demacker, P.N.M., Assen, N.A., Sloots, L.M., Katan, M.B. and Stalenhoef, A.F.H. (1996) Red wine consumption does not effect oxidizability of low density lipoproteins in volunteers. *American Journal of Clinical Nutrition* 63, 329–334.

Frankel, E.N., Kanner, J., German, J.B., Parks, E. and Kinsella, J.E. (1993) Inhibition of oxidation of human low density lipoprotein by phenolic substances in red wine. *Lancet* 341, 454–457.

Frankel, E.N., Waterhouse, A.L. and Teissedre, P.L. (1995) Principle phenolic phytochemicals in selected Californian wines and their antioxidant activity in inhibiting oxidation of human low-density lipoproteins. *Journal of Agricultural and Food Chemistry* 43, 890–894.

Fuhrman, B., Lavy, A. and Aviram, M. (1995) Consumption of red wine with meals reduces the susceptibility of human plasma and low density lipoprotein to lipid peroxidation. *American Journal of Clinical Nutrition* 61, 549–554.

Griffiths, L. (1982) Mammalian metabolism of flavonoids. In: Harborne, J. and Mabry, T. (eds) *The Flavonoids: Advances in Research*. Chapman and Hall, London, pp. 681–718.

Hackett, A.M. (1983) The metabolism and excretion of (+)- 14C-cyanidenol-3 in man following oral administration. *Xenobiotica* 13, 279–286.

Halliwell, B. (1994) Free radicals, antioxidants and human disease: curiosity, cause or consequence? *Lancet* 344, 721–724.

Halliwell, B. (1996) Oxidative stress, nutrition and health. Experimental strategies for optimization of nutritional antioxidant intake in humans. *Free Radical Research* 25, 57–74.

Halliwell, B. and Gutteridge, J.M.C. (1990) The antioxidants of human extracellular fluids. *Archives of Biochemistry and Biophysics* 280, 1–8.

Halliwell, B., Gutteridge, J.M.C. and Cross, C.E. (1992) Free radicals, antioxidants and human disease: where are we now? *Journal of Laboratory Clinical Medicine* 119, 598–620.

Halliwell, B., Aeschbach, R., Loliger, J. and Aruoma, O.I. (1995) The characterization of antixoidants. *Food Chemical Toxicity* 33, 601–617.

Hertog, M.G.L., Feskens, E.J.M., Hollman, P.C.H., Katan, M.B. and Kromhout, D. (1993) Dietary antioxidant flavonoids and risk of coronary heart disease. The Zutphen elderly study. *Lancet* 342, 1007–1011.

Hollman, P.C.H. (1997) Bioavailability of flavonoids. *European Journal of Clinical Nutrition* 51, S66–S69.

Hollman, P.C.H., de Vries, J.H., van Leeuwen, S.D., Mengelers, M.J. and Katan, M.B. (1995) Absorption of dietary quercetin glycosides and quercetin in healthy ileostomy volunteers. *American Journal of Clinical Nutrition* 62, 1276–1282.

Kandaswami, G., Perkins, E., Soloniuk, D.S., Drzewiecki, G. and Middleton, E. (1993) Ascorbic acid enhanced antiproliferative effect of flavonoids on squamous cell carcinoma *in vitro*. *Anticancer Drugs* 4, 91–96.

Kato, Y., Ogino, Y., Aoki, T., Uchida, K., Kawakishi, S. and Osawa, T. (1997) Phenolic antioxidants prevent peroxynitrite-derived collagen modification *in vitro. Journal of Agricultural and Food Chemistry* 45, 3004–3009.

Laranjinha, J.A.N., Almeida, L.M. and Madeira, V.M.C. (1994) Reactivity of dietary phenolic acids with peroxyl radicals: antioxidant activity upon low density lipoprotein peroxidation. *Biochemical Pharmacology* 48, 487–494.

Lee, M.J., Wang, Z.Y., Li, H., Chen, L., Sun, Y., Gabbo, S., Balentine, D.A. and Yang, C.S. (1995) Analysis of plasma and urinary tea polyphenols in human subjects. *Cancer Epidemiology, Biomarkers and Preventors* 4, 393–399.

Lin, T.-J., Zhang, K.-J. and Liu, G.-T. (1996) Effects of salvianolic acid A on oxygen radicals released by rat neutrophils and on neutrophil function. *Biochemical Pharmacology* 51, 1237–1241.

Mann, J. (1978) *Secondary Metabolism.* Oxford Chemistry Series, Clarendon Press, Oxford.

Morrow, J.D. and Roberts, L.J. (1996) The isoprostanes: current knowledge and directions for future research. *Biochemical Pharmacology* 51, 1–9.

Nardini, M., D'Aquino, M., Tomassi, G., Gentili, V., Di Felice, N. and Scaccini, C. (1995) Inhibition of human LDL oxidation by caffeic acid and other hydroxycinnamic acid derivatives. *Free Radical Biology and Medicine* 19, 541–552.

Natarajan, K., Singh, S., Burke, T.R., Grunberger, D. and Aggarwal, B.B. (1996) Caffeic acid phenethyl ester is a potent and specific inhibitor of activation of nuclear transcription factor NF-κB. *Proceedings of the National Academy of Sciences, USA* 93, 9090–9095.

Pace-Asciak, C.R., Hahn, S., Diamandis, E., Soleas, G. and Goldberg, D.M. (1995) The red wine phenolics trans-resveritrol and quercetin block human platelet aggregation and eicosanoid synthesis: implications for protection against coronary heart disease. *Clinica Chimica Acta* 235, 207–219.

Paganga, G. and Rice-Evans, C.A. (1997) The identification of flavonoids as glycosides in human plasma. *FEBS Letters* 401, 78–82.

Puddey, I.B. and Croft, K.D. (1997) Alcoholic beverages and lipid peroxidation: relevance to cardiovascular disease. *Addiction Biology* 2, 269–276.

Rice-Evans, C.A., Miller, N.J. and Paganga, G. (1996) Structure–antioxidant activity relationships of flavonoids and phenolic acids. *Free Radical Biology and Medicine* 20, 9.

Shahidi, F. and Wanasundara, P.K.J.P.D. (1992) Phenolic antioxidants. *Critical Review of Food Science and Nutrition* 32, 67–103.

Sharpe, P.C., McGrath, L.T., McLean, E., Yound, I.S. and Archibold, G.P. (1995) Effect of red wine consumption on lipoprotein (a) and other risk factors for atherosclerosis. *Quarterly Journal of Medicine* 88, 101–108.

Smith, C., Mitchinson, M.J., Arudma, O.I. and Halliwell, B. (1992) Stimulation of lipid peroxidation and hydroxyl radical generation by the contents of human atherosclerotic lesions. *Biochemical Journal* 286, 901–905.

Soleas, G.J., Goldberg, D.M. and Diamandis, E.P. (1997) Towards the fingerprinting of wines: cultivar-related patterns of polyphenolic constituents in Ontario wines. *Journal of Agricultural and Food Chemistry* 45, 3871–3880.

Stagg, G.V. and Millin, D.J. (1975) The nutritional and therapeutic value of tea – a review. *Journal of Science, Food and Agriculture* 26, 1439–1459.

Thomas, S.R., Witting, P.K. and Stocker, R. (1996) 3-Hydroxyanthranilic acid is an efficient, cell-derived co-antioxidant for α-tocopherol, inhibiting human low density lipoprotein and plasma lipid peroxidation. *Journal of Biological Chemistry* 271, 32714–32721.

Van Acker, S.A.B.E., Van Denberg, D.J., Tromp, M.N.J.L., Griffioen, D.H., Van Bennekom, W.P., Van Dervijgh, W.J.F. and Bast, A. (1996) Structural aspects of antioxidant activity of flavonoids. *Free Radical Biology and Medicine* 20, 331–342.

Vieira, O., Laranjinha, J., Madeira, V. and Almeida L. (1998a) Cholesteryl ester hydroperoxide formation in myoglobin-catalysed low density lipoprotein oxidation; concerted antioxidant activity of caffeic and courmaric acids with ascorbate *Biochemical Pharmacology* 55, 333–340.

Vieira, O., Escargueil-Blanc, I., Meilhac, O., Basile, J.-P., Laranjinha, J., Almeida, L., Salvayre, R. and Negre-Salvayre, A. (1998b) Effect of dietary phenolic compounds on apoptosis of human cultured endothelial cells induced by oxidized LDL. *British Journal of Pharmacology* 123, 565–573.

Visioli, F. and Galli, C. (1994) Oleuropein protects low density lipoprotein from oxidation. *Life Science* 55, 1965–1971.

Wang, Z., Ciabattoni, G., Creminon, C., Lawson, J., Fitzgerald, G.A., Patrono, C. and Maclouf, J. (1995) Immunological characterization of urinary 8-epi-prostaglandin F2α excretion in man. *Journal of Pharmacology and Experimental Therapy* 275, 94–100.

Xu, X., Wang, H.J., Murphy, P.A., Cook, L. and Hendrich, S. (1994) Diadzin is a more bioavailable soymilk isoflavone than is genestein in adult women. *Journal of Nutrition* 124, 825–832.

Yamanaka, N., Oda, O. and Nagao, S. (1997) Pro-oxidant activity of caffeic acid, dietary non-flavenoid phenolic acid, on Cu^{2+}-induced low density lipoprotein oxidation. *FEBS Letters* 405, 186–190.

Antioxidant Effects of Soybean Isoflavones 10

GAOLI ZHENG[1] AND SHOUMIN ZHU[2]

[1]*Department of Pharmacology, Zhejiang Academy of Medical Sciences, Zhejiang, People's Republic of China;* [2]*Research Centre of Nutrition and Food, Zhejiang Medical University, Zhejiang, People's Republic of China*

Presence of Isoflavones in Soybeans and Soyfoods

Soybean has a high protein content (about 40%) and as such plays an important role in guarding against malnutrition, especially in parts of Asia. In recent years scientists have paid greater attention to soybeans not only for the substantial amount and high quality of their protein, but also for their many other apparently beneficial constituents. These include isoflavones, phytic acid, saponins, oligosaccharides and trypsin inhibitors (Anderson and Wolf, 1995). Among them, isoflavones have attracted particular interest.

Isoflavones are a type of natural flavonoid and possess oestrogen-like properties; hence they are sometimes referred to as phytoestrogens. Figure 10.1 shows the general structure of the main isoflavones in soybeans. In contrast with flavones, which exist widely in the plant kingdom, isoflavones are found predominately in a limited number of plants, such as legumes, particularly the soybeans. Soyfoods are the most important source of dietary isoflavones. Isoflavones are not essential nutrients, but they seem to play an important role in health maintenance.

Soybean isoflavones (SOYISO) are composed of three major forms, each of which has four derivatives; these are aglycones (genistein, daidzein, and glycitein), and the glucoside, malonyl and acetyl derivatives of genistin, daidzin and glycetin. In intact seeds, SOYISO are mainly present in the form of glucosides. The concentrations of total isoflavones are about $1–4$ g kg^{-1} dry weight in intact soybeans and as high as 17 g kg^{-1} in the hypocotyl (Eldridge and Kwolek, 1983). The concentration varies among different kinds of soybean and even in the same kind produced from different areas or during different years (Wang and Murphy, 1994). The concentration of

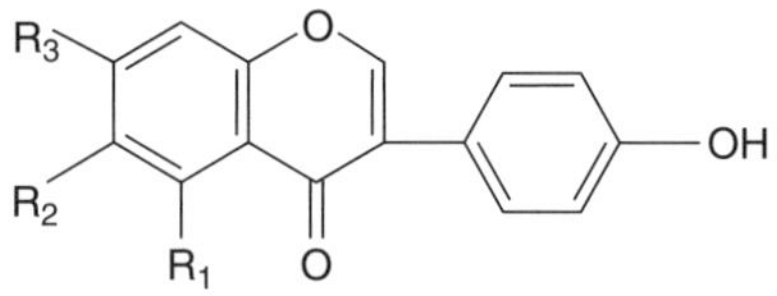

	R_1	R_2	R_3
Genistein	OH	H	OH
Genistin	OH	H	O-Glucose
Daidzein	H	H	OH
Daidzin	H	H	O-Glucose
Glycitein	H	OCH_3	OH
Glycitin	H	OCH_3	O-Glucose

Fig. 10.1. The chemical structure of soybean isoflavones.

genistin is about 330–2000 mg kg^{-1}, daidzin about 150–800 mg kg^{-1}, glycetin about 50–100 mg kg^{-1} and about 10–40 mg kg^{-1} of daidzein, genistein and glycetein (Wang and Murphy, 1994). Their concentrations vary greatly with different processing methods. For example, fermented soyfoods such as tempeh and miso contain greater amounts of aglycones because of enzymatic hydrolysis during fermentation, while non-fermented soyfoods contain greater levels of glucosides. Much of the isoflavones is lost in some processing methods because their glucosides are soluble in water. For instance, we estimate that about half of the total isoflavones in soybeans are lost in tofu processing (Zheng *et al.*, 1997a).

Antioxidant Activity of SOYISO

SOYISO have two (daidzein and glycitein) or three (genistein) phenol hydroxyl groups. Phenol hydroxyl groups can scavenge free radicals *in vivo* and *in vitro*. Generally, the more hydroxyl groups, the greater the antioxidant capacity (Cao *et al.*, 1997), suggesting that these groups are the chemical basis for the antioxidant properties of isoflavones.

Antioxidant activity of SOYISO: *in vitro* and *ex vivo* studies

There are many reports dealing with the antioxidant activity of SOYISO *in vitro*, at the level of the cell, in enzyme systems and in non-biological systems.

Isoflavones can significantly inhibit lipid peroxidation of rat liver microsomes stimulated by the Fe^{2+}-ADP–NADPH complex (Jha *et al.*, 1985). The IC$_{50}$ of genistein, daidzein and glycitein is 1.8×10^{-4}, 6.0×10^{-4} and 1.6×10^{-3} mol l^{-1}, respectively. Using this method to measure total antioxidant activity assay, Ruiz-Larrea *et al.* (1997) determined the order of antioxidant activity of several isoflavones to be as follows: genistein > daidzein = genistin = biochanin A = daidzin > formononetin = ononin. However, using a similar method to that used above but measuring production of thiobarbituric acid-reactive substances (TBARS), Mitchell *et al.* (1998) observed only weak antioxidant activity by genistein and daidzein. Soybean extract rich in isoflavones can inhibit lipid peroxidation formation in ox brain phospholipid stimulated by Fe^{3+}/vitamin C (Wiseman *et al.*, 1996).

Genistein, in a dose-dependent manner, inhibits the formation of 8-hydroxy-2'-deoxyguanosine (8-OHdG) of calf thymus activated by ultraviolet (UV) radiation or by the Fenton reaction (H_2O_2/$FeCl_2$) (Wei *et al.*, 1996). The IC_{50} is 0.25×10^{-6} mol l^{-1} for UV radiation and 25×10^{-6} mol l^{-1} for the Fenton reaction. It was found that 8-OHdG is increased in cancerous tissues and is responsible for DNA base mutation. 8-OHdG may activate certain oncogenes such as H-*ras* and K-*ras*. Inhibition of 8-OHdG formation by isoflavones suggests a potential anticarcinogenic action against photocarcinogenesis.

H_2O_2 is present in normal tissues and induces damage if the concentration rises because it generates hydroxyl radicals which are the most reactive free radicals found in the body. Isoflavones can inhibit the formation of active oxygen induced by some chemicals. Wei *et al.* (1995) used 12-O-tetradecanoylphorbol-13-acetate (TPA, a tumour promoter) to stimulate HL-60 cells to produce H_2O_2. Both genistein and, to a lesser extent, daidzein inhibited H_2O_2 formation in this system. Wei *et al.* (1995) also showed that various isoflavones are able to suppress $O_2^-\cdot$ production by xanthine/xanthine oxidase. Genistein (20 μmol l^{-1}) almost completely inhibited the production of $O_2^-\cdot$, while daidzein inhibited it by 80% at the same concentration.

Genistein can also prevent some of the damage done by H_2O_2 to cells. Genistein, like the hydroxyl scavenger dimethylthiourea, can reduce the induction of adenylyl cyclase activity by H_2O_2 in A10 cells (a murine vascular smooth muscle cell line) (Tan *et al.*, 1995) and prevent haemolysis of sheep red blood cells by dialuric acid or H_2O_2 *in vitro* (Pratt *et al.*, 1981).

Collagen can induce platelet aggregation and produce reactive oxygen species (ROS). Schoene and Guidry (1996) found that a collagen-stimulated rat blood sample will produce a much lower concentration of ROS and platelet aggregation if pretreated with genistein. Gaudette and Holub (1990) previously reported that genistein possesses anti-platelet activity. It is not clear whether this comes from its inhibiting ROS formation in platelets.

Chait (1996) reported that low-density lipoprotein (LDL) oxidation stimulated by copper ions was prevented by genistein and daidzein in a concentration-dependent manner. It was also shown that genistein suppresses the oxidation of LDL induced by copper ions or free radicals (superoxide/nitric oxide radicals) (Kapiotis *et al.*, 1997).

Kanazawa *et al.* (1995) reported that when patients with cerebro-vascular disease were given a soybean supplement in their diets for 6 months, their lipoproteins were less susceptible to peroxidation by copper ions than lipoproteins from unsupplemented subjects. There was a much greater suppression of oxidation of very-low-density lipoproteins and LDL than of high-density lipoproteins. In a similar study, healthy subjects were given a supplement containing 12 mg genistein and 7 mg daidzein daily for 2 weeks. This increased the resistance of their LDL to oxidation (Tikkanen *et al.*, 1998).

Antioxidant activity of SOYISO: *in vivo* studies

Cai and Wei (1996) observed the effects of genistein on the activities of antioxidant enzymes in mice. They fed Sencar mice with a diet containing 0, 50 and 250 mg kg^{-1} genistein for 1 month. Results showed that although some antioxidant enzymes (superoxide dismutase (SOD), chloramphenicol acetyl transferase, glutathione peroxidase (GSH-Px), glutathione reductase and glutathione-*S*-transferase) were increased in some tissues (liver, kidney, lung, small intestine and skin), this was generally by no more than 10–20%.

Another report showed that genistein and daidzein can inhibit sister-chromatid exchanges of bone marrow cells and DNA adduct formation in mouse liver induced by 7,12-dimethylbenz[*a*]anthracene, a carcinogen (Giri and Lu, 1995).

The relatively low antioxidant activity of SOYISO in normal animals is not consistent with its potent activity *in vitro*. This possibly results from using normal, young rats possessing relatively high levels of antioxidant enzymes, which are resistant to further increase. Moreover, the normal tissue levels of free radicals are essential to physiological and immune functioning. For these reasons we designed an experiment to measure the antioxidant activity of SOYISO extract (SIE) in animal models of oxidative stress. This extract contains 41% genistein, 52% daidzein and very little glucoside (genistin and daidzin).

Adriamycin (ADR) is a drug used for treating cancer. Its usage is often limited by severe cardiac toxicity which is generally considered to be a result of oxidative damage. In our study we used ADR to produce oxidative stress in mice and we then monitored the effect of treatment with SIE (Table 10.1). Mice were treated with ADR (20 mg kg^{-1} intraperitoneally as four doses over 12 days). It induced a decrease in the levels of two antioxidant enzymes (SOD and GSH-Px) in red blood cells, liver and heart tissues and an increase in LPO in these tissues. The toxicity of ADR appears to be unrelated to its anticancer action as indicated by the fact that antioxidants, namely vitamin E and probucal, can prevent ADR-induced cardiomyopathy without reducing its antitumour properties (Perez Ripoll *et al.*, 1986; Siveski-Iliskovic *et al.*, 1995). SIE at doses of total isoflavone of 10 and 40 mg kg^{-1} body weight daily for 2 weeks significantly increased the activities of the

Table 10.1. The effect of SIE on antioxidases and lipid peroxidation (LPO) levels in adriamycin-treated mouse (from Zheng *et al.*, 1997b).

	SOD[a]	GSH-px[b]	LPO[c]
Blood[a]			
Normal control	307±16.8		11.6±3.98
ADR	152±46.2		19.9±3.43
ADR+SIE 10 mg kg^{-1}	270±8.5**		17.4±2.90*
ADR+SIE 40 mg kg^{-1}	300±30.7**		14.8±2.75**
Liver			
Normal control	257±25	10.55±1.42	262±30
ADR	190±46	8.23±1.90	343±21
ADR+SIE 10 mg kg^{-1}	285±38.4**	8.89±2.25	328±27
ADR+SIE 40 mg kg^{-1}	154±35**	9.12±1.42	274±21**
Heart			
Normal control	129±30	3.61±0.59	76±7.7
ADR	78±25	1.84±0.59	100±5.6
ADR+SIE 10 mg kg^{-1}	114±25**	3.67±0.47**	84±7.0**
ADR+SIE 40 mg kg^{-1}	253±25**	4.09±0.368**	82±8.4**

Data show mean ± SD, *n* = 10. ADR, adriamycin; SIE, soybean isoflavone extract.
Significance based on comparison with ADR group. *$P<0.05$; **$P<0.01$.
[a] Expressed as U g^{-1} wet tissue or U ml^{-1} erythrocyte.
[b] Expressed as U g^{-1} wet tissue.
[c] Expressed as 10^{-9} mol g^{-1} tissue or U ml^{-1} plasma.

two antioxidant enzymes and lowered LPO in comparison with ADR-treated mice not given SIE. Effects were generally more pronounced with the higher dose of SIE. The results therefore indicate that SIE helped to reverse the effects of ADR. Moreover, SIE also prevented myocardial damage by ADR. The results demonstrate the antioxidant action of SOYISO.

Potential of SOYISO in the Prevention of Cardiovascular Disease and Cancer

Animal experiments have revealed the anticarcinogenic properties of SOYISO and soybean products (Messina *et al.*, 1994; Helms and Gallaher, 1995; Lamartiniere *et al.*, 1995). Genistein arrested the cell cycle at the G2–M phase while daidzein did so at the G1 phase (Jing *et al.*, 1993; Matsukawa *et al.*, 1993). Proposed mechanisms include oestrogenic and anti-oestrogenic effects (Adlercreutz, 1990; Messina and Barnes, 1991), induction of cancer cell differentiation, inhibition of tyrosine kinase in cell signalling (Messina and Barnes, 1991) and DNA topoisomerases in DNA replication (Markovits *et al.*, 1989), and suppression of angiogenesis. But, as stated earlier,

SOYISO can protect DNA from oxidative damage caused by UV or $H_2O_2/FeCl_2$ and inhibit the H_2O_2 formation induced in cancer cell lines by the tumour promoter, TPA. These data demonstrate that the antioxidant activity of SOYISO may play an important role in their anticancer activity. It must be stressed that soybeans contain a variety of compounds in addition to SOYISO which may have anticarcinogenic activity (Kennedy, 1995).

LDL oxidation is a critical event in atherogenesis; it promotes the formation of foam cells and proliferation of smooth muscle cells. This suggests that suppression of LDL oxidation by SOYISO may help prevent atherosclerosis. This possibility is supported by recent reports indicating that SOYISO can reduce the levels of blood lipids including total cholesterol, LDL and apolipoprotein B (Anthony *et al.*, 1996). However, there are as yet no reports demonstrating that SOYISO prevent atherosclerosis *in vivo*.

Research in recent years has supported the concept linking free radicals with many diseases and symptoms, such as cancer, atherosclerosis, inflammation, impaired mental functioning and ageing. Experimental studies have supported the potential value of antioxidant treatment. For example, flavone extracts of *Ginkgo biloba* have been used in the treatment of cardiovascular diseases for several decades. In this regard natural antioxidants may be preferable, as synthetic agents often have side effects. SOYISO may prove to be a family of compounds well worthy of further investigation.

References

Adlercreutz, H. (1990) Western diet and western diseases: some hormonal and biochemical mechanisms and associations. *Scandinavian Journal of Clinical and Laboratory Investigation* 50 (Suppl. 201), 3–23.

Anderson, R.L. and Wolf, W.J. (1995) Compositional changes in trypsin inhibitors, phytic acid, saponins and isoflavones related to soybean processing. *Journal of Nutrition* 125, 581S–588S.

Anthony, M.S., Clarkson, T.B., Hughes, C.L., Morgan, T.M. and Burke, G.L. (1996) Soybean isoflavones improves cardiovascular risk factors without effecting the reproductive system of peripubertal rhesus monkeys. *Journal of Nutrition* 126, 43–50.

Cai, Q. and Wei, H. (1996) Effect of dietary genistein on antioxidant enzyme activities in SENCAR mice. *Nutrition and Cancer* 25, 1–7.

Cao, G.H., Sofic, E. and Prior, R. (1997) Antioxidant and prooxidant behavior of flavonoids: structure–activity relationships. *Free Radical Biology and Medicine* 22, 749–760.

Chait, A. (1996) Effects of isoflavones on LDL-cholesterol *in vitro* but not *in vivo*. *Second International Symposium on the Role of Soy in Preventing and Treating Chronic Disease*. Protein Technologies International, St Louis, Missouri.

Eldridge, A.C. and Kwolek, W.F. (1983) Soybean isoflavones: effect of environment and variety on composition. *Journal of Agricultural and Food Chemistry* 31, 394–396.

Gaudette, D.C. and Holub, B.J. (1990) Effect of genistein, a tyrosine kinase inhibitor, on U46619-induced phosphoinositide phosphorylation in human platelets. *Biochemical and Biophysical Research Communications* 170, 238–242.

Giri, A.K. and Lu, L.J. (1995) Genetic damage and the inhibition of 7,12-dimethyl-benz(a)anthracene-induced genetic damage by the phyoestrogens, genistein and daidzein in female ICR mice. *Cancer Letters* 95, 125–133.

Helms, J.R. and Gallaher, D.D. (1995) The effect of dietary soy protein isolate and genistein on the development of proneoplastic lesions (aberrant crypts) in rats. *Journal of Nutrition* 125, 802S.

Jha, H.C., von Recklinghausen, G. and Zilliken, F. (1985) Inhibition of *in vitro* microsomal lipid peroxidation by isoflavonoids. *Biochemical Pharmacology* 34, 1367–1369.

Jing, Y., Nakaya, K. and Han, R. (1993) Differentiation of promyelocytic leukemia cells HL-60 induced by daidzein *in vitro* and *in vivo*. *Anticancer Research* 13, 1049–1054.

Kanazawa, T., Osanai, T., Zhang, X.S., Uemura, T., Yin, X.Z., Onodera, K., Oike, Y. and Ohkubo, K. (1995) Protective effects of soy protein on the peroxidizability of lipoproteins in cerebrovascular diseases. *Journal of Nutrition* 125, 639S–646S.

Kapiotis, S., Hermann, M., Held, I., Seelos, C., Ehringer, H. and Gmeiner, B.M.K. (1997) Genistein, the dietary-derived angiogenesis inhibitor, prevents LDL oxidation and protects endothelial cells from damage by atherogenic LDL. *Arteriosclerosis, Thrombosis and Vascular Biology* 17, 2868–2874.

Kennedy, A.R. (1995) The evidence for soybean products as cancer preventive agents. *Journal of Nutrition* 125, 733S–743S.

Lamartiniere, C.A., Moore, J.B., Brown, N.M., Thompson, R., Hain, M.J. and Barnes, S. (1995) Genistein suppresses mammary cancer in rats. *Carcinogenesis* 6, 2833–2840.

Markovits, J., Limassier, C. and Fosse, P. (1989) Inhibitory effects of the tyrosine kinase inhibitor genistein on mammalian DNA topoisomerase II. *Cancer Research* 49, 5111–5117.

Matsukawa, Y., Marui N., Sakai, T., Satomi, Y., Yoshida, M., Matsumoto, K., Nishino, H. and Aoike, A. (1993) Genistein arrests cell cycle progression at G2-M. *Cancer Research* 53, 1328–1331.

Messina, M.J. and Barnes, S. (1991) The role of soy products in reducing risk of cancer. *Journal of the National Cancer Institute* 83, 541–546.

Messina, M.J., Persky, V.P., Setchell, K.D.R. and Barnes, S. (1994) Soy intake and cancer risk: a review of the *in vitro* and *in vivo* data. *Nutrition and Cancer* 21, 113–131.

Mitchell, J.H., Morrice, P.C., Collins, A.R. and Duthie, G.G. (1998) Inhibition of peroxidation of vitamin E-deficient microsomes by phyoestrogens. *Proceedings of the Royal Society of Chemistry*, London (in press).

Perez Ripoll, E.A., Rama, B.N. and Weber, M.M. (1986) Vitamin E enhances the chemotherapeutic effects of adriamycin on human prostatic carcinoma cells *in vitro*. *Journal of Urology* 136, 529–531.

Pratt, D.E., Di Pieteo, C., Porter, W.L. and Giffee, J.W. (1981) Phenolic antioxidants of soy protein hydrolyzates. *Journal of Food Science* 47, 24–25.

Ruiz-Larrea, M.B., Mohan, A.R., Paganga, G., Miller, N.J., Bolwell, G.P. and Rice-Evans, C.A. (1997) Antioxidant activity of phytoestrogenic isoflavones. *Free Radical Research* 26, 63–70.

Schoene, N.W. and Guidry, C.A. (1996) Genistein reactive oxygen species (ROS) formation during activation of rat platelets in while blood. In: *The Second International Symposium on the Role of Soy in Preventing and Treating Chronic Disease*. Protein Technologies International, St Louis, Missouri.

Siveski-Iliskovic, N., Hill, M., Chow, D.A. and Singal, P.K. (1995) Probucol protects against adriamycin cardiomyopathy without interfering with its antitumor effect. *Circulation* 91, 10–15.

Tan, C.M., Xenoyannis, S. and Feldman, R.D. (1995) Oxidant stress enhances adenylyl cyclase activation. *Circulation Research* 77, 710–717.

Tikkanen, M.J., Wahala, K., Ojala, S., Vihma, V. and Adlercreutz, H. (1998) Effect of soybean phytoestrogen intake on low density lipoprotein oxidation resistance. *Proceedings of the National Academy of Sciences, USA* 95, 3106–3110.

Wang, H. and Murphy, P.A. (1994) Isoflavone composition of American and Japanese soybeans in Iowa: effects of variety, crop year, and location. *Journal of Agricultural and Food Chemistry* 42, 1674–1677.

Wei, H., Bowen, R., Cai, Q., Barnes, S. and Wang, Y. (1995) Antioxidant and antipromotional effects of the soy bean isoflavone genistein. *Proceedings of the Society for Experimental Biology and Medicine* 208, 124–130.

Wei, H., Cai, Q. and Ronald, R. (1996) Inhibition of UV light- and Fenton reaction-induced oxidative DNA damage by the soybean isoflavone genistein. *Carcinogenesis* 17, 73–77.

Wiseman, H., Lim, P. and O'Reilly, J. (1996) Inhibition of liposomal lipid peroxidation by isoflavonoid type phyto-oestrogens from soybeans of different countries of origin. *Biochemical Society Transactions* 24, 392S.

Zheng, G.L., Zhou, Y.G. and Gong, W.G. (1997a) Isolation of soybean isoflavones from Tofu wastewater. *ACTA Academiae Medicinae Zhejang* 8, 23–25.

Zheng, G.L., Zhu, S.M. and Liu, Z.Y. (1997b) Antioxidant effect of soybean isoflavone extract on adriamycin-treated mouse. *Journal of Zhejiang Medical University* 26, 23–26.

Action of *Ginkgo biloba* Extract as an Antioxidant

11

NORIKO NOGUCHI, KIMIHIRO NISHINO, EIICHI WASHIO, HONGLIAN SHI AND ETSUO NIKI

Research Center for Advanced Science and Technology, University of Tokyo, Tokyo, Japan

Introduction

With increasing evidence showing the involvement of free radicals and active oxygen species in a variety of diseases and even ageing, the role of anti-oxidants has received much attention (Sies, 1991). For example, it is now accepted that oxidative modification of low-density lipoprotein (LDL) is the key initial event in the development of atherosclerosis. Many kinds of natural and synthetic compounds have been found to have antioxidant activities and to inhibit the oxidation of LDL (Esterbauer *et al.*, 1989; Noguchi *et al.*, 1994). For instance, the antioxidant effects of phenolic compounds in red wine may help to explain the French paradox (Kondo *et al.*, 1994), while many natural antioxidants in green tea and spices have also received much attention (Salah *et al.*, 1991; Kuo *et al.*, 1996); a leaf of *Gingko biloba* has been one of the most popular traditional Chinese medicines for several thousand years (Hsu, 1986; Kleijnen and Kripschild, 1992). In Europe, recently, the inhibitory effect of *Gingko biloba* extract (GBE) on diseases of peripheral vessels and cerebellar vessel dysfunctions has been reported (Rong *et al.*, 1996). In connection with this, antioxidant activity has received attention. In this chapter we describe the antioxidant activity of GBE against lipid peroxidation.

Reactivity of GBE Towards Galvinoxyl

GBE is a yellow powder which was supplied by Takehaya Co. (Tokyo, Japan) and was prepared according to Sticker (1993). It contained flavonoid

(24%) and terpenoid (6%). The galvinoxyl radical has often been used in the estimation of the reactivity of antioxidants toward radicals. The interactions of GBE or 2,6-di-*tert*-butyl-4-methylphenyl (BHT) with galvinoxyl were measured with a spectrophotometer (UV-2200, Shimadzu, Kyoto, Japan) equipped with a rapid-mixing stopped-flow apparatus (RX-1000, Applied Photophysics, Leatherhead, UK). The galvinoxyl radical has a maximum absorption at 429 nm and is not interrupted by the absorption spectrum of GBE (Fig. 11.1a). The rate of consumption of galvinoxyl was followed by measuring the decrease in its maximum absorption at 429 nm. It was found that GBE reduces galvinoxyl in a concentration-dependent manner (Fig. 11.1b) and much faster than BHT when compared at the same concentration (in $\mu g\ ml^{-1}$) (Fig. 11.1c). This suggests that GBE has a high reactivity toward radicals by donating hydrogen.

Reactivity of GBE Towards Peroxyl Radical

The reactivities of GBE towards peroxyl radicals were estimated as follows. One molecule of *N,N'*-diphenyl-1,4-phenylenediamine (DPPD) reacts rapidly with two molecules of peroxyl radicals to give *N,N'*-diphenyl-1,4-benzoquinone diimine (DPBQ), which has a strong absorption at 440 nm (Takahashi *et al.*, 1989; Noguchi *et al.*, 1997).

When appropriate amounts of DPPD and 2,2'-azobis(2,4-dimethyl-valeronitrile) (AMVN) were incubated in methanol at 37°C under air, DPBQ was formed at a constant rate (Fig. 11.2). The reactivity of the GBE toward peroxyl radicals was assessed from the extent of reduction of formation of DPBQ by GBE. It was found that GBE added to this mixture suppressed the formation of DPBQ in a concentration-dependent manner, implying that GBE competed with DPPD in scavenging peroxyl radicals derived from AMVN.

Inhibition of Oxidation of Methyl Linoleate by GBE

The rate and mechanism of the oxidation of methyl linoleate induced by free radicals in organic homogeneous solution has been well described (Burton and Ingold, 1981; Niki *et al.*, 1984; Cosgrove *et al.*, 1987; Barclay, 1993). The reaction generates methyl linoleate hydroperoxides (MeLOOH) which have a conjugated diene and the reaction is suitable for measuring the chemical activity of antioxidants. The antioxidant activity of GBE was assessed in the

---

Fig. 11.1. (opposite) (a) Absorption spectra at 429 nm of galvinoxyl (5 μM) and GBE (50 $\mu g\ ml^{-1}$) in methanol. (b) and (c) Decrease in absorption at 429 nm of 5 μM galvinoxyl by reaction with GBE (b) or BHT (c) in methanol under air at 37°C. The numbers in the figure show the concentration of GBE or BHT in $\mu g\ ml^{-1}$.

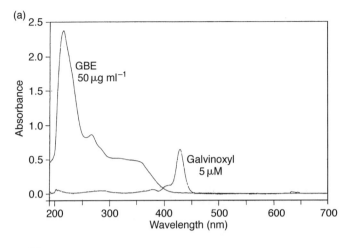

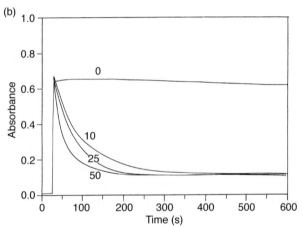

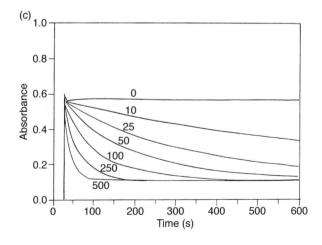

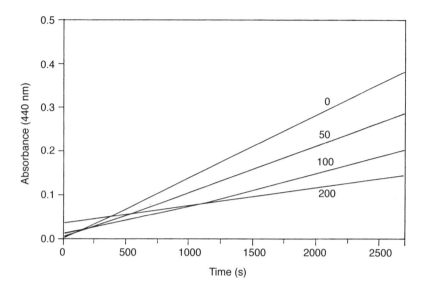

Fig. 11.2. Increase in the absorption at 440 nm due to DPBQ formed during the incubation of DPPD with AMVN in the absence and presence of GBE at 37°C in methanol under air. The numbers show the concentration of GBE in $\mu g\ ml^{-1}$.

oxidation of methyl linoleate induced by AMVN in *tert*-butyl alcohol solution. The rate of spontaneous oxidation of methyl linoleate in this solvent at 37°C under air is low (data not shown), but the addition of AMVN causes the accumulation of MeLOOH without any appreciable induction period. GBE suppresses the reaction in a concentration-dependent manner (Fig. 11.3), but a clear induction period was not observed at the concentration used.

The reaction mixture was treated with triphenylphosphine and the resulting methyl linoleate hydroxides (MeLOH) were analysed by high performance liquid chromatography (HPLC). As shown in Fig. 11.4, methyl linoleate is oxidized to give four types of conjugated diene hydroperoxides. The higher the concentration of hydrogen donors such as substrates and antioxidants, the larger the amount of *cis*, *trans*-hydroperoxides that are formed. Table 11.1 shows that the ratio of *cis,trans-* : *trans,trans-* was 1:4 without or with a low concentration of GBE and changed to 1:2 with 50 μg ml^{-1} of GBE, suggesting that GBE acts as a hydrogen-donating antioxidant.

Inhibition of Oxidation of Soybean PC Liposomal Membranes by GBE

The oxidation of soybean phosphatidylcholine (PC) liposomal membranes induced by either a hydrophilic radical initiator, 2,2′-azobis(2-amidinopropane) dihydrochloride (AAPH), or a lipophilic radical initiator (AMVN) proceeds by

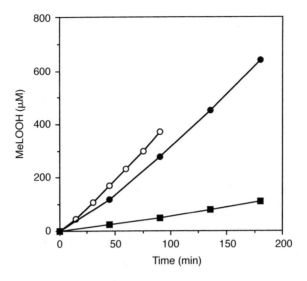

Fig. 11.3. Effect of GBE on the oxidation of methyl linoleate (151 mM) in *tert*-butyl alcohol solution induced by AMVN (0.5 mM) at 37°C under air. The concentration of GBE was: ○, 0; ●, 10; ■, 50 μg ml^{-1}.

a free radical-mediated chain mechanism to give phosphatidylcholine hydroperoxide (PCOOH) as the major primary product (Gotoh *et al.*, 1992). The unilamellar PC liposomal membranes were prepared by sonicating multilamellar vesicles with a Branson Sonifier 250 as reported previously (Komuro *et al.*, 1990). PC, AMVN and antioxidants, when used, were

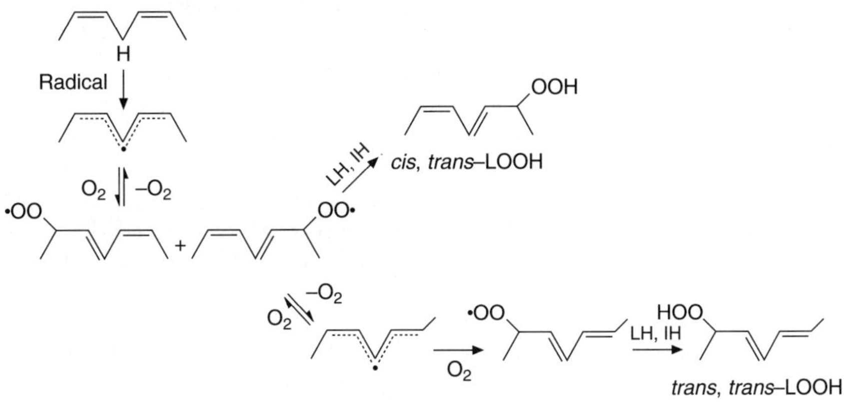

Fig. 11.4. Scheme of free radical-mediated oxidation of linoleic acid and its esters. LH, substrate (lipid); IH, antioxidant.

Table 11.1. Effect of GBE on the isomer distribution of the oxidation products from methyl linoleate[a].

	GBE (μg ml^{-1})		
	0	10	50
13-c, t-MeLOH	10	10	16
13-t, t-MeLOH	40	40	34
9-c, t-MeLOH	10	10	16
9-t, t-MeLOH	40	40	34

[a] Methyl linoleate was oxidized as shown in Fig. 11.3 and the four isomers of methyl linoleate hydroperoxides were analysed by HPLC after reduction by triphenylphosphine to methyl linoleate hydroxide (MeLOH).

incorporated into the membranes simultaneously by dissolving them in the solvent before preparation of the membranes. AAPH and GBE were added as an aqueous solution and a methanol solution, respectively, after preparation of unilamellar vesicles. The PC hydroperoxides (PCOOH) were analysed by absorption at 234 nm with HPLC. As observed previously, in the absence of antioxidant PCOOH is formed at a constant rate without any induction period (Yamamoto *et al.*, 1984; Gotoh *et al.*, 1992). GBE suppresses the formation of PCOOH in a concentration-dependent manner in the oxidation of PC induced by both AAPH (Fig. 11.5a) and AMVN (Fig. 11.5b). It was found that GBE, which was added to liposomal suspension as a solution in methanol, can scavenge radicals within a membrane. However, the clear induction period which is shown in the presence of a potent antioxidant such as α-tocopherol was not observed.

Inhibition of Oxidation of LDL by GBE

LDL was isolated from human plasma as described in the literature (Ramos *et al.*, 1995) and was oxidized with AAPH at 37°C under air. Twenty-five μg ml^{-1} GBE retarded consumption of α-tocopherol and the higher concentration of GBE inhibited it almost completely during a 6 h incubation (Fig. 11.6a). In the absence of GBE, a remarkable accumulation of cholesteryl ester hydroperoxide (CEOOH) was observed, as reported previously (Noguchi *et al.*, 1996); this was significantly inhibited by GBE (Fig. 11.6b).

Inhibition of Lipid Peroxidation by a Combination of GBE and α-Tocopherol

The above results suggest that GBE exerts a weaker antioxidant effect than α-tocopherol against lipid peroxidation in organic solution and in liposomal

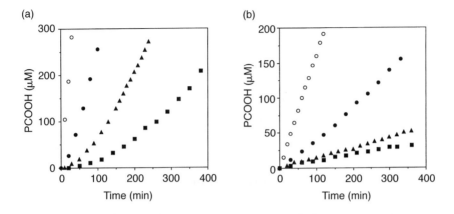

Fig. 11.5. Effect of GBE on the oxidation of soybean PC (5.15 mM) liposomal membranes induced by (a) aqueous AAPH (5 mM) or (b) lipophilic AMVN (1 mM) incorporated into liposomal membranes at 37°C under air. The concentration of GBE was: ○: 0; ●: 10; ▲: 25; ■: 50 μg ml^{-1}.

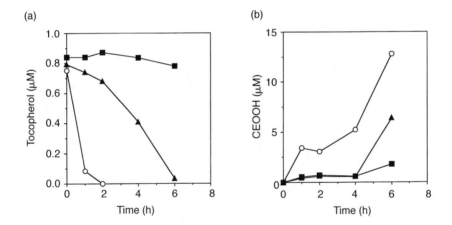

Fig. 11.6. Effect of GBE on the oxidation of human LDL. Human LDL (0.25 mg protein ml^{-1}) was oxidized in phosphate-buffered saline (pH 7.4) with AAPH (3 mM) at 37°C under air and (a) the consumption of endogenous α-tocopherol and (b) formation of cholesteryl ester hydroperoxide (CEOOH) were followed with an HPLC. The concentration of GBE was: ○, 0; ▲, 25; ■, 50 μg ml^{-1}.

membranes but spares α-tocopherol in the oxidation of LDL. To investigate this further, the action of GBE against lipid peroxidation in homogeneous solution was studied in the presence of α-tocopherol. The oxidation of methyl linoleate was induced by AMVN in *tert*-butyl alcohol in the absence and presence of α-tocopherol and GBE (Fig. 11.7). In the presence of α-tocopherol, the formation of MeLOOH was inhibited significantly and it proceeded at a similar rate after depletion of α-tocopherol as that without antioxidant. It was found that GBE retarded consumption of α-tocopherol, resulting in the inhibition of the formation of MeLOOH. We observed that the electron spin resonance (ESR) signal of α-tocopheroxyl radical was diminished rapidly by GBE (data not shown). These data imply that GBE reduces the α-tocopheroxyl radical and thereby spares α-tocopherol as well as scavenging radicals competitively with α-tocopherol.

Conclusions

The above results show that GBE possesses a potent antioxidant activity by acting as a hydrogen donor towards chain-carrying peroxyl radicals to break chain propagation and also towards α-tocopheroxyl radicals to regenerate and spare α-tocopherol. GBE inhibits lipid peroxidation effectively in homogeneous solution, liposomal membranes, and also LDL. Therefore,

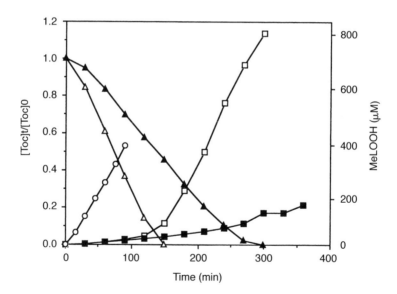

Fig. 11.7. Inhibition of oxidation of methyl linoleate by a combination of GBE and α-tocopherol. Methyl linoleate (151 mM) was oxidized in *tert*-butyl alcohol with AMVN (0.5 mM) in the absence (○) and presence (5 μM) of α-tocopherol and GBE (0, 50 μg ml^{-1}) and formation of methyl linoleate hydroperoxide (MeLOOH) (○, □, ■) and consumption of α-tocopherol (△, ▲) were measured. Open and solid symbols show the results without and with GBE, respectively. [Toc]t/[Toc]0 shows remaining α-tocopherol.

GBE is supposed to prevent development of atherosclerosis *in vivo*. This should be addressed in experiments with animal models in the near future.

References

Barclay, L.R.L. (1993) Model biomembranes: quantitative studies of peroxidation, antioxidant action, partitioning, and oxidative stress. *Canadian Journal of Chemistry* 71,1–16.

Burton, G.W. and Ingold, K.U. (1981) Autoxidation of biological molecules. 1. The antioxidant activity of vitamin E related chain-breaking phenolic antioxidants *in vitro*. *Journal of the American Chemical Society* 103, 6472–6477.

Cosgrove, J.P., Church, D.F. and Pryor, W.A. (1987) The kinetics of the autoxidation of polyunsaturated fatty acids. *Lipids* 22, 299–304.

Esterbauer, H., Rotheneder, M., Striegl, G., Waeg, G., Ashy, A., Sattler, W. and Jurgens, G. (1989) Vitamin E and other lipophilic antioxidants protect LDL against oxidation. *Fat Science and Technology* 91, 316–324.

Gotoh, N., Shimizu, K., Komuro, E., Tsuchiya, J., Noguchi, N. and Niki, E. (1992) Antioxidant activities of probucol against lipid peroxidations. *Biochimica et Biophysica Acta* 1128, 147–154.

Hsu, H.Y. (1986) *Oriental Materia Medica*. Oriental Healing Arts Institute, Long Beach, California.

Kleijnen, J. and Knipschild, P. (1992) Ginkgo biloba. *Lancet* 340, 1136–1139.

Komuro, E., Takahashi, M., Morita, M., Tsuchiya, J., Arakawa, Y., Yamamoto, Y., Niki, E., Sugioka, K. and Nakano, M. (1990) Inhibition of peroxidations of lipids and membranes by estrogens. *Journal of Physical and Organic Chemistry* 3, 309–315.

Kondo, K., Matsumoto, A., Kurata, H., Tanahashi, H., Koda, H., Amachi, T. and Itakura, H. (1994) Inhibition of oxidation of low-density lipoprotein with red wine. *Lancet* 344, 1152.

Kuo, M.L., Huang, T.S. and Lin, J.K. (1996) Curcumin, an antioxidant and anti-tumor promoter, induces apoptosis in human leukemia cells. *Biochimica et Biophysica Acta* 1317, 95–100.

Niki, E., Saito, T., Kawakami, A. and Kamiya, Y. (1984) Inhibition of oxidation of methyl linoleate in solution by vitamin E and vitamin C. *Journal of Biological Chemistry* 259, 4177–4182.

Noguchi, N., Gotoh, N. and Niki, E. (1994) Effects of ebselen and probucol on oxidative modifications of lipid and protein of low density lipoprotein induced by free radicals. *Biochimica et Biophysica Acta* 1213, 176–182.

Noguchi, N. Sakai, H., Kato, Y., Yamamoto, Y., Niki, E., Horikoshi, H. and Kodama, T. (1996) Inhibition of oxidation of low density lipoprotein by troglitazone. *Atherosclerosis* 123, 227–234.

Noguchi, N., Yamashita, H., Gotoh, N., Yamamoto, Y., Numano, R. and Niki, E. (1997) 2,2'-Azobis(4-methoxy-2,4-dimethylvaleronitrile), a new lipid-soluble azo initiator: application to oxidations of lipids and low density lipoprotein in solution and in aqueous dispersions. *Free Radical Biology and Medicine* 24, 259–268.

Ramos, P., Gieseg, S.P., Schuster, B. and Esterbauer, H. (1995) Effect of temperature and phase transition on oxidation resistance of low density lipoprotein. *Journal of Lipid Research* 36, 2113–2128.

Rong, Y., Geng, Z. and Lau, B.H. (1996) Ginkgo biloba attenuates oxidative stress in macrophages and endothelial cells. *Free Radical Biology and Medicine* 20, 121–127.

Salah, N., Miller, N.J., Paganga, G., Tijburg, L., Bolwell, G.P. and Rice-Evans, C. (1991) Polyphenolic flavanols as scavengers of aqueous phase radicals and as chain-breaking antioxidants. *Archives of Biochemistry and Biophysics* 322, 339–346.

Sies, H. (1991) *Oxidative Stress, Oxidants and Antioxidants.* Academic Press, London.

Sticker, O. (1993) Quality of Ginkgo preparations. *Planta Medica* 59, 2–11.

Takahashi, M., Tsuchiya, J. and Niki, E (1989) Oxidation of lipids. XVI. Inhibition of autoxidation of methyl linoleate in solution. *Bulletin of the Chemistry Society of Japan* 62, 1881–1884.

Yamamoto, Y., Niki, E., Kamiya, Y. and Shimasaki, H. (1984) Oxidation of lipids. VII. Oxidation of phosphatidylcholines in homogeneous solution and in water dispersion. *Biochimica et Biophysica Acta* 795, 332–340.

Whole Foods, Antioxidants and Health 12

TED WILSON

*La Crosse Exercise and Health Program and
Department of Biology, University of
Wisconsin-La Crosse, La Crosse, Wisconsin, USA*

Introduction

The capacity of whole foods to improve antioxidant defences and our quality of life is poorly understood. Understanding how antioxidants from whole foods affect our health is very important in controlling the epidemic of heart disease and cancer observed today. The use of specific antioxidant supplements such as ascorbate, α-tocopherol and β-carotene has increased as the public has become more familiar with antioxidant concerns. Because their use has increased, the potential for increased risks associated with their misuse has also increased. For most persons in the developed nations, whole-food products remain the *primary* source of dietary antioxidants, but for poor persons in non-developed nations, whole foods are the *only* source of antioxidants.

For the purpose of this paper a whole food is considered to represent a foodstuff that undergoes no or minimal processing. The term 'whole food' is also meant to include beverages made from whole foods. This review will focus on the contribution of antioxidant activities to health promotion. Most whole-food antioxidant activity is derived from phenolic phytochemicals, including polyphenols and flavonoids. These molecules have antioxidant activity due to the strong reduction potentials of hydroxyls attached to their phenyl rings (Rice-Evans *et al.*, 1996).

This review seeks to clarify some of the factors that are important in determining the value of a whole-food product to human antioxidant status. Specifically, this chapter seeks to describe whole-food antioxidants with respect to: (i) links between whole-food antioxidants and heart disease, cancer and vision loss; (ii) problems associated with dependence on any one antioxidant; (iii) factors influencing whole-food antioxidant content and bioavailability; and (iv) problems related to the evaluation of whole-food antioxidant consumption studies.

© CAB *International* 1999. *Antioxidants in Human Health*
(eds T.K. Basu, N.J. Temple and M.L. Garg)

Links Between Whole-food Antioxidants and Heart Disease, Cancer and Vision Loss

Antioxidant deficiencies have well-established links to the promotion of specific diseases. This is discussed more fully in other chapters. Antioxidant compounds are accumulated from the diet or synthesized in the body and prevent the chemical oxidation of proteins, lipids and other essential compounds. Industrialization has led to increased environmental pollutants in our air, food and water. Many of these pollutants have the capacity to deplete the body's antioxidant reserves. Antioxidant deficiencies resulting from dietary deficiencies and/or increased environmental oxidant stress may be linked to the development of many diseases including heart disease, cancer and vision loss.

Red wine is a whole-food product that has been widely associated with antioxidant effects (Renaud and de Lorgeril, 1992; Frankel *et al.*, 1993). It was one of the first whole-food products shown to have measurable antioxidant effects *in vivo*, including increased resistance of low-density lipoproteins (LDL) to oxidation (Fuhrman *et al.*, 1995; Whitehead *et al.*, 1995; Miyagi *et al.*, 1997). LDL oxidation can also be inhibited *in vitro* by many other whole-food products including: broccoli (Plumb *et al.*, 1997), grape juice (Lanningham-Foster *et al.*, 1995; Miyagi *et al.*, 1997), soybean isoflavonoids (Tikkanen *et al.*, 1998), garlic (Ide *et al.*, 1997), blueberries (Laplaud *et al.*, 1997) and cranberry extracts (Wilson *et al.*, 1998).

Antioxidants may also promote arterial vasodilation and improve blood flow. In humans, antioxidants such as ascorbate have been suggested to promote arterial vasodilation *in vivo* (Heitzer *et al.*, 1996; Solzbach *et al.*, 1997). Vasodilation may be promoted by flavonoids from whole foods serving as antioxidants that increase the half-life of endothelially derived relaxing factor (EDRF), or these flavonoids may activate EDRF-activated receptors directly.

Damage to cellular regulatory proteins and DNA is central to the promotion of cancer in humans. Oxidation is a primary means by which this damage occurs and antioxidants from our food may have the ability to protect against cancer promotion. Analysis of antiproliferative effects of whole-food products also suggests that an anticancer role may exist. Genistein and other flavonoids derived from soybean products have been found to have antiproliferative effects on breast cancer cells *in vitro* (Tikkanen *et al.*, 1998). Flavonoid-rich extracts from two members of the *Vaccinium* genus, cranberries and blueberries, have also been shown to have potent antiproliferative effects on cancer cells *in vitro* (Bomser *et al.*, 1996).

Block *et al.* (1992) evaluated the cancer protection linked to fruit and vegetable consumption. The relative risk ratios of 128 of the 158 studies reviewed suggest that consumption of low amounts of fruits and vegetables is associated with an approximate doubling of the risk for several types of cancer.

Because fruits and vegetables remain the primary source of anti-oxidants, it is probable that the protective effects are due to the antioxidant activities associated with the fruits and vegetables we consume (Block *et al.*, 1992). Compared with today's diet the Paleolithic diet was relatively rich in fruits and vegetables. That diet was evaluated by Eaton *et al.* (1997), who estimated that it contained 604 mg ascorbate and 33 mg α-tocopherol; this is much more than the typical American diet, which contains 77–109 mg ascorbate and 7–10 mg α-tocopherol. In the developed nations, the relatively high incidence of oxidation-related diseases such as heart disease and cancer may reflect a deficiency in total dietary antioxidants relative to the diet of our ancestors.

Vision loss can result from oxidative damage to the macula of the eye (Seddon *et al.*, 1994). Consumption of foods rich in antioxidants may slow or prevent the development of age-related macular degeneration (see Chapter 22). By reducing oxidative damage to the macula, antioxidants from red wine apparently delay or prevent vision loss at consumption levels as low as one glass per month (Obisesan *et al.*, 1998). Similar processes may prove to be useful for preventing oxidation of proteins in the lens of the eye. Future studies will certainly yield interesting developments in this field because with increased life expectancies we need to maintain quality vision for longer. If antioxidants from whole foods can be shown to be effective in this regard, the quality of life for millions of the elderly could be improved worldwide.

Problems Associated with Dependence on One Antioxidant

Over 4000 flavonoids from plant sources have been identified (Kandaswami and Middleton, 1994), in addition to countless non-flavonoid compounds with antioxidant capacities. Indeed, in the 1930s investigators suggested that flavones might be essential to the human diet and they were termed vitamin P (Rusznyak and Szent-Gyorgyi, 1936). The substances that make up this bewildering variety of compounds differ widely in their antioxidant activities and their ability to affect both enzyme function and blood clotting activities. Synergistic effects of a balanced mixture of different antioxidants obtained from the diet may be required by the body for optimal health maintenance.

About half of the plasma antioxidant capacity comes from albumin and urate, the remainder represents the antioxidant gap (Miller and Rice-Evans, 1996). This gap is filled by the activities of single molecules, for example the vitamins α-tocopherol and ascorbate, flavonoids such as quercetin, isoflavonoids such as diadzein, and by the activity of antioxidant enzymes including superoxide dismutase and peroxidase. Furthermore, within the antioxidant system constant recycling of antioxidants such as α-tocopherol also occurs (Bieri, 1972). The importance of whole-food antioxidants in terms of promoting antioxidant recycling in the body is poorly understood.

Supplementation of diets with any single molecule showing *in vitro* antioxidant capacity does not necessarily promote health improvement. Recent studies of β-carotene have revealed that there may be risks associated with antioxidant supplementation. In the Alpha-Tocopherol, Beta-Carotene Cancer Prevention Study (1994) and the CARET study (Omenn *et al.*, 1996) the risk ratio for lung cancer in smokers receiving β-carotene increased. Protective effects of a diet rich in fruit and vegetable have recently been shown to reduce lung cancer independently of the effects of single-vitamin supplements (Yong *et al.*, 1997).

Problems with single supplements have also been observed in animal models. Resveratrol is a polyphenolic compound from red wine with an antioxidant capacity *in vitro* (Siemann and Creasy, 1992) and has received much attention. Resveratrol may inhibit cancer in mice (Jang *et al.*, 1997), however dietary supplementation with it is not associated with reduced lipid peroxidation in rats (Turrens *et al.*, 1997) and may even be associated with increased atherogenesis (Wilson *et al.*, 1996).

Part of the reason for these confusing results may be related to the fact that supplementation studies often use antioxidant amounts that are larger than could be encountered in a normal diet. Occasionally, when very high concentrations of antioxidants are reached, an antioxidant can promote oxidation; this observation has been called a pro-oxidant effect (Otero *et al.*, 1997; Podmore *et al.*, 1998). The popularity of antioxidant neutraceuticals coupled with a 'more is better' mentality may make pro-oxidant considerations important.

Factors Influencing Whole-food Antioxidant Content and Bioavailability

Differences in the distribution of flavonoids within a particular type of plant or fruit affect the antioxidant capacity of whole foods. In grapes, polyphenolic compounds are distributed unequally in the different tissues. The skin is generally much richer in flavonoid content than the pulp (Creasy and Coffee, 1988). As a result, wine can be produced from an antioxidant-rich grape and still be relatively poor in antioxidant content if the skin is not included in the fermentation process. This observation becomes important in describing the wide range observed in wine polyphenol content and antioxidant capacity (Siemann and Creasy, 1992; Frankel *et al.*, 1995). This observation may also be important for interpreting the outcomes of food consumption surveys, as may arise, for example, if apples were eaten after being peeled.

Environmental factors affect plant tissue growth and complicate the study of whole-food antioxidant capacities; for example by altering the antioxidant content of a fruit from year to year or from field to field (Siemann and Creasy, 1992). Polyphenols such as resveratrol are invariably present in grape skin. However, plant exposure to fungal attack and ultraviolet (UV) radiation is associated with dramatic increases in the production of resveratrol and other polyphenolic compounds as part of the immune defence strategy of grapes (Creasy and Coffee, 1988). In foods such as the cranberry, UV exposure is also associated with increased production of flavonoid pigments and potentially with antioxidant capacity.

Whole-food antioxidant content is also modified by a wide range of factors related to the processing of the food prior to consumption. Food processing can reduce antioxidant value by dilution and exposure of the contents to oxidative stress. Antioxidants in food can be oxidized by chemicals used as food preservatives, such as nitrites, intended to inhibit bacterial growth. Conversely, antioxidant capacity can be increased by the food preservative butylated hydroxytoluene (BHT), which is used to prevent the peroxidation of food lipids and the development of rancidity.

Flavonoid absorption and bioavailability is an important concern regarding whole-food antioxidant studies. In humans, the flavonoid catechin has been shown to be absorbed intact from the gastrointestinal tract, with complete clearance at around 48 h (Das, 1971). In plants, flavonoids are typically conjugated to sugars. Both conjugated and unconjugated forms of the flavonoid quercetin are absorbed following consumption of onions by humans (Hollman *et al.*, 1995; Papanga and Rice-Evans, 1997). Absorption appears to be greatest for quercetin conjugated to sugars due to transport by sugar-dependent transporters (Hollman *et al.*, 1996). Absorption of other flavonoids such as phloridzin and anthocyanins has also been detected (Papanga and Rice-Evans, 1997). Quercetin absorption from the gut and plasma concentrations are similar to those observed for β-carotene (Hollman *et al.*, 1996). Accordingly, flavonoids such as quercetin are probably also physiologically active antioxidants in the body.

Problems with the Evaluation of Whole-food Antioxidant Consumption Studies

Evaluation of *in vivo* study outcomes is complicated by many factors that are difficult to objectively address. Given the low baseline incidence of heart disease, cancer and macular degeneration, large long-term interventional studies may be required to fully appreciate whole-food effects on these diseases. Furthermore, the same whole-food products can differ widely in their antioxidant content because of environmental influences and food processing techniques, so surveys of antioxidant intake may not reflect true intake levels. Possible genetic differences influencing human antioxidant status have not been investigated but may also be found to play a role in explaining why individual effects of whole-food antioxidants vary. One of the greatest problems surrounding the study of whole-food effects on *in vivo* antioxidant capacity has been the lack of assays for complete quantification of plasma antioxidant capacity.

A problem with testing the concentrations of individual antioxidants is the amount of labour required. While the chemical antioxidant potential of many flavonoid and phenolic compounds has been determined, the relative physiological importance of each individual antioxidant has not been determined. Given that over 4000 flavonoids are known to exist, and given that flavonoid metabolites also have the potential to serve as antioxidants, it will clearly not be practicable to assay the relative concentrations and activities of all the antioxidants in the body.

Tests have been developed which compare the oxidative resistance of plasma to α-tocopherol analogues. The test rates the antioxidant capacity of a plasma sample as being greater, equal to or less than a given concentration of standard. Problems with the method are reproducability and equipment needs (Cao and Prior, 1997). Plasma antioxidant capacity can be estimated by exposing the plasma to an oxidant followed by measurement of thiobarbituric acid-reactive substances (TBARS) produced by oxidative stress. This method has been applied to studies of red wine and suggests that it has the ability to increase the oxidative resistance of plasma lipids (Fuhrman et al., 1995), although the results are not universally accepted (de Rijke et al., 1996). Finally, isoprostanes are produced as a result of LDL lipid peroxidation (Morrow et al., 1990). Recently developed immunoassays for isoprostane may become useful for evaluating long-term changes in antioxidant protection from whole-food consumption (see Chapter 28).

Discussion

Our understanding of connections between antioxidants in whole foods, antioxidant capacity, and the body's ability to resist oxidative damage is poorly understood (Fig. 12.1). We are beginning to understand that deficiencies in antioxidants are often associated with the promotion of disease. The development of techniques for objective plasma oxidant assessment will increase our ability to understand how whole-food antioxidants affect our health.

The nutraceutical industry has popularized single-supplement antioxidants. While they may indeed provide measurable health benefits, the cost of supplements and their inaccessibility to poor persons in developing countries poses a problem to their utility. Considered individually, antioxidants differ from one another with respect to their individual and possible synergistic effects. Whole foods, by contrast, have the potential to provide humans with a broad range of antioxidant compounds. It is probable that we will determine that consumption of such a mixture of antioxidants with their diverse physiological activities is associated with the best promotion of health.

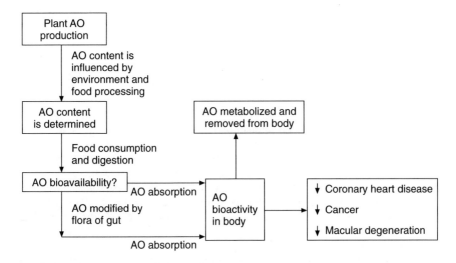

Fig. 12.1. Review of the factors determining the effect of whole-food antioxidants on health. AO, antioxidants from whole food.

Acknowledgements

The author appreciates assistance from Gail Rogers R.D., Dr John Porcari, Dr Margaret Maher and Dr Scott Cooper.

References

Alpha-Tocopherol, Beta-Carotene Cancer Prevention Study Group (1994) The effect of vitamin E and beta carotene on the incidence of lung cancer and other cancers in male smokers. *New England Journal of Medicine* 330, 1029–1035.

Bieri, G. (1972) Kinetics of tissue α-tocopherol depletion and repletion. *Annals of the New York Academy of Science* 203, 181–191.

Block, G., Patterson, B. and Subar, A. (1992) Fruit, vegetables and cancer prevention: a review of the epidemiological evidence. *Nutrition and Cancer* 18, 1–29.

Bomser, J., Madhavi, D.L., Singletary, K. and Smith, M.A.L. (1996) *In vitro* anticancer activity of fruit extracts from *Vaccinium* species. *Planta Medica* 62, 212–216.

Cao, G. and Prior, R.L. (1997) Total antioxidant capacity of human serum determined by three different analytical methods. *FASEB Journal* 11, A585.

Creasy, L.L. and Coffee, M. (1988) Phytoalexin production potential of grape berries. *Journal of the American Society of Horticultural Science* 113, 230–234.

Das, N.P. (1971) Studies of flavonoid metabolism: absorption and metabolism of (+)-catechin in man. *Biochemical Pharmacology* 20, 3435–3445.

Eaton, S.B., Eaton, S.B. III and Konner, M.J. (1997) Paleolithic nutrition revisited: a twelve-year retrospective on its nature and implications. *European Journal of Clinical Nutrition* 51, 206–216.

Frankel, E.N., Kanner, J., German, J.B., Parks, E. and Kinsella, J.E. (1993) Inhibition of oxidation of human low-density lipoprotein by phenolic substances in red wine. *Lancet* 341, 454–457.

Frankel, E.N., Waterhouse, A.L. and Teissedre, P.L. (1995) Principal phenolic phytochemicals in selected California wines and their antioxidant activity in inhibiting oxidation of human low-density lipoproteins. *Journal of Agricultural Food Chemistry* 43, 890–894.

Fuhrman, B., Lavy, A. and Aviram, M. (1995) Consumption of red wine with meals reduces the susceptibility of human plasma and low-density lipoprotein to lipid peroxidation. *American Journal of Clinical Nutrition* 61, 549–554.

Heitzer, T., Hanjorg, J. and Munzel, T. (1996) Antioxidant vitamin C improves endothelial dysfunction in chronic smokers. *Circulation* 94, 6–9.

Hollman, P.C.H., de Vreis, J.H.M., van Leeuwen, S.D., Mengelers, M.J.B. and Katan, M.B. (1995) Absorption of dietary quercetin glycosides and quercetin in healthy ileostomy volunteers. *American Journal of Clinical Nutrition* 62, 1276–1282.

Hollman, P.C.H., Gaag, M.V.D., Mengelers, M.J.B., van Trijp, J.M.P., de Vreis, J.H.M. and Katan, M.B. (1996) Absorption and disposition kinetics of the dietary antioxidant quercetin in man. *Free Radical Biology and Medicine* 21, 703–707.

Ide, N., Nelson, A.B. and Lau, B.H. (1997) Aged garlic extract and its constituents inhibit Cu^{+2}-induced oxidative modification of low density lipoprotein. *Planta Medica* 63, 263–264.

Jang, M., Cai, L., Udeani, G.O., Slowing, K.V., Thomas, C.F., Beecher, C.W.W., Fong, H.H.S., Farnsworth, N.R., Kinghorn, A.D., Mehta, R.G., Moon, R.C. and Pezzuto, J.M. (1997) Cancer chemopreventative activity of resveratrol, a natural product derived from grapes. *Science* 275, 218–220.

Kandaswami, C. and Middleton, E. (1994) Free radical scavenging and antioxidant activity of plant flavonoids. *Free Radicals in Diagnostic Medicine* 366, 351–376.

Lanningham-Foster, L., Chen, C., Chance, D.S. and Loo, G. (1995) Grape extract inhibits lipid peroxidation of human low density lipoprotein. *Biological Pharmacology Bulletin* 18, 1347–1351.

Laplaud, P.M., Lelubre, A. and Chapman, M.J. (1997) Antioxidant action of *Vaccinium myrtillus* extract on human low density lipoproteins *in vitro*: initial observations. *Fundamental and Clinical Pharmacology* 11, 35–40.

Miller, N.J. and Rice-Evans, C.A. (1996) Spectrophotometric determination of antioxidant activity. *Redox Report* 2, 161–171.

Miyagi, Y., Kunihisa, M. and Inoue, H. (1997) Inhibition of human low-density lipoprotein oxidation by flavonoids in red wine and grape juice. *American Journal of Cardiology* 80, 1627–1631.

Morrow, J.D., Hill, K.E., Burk, R.F., Nammour, T.K., Badr, K.F. and Roberts, L.J. II (1990) A series of prostaglandin F_2-like compounds are produced *in vivo* in humans by a non-cyclooxygenase, free radical-catalyzed mechanism. *Proceedings of the National Academy of Sciences, USA* 87, 9383–9387.

Obisesan, T.O., Hirsch, R., Kosoko, O., Carlson, L. and Parrott, M. (1998) Moderate wine consumption is associated with decreased odds of developing age-related macular degeneration in NHANES-1. *Journal of the American Geriatrics Society* 46, 1–7.

Omenn, G.S., Goodman, G.E., Thornquist, M.D., Balmes, J., Cullen, M.R., Glass, A., Keogh, J.P., Meyskens, F.L., Valanis, B., Williams, J.H., Barnhart, S. and Hammar, S. (1996) Effects of a combination of beta carotene and vitamin A on lung cancer and cardiovascular disease. *New England Journal of Medicine* 334, 1150–1155.

Otero, P., Vianna, M., Herrera, E. and Bonet, B. (1997) Antioxidant and prooxidant effects of ascorbic acid, dehydroascobic acid and flavonoids on LDL submitted to different degrees of oxidation. *Free Radical Research* 27, 619–626.

Papanga, G. and Rice-Evans, C.A. (1997) The identification of flavonoids as glycosides in human plasma. *FEBS Letters* 401, 78–82.

Plumb, G.W., Price, K., Rhodes, M.J.C. and Williamson, G. (1997) Antioxidant properties of the major polyphenolic compounds of broccoli. *Free Radical Research* 27, 429–435.

Podmore, I.D., Griffins, H.R., Herbert, K.E., Mistry, N., Mistry, P. and Lunec, J. (1998) Vitamin C exhibits pro-oxidant properties. *Nature* 392, 559.

Renaud, S. and de Lorgeril, M. (1992) Wine, alcohol, platelets and the French Paradox for coronary heart disease. *Lancet* 339, 1523–1526.

Rice-Evans, C.A., Miller, N.J. and Papanga, G. (1996) Structure–antioxidant activity relationships of flavonoids and phenolic acids. *Free Radical Biology and Medicine* 20, 933–956.

de Rijke, T.B., Demacker, P.N.M., Assen, N.A., Sloots, L.M., Katan, M.B. and Stalenhoef, A.F.H. (1996) Red wine consumption does not affect oxidizability of low-density lipoprotein in volunteers. *American Journal of Clinical Nutrition* 63, 329–334.

Rusznyak, S. and Szent-Gyorgyi, A. (1936) Vitamin P: flavonols as vitamins. *Nature* 138, 27.

Seddon, J.M., Ajani, U.A., Sperduto, R.D., Hiller, R., Blair, N., Burton, T.C., Farber, M.D., Gragoudas, E.S., Haller, J., Miller, D.T., Yannuzzi, L.A. and Willett, W. (1994) Dietary carotenoids, vitamins A, C and E and advanced age related macular degeneration. *Journal of the American Medical Association* 272, 1413–1420.

Siemann E.H. and Creasy, L.L. (1992) Concentration of the phytoalexin resveratrol in wine. *American Journal of Enology and Viticulture* 43, 49–52.

Solzbach, U., Burkhard, H., Jeserich, M and Just, H. (1997) Vitamin C improves endothelial dysfunction of epicardial coronary arteries in hypertension patients. *Circulation* 96, 1513–1519.

Tikkanen, M.J., Wahala, K., Ojala, S., Vihma, V and Adlercreutz, H. (1998) Effect of soybean phytoestrogen intake on low density lipoprotein oxidation resistance. *Proceedings of the National Academy of Sciences, USA* 95, 3106–3110.

Turrens, J.L., Lariccia, J. and Nair, M.G. (1997) Resveratrol has no effect on lipoprotein profile and does not prevent peroxidation of serum lipids in normal rats. *Free Radical Research* 27, 557–562.

Whitehead, T.P., Robinson, D., Allaway, S., Syms, J. and Hale, A. (1995) Effect of red wine on the antioxidant capacity of serum. *Clinical Chemistry* 41, 32–35.

Wilson, T., Knight, T.J., Beitz, D.C., Lewis, D.S. and Engen, R.L. (1996) Resveratrol promotes atherosclerosis in hypercholesterolemic rabbits. *Life Sciences* 59, 15–21.

Wilson, T., Porcari, J.P. and Harbin, D. (1998) Cranberry extract inhibits low density lipoprotein oxidation. *Life Sciences* 62, PL381–386.

Yong, L.-C., Brown, C.C., Schatzkin, A., Dresser, C.M., Slesinski, J.M., Cox, C.S. and
     Taylor, P.R. (1997) Intakes of vitamins E, C, and A and risk of lung cancer: the
     NHANES I epidemiologic followup study. *American Journal of Epidemiology*
     146, 231–243.

Antioxidants and Their Role in Coronary Heart Disease Prevention

13

DAVID KRITCHEVSKY[1] AND STEPHEN B. KRITCHEVSKY[2]

[1]The Wistar Institute of Anatomy and Biology, Philadelphia, Pennsylvania; [2]Department of Preventive Medicine, University of Tennessee-Memphis, Memphis, Tennessee, USA

Introduction

One hundred and fifty years have elapsed since Vogel identified cholesterol as a component of the atherosclerotic plaque (Vogel, 1847). Over 80 years have passed since Anitschkow (1913) demonstrated the atherogenic potential of dietary cholesterol. The presence of cholesterol and its oxidized derivatives in arterial deposits was demonstrated early this century. The nature of the initiating event(s) is part of the more recent history of this disease.

The work pioneered by Gofman and his colleagues (1950) demonstrated that cholesterol and other lipids were transported in the blood as a lipid–protein continuum which could be separated into classes of lipoproteins based on their hydrated densities. The class of lipoproteins identified as LDL (low-density lipoproteins) was shown to be the major transporter of cholesterol and was also shown to be most closely correlated with risk of cardiovascular disease. The lipoprotein story is continuing as can be seen from the discoveries of the extra-atherogenic nature of lipoprotein(a) (Lp(a)) (Berg, 1963) and the finding of a spectrum of LDL aggregates of different sizes and atherogenic potential (Krauss, 1991).

Twenty years ago Davignon (1978) presented a unified picture of the process of atherosclerosis. He showed the participation of environmental influences (diet and smoking, among others), humoral influences (circulating lipoproteins, hormones, etc.) and arterial metabolic effects, all of which combined to form the atherosclerotic plaque. The environmental and humoral areas have been worked over pretty thoroughly, although new observations continue to amend the picture. The mode of cholesterol accumulation in the arterial wall is complex and is only now beginning to be understood.

Currently it is believed that blood monocytes adhere to the endothelial lining, migrate through endothelial junctions and differentiate to become macrophages (Ross, 1986). The macrophages take up lipoproteins and become cholesteryl ester-rich foam cells which make up the fatty streak found beneath an unbroken layer of endothelial cells. Foam cells may also arise from smooth muscle cells that migrate into the subendothelial space. The fatty streak proliferates to form complex lesions and fibrous plaques by mechanisms, as yet undelineated, which involve an array of growth factors (Pomerantz *et al.*, 1995).

Oxidized Lipid and Atherosclerosis

The macrophages and foam cells can continue to take up LDL. One might expect that incubation of these moieties (monocytes, macrophages, smooth muscle cells) with concentrated sources of cholesterol (LDL) would convert them to foam cells but this is not the case. However, another form of LDL, oxidized LDL, has been identified *in vivo* and has been shown to be taken up when incubated with the various cell types found in atherosclerotic lesions (Henriksen *et al.*, 1981). Oxidatively modified LDL is also taken up by the scavenger receptor. This observation is the basis of the oxidized-LDL hypothesis used to explain the early steps in the atherosclerotic process.

The possible involvement of oxidized lipid in the atherosclerotic process was considered long before the experiments cited above. About 50 years ago Dam and his colleagues (Jessen *et al.*, 1951; Glavind *et al.*, 1952) reported on the isolation of peroxidized lipid from atherosclerotic arteries. Altschul (1946) suggested that heated (i.e. oxidized) cholesterol might be more atherogenic for rabbits than pure cholesterol. Analysis of atherosclerotic arteries carried out in 1943 revealed the presence of cholesta-3,5-diene-7-one, cholesta-4,6-diene-3-one, and 3β, cholestane 3β, 5α, 6β-triol (Hardegger *et al.*, 1943).

Imai *et al.* (1976) fed rabbits recrystallized cholesterol or impure cholesterol (USP-cholesterol that had been in their laboratory for some years and had become yellowed and rancid). The aortas were examined by electron microscopy 24 h later. The old cholesterol led to 73% more degenerated cells than the recrystallized material. The major autooxidation products were cholesta-3,5-diene-7-one, 25-hydroxycholesterol, 7-keto-cholesterol, 7α and 7β-hydroxycholesterol and cholestane-3β, 5α, 6β-triol (Peng *et al.*, 1978). The oxidation products, especially 25-hydroxycholesterol and the triol, are toxic to cultured rabbit arterial smooth muscle cells (Peng *et al.*, 1978, 1979) and cause arterial injury to rabbits (Cook and MacDougal, 1968). Cholesterol oxidation products are transported in rabbit lipoproteins (Peng *et al.*, 1987).

Comparison of atherogenicity of crystalline and amorpous cholesterol showed the latter to be less cholesterolaemic but more atherogenic. The broad melting point of amorphous cholesterol suggests the presence of impurities (Kritchevsky *et al.*, 1969). The angiotoxicity and atherogenicity of cholesterol oxides has been reviewed by Peng *et al.* (1991). Hodis *et al.* (1991) reported that normal rabbit plasma contains 81 μmol l^{-1} of cholesterol oxides. After feeding a high cholesterol diet to rabbits for 6 weeks the level of plasma cholesterol oxides rose by a factor of 5, while total plasma cholesterol rose by a factor of 64. Aortic levels of total cholesterol oxides rose 150%. Several compounds that had not been present in arteries of the control group were isolated from arteries of cholesterol-fed rabbits, namely, cholesterol β-oxide, 7-ketocholesterol and 25-hydroxy-cholesterol. There have been earlier reports of isolation of 26-hydroxy-cholesterol (Smith and vanLier, 1970) and polar sterol esters have been shown to be present in human atherosclerotic plaques (Brooks *et al.*, 1971). The data suggest that cholesterol oxidation occurs *in vivo*.

Probucol [4,4'-(isopropylidenedithio)bis(2,6-di-t-butylphenol)] is one of a series of potential antioxidants initially synthesized by chemists at the Ethyl Corporation. It was developed by the Dow Chemical Co. and, under the code number of DH-581, was found to reduce significantly the severity of cholesterol-induced atherosclerosis in rabbits (Kritchevsky *et al.*, 1971) and to lower cholesterol levels in humans (Tedeschi *et al.*, 1980). Its precise mode of action was unclear (Kritchevsky, 1980) but a role as an antioxidant was not considered. Since it is transported in the lipoproteins of the serum it is in the right place to exert its antioxidant properties.

Steinberg and his colleagues (1989) have conducted a series of elegant studies to demonstrate that LDL oxidation may indeed play a crucial role in atherogenesis. They showed that probucol, a hypocholesterolaemic agent, could prevent oxidation of LDL *in vitro* and *in vivo* and could prevent progression of atherosclerosis in the Watanabe heritable hyperlipidaemic (WHHL) rabbit and that this action was due to its antioxidant properties and independent of its hypolipidaemic properties (Parthasarathy *et al.*, 1986; Carew *et al.*, 1987). They have also shown that macrophage foam cells isolated from atherosclerotic lesions of rabbits degrade modified lipoproteins and promote oxidation of LDL *in vitro* (Rosenfeld *et al.*, 1991). The oxidation hypothesis has been discussed elsewhere in detail (Steinberg *et al.*, 1989; Esterbauer *et al.*, 1997).

Oxidation of lipoproteins plays a significant role in atherogenesis. That knowledge offers an opportunity to test effects of antioxidants as inhibitors of atherogenesis, which can be done in experimental animals. They can also be studied as inhibitors of lipoprotein oxidation or reducers of risk of cardiovascular disease.

Antioxidants and Arterial Disease

Vitamin E effects on experimental atherosclerosis have been investigated since the 1940s. In early studies conducted using the cholesterol-fed rabbit model, Dam (1994) found that dietary α-tocopherol did not affect atherosclerosis, and Bruger (1945) and Moses *et al.* (1952) reported the intramuscular administration of vitamin E did not inhibit experimentally induced atherosclerosis. More recently, several authors have found that vitamin E may inhibit atherosclerosis in rabbits (Brattsand, 1975; Wilson *et al.*, 1978) and chickens (Smith and Kummerow, 1989). Bocan *et al.* (1992), working with rabbits, found antioxidant therapy (vitamins C and E) to alter progression of diet-induced fatty streaks but to have no effect on progression as regression of more complicated iliac femoral lesions. Singh *et al.* (1995) fed rabbits a high-fat diet for 12 weeks then randomized them to treatment with fruits, vegetables and mustard oil, vitamins C, E, and β-carotene, a high-fat diet or a low-fat diet. After 12 weeks, rabbits in the first two groups exhibited significantly lower plaque size in the aorta and coronary arteries than did those fed the unsupplemented diet. Aortic plaque size was fourfold higher in the fat-fed groups and coronary artery plaque size was about double that of the fruit- or vitamin-fed groups. Verlangieri and Bush (1992) studied atherosclerosis progression and regression in the carotid arteries of monkeys using ultrasound. Addition of α-tocopherol to the diet inhibited atherogenesis and enhanced regression. Godfried *et al.* (1989) reported that very high dietary levels of vitamin E potentiated atherosclerotic lesions in rabbits.

In assessing the efficacy of antioxidants *vis-à-vis* their effects on actual coronary events, we can examine epidemiological studies (observational or case–control) or intervention studies. As we will see, the findings are surprisingly different. Gey *et al.* (1991) has attempted to correlate mortality from ischaemic heart disease (IHD) in 16 European populations being examined in the WHO/MONICA Core Study. In the 12 populations with similar blood pressure and plasma cholesterol levels (5.69–6.21 mmol l^{-1}) he found no significant correlation between those parameters and IHD mortality but levels of vitamin E exhibited a strong inverse correlation (P=0.002). When all 16 populations were evaluated, correlation of IHD mortality with serum cholesterol levels was associated moderately, but the correlation with vitamin E levels was much stronger (Gey *et al.*, 1991). The protective effects of dietary antioxidants were evaluated in a later study with more subjects and the rating for the individual factors was: vitamin E > carotene = vitamin C > vitamin A (Gey *et al.*, 1993a). Gey (1995) has recently reviewed this field in depth.

The effects of vitamin C have also been considered (Frei *et al.*, 1989). Enstrom *et al.* (1992) found a strong inverse relationship between vitamin C intake and cardiovascular mortality. They assessed data from over 11,000 people in the NHANES I and the 10-year follow-up. The NHANES was a national study of diet and health conducted in various populations in the USA. Low plasma levels of vitamin C may increase risk for stroke (Gey *et al.*, 1993b). Vitamin C also protects human LDL against atherogenic modification (Retsky *et al.*, 1993). A diet high in these substances, especially vitamin C and carotenes, is really a diet high in fruits and vegetables.

There have been a number of observational studies examining dietary antioxidant intakes and risk of coronary disease. In an examination of participants in the LRC-CPPT Study (Lipid Research Clinics Coronary Primary Prevention Trial) a decreased risk of coronary heart disease was seen in participants with higher serum carotenoid levels (Morris *et al.*, 1994). Stampfer *et al.* (1993), in analysing dietary and health data from 87,245 female nurses, observed a highly significant trend for coronary risk reduction with increasing vitamin E intake (diet plus supplements). The association was not significant if the contribution of the supplements was not included. Rimm *et al.* (1993) found a similar pattern in 39,910 male health professionals. Namely, there was a highly significant association between trend towards reduction of risk and intake of vitamin E from food plus supplements. When the contributions of either food or supplements alone were analysed neither provided a significant trend. Knekt *et al.* (1994) analysed the correlations between reported antioxidant intake and cardiovascular mortality in 5133 Finnish subjects (2748 men and 2385 women). A significant trend towards protection by vitamin E was only observed in the female cohort. A study of dietary antioxidant intake and carotid artery wall thickness in 11,307 subjects suggested a protective effect for dietary α-tocopherol and vitamin C (Kritchevsky *et al.*, 1995). A subsequent examination of this population in which carotid artery plaque was quantitated showed a protective effect of carotenoids (Kritchevsky *et al.*, 1995).

In a comparison of 50-year-old men in Sweden and Lithuania, Kristenson *et al.* (1997) found the Swedish cohort, who exhibit one-fourth the heart disease mortality, to be significantly taller, to have lower systolic blood pressure and to be significantly more active physically. Their plasma total and LDL-cholesterol levels were significantly higher. Assay of the plasma concentration of lipid-soluble antioxidants showed the Swedish subjects to have significantly more β-carotene (by 35%), lycopene (by 88%) and α-tocopherol (by 84%). Cleary *et al.* (1997) also found levels of lipophilic antioxidants not to be depleted in men with severe atherosclerosis.

Kushi *et al.* (1996) followed 34,486 post-menopausal women free of coronary disease at the initial screen for 7 years. In that period, 242 of the women (0.70%) died of coronary disease. Intake of vitamin E was associated inversely with risk of death but intake of vitamins A and C was not. Riemersma *et al.* (1991) found plasma concentrations of vitamins C, E and carotene to be associated inversely with risk of angina. After adjustment for smoking only the inverse relationship with vitamin E remained. Adipose tissue levels of β-carotene have been found to be associated with reduced risk of myocardial infarction (MI) but there was no association with α-tocopherol levels (Kardinaal *et al.*, 1993). In a population-based, nested case–control study Street *et al.* (1994) found that serum levels of a variety of carotenoids were inversely associated with risk of MI, especially among smokers.

One of the early clinical trials involving use of vitamin E was carried out by Gillilan *et al.* (1977) who found it not to be effective in the treatment of angina. Two well-publicized trials of the effect of vitamins E or A and β-carotene on incidence of lung cancer in smokers have also obtained data relating to cardiovascular disease. Omenn *et al.* (1996) found slightly higher cardiovascular mortality in the group given vitamin A and β-carotene supplements. The Alpha-Tocopherol, Beta-Carotene Cancer Prevention Study (ATBC) Group (1994) found 5% fewer coronary deaths in men who had taken α-tocopherol and 11% more deaths in those who received β-carotene supplements. Subjects who received α-tocopherol exhibited a very slight decrease in incidence of angina pectoris whereas those receiving β-carotene showed a slight increase. Major coronary events were studied during the follow-up period (median 5.3 years). The totals of non-fatal MI and fatal coronary events in the four groups were: α-tocopherol, 94; β-carotene, 113; α-tocopherol and β-carotene, 123; and placebo, 94. The ratio of fatal events to total events was: α-tocopherol, 57.4%; β-carotene, 65.5%; α-tocopherol plus β-carotene, 54.5%; and placebo, 41.5% (Rapola *et al.*, 1996, 1997). Hennekens *et al.* (1996) carried out a randomized, double-blind, placebo-controlled trial of β-carotene in 22,071 male physicians aged 40–84 years. After 12 years they found no difference in the rate of cardiovascular events.

Hodis *et al.* (1995) have demonstrated a reduction in angiographically measured coronary artery disease progression in men given 100 IU or more of vitamin E daily. No benefit was found for supplementary vitamin C. Singh *et al.* (1996) found that a combination of vitamins A, C and E, and β-carotene administered within a few hours after acute MI and continued for 28 days led to significantly fewer cardiac events. Incidence of angina pectoris was significantly lower in the group receiving antioxidants. Cardiac deaths plus non-fatal infarction numbered 13 (20% of subjects) in the patients given antioxidants and 19 (30.6% of subjects) in the control group ($P < 0.05$).

The Cambridge Heart Antioxidant Study (CHAOS) carried out a double-blind, placebo-controlled study in 2002 patients with proven coronary atherosclerosis (Stephens *et al.*, 1996). The test group of 1035 subjects was given α-tocopherol (400 or 800 IU per day) and 967 controls were given a placebo. After 510 days, non-fatal MI numbered 14 in the α-tocopherol group and 41 in the placebo group. MI fatalities were higher in the test group (18 vs. 13) as were total cardiovascular deaths (27 vs. 23). Deaths from all causes were 38% higher in the α-tocopherol group (36 vs. 26). The difference in fatal MI was due, in part, to an excess of early deaths and the authors suggest that α-tocopherol had not yet had time to exert its effects. The treatment had no effect on serum cholesterol.

Greenberg *et al.* (1996) studied mortality associated with low plasma levels of β-carotene and the effect of oral supplementation (50 mg day^{-1}). There were a total of 1720 subjects (1188 men and 532 women). The treatment was carried out for a median period of 4.3 years and the median follow-up was 8.2 years. Subjects whose plasma levels of β-carotene were in the highest quartile at the beginning of the study had the lowest risk of death from all causes compared with those in the lowest quartile. Ingestion of the β-carotene supplement did not reduce all-cause or cardiovascular mortality. Total deaths were 5% higher in the supplemented group (146 vs. 139); cardiovascular deaths were 15% higher in this group (68 vs. 59) and cancer deaths were 14% lower (38 vs. 44).

The effects of another group of dietary antioxidants, flavonoids, on coronary mortality or stroke have also been evaluated. In the Netherlands a group of 552 men was followed between 1970 and 1985. The authors concluded that habitual flavonoid intake might be protective against stroke (Keli *et al.*, 1996). In a Finnish study, the total and coronary mortality in men were both higher in the subjects with lowest flavonoid intake than in those in the highest intake (Knekt *et al.*, 1996). Relative risk for all-cause mortality was reduced significantly in both men and women. Relative risk for coronary mortality was reduced significantly in women and was reduced from 14.4 to 8.3% in men, but the difference did not reach statistical significance. In the Male Health Professionals Study, on the other hand, the investigators found no strong inverse relationship between total flavonoid intake and coronary disease incidence (Rimm *et al.*, 1996).

Dilemma about Antioxidants

We are left with this dilemma – consumption of a diet containing appreciable amounts of antioxidants and high plasma levels of antioxidants appeared to be protective in relation to CHD and yet trials in which selected single antioxidants are added to the diet provide scant and inconsistent evidence of a protective effect. Several possible explanations come to mind. First, consumption of a diet high in vitamins, carotenes, and flavonoids reflects intake of a wide variety of these substances, some of which may still be unidentified. It could be that several of these compounds work in concert whereas single components fed individually are without effect. It is also possible that other dietary components (trace minerals, for instance) may be effectors of carotenoid action. Virtually all nutritional studies are based on replacing one component of the diet with another without considering how these specific substances may interact with the rest of the diet. As an example from fibre research, in an atherogenic rabbit diet in which the fibre is cellulose, casein is more cholesterolaemic and atherogenic than soy protein; when cellulose is replaced by lucerne the two proteins become equivalent (Kritchevsky *et al.*, 1977).

Could it be that the intervention trials have not been carried out for sufficiently long periods? Habitual intake of a wide variety of antioxidants provides a greater source of vitamins or carotenoids over a longer time than administration of one or two compounds for a relatively short time to subjects who have already compromised their level of risk by inappropriate behaviour, e.g. smoking.

Lifestyle may be one of the determinants of the picture presented to the investigators. Heart disease and cancer are generally described as lifestyle disease but the research approach focuses on only one aspect of lifestyle. Slattery *et al.* (1995) examined dietary antioxidants and plasma lipids in participants in the Coronary Artery Risk Development in Young Adults (CARDIA) study and found that higher intake of dietary antioxidants is associated with other lifestyle factors such as physical activity and non-smoking. In Britain, plasma concentrations of antioxidants are related to social class, being higher in the better educated and more affluent (Gregory *et al.*, 1990). If protective levels of antioxidants such as carotenoids, tocopherols, and others are part of a life-long behavioural pattern, we cannot expect too much if we influence one aspect of risk by dietary supplements without addressing other behaviours.

Most studies have been carried out in men. Knekt *et al.* (1996) found flavonoid intake to be significantly associated with reduced coronary risk in women. The risk was lowered non-significantly in men. It is well established that pre-menopausal women are relatively protected against coronary disease and that the protection may be due to circulating oestrogens which affect positively the LDL/HDL (high-density lipoprotein) cholesterol ratio. The protection is lost in post-menopausal women. Could antioxidant protection by oestrogen be another factor in lowering risk in young women? Shwaery *et al.* (1997) have reported that 17β-oestradiol protects LDL against copper-mediated oxidation *in vitro*. In another context, we showed many years ago that oestradiol inhibited ascorbic acid-catalysed oxidation of methyl linoleate (Kritchevsky and Tepper, 1964). White *et al.* (1997) have summarized results from other studies in which oestrogens influenced rates of LDL oxidation.

Accumulating data lend validity to the hypothesis involving oxidized LDL as a major factor in atherogenesis and protection being offered by antioxidant vitamins. Questions relating to *in vivo* initiation of LDL oxidation remain to be answered (Halliwell, 1995) and randomized trials with antioxidant vitamins are needed (Hennekens *et al.*, 1995).

Acknowledgements

Supported, in part, by a Research Career Award (HL-00734) from the National Institutes of Health (DK) and a research grant (N-01-AG-6–2103) from the National Institute on Aging, National Institutes of Health (SBK).

References

The Alpha-Tocopherol Beta-Carotene Cancer Prevention Study Group (1994) The effect of vitamin E and beta carotene on the incidence of lung cancer and other cancers in male smokers. *New England Journal of Medicine* 330, 1029–1035.

Altschul, R. (1946) Experimental cholesterol arteriosclerosis. Changes produced in skeletal muscle. *Archives of Pathology* 42, 277–284.

Anitschkow, N. (1913) Über die veranderung der kaninchenaorta by experimenteller cholesterinsteatose. *Beitrage zur Patholischen Anatomie und zur Allgemeinen Pathologie* 56, 379–404.

Berg, K. (1963) A new serum type system in man: the Lp(a) system. *Acta Pathologica et Microbiologica Scandinavica* 59, 369–382.

Bocan, T.M.A., Mueller, S.B., Brown, E.Q., Uhlendorf, P.D., Mazur, M.J. and Newton, R.S. (1992) Antiatherosclerotic effects of antioxidants are lesion-specific when evaluated in hypercholesterolemic New Zealand White rabbits. *Experimental and Molecular Pathology* 57, 70–83.

Brattsand, R. (1975) Actions of vitamins A and E and some nicotinic acid derivatives on plasma lipids on lipid infiltrations of aorta in cholesterol-fed rabbits. *Atherosclerosis* 22, 47–61.

Brooks, C.J.W., Steel, G., Gilbert, J.D. and Harland, W.A. (1971) Characterization of a new group of polar sterol esters from human atherosclerotic plaques. *Atherosclerosis* 13, 223–237.

Bruger, M. (1945) Experimental atherosclerosis. VII. Effect of vitamin E. *Proceedings of the Society for Experimental Biology and Medicine* 59, 56–57.

Carew, T.E., Schwenke, D.C. and Steinberg, D. (1987) Antiatherogenic effect of probucol unrelated to its hypocholesterolemic effect: evidence that antioxidants *in vivo* can selectively inhibit low density lipoprotein degradation in macrophage-rich fatty streaks and slow the progression of atherosclerosis in the Watanabe heritable hyperlipidemic rabbit. *Proceedings of the National Academy of Sciences, USA* 84, 7725–7729.

Cleary, J., Mohr, D., Adams, M.R., Celermayer, D.S. and Stocker, R. (1997) Plasma and LDL levels of major lipophilic antioxidants are similar in patients with advanced atheroscleroris and age-matched controls. *Free Radical Research* 26, 175–182.

Cook, R.P. and MacDougal, J.D.B. (1968) Experimental atherosclerosis in rabbits after feeding cholestanetriol. *British Journal of Experimental Pathology* 49, 265–271.

Dam, H. (1944) Ineffectiveness of vitamin E in preventing cholesterol deposition in the aorta. *Journal of Nutrition* 28, 289–295.

Davignon, J. (1978) The lipid hypothesis: pathophysiological basis. *Archives of Surgery* 113, 28–34.

Enstrom, J.E., Kanim, L.E. and Klein, M.A. (1992) Vitamin C intake and mortality among a sample of the United States population. *Epidemiology* 3, 194–202.

Esterbauer, H., Schmidt, R. and Hayn, M. (1997) Relationships among oxidation of low density lipoprotein, antioxidant protection and atherosclerosis. *Advances in Pharmacology* 38, 425–455.

Frei, B., England, L. and Ames, B.N. (1989) Ascorbate is an outstanding antioxidant in human blood plasma. *Proceedings of the National Academy of Sciences, USA* 86, 6377–6381.

Gey, K.F. (1995) Ten-year retrospective on the antioxidant hypothesis of arteriosclerosis. Threshold plasma levels of antioxidant micronutrients related to minimum cardiovascular risk. *Journal of Nutritional Biochemistry* 6, 206–236.

Gey, K.F., Puska, P., Jordan, P. and Moser, U.K. (1991) Inverse correlation between plasma vitamin E and mortality from ischemic heart diease in cross cultural epidemiology. *American Journal of Clinical Nutrition* 53, 326S–334S.

Gey, K.F., Moser, U.K., Jordan, P., Stähelin, H.B., Eichholzer, M. and Lüdin, E. (1993a) Increased risk of cardiovascular disease at suboptimal plasma concentrations of essential antioxidants: an epidemiological update with special attention to carotene and vitamin C. *American Journal of Clinical Nutrition* 57, 787S–797S.

Gey, K.F., Stähelin, H.B. and Eichholzer, M. (1993b) Poor plasma status of carotene and vitamin C is associated with higher mortality from ischemic heart disease and stroke: Basel Prospective Study. *Clinical Investigation* 71, 3–6.

Gillilan, R.E., Mondell, B. and Warbasse, J.R. (1977) Quantitative evaluation of vitamin E in the treatment of angina pectoris. *American Heart Journal* 93, 444–449.

Glavind, J., Hartmann, S., Clemmesen, J., Jessen, K.E. and Dam, H. (1952) Studies on the role of lipoperoxides in human pathology. II. The presence of peroxidized lipids in the atherosclerotic aorta. *Acta Pathologica et Microbiologica Scandinavica* 30, 1–6.

Godfried, S.L., Combs, G.F. Jr, Saroka, J.M. and Dillingham, L.A. (1989) Potentiation of atherosclerotic lesions in rabbits by a high dietary level of vitamin E. *British Journal of Nutrition* 61, 607–617.

Gofman, J.W., Lindgren, F., Elliott, H., Mantz, W., Hewitt, J., Strisower, B., Herring, V. and Lyon, T.P. (1950) The role of lipids and lipoproteins in atherosclerosis. *Science* 111, 166–171.

Greenberg, E.R., Baron, J.A., Karagas, M.R., Stukel, T.A., Merenberg, D.W., Stevens, M.M., Mandel, J.S. and Haile, R.W. (1996) Mortality associated with low plasma concentration of beta carotene and the effect of oral supplementation. *Journal of the American Medical Association* 275, 699–703.

Gregory, J., Foster, K., Tyler, H. and Wiseman, M. (1990) *The Dietary and Nutritional Survey of British Adults*. HMSO, London.

Halliwell, B. (1995) Oxidation of low-density lipoproteins: questions of initiation, propagation and the effect of antioxidants. *American Journal of Clinical Nutrition* 61, 670S–677S.

Hardegger, E., Ruzicka, L. and Tagmann, E. (1943) Untersuchungen über organextrakte. Zur kenntnis der unverseifbaren lipoide aus arteriosklerotischen aorten. *Helvetica Chimrurgica Acta* 30, 2205–2221.

Hennekens, C.H., Gaziano, J.M., Manson, J.E. and Buring, J.E. (1995) Antioxidant vitamin-cardiovascular disease hypothesis is still promising, but still unproven: the need for randomized trials. *American Journal of Clinical Nutrition* 62, 1377S–1380S.

Hennekens, C.H., Buring, J.E., Manson, J.E., Stampfer, M., Rosner, B., Cook, N.R., Belanger, C., La Motte, F., Gaziano, J.M., Ridker, P.M., Willett, W. and Peto, R. (1996) Lack of effect of long-term supplementation with beta carotene on the incidence of malignant neoplasms and cardiovascular disease. *New England Journal of Medicine* 334, 1145–1149.

Henriksen, T., Mahoney, E.M. and Steinberg, D. (1981) Enhanced macrophage degradation by low density lipoprotein previously incubated with cultured endothelial cells: recognition by receptors for acetylated low-density lipoprotein. *Proceedings of the National Academy of Sciences, USA* 78, 6499–6503.

Hodis, H.N., Crawford, D.W. and Sevanian, A. (1991) Cholesterol feeding increases plasma and aortic tissue cholesterol oxide levels in parallel: further evidence for the role of cholesterol oxidation in atherosclerosis. *Atherosclerosis* 89, 117–126.

Hodis, H.N., Mack, W.J., LaBrec, L., Cashin-Hemphill, L., Sevanian, A., Johnson, R. and Azen, S.P. (1995) Serial coronary angiographic evidence that antioxidant vitamin intake reduces progression of coronary artery atherosclerosis. *Journal of the American Medical Association* 273, 1849–1854.

Imai, H., Werthessen, N.T., Taylor, C.B. and Lee, K.T. (1976) Angiotoxicity and atherosclerosis due to contaminants of U.S.P. grade cholesterol. *Archives of Pathology and Laboratory Medicine* 100, 565–572.

Jessen, K.E., Glavind, J., Hartmann, S. and Dam, H. (1951) Peroxidation of human adipose in peripheral venous disease. *Acta Pathologica et Microbiologica Scandinavica* 29, 73–76.

Kardinaal, A.F.M., Kok, F.J., Ringstad, J., Gomez-Aracena, J., Mazaev, V.P., Kohlmeier, L., Martin, B.C., Aro, A., Karle, J.D., Delgado-Rodriquez, M., Riemersma, R.A., van't Veer, P., Huttunen, J.K. and Martin-Moreno, J.M. (1993) Antioxidants in adipose tissue and risk of myocardial infarction: the EURAMIC Study. *Lancet* 342, 1379–1384.

Keli, S.O., Hertog, M.G.L., Feskens, E.J.M. and Kromhout, D. (1996) Dietary flavonoids, antioxidant vitamins and incidence of stroke. *Archives of Internal Medicine* 154, 637–642.

Knekt, P., Reunanen, A., Jarvinen, R., Seppanen, R., Helivaara, M. and Aromaa, A. (1994) Antioxidant vitamin intake and coronary mortality in a longitudinal population study. *American Journal of Epidemiology* 139, 1180–1189.

Knekt, P., Jarvinen, R., Reunanen, A. and Maatela, J. (1996) Flavonoid intake and coronary mortality in Finland: a cohort study. *British Medical Journal* 312, 478–481.

Krauss, R.M. (1991) Low density lipoprotein subclasses and risk of coronary artery disease. *Current Opinions in Lipidology* 2, 248–252.

Kristenson, M., Zieden, B., Kucinskienė, Z., Schäfer-Elender, L., Bergdahl, B., Elwing, B., Abaravicus, A., Razinkovenė, L., Calkauskas, H. and Olsson, A.G. (1997) Antioxidant state and mortality from coronary heart disease in Lithuanian and Swedish men: concomitant cross sectional study of men aged 50. *British Medical Journal* 314, 629–653.

Kritchevsky, D. (1980) Pharmacology of probucol. In: Noseda, G., Lewis, B. and Paoletti, R. (eds) *Diet and Drugs in Atherosclerosis*. Raven Press, New York, pp. 143–149.

Kritchevsky, D. and Tepper, S.A. (1964) Autoxidation of methyl linoleate: effect of sex hormones and of nicotinic acid and related compounds. *Proceedings of the Society for Experimental Biology and Medicine* 115, 841–843.

Kritchevsky, D., Marcucci, A.M., Sallata, P. and Tepper, S.A. (1969) Comparison of amorphous and crystalline cholesterol in the establishment of atherosclerosis in rabbits. *Medicina Experimentalis* 19, 185–193.

Kritchevsky, D., Kim, H.K. and Tepper, S.A. (1971) Influence of 4-4'-(Isopropylidenedithio)bis(2,6-di-t-butylphenol) (DH-581) on experimental atherosclerosis in rabbits. *Proceedings of the Society for Experimental Biology and Medicine* 136, 1216–1221.

Kritchevsky, D., Tepper, S.A., Williams, D.E. and Story, J.A. (1977) Experimental atherosclerosis in rabbits fed cholesterol-free diets. 7. Interaction of animal or vegetable protein with fiber. *Atherosclerosis* 26, 397–403.

Kritchevsky, S.B., Shimakawa, T., Tell, G.S., Dennis, B., Carpenter, M., Eckfeldt, J.H., Preacher-Ryan, H. and Heiss, G. (1995) Dietary antioxidants and carotid artery wall thickness. The ARIC Study. *Circulation* 92, 2142–2150.

Kushi, L.H., Folsom, A.R., Prineas, R.J., Mink, P.J., Wu, Y. and Bostick, R.M. (1996) Dietary oxidant vitamins and death from coronary heart disease in postmenopausal women. *New England Journal of Medicine* 334, 1156–1162.

Morris, D.L., Kritchevsky, S.B. and Davis, C.E. (1994) Serum carotenoids and coronary heart disease. The Lipid Research Clinics Coronary Primary Prevention Trial and follow-up study. *Journal of the American Medical Association* 272, 1439–1441.

Moses, C., Rhodes, G.L. and Levinson, J.P. (1952) The effect of alpha tocopherol on experimental atherosclerosis. *Angiology* 3, 397–398.

Omenn, G.S., Goodman, G.E., Thornquist, M.D., Balmes, J., Cullen, M.R., Glass, A., Keogh, J.P., Meyskens, F.L. Jr, Valanis, B., Williams, J.H. Jr, Barnhart, S. and Hammar, S. (1996) Effects of a combination of beta carotene and vitamin A on lung cancer and cardiovascular disease. *New England Journal of Medicine* 334, 1150–1155.

Parthasarathy, S., Young, S.G., Witztum, J.L., Pittman, R.C. and Steinberg, D. (1986) Probucol inhibits oxidative modification of low density lipoproteins. *Journal of Clinical Investigation* 77, 641–644.

Peng, S.-K., Taylor, C.B., Tham, P., Werthessen, N.T. and Mikkelson, B. (1978) Effect of auto-oxidation products from cholesterol on aortic smooth muscle cells. *Archives of Pathology and Laboratory Medicine* 102, 57–61.

Peng, S.-K., Tham, P., Taylor, C.B. and Mikkelson, B. (1979) Cytotoxicity of oxidation derivatives of cholesterol on cultured aortic smooth muscle cells and their effect on cholesterol biosynthesis. *American Journal of Clinical Nutrition* 32, 1033–1042.

Peng, S.-K., Phillips, G.A., Xia, G.Z. and Morin, R.J. (1987) Transport of cholesterol autoxidation products by rabbit lipoproteins. *Atherosclerosis* 64, 1–6.

Peng, S.-K., Hu, B. and Morin, R.J. (1991) Angiotoxicity and atherogenicity of cholesterol oxides. *Journal of Clinical Laboratory Analysis* 5, 144–152.

Pomerantz, K.B., Nicholson, A.C. and Hajjar, D.P. (1995) Signal transduction in atherosclerosis: second messengers and regulation of cellular cholesterol trafficking. *Advances in Experimental Medicine and Biology* 369, 49–64.

Rapola, J.M., Virtamo, J., Haukka, J.K., Heinonen, U.P., Albanes, D., Taylor, P.R. and Huttinen, J.K. (1996) Effect of vitamin E and beta carotene on the incidence of angina pectoris. A randomized, double-blind controlled trial. *Journal of the American Medical Association* 275, 693–698.

Rapola, J.M., Virtamo, J., Ripatti, S., Huttunen, J.K., Albanes, D., Taylor, P.R. and Heinonen, O.P. (1997) Randomised trial of α-tocopherol and β-carotene supplements on incidence of major coronary events in men with previous myocardial infarction. *Lancet* 349, 1715–1720.

Retsky, K.L., Freeman, M.W. and Frei, B. (1993) Ascorbic acid oxidation product(s) protect human low density lipoprotein against atherogenic modification. Antirather than prooxidant activity of vitamin C in the presence of transition metal ions. *Journal of Biological Chemistry* 268, 1304–1309.

Riemersma, R.A., Wood, D.A., Macintyre, C.C.A., Elton, R.A., Gey, K.F. and Oliver, M.F. (1991) Risk of angina pectoris and plasma concentrations of vitamins A, C, E and carotene. *Lancet* 337, 1–5.

Rimm, E.B., Stampfer, M.J., Ascherio, A., Giovannucci, E., Colditz, G.A. and Willett, W.C. (1993) Vitamin E consumption and the risk of coronary heart disease in men. *New England Journal of Medicine* 328, 1450–1456.

Rimm, E.B., Katan, M.B., Ascherio, A., Stampfer, M.J. and Willett, W.C. (1996) Relation between intake of flavonoids and risk of coronary disease in male health professionals. *Archives of Internal Medicine* 125, 384–389.

Rosenfeld, M.E., Khoo, J.C., Miller, E., Parthasarathy, S., Palinski, W. and Witztum, J.L. (1991) Macrophage-derived foam cells freshly isolated from rabbit atherosclerotic lesions degrade modified lipoproteins, promote oxidation of low-density lipoproteins, and contain oxidation-specific lipid–protein adducts. *Journal of Clinical Investigation* 87, 90–99.

Ross, R. (1986) The pathogenesis of atherosclerosis – an update. *New England Journal of Medicine* 314, 488–500.

Shwaery, G.T., Vita, J.A. and Keaney, J.F. Jr (1997) Antioxidant protection of LDL by physiological concentrations of 17β-estradiol. Requirement for estradiol modification. *Circulation* 95, 1378–1385.

Singh, R.B., Niag, A.M., Ghosh, S., Agarwal, P., Ahmad, S., Begum, R., Onouchi, Z. and Kummerow, F.A. (1995) Randomized controlled trial of antioxidant vitamins and cardioprotective diet on hyperlipidemia, oxidative stress and development of experimental atherscelerosis: the diet and antioxidant trial on atherosclerosis (DATA). *Cardiovascular Drugs and Therapy* 9, 763–771.

Singh, R.B., Niaz, M.A., Rastogi, S.S. and Rastogi, S. (1996) Usefulness of antioxidant vitamins in suspected acute myocardial infarction (The Indian Experiment of Infarct Survival-3). *American Journal of Cardiology* 77, 232–236.

Slattery, M.L., Jacobs, D.R. Jr, Dyer, A., Benson, J., Hilmer, J.E. and Caan, B.J. (1995) Dietary antioxidants and plasma lipids: the CARDIA Study. *Journal of the American College of Nutrition* 14, 635–642.

Smith, L.L. and vanLier, J.E. (1970) Sterol metabolism IX. 26-hydroxycholesterol levels in the human aorta. *Atherosclerosis* 12, 1–4.

Smith, T.L. and Kummerow, F.A. (1989) Effect of dietary vitamin E on plasma lipids and atherogenesis in restricted ovulator chickens. *Atherosclerosis* 75, 105–109.

Stampfer, M.J., Hennekens, C.H., Manson, J.E., Colditz, G.A., Rosner, B. and Willett, W.C. (1993) Vitamin E consumption and the risk of coronary disease in women. *New England Journal of Medicine* 328, 1444–1449.

Steinberg, D., Parthasarathy, S., Carew, T.E., Khoo, J.C. and Witztum, J.L. (1989) Beyond cholesterol. Modifications of low-density lipoprotein that increase its atherogenicity. *New England Journal of Medicine* 320, 915–924.

Stephens, N.G., Parsons, A., Schofield, P.M., Kelly, F., Cheeseman, K., Mitchison, M.J. and Brown, J. (1996) Randomised controlled trial of vitamin E in patients with coronary diease: Cambridge Heart Antioxidant Study. *Lancet* 347, 781–786.

Street, D.A., Comstock, G.W., Salkeld, R.M., Schüep, W. and Klag, M.J. (1994) Serum antioxidants and myocardial infarction are low levels of carotenoids and alpha tocopherol risk factors for myocardial infarction? *Circulation* 90, 1154–1161.

Tedeschi, R.E., Taylor, H.L. and Martz, B.L. (1980) Clinical experience of the safety and cholesterol-lowering action of probucol. In: Noseda, G., Lewis, B. and Paoletti, R. (eds) *Diet and Drugs in Atherosclerosis*. Raven Press, New York, pp. 199–207.

Verlangieri, A.J. and Bush, M.J. (1992) Effects of d-α-tocopherol supplementation on experimentally induced primate atherosclerosis. *Journal of the American College of Nutrition* 11, 131–138.

Vogel, J. (1847) *The Pathological Anatomy of the Human Body*. Lea and Blanchard, Philadelphia, Pennsylvania.

White, C.R., Darley-Usmar, V. and Oparil, S. (1997) Gender and cardiovascular disease. Recent insights. *Trends in Cardiovascular Medicine* 7, 94–100.

Wilson, R.B., Middleton, C.C. and Sun, G.Y. (1978) Vitamin E, antioxidants and lipid peroxidation in experimental atherosclerosis of rabbits. *Journal of Nutrition* 108, 1858–1867.

Effect of Antioxidants on Atherogenesis   **14**

FRED A. KUMMEROW, MOHAMEDAIN M. MAHFOUZ AND QI ZHOU

Burnsides Research Laboratory, University of Illinois, Urbana, Illinois, USA

Introduction

This chapter discusses three experimental models which were used to examine the influence of antioxidants on atherogenesis. The models include restricted-fed ovulatory (RO) hens, cholesterol-fed rabbits and cigarette smokers.

Restricted Ovulatory Hens

Restricted Ovulator (RO) hens carry a genetic defect which results in the cessation of egg laying when these hens were exposed to a prolonged photoperiod (Smith and Kummerow, 1989). Such hens developed an extreme hyperlipidaemia compared with laying hens. The plasma cholesterol concentration increased to 1380 compared with 118 mg dl^{-1} for laying hens (Table 14.1). The triglycerides concentration increased to 8160 mg dl^{-1} and the oxidized lipids, as measured by thiobarbituric acid reaction (TBAR) concentration, increased to 40.9 μmol ml^{-1}. When the diet of RO hens was supplemented with vitamin E (1000 IU kg^{-1}), the plasma level of triglycerides and cholesterol did not decrease significantly, but the TBAR level and the intimal thickness of the coronary arteries did decrease by 79% and 37%, respectively. Therefore, hyperlipidaemia without lipid peroxidation either did not promote atherogenesis or did so at a much reduced rate.

Table 14.1. Plasma lipid and TBAR concentrations and intimal thickness in laying and Restricted Ovulator (RO) hens with and without dietary vitamin E supplementation (from Smith and Kummerow (1989)).

	Without vitamin E	With vitamin E
Triglycerides (mg dl^{-1})		
Layer	570 ± 290[b]	640 ± 140[b]
RO	8160 ± 2320[c]	7160 ± 4850[c]
Cholesterol (mg dl^{-1})		
Layer	118 ± 20[d]	180 ± 4[d]
RO	1380 ± 160[e]	1520 ± 150[e]
TBAR (μmol l^{-1})		
Layer	12.2 ± 2.8[f]	7.7 ± 1.4[f]
RO	40.9 ± 6.3	8.4 ± 2.0[f]
Intimal thickness (μm)		
Layer	18 ± 1[g]	15 ± 3[g]
RO	24 ± 1	15 ± 2[g]

Values are mean ± SD.
[b-g] Means with the same superscripts are not statistically different by Tukeys test, $\alpha = 0.05$.

Hypercholesterolaemic Rabbits

This experimental model involved cholesterol-fed rabbits (Mahfouz *et al.*, 1997). Four groups of rabbits were fed for 11 weeks: (i) a Purina stock diet; (ii) this stock diet plus 0.5% cholesterol containing cholesterol oxides; (iii) the stock diet plus 0.5% pure cholesterol; (iv) diet (iii) plus 1000 mg vitamin E and 500 mg vitamin C kg^{-1} of diet (Table 14.2). The pure cholesterol was prepared by six recrystallizations of USP cholesterol from 95% ethanol and was kept under nitrogen at -20°C. Its purity was checked by gas chromatography, which indicated that it contained traces of cholesterol oxides.

The diet containing oxidized cholesterol or pure cholesterol increased the plasma cholesterol concentration by 66- and 70-fold, respectively. Supplementation of the pure cholesterol diet with vitamins E and C significantly reduced the plasma cholesterol concentration by 40%. HDL concentration in the plasma did not differ between the four groups, indicating that the large increase in plasma cholesterol in the cholesterol-fed rabbits was within the low-density lipoproteins (LDL and VLDL) fractions.

The diets containing oxidized cholesterol or pure cholesterol increased the plasma triglyceride concentration about 2.7- and 2.3-fold, respectively, while the pure cholesterol plus antioxidant diet increased it only 1.5-fold compared with the control group. The plasma phospholipid concentration increased about tenfold on the oxidized cholesterol and the pure cholesterol diet but increased only sixfold on the pure cholesterol plus antioxidants.

Table 14.2. Plasma lipid, vitamin C and TBAR concentrations in rabbits fed control, oxidized cholesterol, pure cholesterol or pure cholesterol plus antioxidants diets[*] (from Mahfouz *et al.*, 1997).

	Control diet (n = 6)	Oxidized cholesterol diet (n = 6)	Pure cholesterol diet (n = 6)	Pure cholesterol plus antioxidants diet (n = 6)
Total cholesterol (nmol l[−1])	0.58 ± 0.22[a]	37.7 ± 15.28[b,e,f]	40.0 ± 6.26[c,e]	23.8 ± 4.4[d,f]
HDL cholesterol (nmol l[−1])	0.48 ± 0.12	0.51 ± 0.30	0.53 ± 0.13	0.57 ± 0.10
Triglyceride (nmol l[−1])	0.51 ± 0.08[a]	1.41 ± 0.67[b,e,f]	1.17 ± 0.36[c,e]	0.76 ± 0.136[d,f]
Phospholipids (nmol l[−1])	0.64 ± 0.08[a]	6.95 ± 2.49[b,e,f]	6.56 ± 1.64[c,e]	3.83 ± 0.6[d,f]
Vitamin C (μmol l[−1])	22.4 ± 5.1[a]	26.6 ± 4.3[a,d]	31.1 ± 6.1[b,d]	59.0 ± 16.3[c]
TBAR (nmol MDA l[−1])	617 ± 121[a]	2650 ± 497[b,e]	2667 ± 537[c,e]	1280 ± 299[d]

[*] x ± SD. Means with different superscript letters are significantly different, $P < 0.05$. MDA, malondialdehyde.

These results indicate that the oxidized cholesterol and the pure cholesterol were equally hyperlipidaemic, but the addition of vitamins E and C to the pure cholesterol diet attenuated this.

The plasma TBAR level was significantly increased in all the rabbits fed cholesterol. The increase was more than fourfold on the oxidized cholesterol and the pure cholesterol diet but only twofold on the pure cholesterol plus antioxidants. The addition of the antioxidants to the pure cholesterol diet, therefore, decreased the TBAR concentration by 50%. The plasma vitamin C concentration was significantly increased in the rabbits fed pure cholesterol plus vitamins E and C.

The free and the total amounts of cholesterol deposited in the liver of rabbits fed high cholesterol diets were increased six- and ninefold, respectively, compared to the control group (Table 14.3). Cholesterol esters represented more than 55% of the total liver cholesterol in the cholesterol-fed rabbits compared to 28% in the control group indicating that cholesterol esterification was enhanced in the livers of the cholesterol-fed rabbits. The phospholipid content was increased by 20–30% in the livers of the rabbits fed cholesterol, but the liver triglyceride concentration did not differ significantly from the control group of rabbits.

Collectively, these results indicate that all cholesterol-rich diets cause an accumulation of cholesterol, mainly as cholesterol ester in the liver, and feeding the pure cholesterol and the pure cholesterol plus antioxidants does not reduce the amount of lipids in the liver compared with the diet containing oxidized cholesterol. The accumulation of lipids in the liver tissues is, therefore, independent of cholesterol oxides or antioxidants. The liver membranes were highly enriched with cholesterol in rabbits fed cholesterol reaching a concentration of 270, 280 and 310 μmol g^{-1} of liver membrane protein in the oxidized cholesterol, pure cholesterol, and pure cholesterol plus antioxidants, respectively, as compared to 64 μmol g^{-1} in the control group.

The plasma of the control rabbits contained the following cholesterol oxides: 7α- and 7β-hydroxycholesterols, β-epoxide, cholestanetriol, 7-ketocholesterol and 25-, as well as 26-hydroxycholesterols (Table 14.4). After 11 weeks on the respective diets, the cholesterol oxide concentration significantly increased in the plasma of all the cholesterol-fed rabbits. However, the cholesterol oxide concentration was significantly lower in rabbits fed the pure cholesterol diet as compared to those fed the diet containing oxidized cholesterol. Moreover, the concentration was reduced by about half by addition of vitamins E and C to the pure cholesterol diet.

Stained sections of aorta from the rabbits fed the control diet revealed a normal intima. However, when given oxidized cholesterol there was intimal thickening (atherosclerosis). The extent of this was less in rabbits given pure cholesterol. Rabbits fed pure cholesterol plus antioxidants showed little intimal thickening and little atherosclerosis.

Table 14.3. Lipid contents in liver of rabbits fed control, oxidized cholesterol, pure cholesterol, or pure cholesterol plus antioxidants diets* (from Mahfouz et al., 1997).

	Control diet (n = 6)	Oxidized cholesterol diet (n = 6)	Pure cholesterol diet (n = 6)	Pure cholesterol plus antioxidants diet (n = 6)
Total cholesterol (μmol g^{-1} liver)	8.0 ± 1.6[a]	80.3 ± 26.6[b,e]	75.1 ± 22.8[c,e]	70.2 ± 11.7[d,e]
Free cholesterol (μmol g^{-1} liver)	5.8 ± 1.1[a]	30.1 ± 4.7[b,e]	33.9 ± 5.7[c,e]	31.1 ± 3.1[d,e]
Esterification of cholesterol (%)	28.4 ± 8.0[a]	55.1 ± 8.6[b,e]	57.4 ± 6.4[c,e]	56.4 ± 7.5[d,e]
Triglyceride (μmol g^{-1} liver)	6.1 ± 1.5	5.1 ± 0.8	5.8 ± 1.1	5.5 ± 0.8
Phospholipid (μmol g^{-1} liver)	34.4 ± 3.6[a]	41.6 ± 3.1[b,e,f]	44.5 ± 3.0[c,e]	40.0 ± 1.9[d,f]
Cholesterol in membrane (μmol g^{-1} protein)	64	270	280	310

* Values are mean ± SD. Means with different superscript letters are significantly different, $P < 0.05$.

Under oxidative stress, a combination of moderate levels of vitamins E and C may be more beneficial than a high level of vitamin E alone (Godfried *et al.*, 1989). Our results show that supplementation of a cholesterol-rich diet with vitamins E and C still produces hypercholesterolaemia in rabbits but the vitamins act as effective blood antioxidants, thereby significantly reducing the level of lipid peroxidation, cholesterol oxidation and decreasing the severity of atherosclerosis.

Cigarette Smokers

This experimental model related to cigarette smokers compared with non-smokers (Hulea *et al.*, 1995). Smokers generally had a higher plasma lipid peroxide concentration (TBAR) but a lower total antioxidant capacity (Table 14.5). This was significant at ages 46–80 (groups C and D). These subjects had smoked at least 12 cigarettes per day for more than 2 years.

It was shown in an *in vitro* study (Mahfouz *et al.*, 1995) that smoking increased the concentration of lipid peroxides. We used the apparatus shown in Fig. 14.1. The level of TBAR in isolated LDL which had been exposed to six puffs of cigarette smoke and incubated for 20 h at 37°C

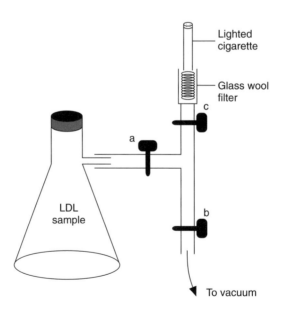

Figure 14.1. Scheme for the system used for LDL exposure to cigarette smoke (CS). Valve c was closed, while valves a and b were opened until a vacuum was established in the flask. Valve b was then closed and valve c was opened to allow a puff of smoke to enter the flask. Valves a and c were closed and the flask was incubated at 37°C in a metabolic shaker. From Mahfouz *et al.* (1995).

Table 14.4. Cholesterol oxide concentrations (mmol cholesterol oxide l^{-1} plasma) in the plasma of rabbits fed control, oxidized cholesterol, pure cholesterol or pure cholesterol plus antioxidants diets[*] (from Mahfouz *et al.*, 1997).

Cholesterol oxides	Control diet ($n = 3$)	Oxidized cholesterol diet ($n = 3$)	Pure cholesterol diet ($n = 3$)	Pure cholesterol plus antioxidants diet ($n = 3$)
7α-Hydroxycholesterol	74 ± 5[a]	1805 ± 175[b]	1078 ± 210[c,e]	729 ± 168[d,e]
7β-Hydroxycholesterol	231 ± 5[a]	5576 ± 1410[b]	3586 ± 1113[c,e]	2306 ± 674[d,e]
β-Epoxide	100 ± 12[a]	578 ± 65[b]	351 ± 24[c,e]	351 ± 67[d,e]
Cholestanetriol	117 ± 7[a]	1367 ± 344[b]	581 ± 131[c]	217 ± 61[d]
25-Hydroxycholesterol	107 ± 12[a]	587 ± 113[b,e]	642 ± 119[c,e]	233 ± 26[d]
7-Ketocholesterol	148 ± 13[a]	2992 ± 156[b]	1767 ± 348[c,e]	395 ± 61[d]
26-Hydroxycholesterol	107 ± 24[a]	936 ± 206[b]	416 ± 84[c]	216 ± 41[d]
Total cholesterol oxides	889 ± 14[a]	13889 ± 1808[b]	8437 ± 1212[c]	4453 ± 562[d]

[*] Values are mean ± SD. Means with different superscript letters are significantly different, $P < 0.05$.

Table 14.5. Plasma concentration of lipid peroxides and total antioxidant capacity (from Hulea *et al.*, 1995).

Parameter	Age group	Non-smokers	Smokers	P value
Lipid peroxides (TBAR) (μmol l^{-1})	A	2.5 ± 0.3	2.8 ± 0.4	NS
	B	2.5 ± 0.3	2.8 ± 0.5	NS
	C	2.7 ± 0.3	3.3 ± 0.4	0.01
	D	3.3 ± 0.2	3.9 ± 0.2	0.0005
Total antioxidant capacity (units l^{-1})	A	21.8 ± 5.9	30.2 ± 6.1	NS
	B	25.3 ± 3.8	20.9 ± 5.3	NS
	C	21.7 ± 4.7	16.5 ± 3.2	0.04
	D	19.1 ± 5.5	14.4 ± 2.4	0.02

Note: A, 18–25 years of age; B, 26–45; C, 46–65; D, 66–80; NS, not significant.

increased significantly compared with LDL exposed to six puffs of air or 10 and 2 nmol malondialdehyde mg^{-1} LDL protein, respectively.

The concentration of five oxysterols normally found in the LDL were increased significantly in the LDL exposed to cigarette smoke (CS-LDL) (Table 14.6). The total oxysterol content was more than double in the LDL exposed to cigarette smoke compared with LDL exposed to air. This study shows that cigarette smoke can increase the atherogenicity as well as the cytotoxicity of LDL by increasing its oxidized cholesterol and lipid peroxidation, as indicated by the elevation of TBAR. Cigarette smoke also modifies the LDL in such a way as to decrease its binding to the hepatic receptors, and this may increase its uptake by scavenger receptors of macrophages as previously reported.

The results of the various experiments described here underline the close association between lipid peroxidation and atherosclerosis. Cigarette smoke, a well-established risk factor for atherosclerosis, leads to lipid peroxidation. We have shown this both *in vivo* and *in vitro*, as has Miller *et al.* (1997), and our animal experiments support this. In both RO hens and rabbits fed a cholesterol-rich diet, we see a combination of hyperlipidaemia, lipid peroxidation and atherosclerosis. Our results from the studies on hens and rabbits also point to the potential value of vitamins E and C as preventatives of both lipid peroxidation and atherosclerosis.

Acknowledgements

The authors thank the Wallace Research Foundation, Cedar Rapids, Iowa, for financial support.

Table 14.6. Comparison of oxysterol concentrations in control and CS-LDL (from Mahfouz *et al.*, 1995).

Oxysterol	Control LDL	CS-LDL	P^a
7α-OH-C	178	356	<0.001
7β-OH-C	224	307	<0.001
α-Epoxy	75	182	<0.001
Triol	127	290	<0.001
7-Keto	157	530	<0.001
Total oxysterols	762	1666	<0.001

Note: the CS-LDL was exposed to six puffs of cigarette smoke then incubated at 37°C for 20 h. Control LDL was exposed to air. Results are expressed as means ± SD of ng oxysterol mg^{-1} LDL protein. 7α-OH-C, 7α-hydroxycholesterol; 7β-OH-C, 7β-hydroxycholesterol; triol, cholestanetriol; 7-keto, 7-ketocholesterol.
[a] Statistically significant differences were calculated by Student *t*-test.

References

Godfried, S.L., Combs, G.F., Saroka, J.M. and Dillingham, L.A. (1989) Potentiation of atherosclerotic lesions in rabbits by a high dietary level of vitamin E. *British Journal of Nutrition* 61, 607–617.

Hulea, S.A., Olinescu, R., Niṭă, S., Crocnan, D. and Kummerow, F.A. (1995) Cigarette smoking causes biochemical changes in blood that are suggestive of oxidative stress: a case control study. *Journal of Environmental Pathology, Toxicology, and Oncology* 14, 173–180.

Mahfouz, M.M., Hulea, S.A. and Kummerow, F.A. (1995) Cigarette smoke increases cholesterol oxidation and lipid peroxidation of human low-density lipoprotein and decreases its binding to the hepatic receptor *in vitro*. *Journal of Environmental Pathology, Toxicology, and Oncology* 14, 181–192.

Mahfouz, M.M., Kawano, H. and Kummerow, F.A. (1997) Effects of cholesterol-rich diets with and without added vitamins E and C on the severity of atherosclerosis in rabbits. *American Journal of Clinical Nutrition* 66, 1240–1249.

Miller, E.R. III, Appel, L.J., Jiang, L. and Risby, T.H. (1997) Association between cigarette smoking and lipid peroxidation in a controlled feeding study. *Circulation* 96, 1097–1101.

Smith, T.L. and Kummerow, F.A. (1989) Effect of dietary vitamin E on plasma lipids and atherogenesis in restricted ovulator chickens. *Atherosclerosis* 75, 105–109.

Flavonoids and Other Phytochemicals in Relation to Coronary Heart Disease

15

SAMIR SAMMAN, PHILIPPA M. LYONS WALL AND EFI FARMAKALIDIS

Human Nutrition Unit, Department of Biochemistry, University of Sydney, Sydney, Australia

Introduction

Antioxidants have been the focus of research on the relationship between diet and disease. The antioxidant hypothesis of coronary heart disease (CHD) stemmed from research on antioxidant nutrients *in vitro*. The large-scale supplementation studies which followed the *in vitro* studies gave disappointing results (Omenn *et al.*, 1996), although α-tocopherol showed the most promise (Stephens *et al.*, 1996) in terms of impacting on a tangible endpoint for CHD, that is, a reduction in the oxidizability of low-density lipoprotein (LDL) (see Chapter 13). However, it became apparent that the dietary sources of the nutrients under investigation were also the sources of a large number of non-nutrients and that the plasma levels of the antioxidant vitamins may be serving as surrogate markers for other dietary components such as flavonoids. Flavonoids have a range of biological effects, including the induction of a favourable lipoprotein profile, a reduction in the oxidizability of LDL and a decrease in platelet aggregation. These effects are exerted through the actions of flavonoids as antioxidants, chelators of divalent cations and via specific interactions with metabolic processes (Samman *et al.*, 1996; Lyons Wall and Samman, 1997).

The basic structural unit of the flavonoid family comprises two benzene rings (A and B) linked through a heterocyclic pyran or pyrone ring (C); variations in the C ring and hydroxylation pattern on the A and B rings define the major classes (Cook and Samman, 1996) (Fig. 15.1). These include flavonols and flavones; the relatively rare chalcones, flavanones and flavanols; the anthocyanidins; and the isoflavones. Discussion in this review will focus on some dietary sources of flavonoids and their reported effects on CHD.

Effect of Flavonoids on Coronary Heart Disease

The association between flavonoid intake and CHD has been examined in several epidemiological studies using estimated intakes of quercetin,

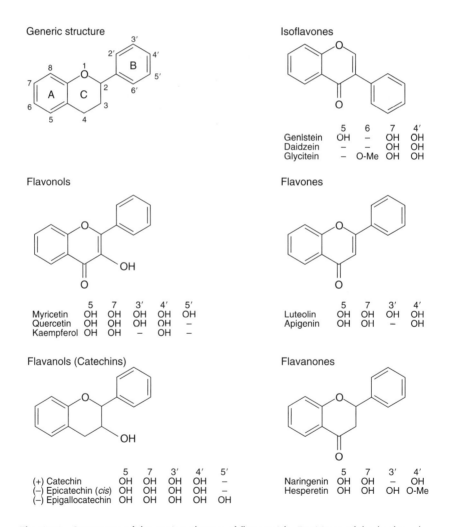

Fig. 15.1. Structures of the major classes of flavonoids. Positions of the hydroxyl groups on the A and B rings are listed for selected examples within each class.

kaempferol, myricetin, luteolin and apigenin. In the Zutphen Elderly Study (Hertog *et al.*, 1993a), a flavonoid intake of greater than 30 mg day^{-1} was associated with a 68% reduction in mortality from CHD and an inverse but weaker relationship with the incidence of myocardial infarction. The major source of flavonoids in this population was black tea, followed by onions and apples, although minor ingredients such as parsley and thyme also made a contribution to the intake of flavones. Keli *et al.* (1996) found a dose-dependent inverse association between the mean intake of flavonoids over 15 years and the risk of stroke, after adjustment for known confounders. In this cohort, tea was again a major contributor to flavonoid intake and men who consumed 4.7 or more cups of tea had a lower incidence of stroke than men who drank less than 2.6 cups per day.

Further support for the cardioprotective effect of flavonoids was obtained from a re-examination of the food records from 16 cohorts in the Seven Countries Study (Hertog *et al.*, 1995). During a 25-year follow-up period, an inverse association was observed between CHD mortality and flavonoid intake, which explained a small (8%) but significant portion of the variance in CHD deaths, independently of intake of alcohol and antioxidant vitamins. CHD mortality was lowest in Japan, with an average flavonoid intake of 61 mg day^{-1}, mainly derived from green tea.

In contrast, other epidemiological studies have shown no significant effects of flavonoid intake, despite large sample sizes (Knekt *et al.*, 1996; Rimm *et al.*, 1996; Hertog *et al.*, 1997). Possible reasons for the discrepancy may include: (i) relatively low flavonoid intakes; (ii) measurement error in the dietary records; (iii) lack of correction for confounding factors; and (iv) the analysis of flavonoids was confined to the five major flavonoids detected in the Dutch diet.

Postulated Mechanisms by Which Flavonoids Exert Their Biological Effects

Several mechanisms have been proposed to explain the protective effect of flavonoids on CHD (Cook and Samman, 1996). Flavonoids could act as antioxidants to protect LDL from oxidation and thereby inhibit atherogenesis. The antioxidant effect appears to increase with increasing number of hydroxyl groups, especially on positions C-5 and C-7 of the A ring and C-3′ and C-4′ of the B ring, as seen with the polyhydroxylated flavonoids: myricetin, quercetin and the catechins (Fig. 15.1).

Flavonoids could also exert protection via their similarity to endogenous oestrogens. Miksicek (1995) showed significant oestrogenic activity in 11 of 38 food flavonoids tested, with greatest activity in genistein followed by kaempferol > apigenin > daidzein > luteolin. The oestrogenic effect required a minimum of two OH groups, in position C-5, 6 or 7 on the A ring and position C-4′ on the B ring – a configuration similar to that of oestradiol-17

OH which permits binding to the oestrogen receptor. Polyhydroxylated flavonoids, such as myricetin, quercetin and the catechins, showed no oestrogenic activity, possibly due to steric hindrance of the additional substitutions.

Dietary Intake, Absorption and Metabolism

Average intakes of flavonols and flavones have ranged from 6 mg day^{-1} in Finland to 64 mg day^{-1} in Japan, with intermediate intakes in the USA (13 mg day^{-1}), Italy (27 mg day^{-1}) and the Netherlands (33 mg day^{-1}). These estimates were based on recent analyses of five flavonoids (quercetin, kaempferol, myricetin, luteolin and apigenin) in composite food samples for populations in the Seven Countries Study (Hertog *et al.*, 1995). Dietary sources of the flavonols and flavones varied between different countries, with major contributions from tea in Japan (90%) and the Netherlands (64%), red wine in Italy (46%), and vegetables and fruits in Finland (100%) and the USA (80%). The main sources of flavonols and flavones in the human diet are shown in Table 15.1. Herbs and spices, although not consumed universally in large quantities, are also rich in phenolic compounds and constitute the largest proportion of known natural antioxidants.

Isoflavones are found in the legume family, mainly soybean. A comprehensive analysis of 49 varieties of dried legumes reported that concentrations of genistein and daidzein, the main dietary isoflavones in the soybean, varied from 38 to 140 mg 100 g^{-1} between different varieties (Mazur *et al.*, 1996). These levels were 50-fold higher than in chick peas (1.1–3.6 mg 100 g^{-1}) and up to 1000-fold higher than in other legumes including kidney beans and lentils (0.08–0.7 mg 100 g^{-1}). The concentrations of genistein and daidzein are influenced by climatic conditions and

Table 15.1. Dietary sources of flavonols and flavones[a,b]. Adapted from Hertog *et al.* (1992, 1993b).

High: 5–35 mg 100 g^{-1}	Medium: 1–4 mg 100 g^{-1}	Low: <1 mg 100 g^{-1}
Onion, kale, celery, broccoli, French bean, broad bean	Apple, black tea, leek, apricot, red wine, grape, strawberry, lettuce, cherry, redcurrant, red capsicum, plum, tomato	Cabbage, white cabbage, cauliflower, mushroom, pea, spinach, beetroot, cucumber, peach, carrot, citrus juices, coffee, white wine

[a] Listed from highest to lowest content within each group.
[b] Quercetin, kaempferol, myricetin, luteolin, apigenin.

seasonal effects, both of which contribute to the wide ranges of isoflavones in traditional and commercial soy products (Table 15.2). The consumption of tofu, miso and tempeh contribute to an average intake of about 50 mg day^{-1} in traditional Asian diets (Wang and Murphy, 1994). By comparison, intake from a typical Western diet is low, about 1–5 mg day^{-1}, although increasing use of soy ingredients in processed food items suggests that intake is rising.

Relatively little is understood about the absorption and metabolism of flavonoids in humans. Aglycone flavonoids can be absorbed from the large intestine and transferred via the portal vein to the liver where they are further metabolized by methylation, or by conjugation with glucuronate or sulphate and excretion in bile to undergo enterohepatic circulation. It is the aglycone flavonoids that appear to exert greatest physiological activity. Flavonoid conjugates are polar and are finally excreted in the urine. In humans, urinary concentrations increase after supplementation with flavonoid-rich foods, but wide unexplained variation is seen between individuals (Fahey and Jung, 1989; Kelly *et al.*, 1995). Dietary constituents, for instance, dietary fibre, could also contribute to the variability, either directly by retarding its absorption (Tew *et al.*, 1996), or indirectly by influencing the composition of colonic bacteria (Xu *et al.*, 1995). The variable response to dietary flavonoids could have important physiological consequences since individual flavonoids and their metabolites have differing biological effects.

Antioxidants from herbs and spices

The consumption of herbs and spices, which is a feature of many dietary practices world-wide, makes a significant contribution to the intake of phytochemicals with biological action (Huang *et al.*, 1994; Plumb *et al.*, 1995). Numerous spices have been shown to exert biological effects by modulating arachidonic acid metabolism and platelet aggregation (Table

Table 15.2. Isoflavone content (mg 100 g^{-1}) in traditional and commercial soy items. Adapted from Samman *et al.* (1996).

Traditional foods		Commercial soy products	
Soybean (dry)	91–160	Defatted soy flour, soy gifts	178–306
Miso	32–92	Textured vegetable protein	104–118
Tempeh	36–43	Soy protein isolates	103–145
Tofu	21–49	Soy protein concentrates: water washed	247–317
Soy drink	25	alcohol washed	21–43
Soy sauce	2	Soy hot dogs, soy bacon, tofu yoghurt	10–13
Soybean oil	0	Soy cheeses	1–7
Soybean sprouts	42		

15.3 and Fig. 15.2). The presence of glycosides of kaempferol, rhamnetin and quercetin and phenolic amides are believed to confer antioxidant activity to pepper (Nakatani *et al.*, 1986). In oregano, among the active components, four flavonoids were identified (Lagouri and Boskou, 1996) while in thyme, compounds have been isolated and identified as dimers of thymol and flavonoids. Similarly, the phenolic antioxidants, *p*-coumaric acid, ferulic acid, curcumin and caffeic acid, which are found in coriander, turmeric, liquorice, oregano, sesame and rosemary, inhibit the formation of 3-nitrotyrosine *in vitro* and may prevent lipid peroxidation *in vivo* (Aruoma *et al.*, 1992, 1996). Caffeic acid and other hydroxycinnamic acids have also been found to have an inhibitory effect on LDL oxidation (Abu-Amsha *et al.*, 1996). Rosmarinic acid also fulfils the requirements for being considered as a potent antioxidant since it is not only capable of scavenging superoxide anions but is also able to chelate iron ions (Houlihan *et al.*, 1985; Aruoma *et al.*, 1996).

The structure and antioxidative properties of several phenolic diterpenes isolated from rosemary have been characterized (Schwarz and Ternes, 1992). From the same plant, compounds such as carnosic acid and carnosol have been identified as antioxidants (Aruoma *et al.*, 1992). Moreover, a number of the compounds found in rosemary have been found in sage and other herbs. Hence, herbs and spices make a significant contribution to the variety of dietary phytochemicals and the many herbs and spices contribute to the total antioxidant capacity of the diet.

Table 15.3. The effect of spices on platelet aggregation and eicosanoid production. Adapted from Srivastava and Mustafa (1989).

Spice	Effects on platelets
Garlic (*Allium sativum*)	Reduced thromboxane formation, reduced incorporation of arachidonic acid (AA) into platelet phospholipids
Onion (*Allium cepa*)	Anti-aggregatory, reduced formation of thromboxane and 12-lipoxygenase products
Ginger (*Zingiber officinale*)	Anti-aggregatory, reduced cyclo-oxygenase products
Cloves (*Eugenia aromatica*)	Anti-aggregatory, reduced cyclo-oxygenase and lipoxygenase products
Omum (*Trachspermum ammi*)	Anti-aggregatory, reduced cyclo-oxygenase products
Cumin (*Cuminum cyminum*)	Inhibits AA-induced aggregation, reduced thomboxane formation
Turmeric (*Curcuma longa*)	Inhibits AA-induced aggregation, reduced release of AA, reduced thromboxane formation, reduced incorporation of AA into platelet phospholipids

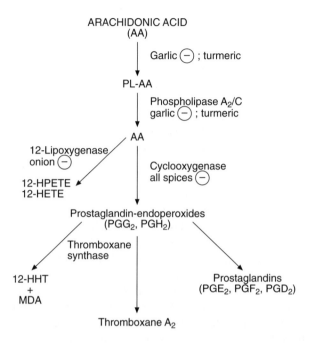

Fig. 15.2. The inhibition by garlic, turmeric and onions of the conversion of arachidonic acid to thromboxane and prostaglandins.

The effect of tea on the risk of coronary heart disease

All varieties of tea (with the exception of herbal preparations) come from the species *Camellia sinensis*. The leaves of this plant are crushed by rolling, and this partly destroys the cell structure and releases enzymes which oxidize the flavonoids, leading to the characteristic colour and flavour of black tea. Harvesting for green tea is similar to that for black tea, except that the fermentation step is eliminated by the leaves being exposed to dry heat (IARC, 1991). Table 15.4 shows the variation of flavonoids in tea. The hydroxyl patterns of these flavonoids fulfil the requirements for antioxidant activity (Cook and Samman, 1996).

Table 15.4. Flavonoid content of tea. Adapted from IARC (1991).

	Fresh leaf tea (%)	Black tea (%)
Epi-gallocatechin gallate	9–13	4.6
Epi-catechin gallate	3–6	3.9
Epi-gallocatechin	3–6	1.1
Epi-catechin	1–3	1.2
Flavonols	3–4	Trace

Tea, or its constituents, are reported to have antioxidant activity *in vitro* which reduces the oxidizability of polyunsaturated fatty acids and of α-tocopherol. There appears to be a hierarchy in antioxidant activity of the flavonoids in tea, with epi-catechin gallate > epi-gallocatechin gallate > epi-gallocatechin > gallic acid > epi-catechin > catechin (Miura *et al.*, 1994; Salah *et al.*, 1995; Luo *et al.*, 1997).

Epidemiological studies support the notion that the consumption of green tea reduces the risk of CHD, possibly by modulating the lipoprotein profile. Stensvold *et al.* (1992) carried out a study in Norway over a 2-year period. Tea consumption was associated with decreased total cholesterol concentration and on follow-up, CHD mortality was higher for those drinking less than one cup per day compared with those drinking more. Similarly, a decrease in cholesterol concentration was associated with increased tea consumption but this did not reach statistical significance after adjusting for known confounders (Green and Harabi, 1992). In Japan, consumption of green tea was associated with a decrease in total cholesterol and triacylglycerol concentrations (Imai and Nakachi, 1995). This substantial decrease in plasma lipids was noted in drinkers who drank ten or more cups of green tea a day. It was also noted that an increased consumption raised the concentration of HDL-C, and decreased the LDL-C and VLDL-C concentration. Support for an effect of green tea consumption on blood lipid concentrations has been obtained from studies in animals. Catechins reduce the plasma cholesterol concentration in rats (Muramatsu *et al.*, 1986), possibly due to a reduction in the absorption of cholesterol (Ikeda *et al.*, 1992).

In contrast with the epidemiologial observations and findings *in vitro*, clinical trials have failed to demonstrate an effect of tea on antioxidant potential, lipoprotein concentrations or platelet activity (Vorster *et al.*, 1996; Bingham *et al.*, 1997; van het Hof *et al.*, 1997; Ishikawa *et al.*, 1997). This suggests that the epidemiological observations are confounded by other factors and that the consumption of tea is a marker for favourable lifestyle activities and dietary patterns, such as a reduced incidence of smoking and higher consumption of fruit and vegetables (Schwarz *et al.*, 1994) (Table 15.5).

The effect of wine on the risk of coronary heart disease

The incongruity between established dietary risk factors and death from CHD was highlighted by the reporting of the French paradox; that is, why the French have a relatively low incidence of CHD while consuming a diet rich in saturated fat, mainly from butter and cream (Renaud and de Longeril, 1992). Epidemiological data from Denmark advanced this hypothesis by demonstrating a lower incidence of cardiovascular disease and stroke in subjects who consumed low or moderate amounts of wine (three glasses per day) (Gronbaek *et al.*, 1995). A possible explanation for this effect is the relatively high consumption of phenolic compounds found in red wine

Table 15.5. Trend analysis of some dietary and lifestyle habits in coffee and tea drinkers. Adapted from Schwarz *et al.* (1994).

	Coffee drinkers	Tea drinkers
Cigarettes	+2.7, $P < 0.000$	−1.3, $P < 0.001$
Fat	+0.04, $P < 0.003$	−0.05, $P < 0.001$
Sausages	+0.06, $P < 0.041$	−0.07, $P < 0.039$
Fish	ns	+0.09, $P < 0.000$
Salad	ns	+0.10, $P < 0.049$
Vegetables	ns	+0.21, $P < 0.000$
Fruit	−0.24, $P < 0.000$	+0.35, $P < 0.001$

Data shown as the association obtained by multiple regression analysis and the level of significance.

(Frankel *et al.*, 1993) which can increase the antioxidant capacity in plasma (Whitehead *et al.*, 1995), reduce the tendency of LDL to oxidation (Frankel *et al.*, 1993; Miyagi *et al.*, 1997) and inhibit platelet aggregation (Demrow *et al.*, 1995).

The majority of experimental studies which have investigated the effect of wine on markers of CHD have yielded favourable results. However, it is unclear whether white or red wine is more effective and to what extent the alcoholic content of the beverage contributes to CHD risk reduction (Klatsky *et al.*, 1997). This aspect has been reviewed in more detail elsewhere (Samman *et al.*, 1997).

Conclusion

Epidemiological data suggest that flavonoids from selected vegetables, fruits, tea and wine contribute to the prevention of cardiovascular disease. One possible mechanism of action relates to the activity of flavonoids as antioxidants. However, controlled clinical trials in humans have failed to confirm these observations possibly because the epidemiological data contained errors introduced by confounding factors and an incomplete database of food composition. Further research is clearly warranted.

References

Abu-Amsha, R., Croft, K.D., Puddey, I.B., Proudfoot, J.M. and Beilin, L.J. (1996) Phenolic content of various beverages determines the extent of inhibition of human serum and low-density lipoprotein oxidation *in vitro*: identification and mechanism of action of some cinnamic acid derivatives from red wine. *Clinical Science* 91, 449–458.

Aruoma, O.I., Halliwell, B., Aeschbach, R. and Loligers, J. (1992) Antioxidant and pro-oxidant properties of active rosemary constituents: carnosol and carnosic acid. *Xenobiotica* 22, 257–268.

Aruoma, O.I., Spencer, J.P., Rossi, R., Aeschbach, R., Khan, A., Mahmood, N., Munoz, A., Murcia, A., Butler, J. and Halliwell, B. (1996) An evaluation of the antioxidant and antiviral action of extracts of rosemary and Provencal herbs. *Food and Chemical Toxicology* 34, 449–456.

Bingham, S.A., Vorster, H., Jerling, J.C., Magee, E., Mulligan, A., Runswick, S.A. and Cummings, J.H. (1997) Effect of black tea drinking on blood lipids, blood pressure and aspects of bowel habit. *British Journal of Nutrition* 78, 41–55.

Cook, N.C. and Samman, S. (1996) Flavonoids – chemistry, metabolism, cardio-protective effects, and dietary sources. *Journal of Nutritional Biochemistry* 7, 66–76.

Demrow, H.S., Slane, P.R. and Folts, J.D. (1995) Administration of wine and grape juice inhibits *in vivo* platelet activity and thrombosis in stenosed canine coronary arteries. *Circulation* 91, 1182–1188.

Fahey, G.C. and Jung, H.-J.C. (1989) Phenolic compounds in forages and fibrous feedstuffs. In: Cheeke, P.R. (ed.) *Toxicants of Plant Origin*, Vol. IV, *Phenolics*. CRC Press, Boca Raton, Florida, pp. 141–148.

Frankel, E.N., Kanner, J., German, J.B., Parks, E. and Kinsella, J.E. (1993) Inhibition of oxidation of human low-density lipoprotein by phenolic substances in red wine. *Lancet* 341, 454–457.

Green, M.S. and Harabi, G. (1992) Association of serum lipoproteins and health-related habits with coffee and tea consumption in free-living subjects examined in the Israeli CORDIS study. *Preventive Medicine* 21, 532–545.

Gronbaek, M., Deis, A., Sorensen, T.I., Becker, U., Schnohr, P. and Jensen, G. (1995) Mortality associated with moderate intakes of wine, beer, or spirits. *British Medical Journal* 310, 1165–1169.

Hertog, M.G.L., Hollman, P.C.H. and Katan, M.B. (1992) Content of potentially anticarcinogenic flavonoid of 28 vegetables and 9 fruits commonly consumed in The Netherlands. *Journal of Agriculture and Food Chemistry* 40, 2379–2383.

Hertog, M.G.L., Feskens, E.J.M., Hollman, P.C.H., Katan, M.B. and Kromhout, D. (1993a) Dietary antioxidant flavonoids and risk of coronary heart disease: the Zutphen Elderly Study. *Lancet* 342, 1007–1011.

Hertog, M.G.L., Hollman, P.C.H. and Van de Putte, B. (1993b) Content of potentially anticarcinogenic flavonoids of tea infusions, wines and fruit juices. *Journal of Agriculture and Food Chemistry* 41, 1242–1246.

Hertog, M.G.L., Kromhout, D., Aravanis, C., Blackburn, H., Buzina, R., Fidanza, F., Giampaoli, S., Jansen, A., Menotti, A. and Nedeljkovic, S. (1995) Flavonoid intake and long-term risk of coronary heart disease and cancer in the Seven Countries Study. *Archives of Internal Medicine* 155, 381–386.

Hertog, M.G.L., Sweetnam, P.M., Fehily, A.M., Elwood, P.C. and Kromhout D. (1997) Antioxidant flavanols and ischaemic heart disease in a Welsh population of men: the Caerphilly Study. *American Journal of Clinical Nutrition* 65, 1489–1494.

van het Hof, K.H., de Boer, S.M., Wiseman, S.A., Lien, N., Weststrate, J.A. and Tijburg, L.B.M. (1997) Consumption of green or black tea does not increase resistance of low density lipoprotein to oxidation in humans. *American Journal of Clinical Nutrition* 66, 1125–1132.

Houlihan, C.M., Ho, C.T. and Chang, S.S. (1985) The structure of rosmariguinone – a new antioxidant isolated from *Rosemarinus officinalis* L. *Journal of the American Oil Chemists Society* 62, 96–98.

Huang, M.T., Ho, C.T., Wang, Z.Y., Ferraro, T., Lou, Y.R., Stauber, K., Ma, W., Georgiadis, C., Laskin, J.D. and Conney, A.H. (1994) Inhibition of skin tumorigenesis by rosemary and its constituents carnosol and ursolic acid. *Cancer Research* 54, 701–708.

Ikeda, I., Imasato, Y., Sasaki, E., Nakayama, M., Nagao, H., Takeo, T., Yayabe, F. and Sugano, M. (1992) Tea catechins decrease micellar solubility and intestinal absorption of cholesterol in rats. *Biochimica et Biophysica Acta* 1127, 141–146.

Imai, K. and Nakachi, K. (1995) Cross sectional study of effects of drinking green tea on cardiovascular and liver diseases. *British Medical Journal* 310, 693–696.

International Agency for Research on Cancer (IARC) (1991) Tea. In: *Coffee, Tea, Mate and Methylxanthines-Methylglyoxyl*. IARC Monographs on the Evaluation of Carcinogenic Risks to Humans, No. 51, IARC, Lyon, France, pp. 207–271.

Ishikawa,T., Suzukawa, M., Ito, T., Yoshida, H., Ayaori, M., Nishiwaki, M., Yonemura, A., Hara, Y. and Nakamura, H. (1997) Effect of tea flavonoid supplementation on the susceptibility of low-density lipoprotein to oxidative modification. *American Journal of Clinical Nutrition* 66, 261–266.

Keli, S.O., Hertog, M.G.L., Feskens, E.J.M. and Kromhout, S. (1996) Dietary flavonoids, antioxidant vitamins and incidence of stroke: the Zutphen Elderly Study. *Archives of Internal Medicine* 154, 637–642.

Kelly, G.E., Joannou, G.E., Reeder, A.Y., Nelson, C. and Waring, M.A. (1995) The variable metabolic response to dietary isoflavones in humans. *Proceedings of the Society of Experimental Biology and Medicine* 208, 40–43.

Klatsky, A.L., Armstrong, M.A. and Friedman, G.D. (1997) Red wine, white wine, liquor, beer, and risk of coronary artery disease hospitalization. *American Journal of Cardiology* 80, 416–420.

Knekt, P., Jarvinen, R., Reunanen, A. and Maatela, J. (1996) Flavonoid intake and coronary mortality in Finland: a cohort study. *British Medical Journal* 312, 478–481.

Lagouri, V. and Boskou, D. (1996) Nutrient antioxidants in oregano. *International Journal of Food Sciences and Nutrition* 47, 493–497.

Luo, M., Kannar, K., Wahlqvist, M.L. and O'Brien, R.C. (1997) Inhibition of LDL oxidation by green tea extract. *Lancet* 349, 360–361.

Lyons Wall, P.M. and Samman, S. (1997) Flavonoids – dietary perpectives and health benefits. *Proceedings of the Nutrition Society of Australia* 21, 106–114.

Mazur, W.M., Duke, J.A., Wahala, K., Rasku, S. and Adlercreutz, H. (1996) Phytoestrogens in legumes. In: *Proceedings of the International Symposium on the Role of Soy in Preventing and Treating Chronic Disease*, Vol. 2, pp. 52–53.

Miksikek, R.J. (1995) Estrogenic flavonoids: structural requirements for biological activity. *Proceedings of the Society of Experimental Biology and Medicine* 208, 44–50.

Miura, S., Watanabe, J., Tomita, T., Sano, M. and Tomita, I. (1994) The inhibitory effects of tea polyphenols (flavan-3-ol derivatives) on Cu^{2+} mediated oxidative modification of low density lipoprotein. *Biological and Pharmaceutical Bulletin* 17, 1567–1572.

Miyagi, Y., Miwa, K. and Inoue, H. (1997) Inhibition of human low density lipoprotein oxidation by flavonoids in red wine and grape juice. *American Journal of Cardiology* 80, 1627–1631.

Muramatsu, K., Fukuyo, M. and Hara, Y. (1986) Effect of green tea catechins on plasma cholesterol level in cholesterol-fed rats. *Journal of Nutritional Science and Vitaminology* 32, 613–622.

Nakatani, N., Inatani, R., Ohta, H. and Nishioka, A. (1986) Chemical constituents of peppers (*Piper* spp.) and application to food preservation: naturally occurring antioxidative compounds. *Environmental Health Perspectives* 67, 135–142.

Omenn, G.S., Goodman, G.E., Thornquist, M.D., Balmes, J., Cullen, M.R., Glass, A., Keogh, J.P., Meyskens, F.L., Valanis, B., Williams, J.H., Barnhart, S. and Hammar, S. (1996) Effects of a combination of beta carotene and vitamin A on lung cancer and cardiovascular disease. *New England Journal of Medicine* 334, 1150–1155.

Plumb, G.W., Chambers, S.J., Lambert, N., Wanigatunga, S., Fenwick, G.R. and Williamson, G. (1995) Evaluation of the antioxidant properties of food extracts. *Biochemical Society Transactions* 23, 254S.

Renaud, S. and de Longeril, M. (1992) Wine, alcohol, platelets and the French Paradox for coronary heart disease. *Lancet* 339, 1523–1526.

Rimm, E.B., Katan, M.B., Ascherio, A., Stampfer, M.J. and Willett, W.C. (1996) Relation between intake of flavonoids and risk of coronary heart disease in male health professionals. *Annals of Internal Medicine* 125, 384–389.

Salah, N., Miller, N.J., Paganga, G., Tijburg, L., Bolwell, G.P. and Rice-Evans, C. (1995) Polyphenolic flavanols as scavengers of aqueous phase radicals and as chain-breaking antioxidants. *Archives of Biochemistry and Biophysics* 322, 339–346.

Samman, S., Lyons Wall, P.M., Cook, N.C. and Naghii, M.R. (1996) Minor dietary factors in relation to coronary heart disease: flavonoids, isoflavones and boron. *Journal of Clinical Biochemistry and Nutrition* 20, 173–180.

Samman, S., Lyons Wall, P.M. and Cook, N.C. (1997) Flavonoids and coronary heart disease: dietary perspectives. In: Rice-Evans, C. and Packer, L. (eds) *Flavonoids in Health and Disease*. Marcel Dekker, New York, pp. 469–481.

Schwarz, B., Bischof, H.P. and Kunze, M. (1994) Coffee, tea, and lifestyle. *Preventive Medicine* 23, 377–384.

Schwarz, K. and Ternes, W. (1992) Antioxidative constituents of *Rosmarinus officinalis* and *Salvia officinalis*. I. Determination of phenolic diterpenes with antioxidative activity amongst tocochromanols using HPLC. *Zeitschrift für Lebensmittel-Untersuchung und -Forschung* 195, 95–98.

Srivastava, K.C. and Mustafa, T. (1989) Spices: antiplatelet activity and prostanoid metabolism. *Prostaglandins Leukotrienes and Essential Fatty Acids* 38, 255–266.

Stensvold, I., Tverdal, A., Solvoll, K. and Per Foss, O. (1992) Tea consumption. Relationship to cholesterol, blood pressure and coronary and total mortality. *Preventive Medicine* 21, 546–553.

Stephens, N.G., Parsons, A., Schofield, P.M., Kelly, F., Cheeseman, K. and Mitchinson, M.J. (1996) Randomised controlled trial of vitamin E in patients with coronary disease: Cambridge Heart Antioxidant Study (CHAOS). *Lancet* 347, 781–786.

Tew, B.-Y., Xu, X., Wang, H.-J., Murphy, P.A. and Hendrich, S. (1996) A diet high in wheat fibre decreases bioavailability of soybean isoflavones in a single meal fed to women. *Journal of Nutrition* 126, 871–877.

Vorster, H., Jerling, J., Oosthuizen, W., Cummings, J., Bingham, S., Magee, L., Mulligan, A. and Runswick, S. (1996) Tea drinking and haemostasis: a randomized, placebo-controlled, crossover study in free-living subjects. *Haemostasis* 26, 58–64.

Wang, H.J. and Murphy, P.A. (1994) Isoflavone content in commercial soybean foods. *Journal of Agriculture and Food Chemistry* 42, 1666–1673.

Whitehead, T.P., Robinson, D., Allaway, S., Syms, J. and Hale, A. (1995) Effect of red wine ingestion on the antioxidant capacity of serum. *Clinical Chemistry* 41, 32–35.

Xu, X., Harris, K.S., Wang, H.-J., Murphy, P.A. and Hendrich, S. (1995) Bioavailability of soybean isoflavones depends upon gut microflora in women. *Journal of Nutrition* 125, 2307–2315.

Antioxidant Vitamins and Coenzyme Q10 in the Prevention and Treatment of Coronary Artery Disease and Diabetes

16

RAM B. SINGH[1], SHANTI S. RASTOGI[2], MAHMOOD MOSHIRI[3] AND HEMMY N. BHAGVAN[4]

[1]Medical Hospital and Research Centre, Civil Lines, Moradabad-10, India; [2]Centre for Diabetes and Clinical Nutrition, Delhi, India; [3]Rajai Cardiovascular Research Centre, Tehran, Iran; [4]Tishcon Corporation, Westbury, New York, USA

Introduction

The incidence of such diseases as cardiovascular disease (CVD), diabetes and cancer show markedly different rates in different countries (WHO, 1990). For instance, populations living in Mediterranean countries and Japan enjoy a longer life expectancy than northern Europeans. Coronary heart disease (CHD) mortality is twofold greater in India than China, whereas stroke mortality is twofold higher in Chinese compared to Indians. Genetic or racial factors do not explain these societal differences as revealed by studies in Japanese migrants (WHO, 1990). These differences appear to depend on varied dietary patterns around the world.

India is clearly one part of the world which poses an enigma for epidemiologists. The prevalence of CHD is about 3–4% in rural Indians and 8–10% in urban north and west Indians. However, in urban south Indians and Indian immigrants to developed countries, the prevalence of CHD is about 14%. These two populations show a similarly high prevalence of diabetes: about 10% in south Indians and about 20% in immigrants to developed countries but with much lower rates in other Indian populations. Similarly wide variations are seen with hypertension. Another important factor has been the massive increase in incidence of these diseases in recent years. There is no clear dietary or lifestyle explanation for these observations (Indian Consensus Group, 1996; Indian Consensus Group for Prevention of Diabetes, 1997). This emphasizes the necessity for investigating such dietary factors as antioxidant vitamins and phytochemicals.

Antioxidant Vitamins and CHD

Oxidized LDL is now known to be more atherogenic than native LDL (see also Chapters 2 and 13). The extent of oxidation of LDL reflects the balance between oxidative stress and antioxidant defence. In the Indian diet, common oxidants include linoleic acid and cholesterol oxide. Although the Indian urban diet contains more fruit and vegetables than the rural diet, it also contains more fat and oxidants.

The Indian Lifestyle and Heart Study in Elderly, comprising 595 subjects aged 50–84 years, showed that 70 patients (11.7%) had diabetes and 72 (12.1%) had CHD (Singh *et al.*, 1995a). This study showed that the consumption of fruits, vegetables and legumes is half of that suggested by the World Health Organization (400 vs. 200 g day^{-1}) (Singh *et al.*, 1995a). One-third of the diabetic patients also had CHD. Dietary intake and plasma levels of vitamins C and E and β-carotene were significantly lower in patients with diabetes or CHD (Table 16.1). Similar observations have been made in other studies (Tables 16.2–16.4). Patients with glucose intolerance generally had intermediate levels of vitamins C and E but normal levels of β-carotene. In 505 patients with suspected acute myocardial infarction (MI), the plasma level of vitamin C was lower than in subjects without MI (Singh *et al.*, 1995c). These data imply that a poor intake of antioxidant vitamins is a risk factor for diabetes and CHD. Indians cook their green leafy vegetables by frying, half of them using open frying pans, and this is likely to destroy much of the antioxidant content (Singh *et al.*, 1995a; Singh and Niaz, 1996). These studies also revealed a raised level of plasma lipid peroxides, an index of free radical stress.

The Indian diet heart study, comprising 800 high-risk patients and those with CVD, showed that feeding a diet containing 600 g day^{-1} of fruit, vegetables, legumes and nuts significantly raises the plasma levels of vitamins A (retinol and β-carotene), E and C. This, in turn, led to a significant reduction in cardiac end-points within 2 years (Singh *et al.*, 1995d). In the Indian Experiment of Infarct Survival on 125 patients with suspected MI, 63 were administered vitamins A, E, C and β-carotene and 62 received the placebo for a period of 28 days (Singh *et al.*, 1996). Plasma levels of these nutrients increased significantly after supplementation. Conversely, plasma lipid peroxides declined in the supplemented group. The latter also had a reduced infarct size and improvements in electro-cardiographic (ECG) QRS score, angina, ventricular ectopics, and left ventricular enlargement and hypertrophy.

Table 16.1. Vitamin status and lipid peroxides in elderly subjects with glucose intolerance, diabetes and CHD. From Singh *et al.* (1995a).

	Glucose intolerance	Diabetes	CHD	Healthy
Vitamin intake				
Vitamin C (mg 1000 kcal^{-1})	34.5 (4)*	32.6 (3.8)*	31.5 (4.1)*	41.6 (4.6)
Vitamin E (mg 1000 kcal^{-1})	3.8 (0.4)*	3.8 (0.6)*	3.3 (0.5)*	4.7 (1.1)
β-Carotene (μg 1000 kcal^{-1})	1115 (95)	1082 (95)**	1086 (86)**	1110 (98)
Plasma level (mmol l^{-1})				
Vitamin C (μmol l^{-1})	32.6 (4.2)*	19.4 (3.1)**	20.3 (3.1)**	37.8 (5.6)
Vitamin E (μmol l^{-1})	18.1 (3.4)	14.2 (3.1)**	15.0 (2.6)**	20.2 (4.2)
β-Carotene (μmol l^{-1})	0.50 (0.08)	0.30 (0.05)**	0.31 (0.05)**	0.48 (0.09)
Lipid peroxides (nmol ml^{-1})	1.61 (0.18)	2.61 (0.21)**	2.61 (0.23)**	1.5 (0.12)

* $P < 0.05$; ** $P < 0.01$.
Values are mean (SD).

Table 16.2. Vitamin status and lipid peroxides in subjects with diabetes and CHD.

	Diabetes	CHD	Healthy
Vitamin intake			
Vitamin C (mg 1000 kcal^{-1})	30.5 (3.2)**	28.8 (3.1)**	37.5 (3.8)
Vitamin E (mg 1000 kcal^{-1})	4.2 (0.4)	3.1 (0.4)*	4.6 (0.6)
β-Carotene (μg 1000 kcal^{-1})	624 (30)*	605 (21)**	693 (38)
Plasma level			
Vitamin C (μg dl^{-1})	20.2 (2.8)**	21.6 (3.3)**	42.5 (4.5)
Vitamin E (μmol l^{-1})	15.6 (2.7)*	15.2 (2.8)*	21.4 (3.2)
β-Carotene (μmol l^{-1})	0.31 (0.05)**	0.33 (0.06)*	0.55 (0.08)
Lipid peroxides (nmol ml^{-1})	2.86 (0.22)	2.82 (0.22)*	1.6 (0.20)

* $P < 0.05$; ** $P < 0.01$.
Values are mean (SD).

Table 16.3. Vitamins status and lipid peroxides in subjects with diabetes. From Singh *et al.* (1995b).

	Diabetes (n=54)	Controls (n=202)
Vitamin intake		
Vitamin C (mg day^{-1})	95 (8.5)*	125 (18)
Vitamin E (mg day^{-1})	7.7 (1.2)*	9.2 (2.1)
β-Carotene (μg day^{-1})	1685 (212)*	2352 (305)
Plasma level		
Vitamin C (μmol l^{-1})	22.5 (3.5)*	27.4 (4.4)
Vitamin E (μmol l^{-1})	16.6 (2.1)*	19.2 (3.8)
β-Carotene (μmol l^{-1})	0.46 (0.1)*	0.51 (0.1)
Lipid peroxides (pmol l^{-1})	2.7 (0.4)*	1.4 (0.2)

* $P < 0.05$.
Values are mean (SD).

Consumption of 600 g day^{-1} of fruits, vegetables, legumes and nuts was associated with a significant reduction in lipid peroxides and a lower level of lactate dehydrogenase in the intervention group compared to the control group. This indicates that a diet rich in antioxidants can decrease cardiac damage during acute myocardial ischaemia and might also decrease atherosclerosis (Singh *et al.*, 1995e).

Coenzyme Q10 and disease

Coenzyme Q10 (CoQ10), also known as ubiquinone, is a naturally occurring compound and is synthesized in all body tissues. Fruit, vegetables, legumes and nuts as well as organ meat and fatty fish such as sardines and

Table 16.4. Vitamin status and lipid peroxides in subjects with diabetes and acute coronary disease. From Singh *et al.* (1994).

Plasma level	Diabetes with coronary disease (*n*=21)	Coronary disease without risk factors (*n*=50)	Diabetes (*n*=16)	Controls (*n*=110)
Vitamin C (μmol l^{-1})	3.0 (0.5)**	6.5 (1.4)*	24.6 (3.8)*	30.8 (4.1)
Vitamin E (μmol l^{-1})	13.0 (3.1)*	14.5 (3.5)*	16.4 (4)	18.3 (4.5)
β-Carotene (μmol l^{-1})	0.12 (0.03)**	0.18 (0.04)*	0.46 (1)*	0.58 (1.2)
Lipid peroxide (pmol l^{-1})	3.41 (0.8)*	2.8 (0.7)*	2.3 (0.3)*	2.3 (0.22)

* $P < 0.05$; ** $P < 0.01$.
Values are mean (SD).

mackerel are important sources of the coenzyme; however, the amount from dietary sources is probably insufficient to produce the clinical effects observed with therapeutic doses (Weber *et al.*, 1997). CoQ10 inadequacy can exist; this may be due to dietary insufficiency, impairment in synthesis, excessive utilization by the body (due to an increased antioxidant demand), or any combination of the three (Greenberg and Frishman, 1990). Most experts agree that the dominant source of CoQ10 is endogenous synthesis. There is increased requirement in several diseases including CHD, diabetes, obesity and cancer. It is likely that depleted body stores can predispose to several of the chronic diseases and that CoQ10 supplementation may be protective (Littarru *et al.*, 1972; Singh *et al.*, 1998a).

CoQ10 is an essential cofactor in the electron transport chain. It appears to possess membrane stabilization properties (Mitchell, 1991). There is also evidence that CoQ10 in a reduced form is a potent free-radical scavenger. In mitochondrial membranes CoQ10 is the first free-radical scavenger to be depleted prior to the onset of lipid peroxidation. The clinical benefits of CoQ10 are mainly due to its ability to improve energy production, its antioxidant activity and its membrane stabilizing properties. These effects are believed to be beneficial in the prevention and treatment of CVD, diabetes, ageing and cancer (Greenberg and Frishman, 1990; Ernster and Dallner, 1995; Singh *et al.*, 1998a).

CoQ10 in heart disease

Patients with more severe cardiac disease show lower cardiac levels of CoQ10 when compared to patients with less severe disease (Mortensen *et al.*, 1984). Decreased CoQ10 in myocardial tissue and in plasma has been reported in patients with heart failure as well as in general cardiac patients (Littarru *et al.*, 1972). This suggests that there is an impairment of CoQ10 synthesis or accelerated catabolism or both. The ubiquinol/ubiquinone ratio as a marker for oxidative stress in CHD has also been described (Lagendijk *et al.*, 1997). In experimental coronary artery ischaemia using a swine model, pretreatment with CoQ10 increased the ventricular fibrillation threshold while minimizing the impairment in contractility and myocardial stunning (Atar *et al.*, 1993).

These findings and the observation of myocardial protection by CoQ10 during ischaemia provided the rationale for the therapeutic use of CoQ10 administration in heart disease. In the mid 1960s it was used for the first time by Yamamura in the treatment of congestive heart failure (Littarru *et al.*, 1996).

Treatment with CoQ10 has been associated with improvement in cardiac energetics, namely a higher ejection fraction, improvement in clinical manifestations, decreased levels of serum catecholamines, better work capacity, decreased frequency of hospitalization and prolonged survival (Littarru, 1994). CoQ10 protects ischaemic tissue from reperfusion damage by its antioxidant and free-radical scavenging activities. The membrane-stabilizing property is distinct from its ability to neutralize free radicals (Mitchell, 1991). Its actions resemble angiotensin-converting enzyme inhibitors, potassium channel activators and trimetazidine.

The beneficial effects of either intravenous or oral CoQ10 in patients with congestive heart failure have been reported in several studies (Soja and Mortensen, 1997). In dilated cardiomyopathy it was reported that patients with a greater inadequacy of CoQ10 at baseline showed a better response to treatment with CoQ10 compared with those with mild inadequacy (Folkers *et al.*, 1985). CoQ10 also appears to be protective against damage to the myocardium during surgery (Takasawa *et al.*, 1991). Its antiarrhythmic effects have been studied in several experiments.

CoQ10 is a potential anti-anginal medication. In a controlled trial, intravenous CoQ10 (1.5 mg kg^{-1} once daily for 7 days) was administered to 18 patients with chronic stable angina. The mean exercise time showed significant increase compared to placebo treatment from a baseline of 4.6 ± 2.0 to 7.2 ± 2.5 min. Heart rate and blood pressure showed little change (Greenberg and Frishman, 1990).

At least five double-blind intervention trials have been published concerning the therapeutic benefit of CoQ10 in CHD. Kamikawa *et al.* (1985) administered oral CoQ10 (150 mg day^{-1}) or placebo for 4 weeks to 12 patients with chronic stable angina. This was followed by a crossover to the opposing treatment regimen for another 4 weeks. Exercise time and time to onset of 1 mm ECG ST–depression were significantly increased in the CoQ10 group compared to the placebo group. Schardt *et al.* (1986) compared the effects of 600 mg day^{-1} of oral CoQ10 with placebo in a double-blind crossover study in 15 patients with chronic stable angina. Treatment with CoQ10 was associated with a significant reduction in cumulative exercise-induced ST-segment depression but no difference was noted compared with conventional anti-anginal drugs. There was a significant reduction in exercise systolic blood pressure during CoQ10 treatment compared to the placebo treatment.

The effect of CoQ10 (150 or 300 mg day^{-1}) was compared with placebo in 37 patients with stable angina (Wilson *et al.*, 1991). CoQ10 caused an increase in exercise duration to onset of angina of 70 s in the 300 mg group and 65 s in the 150 mg group at the end of the first week and of 140 and 127 s, respectively, by week 4. There was a 60% decrease in the frequency of anginal attacks in the 150 mg group.

In postinfarction patients, treatment with CoQ10 caused a significant beneficial effect on work capacity and a significantly lower level of plasma malondialdehyde in the treatment group compared to placebo (Rossi *et al.*, 1991). In one 58-year-old patient with diabetes and unstable angina, addition of CoQ10 (60 mg day^{-1}) to treatment with nitrates and calcium blockers was associated with exercise tolerance and relief of angina within 2 weeks, although no response had been observed during the previous 4 weeks with conventional drugs (Singh *et al.*, 1998a). The exact mechanism of improved exercise capacity after CoQ10 therapy is not clear but is likely to be due to increased energy (ATP) production, direct membrane protection and antioxidant protection. It is also possible that CoQ10 may activate ATP-sensitive potassium channels and modulate calcium channels.

Currently, CoQ10 is being studied in the developed countries for its anti-anginal efficacy. The results of the Indian Experiment of Infarct Survival in 144 patients provide further evidence regarding the role of CoQ10 in MI (Singh *et al.*, 1998c). We also showed that treatment with CoQ10 is associated with a significant decrease in plasma insulin response and lipoprotein (a) (unpublished observations). In one study of 61 patients with MI, treatment with CoQ10 plus selenium was associated with significant benefit (Kuklinski *et al.*, 1994).

Much of a dose of CoQ10 is secreted by the liver in very-low-density lipoprotein. Excretion is via the biliary tract and approximately 63% of the administered dose may be recovered in the stool. During chronic administration, CoQ10 is concentrated in the liver, myocardial and other tissues. It is poorly absorbed because of its very low solubility in lipids. However, hydrosoluble forms of CoQ10 are now available which have vastly superior absorption (Q-Gel, Tishcon Corp., Westbury, New York, USA) and can raise plasma levels to the therapeutic range within 4 h and maximum levels in a few days (Chopra *et al.*, 1998).

CoQ10 in hypertension

The role of CoQ10 in decreasing blood pressure has been known since 1972. Yamagami *et al.* (1977) found low CoQ10 status in 29 patients with hypertension and treatment with CoQ10 (1–2 mg kg^{-1} day^{-1}) caused a decrease in blood pressure. In a pilot study they administered 30–45 mg day^{-1} of CoQ10 to 17 patients with hypertension for 2–16 weeks (Yamagami *et al.*, 1977). This produced a beneficial effect in only four patients. In another study by Yamagami *et al.* (1986), 20 patients having low serum CoQ10 levels were administered either 100 mg CoQ10 or placebo for 12 weeks. Treatment with CoQ10 was associated with a significant decrease in blood pressure. Montaldo *et al.* (1991) administered CoQ10, 100 mg day^{-1} for 3 months, to 15 patients with hypertension. There was a significant reduction in blood pressure, both at rest and during exercise, together with a significant improvement in myocardial stroke work index. Digiesi *et al.* (1994) also studied the role of CoQ10 in hypertension and reported a decrease in total peripheral resistance which may have been due to improvement in arteriolar smooth muscle cell metabolism. In a study by Langsjoen *et al.* (1994) in 109 patients with essential hypertension, CoQ10 (225 mg day^{-1}) improved the effectiveness of antihypertensive drugs. CoQ10 also caused a significant decrease in serum catecholamines and possibly reduced peripheral vascular resistance.

The available data thus indicate that a study should be conducted with higher doses of a more bioavailable form of CoQ10 (Q-Gel, Tishcon Corp.) with a follow-up of at least 12 weeks to further investigate its effectiveness in decreasing blood pressure.

CoQ10 and lipoproteins

The antioxidant content of LDL becomes depleted following exposure to free radicals. Vitamin C is the first antioxidant to be used up followed by reduced levels of CoQ10. When LDL depleted of vitamin C is exposed to a free-radical source, peroxidation remains under control as long as CoQ10 as ubiquinol is present (Merati *et al.*, 1992). However, when ubiquinol is completely oxidized, lipid peroxidation starts despite 95% of the vitamin E and 80% of the carotenoid content still being present.

It is noteworthy that a higher LDL/CoQ10 ratio is associated with CHD. It seems that decreases in this ratio, whether by increasing blood CoQ10, by decreasing the LDL level or both, may be protective against CHD. Plasma ubiquinol-10 may be decreased in patients with hyperlipidaemia (Kontush *et al.*, 1997).

In one experimental study, Singh *et al.* (1997) demonstrated that lovastatin has a modest antioxidant activity. However, statin drugs lead to a reduction in CoQ10 status due to their inhibition of endogenous CoQ10 synthesis. This indicates that treatment of hypercholesterolaemia with these drugs should be combined with CoQ10 to prevent its depletion.

Antioxidant Vitamins and CoQ10 in Diabetes in Relation to Vascular Disease

The evidence concerning the role of antioxidants and free radicals in human diabetes is limited (Oberley, 1988; Packer, 1993; Wolff, 1993). A low intake and plasma level of vitamins C and E and β-carotene has been observed in patients with diabetes compared to control subjects (Tables 16.1–16.4).

Oxidative stress seems to play an important role in the development of diabetes and CVD. In several of our clinical and epidemiological studies, we have reported that plasma levels of lipid peroxides are significantly higher among patients with diabetes and CHD compared to healthy subjects (Tables 16.1–16.3). Those diabetics with vascular complications tend to have higher lipid peroxide levels compared to diabetics without such complications (Table 16.4). Bambolker and Sainani (1995) also reported greater oxidative stress in diabetics with complications compared to those with uncomplicated diabetes.

There is increased utilization of antioxidant vitamins and ubiquinol in diabetes. Plasma copper levels are higher and magnesium and zinc levels are lower in diabetes and CHD (Mateo *et al.*, 1978; Noto *et al.*, 1983). Free copper ions are known to catalyse ascorbate oxidation and substances such as aldos reductase inhibitor may block such reactions by binding free copper ions (Jiang *et al.*, 1991). Zinc deficiency is associated with insulin resistance, and zinc therapy is capable of modulating insulin action (Kinlaw *et al.*, 1983). Zinc may work as an antioxidant through superoxide dismutase. Zinc deficiency may also decrease the zinc/copper ratio and thereby increase the adverse effects of copper ions on oxidant stress in diabetes. There is no evidence that once oxidative damage occurs, it can be reversed. Modification of long-lived extracellular proteins and structural changes in tissues rich in proteins are associated with the development of complications in diabetes such as cataracts, microangiopathy, atherosclerosis and nephropathy.

It is difficult to determine whether increased lipid peroxidation is a cause or an effect of complications in diabetes. It may be more appropriate to consider lipid peroxidation as part of a continuous cycle of oxidative stress and damage. Recent studies indicate an increased oxidative stress and lower plasma level of carotenoids in patients with severe obesity (Ohrvall *et al.*, 1993; Pipek *et al.*, 1996). Obesity is an independent risk factor for diabetes and this finding suggests that oxidative stress in obese subjects may be a risk factor for diabetes.

There are only a few studies showing the role of CoQ10 in diabetes. In a study of 120 diabetic patients, 8.3% showed CoQ10 deficiency compared with 1.9% of healthy subjects (Kishi, 1976). The incidence of CoQ10 deficiency was 20% among patients receiving oral hypoglycaemic agents indicating that these drugs might interfere with CoQ10 metabolism. In another study CoQ7, which is similar to CoQ10, was administered to patients with diabetes at a dosage of 120 mg day^{-1} for 2–18 weeks (Shigeta *et al.*, 1966). Fasting blood glucose decreased by 30% among 12 (31%) of 39 patients. There was a marked reduction (30%) in ketone bodies among 13 (59%) of 22 patients. Cessation of treatment was associated with an increase in blood glucose in a few patients. The mechanism by which CoQ10 modulates blood glucose is not clear. Possibly, it induces synthesis of CoQ10-dependent enzymes which in turn enhance carbohydrate metabolism. CoQ10 also regenerates vitamin E which indicates that CoQ10 might improve insulin sensitivity. This hypothesis is further suggested by the fact that the resistance of peripheral tissues to glucose uptake may be a consequence of permanently high lipid oxidation. The oxidation of lipids could be enhanced if the concentration of lipid-soluble antioxidants such as CoQ10 and vitamin E are low.

There are no published studies on the role of CoQ10 in patients with diabetes associated with vascular disease. However, in several studies CoQ10 has been shown to be beneficial in patients with angina, CHD, heart failure, hypertension and cardiomyopathy (Kuklinski *et al.*, 1994; Karlsson *et al.*, 1996, 1997; Barbiroli *et al.*, 1997; Lagendijk *et al.*, 1997). In one study CoQ was shown to be beneficial in patients with unstable angina (Table 16.5) (Kamikawa, 1985). We have shown its beneficial effects in refractory heart disease, namely a significant decrease in blood glucose levels and an improvement in refractory heart failure in all the subjects (Table 16.6).

There have been few clinical trials on the role of antioxidants in diabetes (Raheja and Sodikot, 1991; Sadikot and Raheja, 1991). In a small, double-blind randomized crossover trial in 15 non-insulin-dependent diabetic and 10 healthy subjects, supplementation with 900 mg vitamin E daily for 4 months reduced oxidative stress and improved insulin action. In a euglycaemic hyperinsulinaemic glucose clamp (Caballero, 1993; Paolisso *et al.*, 1993), treatment with vitamin E reduced the area under the curve of plasma glucose and increased the total body glucose disposal and non-oxidative glucose metabolism in both healthy and diabetic subjects.

Vitamin E (400–800 mg day^{-1}), β-carotene (20–50 mg day^{-1}), vitamin C (500–1000 mg day^{-1}) and CoQ10 (60–300 mg day^{-1}) may be administered to diabetics without any significant side effects. However, long-term follow-up intervention trials are necessary to demonstrate the benefit of antioxidants in the prevention of complications in diabetes and to assess whether the above doses can be safely used. It may be prudent to advise a daily intake of 600 g of fruit, vegetables and legumes (plus vegetable oils rich in omega-3 fatty acids) for primary prevention of diabetes and CVD because these foods are rich sources of antioxidants and phytochemicals (Singh *et al.*, 1995c, d).

Table 16.5. Effect of CoQ10 in patients with unstable angina.

Data (*n*=12)	Baseline	CoQ10	Placebo
Frequency of anginal attacks/2 weeks	4.6 (4.1)	2.5 (3.3)	5.3 (4.9)
Nitroglycerin consumption/2 weeks	2.8 (2.8)	1.3 (1.7)	2.6 (2.8)
Exercise time (s)	340 (126)	406 (114)	345 (102)[*]
Time to onset of 1 mm ECG ST-depression (s)	205 (90)	284 (104)	196 (76)[**]

[*] $P < 0.05$; [**] $P < 0.01$.
Values are mean (SD).

Table 16.6. CoQ10 therapy in refractory heart disease.

Disease	Age	Drug therapy	Duration	CoQ10	FBG (mM) Before	FBG (mM) After
Refractory ventricular ectopics CHD, diabetes	47 male ($n = 1$)	Lignocaine Dysopiramide	4 weeks	20 mg thrice daily × 2 weeks	8.33	7.33
Refractory angina, diabetes	58 male ($n = 1$)	Nitrates, diltiazem	7 weeks	20 mg thrice daily × 3 weeks	8.22	7.67
Refractory heart failure, diabetes, CHD	46 male ($n = 1$)	Digoxin, nitrates, Enalepril, maliate, Furosemide	6 weeks	20 mg thrice daily × 3 weeks	10.56	8.67
Refractory heart failure diabetes, CHD	52 female ($n = 1$)	Digoxin, nitrate, enalepril, maliate, furosemide	5 weeks	20 mg thrice daily × 2 weeks	9.11	8.06
Refractory cardiogenic shock, CHD, diabetes	54 male ($n = 1$)	Dopamine, dobutamine, hydrocortisone hemvisuccinate	48 h	20 mg four times daily × 1 week	7.67	7.50

CAD, coronary artery disease; FBG, fasting blood glucose.

References

Atar, D., Mortensen, S.A., Flachs, H. and Herzog, W.R. (1993) Coenzyme Q10 protects ischemic myocardium in an open chest swine model. *Clinical Investigation* 71, 103–111.

Bambolker, S. and Sainani, G.S. (1995) Evaluation of oxidative stress in diabetics with or without vascular complications. *Journal of the Association of Physicians of India* 43, 10–12.

Barbiroli, B., Frassineti, C., Martinelli, P., Iotti, S., Lodi, R., Corfeth, P. and Montoam, P. (1997) Coenzyme Q10 improves mitochondrial respiration in patients with mitochondrial cytopathies. An *in vivo* study on brain and skeletal muscle by phosphorous magnetic resonance spectroscopy. *Cellular and Molecular Biology* 43, 741–749.

Caballero, B. (1993) Vitamin E improves the action of insulin. *Nutrition Reviews* 51, 339–340.

Chopra, R.K., Goldman, R., Sinatra, S.T. and Bagavan, H.N. (1998) Relative bioavailability of coenzyme Q10 formulations in human subjects. *International Journal of Vitamin and Nutritional Research* 68, 109–113.

Digiesi, V., Cantini, F., Oradei, A., Bisi, G., Guarino, G.C., Brocchi, A., Bellandi, F., Mancini, M. and Littarru, G.P. (1994) Coenzyme Q10 in essential hypertension. *Molecular Aspects of Medicine* 15 (Suppl.), 255–263.

Ernster, L. and Dallner, G. (1995) Biochemical, physiological and medical aspects of ubiquinone function. *Biochimica et Biophysica Acta* 1271, 195–204.

Folkers, K., Vadhanavikit, S. and Mortensen, S.A. (1985) Biochemical rationale and myocardial tissue data on the effective therapy of cardiomyopathy with coenzyme Q10. *Proceedings of the National Academy of Sciences, USA* 82, 901–911.

Greenberg, S. and Frishman, W.H. (1990) Coenzyme Q10; a new drug for cardiovascular disease. *Journal of Clinical Pharmacology* 30, 596–608.

Indian Consensus Group (1996) Indian consensus for prevention of hypertension and coronary artery disease. *Journal of Nutritional and Environmental Medicine* 6, 309–318.

Indian Consensus Group for Prevention of Diabetes (1997) Diet and lifestyle guidelines and desirable levels of risk factors for the prevention of diabetes and its vascular complications in Indians: a scientific statement of the International College of Nutrition. *Journal of Cardiovascular Risk* 4, 201–208.

Jiang, Z.Y., Qiong, L.Z., Eaton, J.W., Hunt, J.V., Koppenol, W.H. and Wolf, S.P. (1991) Spirohydantoin inhibitors of aldose reductase inhibit iron and copper catalysed ascorbic oxidation *in vitro*. *Biochemical Pharmacology* 42, 1273–1278.

Kamikawa, T., Kobayashi, A., Yamashuta, T., Hayashi, H. and Yamasaki, N. (1985) Effects of coenzyme Q10 on exercise tolerance in chronic stable angina pectoris. *American Journal of Cardiology* 56, 247–251.

Karlsson, J. and Semb, B. (1996) Muscle ubiquinone and plasma antioxidants in effort angina. *Journal of Nutritional and Environmental Medicine* 6, 255–266.

Karlsson, J., Lin, L., Gunnes, S., Sylven, C., Astrom, H., Jansson, E. and Semb, B. (1997) Muscle characteristics in effort angina before and after CABG. *Canadian Journal of Cardiology* 13, 577–582.

Kinlaw, W.B., Levine, A.S., Morley, J.E., Silvis, S.E. and McClain, C.J. (1983) Abnormal zinc metabolism in type II diabetes mellitus. *American Journal of Medicine* 75, 273–277.

Kishi, T. (1976) Bioenergetics in clinical medicine. XI. Studies on coenzyme Q and diabetes mellitus. *Journal of Medicine* 7, 307–312.

Kontush, A., Reich, A., Baum, K., Spranger T., Finckh, B., Kohlschutter, A. and Beisiegel, U. (1997) Plasma ubiquinol-10 is decreased in patients with hyperlipidemia. *Atherosclerosis* 129, 119–126.

Kuklinski, B., Weissenbacher, E, and Fahnrich, A. (1994) Coenzyme Q10 and antioxidants in acute myocardial infarction. *Molecular Aspects of Medicine* 15 (Suppl.), 143–147.

Lagendijk, J., Ubbink, J.B. Delport, R., Vermaak W.J. and Human, J.A. (1997) Ubiquinol/ubiquinone ratio as a marker of oxidative stress in coronary artery disease. *Research Communications in Molecular Pathology and Pharmacology* 95, 11–20.

Langsjoen, P., Langsjoen, A., Willis, R. and Folkers, K. (1994) Treatment of essential hypertension with coenzyme Q10. *Molecular Aspects of Medicine* 15 (Suppl.), 265–272.

Littarru, G.P., Ho, L. and Folkers, K. (1972) Deficiency of coenzyme Q10 in human heart disease. Part I and II. *International Journal of Vitamin and Nutritional Research* 42, 291–305, 413–434.

Littarru, G.P., Battino, M. and Folkers, K. (1996) Clinical aspects of coenzyme Q. In: Cadenas, E. and Packer, L. (eds) *Handbook of Antioxidants.* Marcel Dekker, New York, pp. 203–237.

Mateo, M.C.M., Bustamante, J.B. and Cantalapiedra, M.A.G. (1978) Serum, zinc, copper and insulin in diabetes mellitus. *Biomedicine* 29, 56–58.

Merati, G., Pasquali, P., Vergani, C. and Landi, L. (1992) Antioxidant activity of ubiquinone-3 in human low density lipoprotein. *Free Radical Research Communications* 16, 11–17.

Mitchell, P. (1991) The vital protonmotive role of coenzyme Q. In: Folkers, K., Littarru, G.P. and Yamagami, T. (eds) *Biomedical and Clinical Aspects of Coenzyme Q*, Vol. 6. Elsevier, Amsterdam, pp. 3–10.

Montaldo, P.L., Fadda, G., Salis, S., Satta, G., Tronci, M., Dicesare, R., Reina, R. and Concu, A. (1991) Effects of the prolonged administration of coenzyme Q10 in borderline hypertensive patients: a hemodynamic study. In: Folkers, K., Littarru, G.P. and Yamagami, T. (eds) *Biomedical and Clinical Aspects of Coenzyme Q*, Vol. 6. Elsevier, Amsterdam, pp. 417–424.

Mortensen, S.A., Vadhanavikit, S. and Folkers, K. (1984) Deficiency of coenzyme Q10 in myocardial failure. *Journal of Drugs in Experimental and Clinical Research* 10, 497–502.

Noto, R., Alicata, R. and Sfolgliano, L. (1983) A study of cupremia in a group of elderly diabetics. *Acta Diabetologica Latina* 20, 81–85.

Oberley, L. (1988) Free radicals and diabetes. *Free Radical Biology and Medicine* 5, 113–124.

Ohrvall, M., Tengblad, S. and Vessby, B. (1993) Lower tocopherol serum levels in subjects with abdominal obesity. *Journal of Internal Medicine* 234, 53–60.

Packer, L. (1993) The role of antioxidative treatment in diabetes mellitus. *Diabetologia* 36, 1212–1213.

Paolisso, G., D'Amore, A., Giugliano, D., Ceriell, A., Varrichio, M. and D'Onofrio, F. (1993) Pharmacologic doses of vitamin E improve insulin action in healthy subjects and non-insulin dependent diabetic patients. *American Journal of Clinical Nutrition* 57, 650–656.

Pipek, R., Dankner, G., Ben-Amotz, A., Aviram, M. and Levy, Y. (1996) Increased plasma oxidizability in subjects with severe obesity. *Journal of Nutritional and Environmental Medicine* 6, 267–272.

Raheja, B.S. and Sadikot, S.M. (1991) Vitamin C supplementation decreases oxidant stress and free radical damage in diabetes. *Journal of the Diabetes Association of India* 31, 79–81.

Rossi, E., Lombardo, A., Testa, M., Lippa, S., Oradei, A., Littarru, G.P., Lucente, M., Coppola, E. and Manzoli, U. (1991) Coenzyme Q10 is ischaemic cardiopathy. In: Folkers, K., Littarru, G.P. and Yamagami, T. (eds) *Biomedical and Clinical Aspects of Coenzyme Q*, Vol. 6. Elsevier, Amsterdam, pp. 321–326.

Sadikot, S.M. and Raheja, B.S. (1991) Vitamin E supplementation and oxidant stress in diabetes. *Journal of the Diabetes Association of India* 31, 68–70.

Schardt, F., Weizel, D., Schess, W. and Toda, K. (1986) Effect of coenzyme Q10 on ischaemia induced ST-segment depression: a double blind placebo controlled crossover study. In: Folkers, K., Littarru, G.P. and Yamamura, Y. (eds) *Biomedical and Clinical Aspects of Coenzyme Q*, Vol. 5. Elsevier, Amsterdam, pp. 385–394.

Shigeta, Y., Izumi, and Abe, H. (1996) Effect of coenzyme Q7 treatment on blood sugar and ketone bodies of diabetics. *Journal of Vitaminology* 12, 293–297.

Singh, R.B. and Niaz, M.A. (1996) Antioxidants, oxidants and free radical stress in cardiovascular disease. *Journal of the Association of Physicians of India* 44, 43–48.

Singh, R.B., Niaz, M.A., Gupta, S., Ahmad, S., Rastogi, S.S., Raizada, M., Beegom, R., Shoumin, Z., Hong, C. and Sharma, J.P. (1994a) Diet, antioxidant vitamins, oxidative stress and risk of coronary disease. *Acta Cardiologica* 49, 453–467.

Singh, R.B., Niaz, M.A., Sharma, J.P., Rastogi, S.S., Ghosh, S., Kumar, R. and Raizada, M. (1994b) Plasma levels of antioxidant vitamins and oxidative stress in patients with acute myocardial infarction. *Acta Cardiologica* 49, 441–452.

Singh, R.B., Ghosh, S., Niaz, M.A., Singh, R., Beegom, R., Chhibo, H., Shoumin, Z. and Postiglione, A. (1995a) Dietary intakes, plasma levels of antioxidant vitamins and free radical stress in relation to coronary artery disease in the elderly subjects. *American Journal of Cardiology* 76, 1233–1238.

Singh, R.B., Niaz, M.A., Ghosh, S., Beegom, R. and Rastogi, S.S. (1995b) Dietary intakes and plasma levels of antioxidant vitamins in health and disease: a hospital based case control study. *Journal of Nutritional and Environmental Medicine* 5, 235–242.

Singh, R.B., Niaz, M.A., Agarwal, P., Beegom, R. and Rastogi, S.S. (1995c) Effect of antioxidant rich foods on plasma ascorbic acid, cardiac enzyme, lipid peroxides levels in patients hospitalized with acute myocardial infarction. *Journal of the American Dietetic Association* 95, 775–780.

Singh, R.B., Niaz, M.A., Rastogi, S.S. and Beegom, R. (1995d) The influence of antioxidant rich diet on plasma antioxidant vitamins, oxidative stress and mortality and reinfarction in the Indian diet heart study (abstract). Asian Pacific Congress of Cardiology, Indonesia.

Singh, R.B., Niaz, M.A., Ghosh, S., Rastogi, S.S. and Beegom, R. (1995e) Randomized controlled trial of antioxidant vitamins and cardioprotective diet in hyperlipidemia, oxidative stress and development of atherosclerosis. The diet and antioxidant trial in atherosclerosis (DATA). *Cardiovascular Drugs and Therapy* 9, 763–771.

Singh, R.B., Niaz, M.A., Ghosh, S., Rastogi, S.S. and Beegom, R. (1996) Usefulness of antioxidant vitamins A, E and C and beta-carotene in patients with suspected acute myocardial infarction. *American Journal of Cardiology* 77, 232–236.

Singh, R.B., Singh, N.K., Rastogi, S.S., Wander G.S., Aslam, M., Onouchi, Z., Kummerow, F. and Nangia, S. (1997) Antioxidant effects of lovastatin and vitamin E on experimental atherosclerosis in rabbits. *Cardiovascular Drugs and Therapy* 11, 575–580.

Singh, R.B., Niaz, M.A., Rastogi, V. and Rastogi. S.S. (1998a) Coenzyme Q in cardiovascular disease. *Journal of the Association of Physicians of India* 46, 299–306.

Singh, R.B., Wander, G.S., Rastogi, A., Shukla, P.K., Mittal, A., Sharma, J.P., Mehiotra, S.K. and Kapoor, R. (1998b) Randomized, double blind placebo controlled trial of coenzyme Q10 in acute myocardial infarction. *Cardiovascular Drug and Therapy* 12, 347–353.

Soja, A.M. and Mortensen, S.A. (1997) Treatment of congestive heart failure with coenzyme Q10 illuminated by metaanalysis of clinical trials. *Molecular Aspects of Medicine* 18 (Suppl.), 159–168.

Takasawa, K., Fuse, K., Konishi, T. and Watanabe, Y. (1991) Prevention of premature ventricular contractions with coenzyme Q10 after coronary artery bypass grafting. In: Folkers, K., Littarru, G.P. and Yamagami, T. (eds) *Biomedical and Clinical Aspects of Coenzyme Q*, Vol. 4. Elsevier, Amsterdam, pp. 357–359.

Weber, C., Bysted, A. and Hllmer, G. (1997) The coenzyme Q10 content of the average Danish diet. *International Journal of Vitamin and Nutritional Research* 67, 123–129.

Wilson, M.F., Frishman, W.H., Giles, T., Sethi, G., Greenberg, S.M. and Brackett, D.J. (1991) Coenzyme Q10 therapy and exercise duration in stable angina. In: Folkers, K., Littarru, G.P. and Yamagami, T. (eds) *Biomedical and Clinical Aspects of Coenzyme Q*, Vol. 6. Elsevier, Amsterdam, pp. 339–348.

Wolff, S.P. (1993) Diabetes mellitus and free radicals. Free radicals, transition metals and oxidative stress in the aetiology of diabetes mellitus and complications. *British Medical Bulletin* 49, 642–652.

World Health Organization Study Group (1990) *Diet, Nutrition, and the Prevention of Chronic Diseases.* WHO, Geneva.

Yamagami, T., Shibata, N. and Folkers, K. (1977) Study of coenzyme Q10 in essential hypertension. In: Folkers, K. and Yamamura, Y. (eds) *Biomedical and Clinical Aspects of Coenzyme Q*, Vol. 1. Elsevier, Amsterdam, pp. 231–242.

Yamagami, T., Takagi, M., Akagami, H., Kubo, H., Toyama, S., Okamoto, T., Kishi, T. and Folkers, K. (1986) Effect of coenzyme Q10 on essential hypertension, a double blind controlled study. In: Folkers, K., Littarru, G.P. and Yamamura, Y. (eds) *Biomedical and Clinical Aspects of Coenzyme Q*, Vol. 5. Elsevier, Amsterdam, pp. 337–343.

Fruit, Vegetables and Antioxidants: Their Role in the Prevention of Cardiovascular and Other Diseases

17

JAYNE V. WOODSIDE[1],
IAN S. YOUNG[2] AND
JOHN W.G. YARNELL[3]

[1] Department of Surgery, University College London Medical School, London, UK;
[2] Department of Clinical Biochemistry, Institute of Clinical Science, Belfast, UK;
[3] Department of Epidemiology and Public Health, Institute of Clinical Science, Belfast, UK

Introduction

Hypercholesterolaemia is universally accepted as a major risk factor for atherosclerosis. However, at any given concentration of blood cholesterol, there is still great variability in the risk of cardiovascular events. One of the major breakthroughs in atherogenesis research has been the realization that oxidative modification of LDL may be a critically important step in the development of the atherosclerotic plaque (Fig. 17.1). The formation of foam cells from monocyte-derived macrophages in early atherosclerotic lesions is not induced by native LDL but only by LDL modifications such as oxidation (Witztum and Steinberg, 1991).

Evidence for LDL oxidation *in vivo* is now overwhelming. In immunocytochemical studies, antibodies against oxidized LDL stain atherosclerotic lesions but not normal arterial tissue (Palinski *et al.*, 1989). LDL extracted from animal and human lesions has been shown to be oxidized and is rapidly taken up by macrophage scavenger receptors (Yla-Herttuala *et al.*, 1989). In young myocardial infarction (MI) survivors, an association has

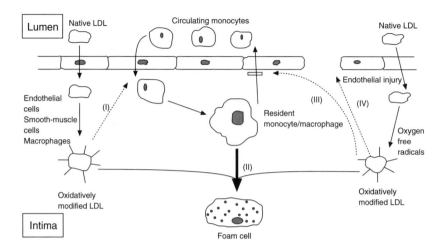

Fig. 17.1. Mechanisms by which oxidation of LDL may contribute to atherogenesis. Oxidized LDL is chemotactic for circulating monocytes (I). These are phenotypically modified and become macrophages. Oxidized LDL is recognized by the scavenger receptor on the macrophage and becomes internalized rapidly. As more lipid is ingested by the macrophage, a foam cell is formed (II). This eventually bursts and a fatty streak, the first phase of an atherosclerotic lesion, results. Oxidized LDL inhibits the motility of resident macrophages and therefore their ability to leave the intima (III). Oxidized LDL is cytotoxic to endothelial cells, leading directly to endothelial cell damage (IV). Oxidation can occur via the effects of reactive oxygen species or due to the oxidation of the cell's own lipids. Adapted from Steinberg *et al.* (1989).

been demonstrated between increased susceptibility of LDL to oxidation and the degree of coronary atherosclerosis (Regnstrom *et al.*, 1992), while the presence of ceroid, a product of lipid peroxidation, has been shown in advanced atherosclerotic plaques (Ball *et al.*, 1987).

Antioxidants and LDL Oxidation

The role of dietary factors in protecting against the change from native to oxidized LDL has received considerable attention. An overview of epidemiological research suggests that individuals with the highest intakes of antioxidant vitamins, whether through diet or supplements, tend to experience 20–40% lower risk of coronary heart disease (CHD) than those with the lowest intake or blood levels (Gaziano, 1994; also see Chapter 13). Vitamin E is the major lipid-soluble antioxidant present in LDL preventing the formation of lipid hydroperoxides from polyunsaturated fatty acids. Vitamin C can scavenge free radicals in the cytoplasm and may also regenerate vitamin E (Leake, 1993). β-Carotene, a vitamin A precursor, does not have a confirmed antioxidant mechanism (Frei, 1995), although it is contained within LDL (Duthie and Wahle, 1990).

The antioxidant vitamins cannot be synthesized from simple precursors. They are derived mainly from fresh fruit and vegetables. Vitamin E is obtained from vegetable oil and polyunsaturated margarine. In addition, it is sometimes added to margarine as an antioxidant. Thus, concentrations of these vitamins in blood and body tissues are determined by dietary intake, absorption, metabolism and storage.

A number of studies have evaluated the effects of vitamin E on copper-catalysed LDL oxidation in healthy volunteers. Men supplemented with 268, 537 or 805 mg of vitamin E per day for 8 weeks showed a decreased susceptibility of LDL to oxidation. There was no significant effect of daily supplementation with 40 or 134 mg (Jialal and Grundy, 1992). In a study of the effects of low-dose vitamin E supplementation (100 mg day^{-1} for 1 week, then 200 mg day^{-1} for 3 weeks), there was a significant increase in lag time before the onset of LDL oxidation and a significant decrease in the propagation rate (Suzukawa *et al.*, 1995). Princen *et al.* (1995) have evaluated the minimal supplementary dose of vitamin E necessary to protect LDL against oxidation *in vitro* in healthy young adults with a stepwise increase of vitamin E supplements. Resistance of LDL to oxidation increased in a dose-dependent manner, with resistance time differing significantly from baseline even after ingestion of only 17 mg day^{-1} of vitamin E. However, the propagation of lipid peroxidation in LDL was only reduced after intake of 268 and 536 mg day^{-1}.

The effect of high-dose vitamin C supplementation (1000 mg day^{-1}) on LDL oxidation was evaluated in a study of 19 smokers. The vitamin C-supplemented group had a significant reduction in the susceptibility of LDL to oxidation after 4 weeks (Fuller *et al.*, 1996). Jialal *et al.* (1991) found that β-carotene (1–2 μmol l^{-1}) inhibited the oxidative modification of LDL *in vitro* in healthy subjects. However, when the effectiveness of β-carotene, vitamin C and vitamin E supplements was assessed by Reaven *et al.* (1993), susceptibility of LDL to oxidation did not change during β-carotene supplementation (60 mg day^{-1}) but decreased by 30–40% with the addition of vitamin E (1600 mg day^{-1}). Addition of vitamin C (2 g day^{-1}) did not further reduce the susceptibility to oxidation. In a group of smokers and non-smokers given vitamin E supplementation (671 mg day^{-1} for 7 days), resistance of LDL to oxidation increased significantly and the rate of LDL oxidation decreased significantly. There was a small but significant increase in resistance of LDL to oxidation in smokers after supplementation with β-carotene (20 mg day^{-1} for 2 weeks, then 40 mg day^{-1} for 12 weeks), but not when the β-carotene-supplemented group was compared as a whole with the placebo group (Princen *et al.*, 1992). Finally, in a study that evaluated the effects of supplements of β-carotene (30 mg day^{-1}), vitamin C (1 g day^{-1}) and vitamin E (530 mg day^{-1}) for 3 months in men, there was a twofold prolongation of the lag phase of LDL oxidation and a 40% reduction in the oxidation rate (Jialal and Grundy, 1993). Similarly, we have recently shown that a combination of low-dose antioxidant vitamins (150 mg ascorbic acid, 67 mg α-tocopherol, 9 mg β-carotene daily) over a period of 8 weeks significantly prolonged the lag time to oxidation (Woodside *et al.*, 1997). In the study by Jialal and Grundy (1993), the effects of combined antioxidant supplementation were not significantly different from the effects of vitamin E supplementation alone.

In summary, experimental evidence suggests that antioxidant vitamins can reduce the susceptibility of LDL to oxidation *in vitro*. Vitamin E would appear to be the most effective antioxidant; both β-carotene and vitamin C have produced extensions in lag time to oxidation only in a minority of studies, although it remains possible that they may have a beneficial effect in individuals with poor baseline status.

Antioxidants and CVD: Intervention Studies

Largely negative results have been produced from intervention studies using antioxidant vitamin supplementation with a clinical endpoint such as a cardiovascular event. These have been considered in Chapter 13. A number of reasons have been put forward for these negative findings. One possibility is that the complex mixture of antioxidant micronutrients found in a diet high in fruit and vegetables may be more effective than large doses of one or two antioxidant vitamins.

There are several trials underway at present to assess the effects of antioxidant vitamin supplementation on cardiovascular disease (CVD). In each of these trials, doses of vitamin E greater than 200 mg day^{-1} are being used, and these should be sufficient to increase serum levels at least two- to threefold. The Women's Health Study is a primary prevention trial investigating the effects of vitamin E, β-carotene and aspirin on CVD and cancer in 40,000 women aged 50 years and over (Buring and Hennekens, 1992). In France, the Supplementation Vitamins, Minerals and Antioxidant (SU.VI.MAX) Trial is testing a combination of antioxidant vitamins including vitamin E, vitamin C and β-carotene in 15,000 healthy men and women (Gaziano, 1994). The Heart Protection Study is investigating the effects of vitamins E and C, and β-carotene in 18,000 subjects with above average risk of future MI (Sleight, 1995) and a secondary prevention trial using the same three vitamins in 8000 women has been established in the USA (Women's Antioxidant Cardiovascular Disease Trial, WACDT) (Manson *et al.*, 1995). The Heart Outcomes Protection Study is also assessing vitamin E in 9000 persons with previous MI, stroke or peripheral vascular disease or who have diabetes (HOPE Investigators, 1995). Finally, the GISSI Prevention Trial in Italy is evaluating vitamin E and fish oil supplements among 11,000 patients after a recent MI (Jha *et al.*, 1995). The results of these trials should provide better evidence about the efficacy and safety of the various antioxidant vitamins.

A trial using supplements of fruit and vegetables would also be useful as the results of the intervention trials so far suggest that any reduction in the risk of disease associated with high antioxidant intake may result from consuming a mix of foods rich in antioxidants rather than consuming antioxidants as single nutrients. A diet rich in fruit and vegetables may represent a more general, favourable promoter of reduced disease risk. Quantification of the relationship between fruit and vegetable intake and cardiovascular risk is important for public health since practical perspectives can be opened for prevention and health education even in the absence of a precise understanding of the underlying mechanism.

Effects of Fruit and Vegetables on Disease

Research examining the effects of a diet rich in fruits and vegetables on disease has been carried out using several types of study.

Observational studies of fruit and vegetable intake

A number of studies of people who eat a diet rich in fruit and vegetables, and therefore rich in antioxidant nutrients, have tried to test the hypothesis that fruit and vegetables lower the risk of CHD (Phillips *et al.*, 1980; Chang-Claude *et al.*, 1992; Thorogood *et al.*, 1994; Key *et al.*, 1996). In general, observational studies of vegetarians and those with diets rich in fruits and vegetables support the hypothesis that such diets might lower the risk of CHD. Vegetarians generally have high intakes of cereals, nuts and vegetable oils, carrots and green vegetables as well as fruit. However, vegetarians differ from the rest of the population in a number of important ways: they tend to smoke less, have a lower body mass index and alcohol intake, and come predominantly from higher social classes, all of which are known to confer a health advantage.

Dietary intervention trials

The Woman's Health Initiative (WHI) is currently evaluating the effectiveness of a dietary modification strategy to reduce the incidence of breast and colorectal cancer and CHD (Eaker and Hahn, 1994). The dietary goals of the WHI are multifactorial and include a reduction of total dietary fat intake to 20% of total energy intake, a reduction of saturated fat intake to 7% of total energy intake, and an increase in the intake of fruit and vegetables (five or more daily servings) and grain products. The effects of fat reduction on disease incidence will be hard to differentiate from the effect of an increase in fruit and vegetable consumption.

Dietary intervention trials and secondary prevention

Clinical trials using dietary intervention with clinical endpoints are, up to the present, from secondary prevention. In a study using an α-linolenic acid-rich diet patients were randomly assigned after first MI to the experimental (*n* = 302) or control group (*n* = 303) (de Lorgeril *et al.*, 1994; Renaud *et al.*, 1995). Subjects in the experimental group were advised to eat more bread, more vegetables and legumes, more fish, less meat (beef, lamb and pork), it being replaced by poultry, to have no day without fruit, and to replace butter and cream with a margarine comparable with olive oil. The experimental group consumed considerably less lipids, saturated fat, cholesterol and linoleic acid, but more oleic acid and α-linolenic acid and had increased plasma concentrations of these nutrients and also of vitamins C and E. The diet was also rich in folic acid. After follow-up of 27 months those in the experimental group had a relative risk of 0.27 (95% CI 0.12–0.59, *P* = 0.001) of MI or cardiac death compared to the control group. These changes were not related to change in cholesterol levels, but to changes in serum fatty acids and an increase in vitamins C and E. A similar study, but in a very different population from India, also produced a fall in mortality after acute MI in patients following a fat-reduced diet rich in soluble dietary fibre and antioxidant vitamins (Singh *et al.*, 1992a). Both placebo and intervention groups were advised to follow a fat-reduced diet but the intervention group were also advised to eat more fruit, vegetables, nuts and grain products.

The feasibility of a long-term randomized study of a diet rich in vegetables to prevent recurrence of breast cancer has been examined (Pierce *et al.*, 1997). The daily diet consisted of five vegetable servings, 16 ounces of fresh vegetable juice, three fruit servings, 15% of energy from fat and 30 g fibre. The juice was added in order to increase micronutrient intake without adding bulk and potential discomfort associated with high fibre intakes.

Therefore, although intervention trials using antioxidant supplements are important in evaluating possible beneficial effects of antioxidants against development or progression of CVD, they have limitations and should be considered as only one component in the totality of available research evidence. It may be that a lifetime of intake is required to show a protective effect, or that a mixture of natural antioxidants, including other bioactive compounds in addition to vitamins C, E and β-carotene, found in fruits and vegetables provide the necessary protective mixture. Further study using diets rich in fruit and vegetables should provide evidence for their beneficial effect on disease.

Effects of Fruit and Vegetables: Biochemical Observations

A recent study asked subjects with normal lipid concentrations who ate three or fewer servings of fruit and vegetables daily to consume eight servings per day (Zino *et al.*, 1997). Plasma concentrations of vitamin C, retinol, α-tocopherol, α- and β-carotene, lipids and lipoproteins were assessed before and after an 8-week intervention period. The plasma vitamin C, α-carotene, and β-carotene concentrations increased, while concentrations of retinol, α-tocopherol, lipids and lipoproteins remained unchanged despite some increase in dietary vitamin E and a small reduction in saturated fat intake. An interesting addition to the results would have been the inclusion of data on the susceptibility of LDL to oxidation. The authors concluded that more specific dietary advice to modify fat intake may be necessary to reduce the risk of CVD.

By contrast, Singh *et al.* (1992b) found over a 12-week period that fruit and vegetable administration in subjects at high risk of CHD lowered total- and LDL-cholesterol and triglyceride levels, and increased HDL-cholesterol (see Chapter 16). Another study by Wise *et al.* (1996) using dehydrated fruit and vegetable extracts over a period of 28 days in 15 healthy adults aged 18–53 years produced increases of the order of 50- to 2000-fold in carotenoid and tocopherol levels, while serum lipid peroxides decreased fourfold during the intervention period, with much of this lowering taking place during the first week.

Dietary Supply of Antioxidants in the Developed World

Vitamin C and β-carotene are available from fruits and/or vegetables, and vitamin E from vegetable oils. Southern European countries consuming the classical Mediterranean diet show that optimal plasma levels of these antioxidants can easily be achieved. This diet is characterized by a preference for fresh products and frequent consumption of fruit/vegetables/ legumes and oils with high vitamin E content. In contrast, major parts of populations in the USA or in northern parts of Europe do not consume optimal amounts of antioxidant nutrients. The availability of lower-priced convenience foods in the USA acts against the consumption of freshly prepared foods. Thus, only 10% of Americans achieved five servings of fruit and vegetables daily (Patterson *et al.*, 1990) as recommended by the United States' national food guide, the Food Guide Pyramid (Achterberg *et al.*, 1994). Only a quarter consumed fruits or vegetables rich in vitamin C or the carotenoids, and 41% had no fruits or vegetables on the day the survey was carried out (Block, 1991). A recent re-analysis of the NHANES II data showed that vitamin supplements are the major contributors of the principal antioxidant micronutrients in the US diet (28% of vitamin C and 46% of vitamin E) (Block *et al.*, 1994).

The requirement for a micronutrient is the minimum quantity necessary to prevent a deficiency. The translation of minimum requirement to a dietary recommendation for population groups necessitates that allowance be made for a number of variables, including: (i) periods of low intake, (ii) increased utilization, (iii) individual variability, and (iv) bioavailability. In the United States, the recommended daily allowances (RDAs) incorporate 'margins of safety' intended to be sufficiently generous to encompass the variability in the minimum requirement among people, and bioavailability from different food sources.

To date, recommendations on micronutrient intake have therefore primarily been intended to prevent clinically overt deficiencies, e.g. scurvy or neural tube defects. If, however, observational and experimental evidence continues to show that the prevention of slow multistage processes such as CVD and cancer might require a higher intake of some essential antioxidants, then a recommended intake should be devised referring to amounts considered sufficient for the avoidance of these disease states. Gey (1995) suggests that the present recommendations will require either an upgrading or an additional term, e.g. a recommended optimum intake (ROI) which will vary with gender, age, with special requirements for smokers, pregnancy and the elderly. The ROI could be defined as sufficient (culture- and/or region-specific) intake to achieve blood levels associated with the observed minimum relative risk of disease (Gey, 1995). A ROI would simply quantify specific dietary constituents of conceivably crucial importance within the still desirable 'five servings of fruit and vegetables daily.'

Conclusion

There is strong scientific evidence to support an increase in intakes of vegetables and fruit in the prevention of disease. Further research is required to clarify which particular components of fruit and vegetables are responsible for their protective effects. Antioxidants have a definite protective effect on the susceptibility of LDL to oxidation, but the relevance of this to CHD incidence, and the possibility of other important bioactive micronutrients in vegetables and fruit requires further research. Only then can dietary recommendations, referring to intakes of these specific micro-nutrients required to avoid disease in addition to the general 'five servings a day', be made possible.

References

Achterberg, C., McDonnell, E. and Bagby, R. (1994) How to put the Food Guide Pyramid into practice. *Journal of the American Dietetic Association* 94, 1030–1035.

Ball, R.Y., Carpenter, K.L. and Mitchinson, M.J. (1987) What is the significance of ceroid in human atherosclerosis? *Archives of Pathology and Laboratory Medicine* 111, 1134–1140.

Block, G. (1991) Dietary guidelines and the results from food consumption surveys. *American Journal of Clinical Nutrition* 53, 356S–357S.

Block, G., Sinha, R. and Gridley, G. (1994) Collection of dietary-supplement data and implications for analysis. *American Journal of Clinical Nutrition* 59 (Suppl.), 232S–239S.

Buring, J.E. and Hennekens, C.H. (1992) The Women's Health Study: rationale and background. *Journal of Myocardial Ischemia* 4, 30–40.

Chang-Claude, J., Frentzel-Beyme, R. and Eilber, U. (1992) Mortality pattern of German vegetarians after 11 years of follow up. *Epidemiology* 3, 395–401.

Duthie, G.G. and Wahle, K.J. (1990) Smoking, antioxidants, essential fatty acids and coronary heart disease. *Biochemical Society Transactions* 18, 1051–1054.

Eaker, E. and Hahn, R.A. (1994) Women's Health Initiative. *New England Journal of Medicine* 330, 70–71.

Frei, B. (1995) Cardiovascular disease and nutrient antioxidants: role of low-density lipoprotein oxidation. *Critical Reviews in Food Science and Nutrition* 35, 83–98.

Fuller, C.J., Grundy, S.M., Norkus, E.P. and Jialal, I. (1996) Effect of ascorbate supplementation on low-density lipoprotein oxidation in smokers. *Atherosclerosis* 119, 139–150.

Gaziano, J.M. (1994) Antioxidant vitamins and coronary artery disease risk. *American Journal of Medicine* 97, 3–18.

Gey, K.F. (1995) Ten year retrospective on the antioxidant hypothesis of arteriosclerosis: threshold plasma levels of antioxidant micronutrients related to minimum cardiovascular risk. *Nutritional Biochemistry* 6, 206–236.

HOPE Investigators (1995) The HOPE (Heart Outcomes Prevention Evaluation) Study. The design of a large, simple randomised trial of an angiotensin converting enzyme inhibitor (ramipril) and vitamin E in patients at high risk of cardiovascular events. *Canadian Journal of Cardiology* 12, 127–137.

Jha, P., Flather, M., Lonn, E., Farkouh, M. and Yusuf, S. (1995) The antioxidant vitamins and cardiovascular disease. A critical review of epidemiologic and clinical trial data. *Annals of Internal Medicine* 123, 860–872.

Jialal, I. and Grundy, S.M. (1992) Effect of dietary supplementation with alpha-tocopherol on the oxidative modification of low-density lipoprotein. *Journal of Lipid Research* 33, 899–906.

Jialal, I. and Grundy, S.M. (1993) Effect of combined supplementation with alpha-tocopherol, ascorbate and beta-carotene on low-density lipoprotein oxidation. *Circulation* 88, 2780–2786.

Jialal, I., Norkus, E.P., Cristol, L. and Grundy, S.M. (1991) Beta-carotene inhibits the oxidative modification of low-density lipoprotein. *Biochimica et Biophysica Acta* 1086, 134–138.

Key, T., Thorogood, M., Appleby, P. and Burr, M. (1996) Dietary habits and mortality in 11,000 vegetarians and health conscious people: results of a 17 year follow up. *British Medical Journal* 313, 775–779.

Leake, D.S. (1993) Oxidised low density lipoproteins and atherogenesis. *British Heart Journal* 69, 476–478.

de Lorgeril, M., Renaud, S., Mamelle, N., Salen, P., Martin, J.L. and Monjaud, I. (1994) Mediterranean alpha-linolenic acid-rich diet in secondary prevention of coronary heart disease. *Lancet* 343, 1454–1459.

Manson, J.E., Gaziano, J.M., Spelsberg, A., Ridker, P.M., Cook, N.R., Buring, J.E., Willett, W.C. and Hennekens, C.H. (1995) A secondary prevention trial of antioxidant vitamins and cardiovascular disease in women: rationale, design and methods. *Annals of Epidemiology* 5, 261–269.

Palinski, W., Rosenfeld, M.E., Yla-Herttuala, S., Gurtner, G.C., Socher, S.S., Butler, S.W., Parthasarathy, S., Carew, T.E., Steinberg, D. and Witztum, J.L. (1989) Low density lipoprotein undergoes oxidative modification *in vivo*. *Proceedings of the National Academy of Sciences, USA* 86, 1372–1376.

Patterson, B., Block, G., Rosenberger, R. and Pee, D. (1990) Fruit and vegetables in the American diet: data from the NHANES II Survey. *American Journal of Public Health* 80, 1443–1449.

Phillips, R.L., Kuzma, J.W., Beeson, W.L. and Lotz, T. (1980) Influence of selection versus lifestyle on risk of fatal cancer and cardiovascular disease among Seventh-Day Adventists. *American Journal of Epidemiology* 112, 296–314.

Pierce, J.P., Faerber, S., Wright, F.A., Newman, V., Flatt, S.W., Kealey, S., Rock, C.L., Hrniuk, W. and Greenberg, E.R. (1997) Feasibility of a randomized trial of a high-vegetable diet to prevent breast cancer recurrence. *Nutrition and Cancer* 28, 282–288.

Princen, H.M., van Poppel, G., Vogelezang, C., Buytenhek, R. and Kok, F.J. (1992) Supplementation with vitamin E but not β-carotene *in vivo* protects low-density lipoprotein from lipid peroxidation *in vitro*. Effect of cigarette smoking. *Arteriosclerosis and Thrombosis* 12, 554–562.

Princen, H.M.G., van Duyvenvoorde, W., Buytenhek, R., van der Laarse, A., van Poppel, G., Leuven, J.A.G. and van Hinsbergh, V.W.M. (1995) Supplementation with low doses of vitamin E protects LDL from lipid peroxidation in men and women. *Arteriosclerosis, Thrombosis and Vascular Biology* 15, 325–333.

Reaven, P.D., Khouw, A., Beltz, W.F., Parthasarathy, S. and Witztum, J.L. (1993) Effect of dietary antioxidant combinations in humans. Protection of LDL by vitamin E but not by β-carotene. *Arteriosclerosis and Thrombosis* 13, 590–600.

Regnstrom, J., Nilsson, J., Tornvall, P., Landou, C. and Hamsten, A. (1992) Susceptibility to low-density lipoprotein oxidation and coronary atherosclerosis in man. *Lancet* 339, 1183–1186.

Renaud, S., de Lorgeril, M., Delaye, J., Guidollet, J., Jacquard, F., Mamelle, N., Martin, J.L., Monjaud, I., Salen, P. and Toubol, P. (1995) Cretan Mediterranean diet for prevention of coronary heart disease. *American Journal of Clinical Nutrition* 61 (Suppl.), 1360S–1367S.

Singh, R.B., Rastogi, S.S., Verma, R., Laxmi, B., Singh, R., Ghosh, S. and Niaz, M.A. (1992a) Randomized controlled trial of cardioprotective diet in patients with recent acute myocardial infarction – results of a one year follow-up. *British Medical Journal* 304, 1015–1019.

Singh, R.B., Rastogi, S.S., Niaz, M.A., Ghosh, S., Singh, R. and Gupta, S. (1992b) Effect of fat-modified and fruit-enriched and vegetable-enriched diets and blood lipids in the Indian Diet Heart Study. *American Journal of Cardiology* 70, 869–874.

Sleight, P. (1995) Can vitamins and cholesterol-lowering drugs help guard against heart disease? *MRC News* 66, 35–39.

Steinberg, D., Parthasarathy, S., Carew, T.E., Khoo, J.D. and Witztum, J.L. (1989) Beyond cholesterol: modifications of low density lipoprotein that increase its atherogenicity. *New England Journal of Medicine* 320, 915–924.

Suzukawa, M., Ishikawa, T., Yoshida, H. and Makamura, H. (1995) Effect of *in vivo* supplementation with low-dose vitamin E on susceptibility of low-density lipoprotein and high density lipoprotein to oxidative modification. *Journal of the American College of Nutrition* 14, 46–52.

Thorogood, M., Mann, J., Appleby, P. and McPherson, K. (1994) Risk of death from cancer and ischaemic heart disease in meat and non-meat eaters. *British Medical Journal* 308, 1667–1671.

Wise, J.A., Morin, R.J., Sanderson, R. and Blum, K. (1996) Changes in plasma carotenoid, alpha-tocopherol, and lipid peroxide levels in response to supplementation with concentrated fruit and vegetable extracts – a pilot study. *Current Therapeutic Research – Clinical and Experimental* 57, 445–461.

Witztum, J.L. and Steinberg, D. (1991) Role of oxidized LDL in atherogenesis. *Journal of Clinical Investigation* 88, 1785–1792.

Woodside, J.V., Yarnell, J.W.G., Young, I.S., McMaster, D., Gey, K.F., Mercer, C., Patterson, C.C., McCrum, E.E. and Evans, A.E. (1997) The effects of oral vitamin supplementation on cardiovascular risk factors. *Proceedings of the Nutrition Society* 56, 149A.

Yla-Herttuala, S., Palinski, W., Rosenfeld, M.E., Parthasarathy, S., Carew, T.E., Butler, S., Witztum, J.L. and Steinberg, D. (1989) Evidence for the presence of oxidatively modified low density lipoprotein in atherosclerotic lesions of rabbit and man. *Journal of Clinical Investigation* 84, 1086–1095.

Zino, S., Skeaff, M., Williams, S. and Mann, J. (1997) Randomised controlled trial of effect of fruit and vegetable consumption on plasma concentrations of lipids and antioxidants. *British Medical Journal* 314, 1787–1791.

Antioxidants and the Prevention of Cancer 18

PETER GREENWALD[1] AND SHARON S. McDONALD[2]

[1]*Division of Cancer Prevention, National Cancer Institute, Bethesda, Maryland, USA;* [2]*The Scientific Consulting Group, Inc., Gaithersburg, Maryland, USA*

Introduction

Oxidative damage to DNA, lipids and proteins in the human body is generally considered to be an important factor in carcinogenesis. Reactive oxygen species such as superoxide, nitric oxide and hydroxyl radicals, formed continuously as a result of biochemical reactions, can cause significant oxidative damage. Also, environmental carcinogens from various sources – for instance, tobacco smoke and industrial pollution – and food contaminants such as heterocyclic aromatic amines (HAAs) contribute to an individual's total burden of oxidative stress (Jacob and Burri, 1996; Loft and Poulsen, 1996). Antioxidant defences – for example, enzymes that continually repair DNA damage – frequently cannot counteract all of the oxidative attack, and the resulting damage may lead to genetic mutations that could contribute to carcinogenesis. Dietary antioxidants, ubiquitous in plant foods where they have evolved to protect the plants against oxidative assault, may be protective to humans, in terms of reducing cancer risk. Reactive oxygen species appear to be involved at all stages of cancer development; consequently, dietary antioxidants may have potential benefits throughout the carcinogenic process (Diplock, 1996; Cozzi *et al.*, 1997).

Epidemiologic data provide strong evidence of a cancer-protective effect for high intakes of vegetables, fruits and whole grains. Many studies indicate that the risk of cancer incidence associated with lowest vegetable and fruit intakes is approximately twice that associated with highest intakes (Block *et al.*, 1992). A review of more than 200 case–control and cohort studies found a probable protective effect for cancers of the breast, colon, endometrium, oral cavity and pharynx, pancreas and bladder, and convincing evidence for inverse associations with cancers of the stomach, oesophagus, and lung (Steinmetz and Potter, 1996). In 85% of the studies, raw vegetables appeared to be protective; highly protective categories included *Allium* vegetables, carrots, green vegetables, cruciferous vegetables, and tomatoes – all protective in 70% or more of the studies. Total fruits and citrus fruit were protective in about 65% of the studies. The cancer-inhibitory effects reported for these plant foods may be attributed in part to various antioxidant constituents, including micronutrients (e.g. β-carotene (provitamin A), vitamins E and C, selenium) and certain phyto-chemicals (e.g. polyphenolics, carotenoids) (Wattenberg, 1992). It is likely that numerous constituents contribute to the overall protective effect. Lung cancer risk, for instance, consistently has been shown to be reduced by high vegetable and/or fruit consumption in both prospective and retrospective epidemiological studies, but the beneficial effect cannot be explained completely by either β-carotene or total provitamin A carotenoid intakes (Ziegler *et al.*, 1996a).

When interpreting the results of epidemiological studies, it must be kept in mind that the effects of dietary factors on cancer risk can be influenced by an individual's genetic susceptibility. Several of the more common variations in susceptibility among individuals result from polymorphisms in specific genes (including *CYP1A1*, *CPY1A2*, *CYP2D6*, *GSTM1* and *NAT2*) that cause differences in metabolic or detoxification activities (Perera, 1996). Increased risk of lung cancer, for example, has been correlated with variant forms of *CYP1A1* (catalyses the oxygenation of polyaromatic hydrocarbons (PAHs) and is induced by cigarette smoke), *CYP2D6* (acts on an unknown substrate, possibly tobacco-specific nitrosamines), and *GSTM1* (detoxifies reactive, electrophilic compounds such as PAHs) (Perera, 1996). The relative prevalence and/or distribution of such polymorphisms in populations targeted in epidemiological studies may affect individual responses to both risk and protective factors, including antioxidants and other dietary constituents, and thus may contribute to confounding in analysis and interpretation of study results.

The Chemoprevention Program developed at the National Cancer Institute (NCI) is systematically carrying out preclinical and clinical studies on numerous potential agents identified by surveying a broad spectrum of epidemiological, laboratory and clinical research for compounds that have demonstrated apparent cancer-protective activity. Since the programme's inception in 1987, more than 400 agents have been entered and more than 250 of these have been tested in animal screens. Based on Phase I pharmacokinetic and clinical safety trials, the most promising agents progress to Phase II and III clinical trials; more than 30 agents, including naturally occurring antioxidant micronutrients and phytochemicals, as well as synthetic antioxidants, are currently being studied.

Micronutrients

β-Carotene

Clinical chemoprevention trials using β-carotene are based on extensive evidence from epidemiological studies. Weighing the evidence from studies conducted in the 1970s, which linked high vegetable and fruit intake – an index of β-carotene intake – with reduced cancer risk, Peto and colleagues (1981) suggested that β-carotene might be the protective factor in these foods. Several possible mechanisms were proposed that supported the biological plausibility of β-carotene as a cancer-protective agent, including antioxidant protection and the differentiating action of vitamin A formed from β-carotene. The encouraging epidemiological evidence, as well as supporting laboratory data, provided a strong scientific rationale for the hypothesis that β-carotene can reduce cancer risk. Randomized, controlled clinical chemoprevention trials, the only definitive way to test such hypotheses, were initiated in the 1980s; results of these trials are described below in the section 'Large-scale, Randomized Intervention Trials'.

Early clinical trials on oral cancer showed evidence of benefit from β-carotene. In Filipino betel nut chewers, who are at very high risk for oral cancer, the percentage of buccal mucosa cells with micronuclei – evidence of genotoxic damage – was significantly lower in people given β-carotene for 9 weeks than in those given canthaxanthin, a carotenoid with no vitamin A activity (Stich *et al.*, 1984). One study that examined the effect of β-carotene on leukoplakia, a precancerous oral lesion, reported that 17 of 24 patients showed significant reversal of lesions after 6 months of treatment (Garewal *et al.*, 1990). In another study, however, low-dose 13-*cis*-retinoic acid was significantly more effective than β-carotene in maintaining the stability of leukoplakia reversed by high-dose 13-*cis*-retinoic acid (Lippman *et al.*, 1993).

Trials to prevent colorectal polyps showed no evidence of benefit from β-carotene. In a study in which 864 people, who previously had polyps removed, received either β-carotene, vitamins C and E, all three antioxidants, or placebo for 4 years, no reduction in polyp incidence – and no evidence of harm – was demonstrated for any of the interventions (Greenberg *et al.*, 1994). Similarly, an Australian polyp prevention trial, in which approximately 400 patients with previous polyps received either β-carotene or placebo along with usual diet, low-fat diet, high-wheat bran diet or low-fat/high-wheat bran diet, found no significant polyp reduction (MacClennan *et al.*, 1995). The data suggested, however, that the low-fat/high-wheat bran diet may inhibit the transition from smaller to larger polyps, which have greater malignant potential.

Numerous epidemiological studies investigating the possible association between β-carotene and the risk of various types of cancer have been conducted since the early 1980s, concurrent with clinical trials. A significant protective effect of dietary β-carotene for lung cancer is strongly supported by epidemiological data. A review by van Poppel and Goldbohm (1995) of approximately 80 retrospective studies and 50 prospective studies reported that associations of either high intakes of β-carotene-rich vegetables and fruits or high blood concentrations of β-carotene with reduced cancer risk were most consistent for lung and stomach cancer. Oesophageal cancer also showed a promising risk reduction, but the number of studies was limited. Reported results for the effects of both β-carotene and vitamin A on prostate cancer have been equivocal, with studies being almost equally divided between inverse and positive associations (Kolonel, 1996). For breast cancer, evidence from case–control studies has indicated a possible protective effect of β-carotene (Hunter and Willett, 1996). For colon cancer, some case–control studies have reported significantly reduced risk at high intakes, but the overall data have suggested only a modest risk reduction (van Poppel and Goldbohm, 1995).

Vitamin E/vitamin C

Vitamin E

Epidemiological studies that have investigated associations of cancer risk at specific sites and diets high in vitamin E (α-tocopherol) are limited in number and data are inconsistent, possibly because estimation of vitamin E intake is difficult (Byers and Guerrero, 1995; Steinmetz and Potter, 1996). A review that examined case–control and cohort studies of vitamin E intake and serum vitamin E levels in relation to breast cancer risk reported that the data were inconclusive (Kimmick et al., 1997). One case–control study that investigated the association between micronutrient intake and colorectal adenomas reported that men in the highest quartile of vitamin E intake, compared with the lowest quartile, were about one-fifth as likely to develop adenomas (OR=0.22 for men and 0.74 for women), after adjustment for possible confounding variables, including other micronutrients (Tseng et al., 1996). Similarly, another case–control study showed decreased risk of adenoma for the highest tertile of vitamin E intake (OR=0.6, men and women combined, adjusted for total energy and physical activity) (Lubin et al., 1997). In the recently completed Alpha-Tocopherol Beta-Carotene (ATBC) Cancer Prevention Study, conducted in Finland in more than 29,000 male cigarette smokers at high risk for lung cancer, 34% fewer cases of prostate cancer and 16% fewer cases of colorectal cancer were diagnosed among men who received daily vitamin E supplements (ATBC Cancer Prevention Study Group, 1994). Although these results suggest a protective effect of vitamin E, prostate and colon cancers were not primary study endpoints. Further research, targeted at these cancers, is needed before conclusions can be drawn about the potential of vitamin E for their preven-tion. A recent review suggests that antioxidant effects of γ-tocopherol may be superior to those of α-tocopherol, and that studies of vitamin E and colorectal cancer should consider all tocopherols (Stone and Papas, 1997).

Vitamin C

Epidemiological evidence for a protective effect of diets high in vegetables and fruits that contain vitamin C is strong and consistent for cancers of the oral cavity, oesophagus and stomach, but moderate and less consistent for colon and lung cancers. The data do not support an association with prostate cancer and the evidence for breast cancer has been conflicting (Block, 1991; Byers and Guerrero, 1995). A review of more than 50 case–control and cohort studies that investigated intakes of vegetables and fruits, vitamin C, and vitamin E, reported that, across studies, individuals in the highest quartile or quintile of vegetable and fruit intake had approximately 40% less risk of gastrointestinal and respiratory tract cancers than those in the lowest intake levels (Byers and Guerrero, 1995). Indices of vitamin C computed from vegetable and fruit intakes also were associated with lower risk.

Selenium

The trace mineral selenium, although not an antioxidant *per se*, functions as a cofactor for glutathione peroxidase, an enzyme that may protect against oxidative tissue damage (Steinmetz and Potter, 1996). Dietary assessment of selenium can be difficult because the selenium content of plant foods depends on the selenium content of the soil in which the plants grow. Thus, selenium status is best determined by biochemical measures, such as blood or toenail selenium levels. Cancer mortality international correlation studies suggest an inverse association between selenium status and cancer incidence (Schrauzer *et al.*, 1977). Also, animal studies strongly support a cancer-protective effect of selenium (Kelloff and Boone, 1996a). Data from most case–control and cohort studies, however, have not been convincing for those cancer sites investigated, including lung, breast and stomach cancers (Hunter and Willett, 1996; Kono and Hirohata, 1996; Ziegler *et al.*, 1996a). Data from a recent prospective study that examined the association between serum selenium levels and development of ovarian cancer indicated that women in the highest tertile, compared with the lowest tertile, were four times less likely to develop ovarian cancer (OR=0.23) (Helzlsouer *et al.*, 1996). A randomized, controlled clinical intervention trial that tested whether a daily 200 μg selenium supplement will decrease incidence of basal cell and squamous cell skin cancers found no protective effect against skin cancer. Secondary endpoint analyses, however, showed significant reductions in total cancer mortality (RR=0.5), total cancer incidence (RR=0.63), and incidences of lung (RR=0.54), colorectal (RR=0.42) and prostate (RR=0.37) cancers, for individuals who received selenium supplements, compared with controls (Clark *et al.*, 1996). These findings support the cancer-protective effect of selenium, but must be confirmed in independent intervention trials.

The effective doses and toxic doses of organoselenium compounds, such as selenomethionine and selenocysteine, are quite close. Synthesis of

1,4-phenylenebis(methylene)-selenocyanate (*p*-XSC) and benzylseleno-cyanate (BSC) has provided effective, less toxic alternatives. Preclinical data indicate that administration of either *p*-XSC or *p*-methoxy-BSC during the postinitiation phase significantly reduces the formation of chemically induced colon tumours in rats fed a high-fat diet (Reddy *et al.*, 1997). In this study, the chemopreventive effects of *p*-XSC were enhanced in animals fed a low-fat diet. The NCI is currently sponsoring preclinical toxicity studies for *p*-XSC; if results are acceptable, a Phase I clinical trial will be considered (Kelloff and Boone, 1996a). Determining the optimal form and dose level of selenium for use in clinical trials, however, is complicated by the fact that toxicity thresholds may differ among individuals.

Phytochemicals

Vegetables, fruits and whole grains contain a wide variety of primarily non-nutritive phytochemical antioxidants, such as phenolic/polyphenolic compounds and carotenoids, that have the potential to modulate cancer development (Wattenberg, 1992). To illustrate, the oil obtained from the first cold pressing of olives can contain as much as 1 g kg^{-1} of poly-phenolic compounds with antioxidant potential, including oleuropein (the principal bitter constituent in olives), (3,4-dihydroxyphenyl)ethanol and (*p*-hydroxyphenyl)ethanol (Visioli *et al.*, 1995). In an experimental model, (3,4-dihydroxyphenyl)ethanol demonstrated a protective effect on Caco-2 human colon cancer cells subjected to chemically induced oxidative stress, suggesting that dietary intake of olive oil polyphenols could protect against damage by reactive oxygen species (Manna *et al.*, 1997).

The NCI has conducted preclinical screening on approximately 100 potential chemopreventive agents that are classified as antioxidants, many of which are naturally occurring, such as fumaric acid, quercetin, (+)-catechin, chlorogenic acid, ellagic acid, ascorbyl palmitate, ethylvanillin, 18-glycyrrhetinic acid and vitamin E acetate (Steele *et al.*, 1996). Several antioxidant phytochemicals that have shown promise in screening and/or epidemiological studies have progressed to early-stage clinical testing. Selected antioxidant phytochemicals that may be beneficial in reducing cancer risk are highlighted below.

Phenolic compounds

Tea extracts/green tea polyphenols (GTP)
Although the data are not wholly consistent, epidemiological studies have suggested a protective effect of black (oxidized) or green (unoxidized) tea consumption against cancers of the breast, colon and rectum, lung, nasopharynx, stomach, uterus, gall bladder, liver and pancreas (Stoner and

Mukhtar, 1995; Yang *et al.*, 1996). For instance, a case–control study in Shanghai, China, recently reported an inverse association for green tea consumption (highest tertile vs. lowest tertile) and cancer risk for colon (men, RR=0.82; women, RR=0.67), rectum (men, RR=0.72; women, RR=0.57), and pancreas (men, RR=0.63; women, RR=0.53), with statistically significant trends for both rectal and pancreatic cancers (Ji *et al.*, 1997). Also, a prospective cohort study in Japan found that consumption of more than ten cups of green tea daily reduced cancer risk among both women (RR = 0.57) and men (RR = 0.68), after adjustment for confounding variables (Imai *et al.*, 1997). A significant delay of cancer onset, about 9 years, was found in women who consumed more than ten cups daily vs. those who consumed less than three cups daily; for men and women combined, this delay, also significant, was 4 years. Most experimental studies examining a possible relationship between tea and cancer risk have focused on extracts of either black or green tea and on GTP, including (−)-epicatechin (EC), (−)-epicatechin-3-gallate (ECG), (−)-epigallocatechin (EGC) and (−)-epigallocatechin-3-gallate (EGCG). EGCG, the major catechin in green tea, accounts for 40% of GTP and possesses the greatest anticarcinogenic activity (Stoner and Mukhtar, 1995). Findings in one recent study suggest that GTP may protect against cancer by causing cell cycle arrest and inducing apoptosis (Ahmad *et al.*, 1997).

Curcumin

Curcumin, the yellow colouring agent in the spice turmeric, has effectively inhibited chemically induced tumours in the skin, forestomach, mammary gland (*in vitro*), colon (*in vitro*) and duodenum of rodents (Kelloff *et al.*, 1994). In combination studies, curcumin plus *N*-(4-hydroxyphenyl)retinamide (4-HPR) appeared to be more effective than either agent alone against rat mammary carcinogenesis (Kelloff and Boone, 1996b). The NCI is sponsoring a Phase I trial of curcumin in normal, healthy subjects to define both its safety and pharmacokinetic characteristics. A Phase II trial of curcumin in dysplastic oral leukoplakia patients, using topical administration, also is being considered.

Ellagic acid

Ellagic acid, found in certain berries and nuts, has exhibited anticarcinogenic effects for chemically induced tumours of the lung, skin, oesophagus and liver in experimental studies (Kelloff *et al.*, 1994; Stoner and Mukhtar, 1995). Pharmacokinetic studies with ellagic acid, however, suggest that its poor bioavailability may adversely affect usefulness in humans (Kelloff *et al.*, 1994).

Carotenoids

Common green, yellow/red and yellow/orange vegetables and fruits contain more than 40 carotenoids, in addition to β-carotene, that can be absorbed and metabolized by humans, including lutein, zeaxanthin, cryptoxanthin, lycopene, α-carotene, phytofluene, phytoene, astaxanthin, canthaxanthin and crocetin (Khachik *et al.*, 1995). As a class, carotenoids exhibit strong antioxidant activity, increase metabolic detoxification, increase cellular communication and have anti-inflammatory properties (Kelloff and Boone, 1994). Preliminary human metabolic studies on lutein and lycopene, two major dietary carotenoids, and zeaxanthin, a dihydroxycarotenoid isomeric to lutein, have established that these compounds undergo oxidation *in vivo*, clearly demonstrating their antioxidant capabilities (Khachik *et al.*, 1995).

Using a carotenoid database compiled for more than 2400 vegetables, fruits and multicomponent foods containing vegetables and fruits (Chug-Ahuja *et al.*, 1993), Ziegler and colleagues (1996b) reanalysed data from a population-based study conducted in New Jersey during 1980 and 1981 to evaluate the hypothesis that β-carotene may be protective against lung cancer. The reanalysis estimated smoking-adjusted risk of lung cancer in white male current and recent cigarette smokers by intakes of α-carotene, β-carotene, β-cryptoxanthin, lutein/zeaxanthin, lycopene, α-carotene + β-carotene + lutein/zeaxanthin and total carotenoids. Men in the lowest quartile of α-carotene intake had more than twice the risk of men in the highest quartile. The corresponding risks associated with intakes of β-carotene and lutein/zeaxanthin were increased only about 60%, suggesting that β-carotene is not the dominant protective factor in vegetables and fruits for lung cancer (Ziegler *et al.*, 1996b). Ecological data suggested that an inverse association with lutein (but not with α- or β-carotene) accounted for 14% of the variation in incidence in Fiji, where lung cancer rates are markedly lower than for other South Pacific islands (Le Marchand *et al.*, 1995). Data from a nested case–control study of serum micronutrient levels (highest vs. lowest tertiles) in a cohort of Japanese–American men indicated that α-carotene (RR = 0.19), β-carotene (RR = 0.10), β-cryptoxanthin (RR = 0.25) and total carotenoids (RR = 0.22) all significantly reduce the risk of aerodigestive tract cancers (Nomura *et al.*, 1997a).

Carotenoids also have been associated with reduced risk for hormone-related cancers. In a case–control study in Italian women, decreased breast cancer risk was associated with dietary intakes of α-carotene (RR=0.58, highest quintile) and β-carotene (RR = 0.68, highest quintile); however, when both α-carotene and β-carotene were introduced into the same model, only α-carotene remained protective. Intakes of β-cryptoxanthin, lycopene, and lutein/zeaxanthin were not related to risk (La Vecchia *et al.*, 1998). Although numerous epidemiological studies have reported inverse associations between either dietary total carotenoids, β-carotene, or other specific carotenoids and cervical cancer risk (Potischman and Brinton, 1996), results from β-carotene chemoprevention trials have not been promising, possibly in part because small sample sizes limited the power of the studies (Giuliano and Gapstur, 1998).

One review of epidemiological studies of vegetable and fruit intake and cancer risk suggested a slightly increased risk of prostate cancer among those with low intake (RR=1.3) (Block *et al.*, 1992). A later review reported inconsistent results for prostate cancer; six prospective studies failed to confirm the inverse association found in three out of five case–control studies (van Poppel and Goldbohm, 1995). Results from one large prospective epidemiological cohort study suggested that significant reduction in prostate cancer may be associated with increased dietary intake levels of lycopene (RR=0.79, highest vs. lowest quintile) and tomato-based foods (RR=0.65), which are high in lycopene (Giovannucci *et al.*, 1995). Results from a study of serum carotenoids in a cohort of American men of Japanese descent, however, did not support a reduced prostate cancer risk for any carotenoid, including lycopene (Nomura *et al.*, 1997b). Analysis of prostate tissue has determined that lycopene is present in biologically active concentrations, supporting the hypothesis that lycopene could have direct cancer-protective effects within the prostate (Clinton *et al.*, 1996).

Large-scale, Randomized Intervention Trials

The randomized, controlled clinical intervention trial is considered the best means available to determine whether antioxidants actually do reduce cancer risk. Selected ongoing and completed NCI-sponsored chemoprevention trials using antioxidants are described briefly below. The laboratory data and epidemiological studies that linked high intakes of β-carotene-containing foods and high blood levels of β-carotene to reduced risk of lung cancer provided strong hypotheses for the interventions used in these chemoprevention trials. Although the results were not as expected, these studies demonstrate the difficulty of isolating a single component of a healthful diet as the one beneficial element and exemplify the need for large-scale clinical trials.

Ongoing trials

The Harvard Women's Health Study (WHS) is a chemoprevention trial designed to evaluate the risks and benefits of low-dose aspirin, β-carotene and vitamin E in the primary prevention of cardiovascular disease and cancer in healthy postmenopausal women in the United States (Buring and Hennekens, 1993a,b). Begun in 1992, the WHS has enrolled approximately 40,000 female nurses, ages 45 and older, without a history of either disease. Participants are randomized to treatment or placebo groups for 2 years following a 3-month non-randomized run-in phase. In response to the lack of benefit for β-carotene seen in completed trials, the WHS removed β-carotene supplementation from its intervention. The study will continue to evaluate aspirin and vitamin E.

Closed trials

This section summarizes five large-scale, randomized trials for which accrual has been either completed or closed and results reported; long-term follow-up is continuing for these trials to determine safety as well as efficacy (Omenn *et al.*, 1996a).

The *Linxian Trials*, conducted by the NCI in collaboration with the Cancer Institute of the Chinese Academy of Medical Sciences, were two randomized, double-blind chemoprevention trials designed to determine whether daily ingestion of vitamin/mineral supplements would reduce incidence and mortality rates for oesophageal cancer in a high-risk population in Linxian, China, where approximately 20% of all deaths result from oesophageal cancer. The General Population Trial began in 1986 and randomized more than 29,000 individuals, who received one of four combinations of supplements, at doses equivalent to one to two times the US recommended daily allowances (RDAs), each day for 5 years. Combinations included retinal and zinc; riboflavin and niacin; vitamin C and molybdenum; and β-carotene, vitamin E and selenium. The second study, the Dysplasia Trial, enrolled 3318 individuals with evidence of severe oesophageal dysplasia; subjects were randomized to receive either a placebo or a daily supplement of 14 vitamins and 12 minerals, at two to three times the US RDAs, for 6 years.

Results of the General Population Trial indicated a significant benefit for those receiving the β-carotene/vitamin E/selenium combination – a 13% reduction in cancer mortality, due largely to a 21% drop in stomach cancer mortality (Blot *et al.*, 1993). Also, this group experienced a 9% reduction in deaths from all causes, a 10% decrease in deaths from strokes, and a 4% decrease in deaths from oesophageal cancer. The effects of the β-carotene/vitamin E/selenium combination began to appear within 1–2 years after the intervention began and continued throughout the study; the three other combinations did not affect cancer risk.

A non-significant, 16% reduction in mortality from oesophageal cancer was reported for the Dysplasia Trial (Li *et al.*, 1993). Analysis of oesophageal dysplasia data, however, showed that supplementation had a significant beneficial effect; individuals receiving supplements were 1.2 times more likely to have no dysplasia after 30 and 72 months of intervention, compared with individuals receiving the placebo (Mark *et al.*, 1994). The results of these trials are encouraging but may not be directly applicable to Western cultures, which tend to be well nourished and not deficient in multiple micronutrients, in contrast with the Linxian community. Even so, valuable information might be gained by determining cancer incidence for the 5 years since the trials ended, including analysis according to baseline nutrient levels (Omenn, 1998).

The *Physicians' Health Study* (*PHS*), a general population trial in 22,000 US physicians that evaluated the effect of aspirin and β-carotene supplementation on the primary prevention of cardiovascular disease and cancer, began in 1982. The dose of β-carotene was 50 mg on alternate days. The aspirin component of PHS ended in 1987, because a benefit of aspirin on risk of first heart attack (44% reduction) was found. The treatment period for β-carotene continued until December 1995; data showed no significant evidence of benefit or harm from β-carotene for either cardiovascular disease or cancer (Hennekens *et al.*, 1996).

The *Alpha-Tocopherol, Beta-Carotene* (*ATBC*) *Cancer Prevention Study* and the *Beta-Carotene and Retinol Efficacy Trial* (*CARET*) both were carried out in populations at high risk for lung cancer. The ATBC Study investigated the efficacy of vitamin E (α-tocopherol, 50 mg) alone, β-carotene alone (20 mg), or a combination of the two compounds in preventing lung cancer among more than 29,000 male cigarette smokers ages 50–69, with an average treatment/followup of 6 years. Unexpectedly, this study showed a 16% higher incidence of lung cancer in the β-carotene group. However, 16% fewer cases of colorectal cancer were diagnosed among men who received vitamin E (ATBC Cancer Prevention Study Group, 1994; Albanes *et al.*, 1996). Further, recent analysis of ATBC followup data found a 36% decrease in prostate cancer incidence and a 41% decrease in mortality from prostate cancer among men receiving vitamin E (Heinonen *et al.*, 1998). In the ATBC Study, the adverse effects of β-carotene were observed at the highest two quartiles of ethanol intake, indicating that alcohol consumption may enhance the actions of β-carotene (Albanes *et al.*, 1996). Also, follow-up data analysis showed a 32% lower incidence of prostate cancer among non-drinkers, whereas the risk among drinkers increased 25%, 42%, and 40% by tertiles (Heinonen *et al.*, 1998). It is not clear how alcohol might influence the protective effect of β-carotene. CARET tested the efficacy of a combination of β-carotene (30 mg) and retinol (25,000 IU as retinyl palmitate) in former and current heavy smokers and in men with extensive occupational asbestos exposure. This trial was terminated in January 1996 after 4 years of treatment, when data showed an overall 28% higher incidence of lung cancer in participants receiving the β-carotene/retinyl palmitate combination (Omenn *et al.*, 1996b). Male current smokers in CARET, excluding those exposed to asbestos, showed a 39% higher incidence (Omenn *et al.*, 1996a), compared with the 16% higher incidence in the ATBC Study (Albanes *et al.*, 1996), suggesting a possible adverse effect for supplemental retinol.

The results of these trials have led some to suggest that β-carotene should no longer be a candidate for inclusion in any future health interventions. Before such an extreme position is taken, however, a better understanding of the reasons for the unanticipated findings from ATBC and CARET is needed, especially considering that no increase in lung cancer incidence was observed in the 11% of men in the PHS who were current smokers (Hennekens *et al.*, 1996). Several possible explanations for the unanticipated outcomes of these β-carotene trials have been considered. The timing of the intervention may have been wrong (Erdmann *et al.*, 1996; Omenn *et al.*, 1996b; Rautalahti *et al.*, 1997). The median follow-up of 6 years may have been too short, either to show any effect on carcinogenesis or to reverse or overcome lung cancer risk factors, particularly in active smokers. The continuing post-trial followup will help to clarify this issue (Omenn *et al.*, 1996b; Rautalahti *et al.*, 1997). Further, many heavy smokers and asbestos-exposed individuals may have developed the initial stages of lung cancer prior to supplementation. Although evidence prior to the trials suggested that β-carotene may be more effective at later stages of carcinogenesis, this might not be the case, and benefit might be minimal once initiation has occurred. Judging by the fact that the β-carotene effect appeared after only 2 years of supplementation, it is probable that the observed effect was related to the growth of cells that had already undergone malignant transformation (Erdmann *et al.*, 1996; Rautalahti *et al.*, 1997).

Inappropriate timing of the intervention, however, does not fully explain the excess risk observed in ATBC and CARET in individuals receiving supplements. Another consideration is that the high doses used (ATBC, 20 mg β-carotene; CARET, 30 mg β-carotene + 25,000 IU preformed vitamin A) may have had pro-oxidant effects rather than cancer-protective effects in combination with cigarette smoke and/or asbestos exposure (Erdmann *et al.*, 1996; Mayne *et al.*, 1996; Rautalahti *et al.*, 1997). Direct oxidative attack on β-carotene by extremely reactive constituents of high-intensity cigarette smoke in the lungs of heavy smokers may induce the formation of β-carotene products that have pro-oxidant activity (Mayne *et al.*, 1996). In asbestos workers, the inflammatory process in the asbestos-exposed lung – characterized by increased amounts of superoxide and hydrogen peroxide, both reactive oxygen species – may provide a favourable environment for the formation of pro-oxidant products of β-carotene (Mayne *et al.*, 1996). Another possibility for the observed results is competitive inhibition by β-carotene of the antioxidant activity of other dietary carotenoids, such as α-carotene and lutein. α-Carotene, for example, has been reported to show higher potency than β-carotene in suppressing tumorigenesis in animal lung and skin models (Nishono, 1995).

It is noteworthy that participants with higher serum β-carotene concentrations at entry into the ATBC Study (Albanes *et al.*, 1996) and CARET (Omenn *et al.*, 1996a) developed fewer lung cancers during the course of the trials, even among those who received β-carotene supplements. Baseline serum concentrations of β-carotene reflect total intake of vegetables and fruits, which contain numerous other antioxidants, as well as many naturally occurring potential anticarcinogens that may exert their effects through diverse mechanisms; the β-carotene serum levels may simply be a marker for the actual protective agents. Thus, this finding is in agreement with epidemiological evidence linking β-carotene-containing foods and lung cancer and re-affirms the importance of including an abundance of plant foods in our diets (Albanes *et al.*, 1996; Mayne *et al.*, 1996).

Future Directions

The cancer-protective effect of vegetables and fruits is not in question. Epidemiological evidence strongly and consistently supports such an effect. What is in question is which particular constituents in vegetables and fruits are responsible for the observed protective effect. Although it may be logical to believe that naturally occurring antioxidants in these plant foods play some role in reducing human cancer risk, it would be presumptuous to assume that antioxidants alone account for the cancer risk reduction. Is it possible to determine which constituents of foods are the effective agents? This question does not have a simple answer. It is likely that many constituents have important, but different roles with respect to carcinogenesis, depending on cancer site, cancer stage and prevailing risk factors (Block, 1993). Also, doses of substances delivered to any specific tissue, and hence their effects, will be determined in part by genetic metabolic profiles that vary across populations and within individuals (Potter, 1996). Considering the variety of phyto-chemicals in commonly consumed plant foods and the possibility that they may act simultaneously, the interactive effects of these substances could be significant, as well as complex and difficult to unravel.

Although sorting out the cancer-related effects of vegetable and fruit constituents and the mechanisms by which they exert these effects may seem overwhelming, the potential benefits of such research endeavours for human health are great and will be well worth the multidisciplinary approaches and collaborative efforts required. Large gaps exist in our basic knowledge of even the most widely studied substances. Carotenoids, including β-carotene, illustrate this point well. As noted by the Carotenoid Research Interactive Group (CARIG) (Erdmann *et al.*, 1996), an international organization of scientists, basic information is lacking about digestion and absorption of carotenoids from foods, carotenoid bioavailability and metabolic fate, the role of *cis*-carotene isomers as provitamin A, effects of carotenoids on cellular metabolism and immunity, gene/carotenoid inter-actions, *in vivo* antioxidant value of carotenoids, composition of carotenoids in foods, and effects of simple food preparation techniques on carotenoid chemistry. Also, inadequate clinical research data are available about which types of cancer might be responsive to carotenoids, optimal carotenoid mixtures and dose levels, timing of dose in relationship to carcinogenic stages, characteristics of individuals who might be responsive, and appropriate pharmacokinetic and safety data (Erdmann *et al.*, 1996). Comprehensive, yet well-targeted, clinical trials and other research approaches that aim to answer such questions for nutritive and non-nutritive

constituents of plant foods, including the carotenoids and other antioxidants, are essential to accelerate progress in cancer prevention research
and to achieve definitive results that can be translated into effective,
practical cancer-preventive applications for the general population.

References

Ahmad, N., Feyes, D.K., Niemenen, A.-L., Agarwal, R. and Mukhtar, H. (1997) Green
    tea constituent epigallocatechin-3-gallate and induction of apoptosis and cell
    cycle arrest in human carcinoma cells. *Journal of the National Cancer Institute*
    89, 1881–1886.
Albanes, D., Heinonen, O.P., Taylor, P.R., Virtamo, J., Edwards, B.K., Rautalahti, M,
    Hartman, A.M., Palmgren, J., Freedman, L.S., Haapakoski, J., Barrett, M.J.,
    Pietinen, P., Malila, N., Tala, E., Liippo, K., Salomaa, E.-R., Tangrea, J.A., Teppo,
    L., Askin, F.B., Taskinen, E., Erozan, Y., Greenwald, P. and Huttunen, J.K. (1996)
    α-Tocopherol and β-carotene supplements and lung cancer incidence in the
    Alpha-Tocopherol, Beta-Carotene Cancer Prevention Study: effects of base-line
    characteristics and study compliance. *Journal of the National Cancer Institute*
    88, 1560–1570.
Alpha-Tocopherol Beta-Carotene Cancer Prevention Study Group (1994) The effect
    of vitamin E and beta carotene on the incidence of lung cancer and other
    cancers in male smokers. *New England Journal of Medicine* 330, 1029–1035.
Block, G. (1991) Vitamin C and cancer prevention: the epidemiologic evidence.
    American Journal of Clinical Nutrition 53, 270S–282S.
Block, G. (1993) Micronutrients and cancer: time for action? (editorial). *Journal of
    the National Cancer Institute* 85, 846–848.
Block, G., Patterson, B.H. and Subar, A.F. (1992) Fruit, vegetables, and cancer
    prevention: a review of the epidemiological evidence. *Nutrition and Cancer* 18,
    1–29.
Blot, W.J., Li, J.-Y., Taylor, P.R., Guo, W., Dawsey, S.M., Wang, G.-Q., Yang, C.S.,
    Zheng, S.-F., Gail, M.H., Li, G.-Y., Yu, Y., Liu, B.-Q., Tangrea, J.A., Sun, Y.-H.,
    Liu, F., Fraumeni, J.F. Jr, Zhang, Y.-H. and Li. B. (1993) Nutrition intervention
    trials in Linxian: supplementation with specific vitamin/mineral combinations,
    cancer incidence, and disease-specific mortality in the general population.
    Journal of the National Cancer Institute 85, 1483–1492.
Buring, J.E. and Hennekens, C.H. (1993a) The Women's Health Study: summary of
    the study design. *Journal of Myocardial Ischemia* 4, 27–29.
Buring, J.E. and Hennekens, C.H. (1993b) The Women's Health Study: rationale and
    background. *Journal of Myocardial Ischemia* 4, 30–40.
Byers, T. and Guerrero, N. (1995) Epidemiologic evidence for vitamin C and vitamin
    E in cancer prevention. *American Journal of Clinical Nutrition* 62, 1385S–1392S.
Chug-Ahuja, J.K., Holden, J.M., Forman, M.R., Mangels, A.R., Beecher, G.R. and
    Lanza, E. (1993) The development and application of a carotenoid database for
    fruits, vegetables, and selected multicomponent foods. *Journal of the American
    Dietetic Association* 93, 318–323.
Clark, L.C., Combs, G.F. Jr, Turnbull, B.W., Slate, E.H., Chalker, D.K., Chow, J., Davis,
    L.S., Glover, R.A., Graham, G.F., Gross, E.G., Krongrad, A., Lesher, J.L. Jr, Park,

H.K., Sanders, B.B. Jr, Smith, C.L. and Taylor, J.R. (1996) Effects of selenium supplementation for cancer prevention in patients with carcinoma of the skin. *Journal of the American Medical Association* 276, 1957–1963.

Clinton, S.K., Emenhiser, C., Schwartz, S.J., Bostwick, D.G., Williams, A.W., Moore, B.J. and Erdman, J.W. Jr (1996) *cis-trans* lycopene isomers, carotenoids, and retinol in the human prostate. *Cancer Epidemiology, Biomarkers and Prevention* 5, 823–833.

Cozzi, R., Ricordy, R., Aglitti, T., Gatta, V., Perticone, P. and De Salvia, R. (1997) Ascorbic acid and β-carotene as modulators of oxidative damage. *Carcinogenesis* 18, 223–228.

Diplock, A.T. (1996) Antioxidants and disease prevention. *Food and Chemical Toxicology* 34, 1013–1023.

Erdman, J.W. Jr, Russell, R.M., Mayer, J., Rock, C.L., Barua, A.B., Bowen, P.E., Burri, B.J., Curran-Celentano, J., Furr, H., Mayne, S.T. and Stacewicz-Sapuntzakis, M. (1996) Beta-carotene and the carotenoids: beyond the intervention trials. *Nutrition Reviews* 54, 185–188.

Garewal, H.S., Meyskens, F.L. Jr, Killen, D., Reeves, D., Kiersch, T.A., Elletson, H., Strosberg, A., King, D. and Steinbronn, K. (1990) Response of oral leukoplakia to beta-carotene. *Journal of Clinical Oncology* 8, 1715–1720.

Giovannucci, E., Ascherio, A., Rimm, E.B., Stampfer, M.J., Colditz, G.A. and Willett, W.C. (1995) Intake of carotenoids and retinol in relation to risk of prostate cancer. *Journal of the National Cancer Institute* 87, 1767–1776.

Giuliano, A.R. and Gapstur, S. (1998) Can cervical dysplasia and cancer be prevented with nutrients? *Nutrition Reviews* 56, 9–16.

Greenberg, E.R., Baron, J.A., Tosteson, T.D., Freeman, D.H. Jr, Beck, G.J., Bond, J.H., Colacchio, T.A., Coller, J.A., Frankl, H.D., Haile, R.W., Mandel, J.S., Nierenberg, D.W., Rothstein, R., Snover, D.C., Stevens, M.M., Summers, R.W. and van Stolk, R.U. (1994) A clinical trial of antioxidant vitamins to prevent colorectal adenoma. *New England Journal of Medicine* 331, 141–147.

Heinonen, O.P., Albanes, D., Virtamo, J., Taylor, P.R., Huttenen, J.K., Hartman, A.M., Haapakoski, J., Malila, N., Rautalahti, M., Ripatti, S., Mäenpää, H., Teerenhovi, L., Koss, L., Virolainen, M. and Edwards, B.K. (1998) Prostate cancer and supplementation with α-tocopherol and β-carotene: incidence and mortality in a controlled trial. *Journal of the National Cancer Institute* 90, 440–446.

Helzlsouer, K.J., Alberg, A.J., Norkus, E.P., Morris, J.S., Hoffman, S.C. and Comstock, G.W. (1996) Prospective study of serum micronutrients and ovarian cancer. *Journal of the National Cancer Institute* 88, 32–37.

Hennekens, C.H., Buring, J.E., Manson, J.E., Stampfer, M., Rosner, B., Cook, N.R., Belanger, C., LaMotte, F., Gaziano, J.M., Ridker, P.M., Willett, W. and Peto, R. (1996) Lack of effect of long-term supplementation with beta carotene on the incidence of malignant neoplasms and cardiovascular disease. *New England Journal of Medicine* 334, 1145–1149.

Hunter, D.J. and Willett, W.C. (1996) Nutrition and breast cancer. *Cancer Causes and Control* 7, 56–68.

Imai, K., Suga, K. and Nakachi, K. (1997) Cancer-preventive effects of drinking green tea among a Japanese population. *Preventive Medicine* 26, 769–775.

Jacob, R.A. and Burri, B.J. (1996) Oxidative damage and defense. *American Journal of Clinical Nutrition* 63, 985S–990S.

Ji, B.-T., Chow, W.-H., Hsing, A.W., McLaughlin, J.K., Dai, Q., Gao, Y.-T., Blot, W.J. and Fraumeni, J.F. Jr. (1997) Green tea consumption and the risk of pancreatic and colorectal cancers. *International Journal of Cancer* 70, 255–258.

Kelloff, G.J. and Boone, C.W. (eds) (1994) Clinical development plan: β-carotene and other carotenoids. *Journal of Cellular Biochemistry* 20S, 110–140.

Kelloff, G.J. and Boone, C.W. (eds) (1996a) Clinical development plan: 1,4-phenylenebis-(methylene) selenocyanate. *Journal of Cellular Biochemistry* 26S, 219–226.

Kelloff, G.J. and Boone, C.W. (eds) (1996b) Clinical development plan: curcumin. *Journal of Cellular Biochemistry* 26S, 72–85.

Kelloff, G.J., Boone, C.W., Crowell, J.A., Steele, V.E., Lubert, R. and Sigman, C.C. (1994) Chemopreventive drug development: perspectives and progress. *Cancer Epidemiology, Biomarkers and Prevention* 3, 85–98.

Khachik, F., Beecher, G.R. and Smith, J.C. Jr (1995) Lutein, lycopene, and their oxidative metabolites in chemoprevention of cancer. *Journal of Cellular Biochemistry* 22S, 236–246.

Kimmick, G.G., Bell, R.A. and Bostick, R.M. (1997) Vitamin E and breast cancer: a review. *Nutrition and Cancer* 27, 109–117.

Kolonel, L.N. (1996) Nutrition and prostate cancer. *Cancer Causes and Control* 7, 83–94.

Kono, S. and Hirohata, T. (1996) Nutrition and stomach cancer. *Cancer Causes and Control* 7, 41–55.

La Vecchia, C., Ferraroni, M., Negri, E. and Franceschi, S. (1998) Role of various carotenoids in the risk of breast cancer. *International Journal of Cancer* 75, 482–483.

Le Marchand, L., Hankin, J.H., Bach, F., Kolonel, L.N., Wilkens, L.R., Stacewicz-Sapuntzakis, M., Bowen, P.E., Beecher, G.R., Laudon, F., Baque, P., Daniel, R., Seruvatu, L. and Henderson, B.E. (1995) An ecological study of diet and lung cancer in the South Pacific. *International Journal of Cancer* 63, 18–23.

Li, J.-Y., Taylor, P.R., Dawsey, S.M., Wang, G.-Q., Ershow, A.G., Guo, W., Liu, S.-F., Yang, C.S., Shen, Q., Wang, W., Mark, S.D., Zou, X.-N., Greenwald, P., Wu, Y.-P. and Blot, W.J. (1993) Nutrition intervention trials in Linxian, China: multiple vitamin/mineral supplementation, cancer incidence, and disease-specific mortality among adults with esophageal dysplasia. *Journal of the National Cancer Institute* 85, 1492–1498.

Lippman, S.M., Batsakis, J.G., Toth, B.B., Weber, R.S., Lee, J.J., Martin, J.W., Hays, G.L., Goepfert, H. and Hong, W.K. (1993) Comparison of low-dose isotretinoin with beta carotene to prevent oral carcinogenesis. *New England Journal of Medicine* 328, 15–20.

Loft, S. and Poulsen, H.E. (1996) Cancer risk and oxidative DNA damage in man. *Journal of Molecular Medicine* 74, 297–312.

Lubin, F., Rozen, P., Arieli, B., Farbstein, M., Knaani, Y., Bat, L. and Farbstein, H. (1997) Nutritional and lifestyle habits and water–fiber interaction in colorectal adenoma etiology. *Cancer Epidemiology, Biomarkers and Prevention* 6, 79–85.

MacClennan, R., Macrae, F., Bain, C., Battistutta, D., Chapuis, P., Gratten, H., Lambert, J., Newland, R.C., Ngu, M., Russell, A., Ward, M. and Wahlqvist, M.L. (1995) Randomized trial of intake of fat, fiber, and beta carotene to prevent colorectal adenomas. *Journal of the National Cancer Institute* 87, 1760–1766.

Manna, C., Galletti, P., Cucciolla, V., Moltedo, O., Leone, A. and Zappia, V. (1997) The protective effect of the olive oil polyphenol (3,4-dihydroxyphenyl)-ethanol counteracts reactive oxygen metabolite-induced cytotoxicity in Caco-2 cells. *Journal of Nutrition* 127, 286–292.

Mark, S.D., Liu, S.-F., Li, J.-Y., Gail, M.H., Shen, Q., Dawsey, S.M., Liu, F., Taylor, P.R., Li, B. and Blot, W.J. (1994) The effect of vitamin and mineral supplementation on esophageal cytology: results from the Linxian Dysplasia Trial. *International Journal of Cancer* 57, 162–166.

Mayne, S.T., Handelman, G.J. and Beecher, G. (1996) β-carotene and lung cancer promotion in heavy smokers – a plausible relationship? *Journal of the National Cancer Institute* 88, 1513–1515.

Nishono, H. (1995) Cancer chemoprevention by natural carotenoids and their related compounds. *Journal of Cellular Biochemistry* 22S, 231–235.

Nomura, A.M.Y., Ziegler, R.G., Stemmermann, G.N., Chyou, P.-H. and Craft, N.E. (1997a) Serum micronutrients and upper aerodigestive tract cancer. *Cancer Epidemiology, Biomarkers and Prevention* 6, 407–412.

Nomura, A.M.Y., Stemmermann, G.N., Lee, J. and Craft, N.E. (1997b) Serum micronutrients and prostate cancer in Japanese Americans in Hawaii. *Cancer Epidemiology, Biomarkers and Prevention* 6, 487–491.

Omenn, G.S. (1998) Interpretation of the Linxian vitamin supplement chemoprevention trials. *Epidemiology* 9, 1–3.

Omenn, G.S., Goodman, G.E., Thornquist, M.D., Balmes, J., Cullen, M.R., Glass, A., Keogh, J.P., Meyskens, F.L. Jr, Valanis, B., Williams, J.H. Jr, Barnhart, S., Cherniack, M.G., Brodkin, C.A. and Hammar, S. (1996a) Risk factors for lung cancer and for intervention effects in CARET, the Beta-Carotene and Retinol Efficacy Trial. *Journal of the National Cancer Institute* 88, 1550–1559.

Omenn, G.S., Goodman, G.E., Thornquist, M.D., Balmes, J., Cullen, M.R., Glass, A., Keogh, J.P., Meyskens, F.L. Jr, Valanis, B., Williams, J.H. Jr, Barnhart, S. and Hammar, S. (1996b) Effects of a combination of beta carotene and vitamin A on lung cancer and cardiovascular disease. *New England Journal of Medicine* 334, 1150–1155.

Perera, F.P. (1996) Molecular epidemiology: insights into cancer susceptibility, risk assessment, and prevention. *Journal of the National Cancer Institute* 88, 496–509.

Peto, R., Doll, R., Buckley, J.D. and Sporn, M.B. (1981) Can dietary beta-carotene materially reduce human cancer rates? *Nature* 290, 201–208.

van Poppel, G. and Goldbohm, R.A. (1995) Epidemiologic evidence for β-carotene and cancer prevention. *American Journal of Clinical Nutrition* 62, 1393S–1402S.

Potter, J.D. (1996) Food and phytochemicals, magic bullets and measurement error: a commentary. *American Journal of Epidemiology* 144, 1026–1027.

Potischman, N. and Brinton, L.A. (1996) Nutrition and cervical neoplasia. *Cancer Causes and Control* 7, 113–126.

Rautalahti, M., Albanes, D., Virtamo, J., Taylor, P.R., Huttunen, J.K. and Heinonen, O.P. (1997) Beta-carotene did not work: aftermath of the ATBC Study. *Cancer Letters* 114, 235–236.

Reddy, B.S., Rivenson, A., El-Bayoumy, K., Upadhyaya, P., Pittman, B. and Rao, C.V. (1997) Chemoprevention of colon cancer by organoselenium compounds and impact of high- or low-fat diets. *Journal of the National Cancer Institute* 89, 506–512.

Schrauzer, G.N., White, D.A. and Schneider, C.J. (1977) Cancer mortality correlation studies. III. Statistical associations with dietary selenium intakes. *Bioinorganic Chemistry* 7, 23–34.

Steele, V.E., Sharma, S., Mehta, R., Elmore, E., Redpath, L., Rudd, C., Bagheri, D., Sigman, C.C. and Kelloff, G.J. (1996) Use of *in vitro* assays to predict the efficacy of chemopreventive agents in whole animals. *Journal of Cellular Biochemistry* 26S, 29–53.

Steinmetz, K.A. and Potter, J.D. (1996) Vegetables, fruit, and cancer prevention: a review. *Journal of the American Dietetic Association* 96, 1027–1039.

Stich, H.F., Stich, W., Rosin, M.P. and Vallejera, M.O. (1984) Use of the micronucleus test to monitor the effect of vitamin A, beta-carotene and canthaxanthin on the buccal mucosa of betel nut/tobacco chewers. *International Journal of Cancer* 34, 745–750.

Stone, W.L. and Papas, A.M. (1997) Tocopherols and the etiology of colon cancer. *Journal of the National Cancer Institute* 89, 1006–1014.

Stoner, G.D. and Mukhtar, H. (1995) Polyphenols as cancer chemopreventive agents. *Journal of Cellular Biochemistry* 22S, 169–180.

Tseng, M., Murray, S.C., Kupper, L.L. and Sandler, R.S. (1996) Micronutrients and the risk of colorectal adenomas. *American Journal of Epidemiology* 144, 1005–1014.

Visioli, F., Bellomo, G., Montedoro, G. and Galli, C. (1995) Low density lipoprotein oxidation is inhibited *in vitro* by olive oil constituents. *Atherosclerosis* 117, 25–32.

Wattenberg, L.W. (1992) Inhibition of carcinogenesis by minor dietary constituents. *Cancer Research* 52, 2085S–2091S.

Yang, C.S., Chen, L., Lee, M.-J. and Landau, J.M. (1996) Effects of tea on carcinogenesis in animal models and humans. In: American Institute for Cancer Research (ed.) *Dietary Phytochemicals in Cancer Prevention and Treatment.* Plenum Press, New York, pp. 51–61.

Ziegler, R.G., Mayne, S.T. and Swanson, C.A. (1996a) Nutrition and lung cancer. *Cancer Causes and Control* 7, 157–177.

Ziegler, R.G., Colavito, E.A., Hartge, P., McAdams, M.J., Schoenberg, J.B., Mason, T.J. and Fraumeni, J.F. Jr. (1996b) Importance of α-carotene, β-carotene, and other phytochemicals in the etiology of lung cancer. *Journal of the National Cancer Institute* 88, 612–615.

The Role of β-Carotene and Vitamin E in the Treatment of Early Gastric Premalignant Lesions: Biochemical and Clinical Aspects

19

YURIY V. BUKIN AND VLADIMIR A. DRAUDIN-KRYLENKO

Cancer Research Center of the Russian Academy of Medical Sciences, Moscow, Russia

Introduction

Although the rate of gastric cancer has decreased substantially in many Western countries during the past several decades, it is still the second most common cancer worldwide (Buiatti and Muñoz, 1996). Unlike Russia, China, Japan and some countries of Latin America, where the gastric cancer incidence reaches 40–150 per 100,000 per year (Parkin *et al.*, 1993), its incidence in the USA is very low, and since 1954 has plateaued at about 25,000 new cases annually (Wanebo *et al.*, 1993). However, even in countries with a low incidence, this disease is a serious medical and public health problem, because the 5-year survival rate after the diagnosis does not exceed, as a rule, 14% (Wanebo *et al.*, 1993). Finding effective ways to prevent gastric cancer must therefore be our number one priority in fighting against it.

So called 'intestinal' type of gastric adenocarcinoma, predominating in high-risk populations, is preceded, according to Correa (1988, 1992), by a sequential chain of events characterized as chronic superficial gastritis, chronic atrophic gastritis (CAG), small intestinal metaplasia (SIM), colonic metaplasia, dysplasia and carcinoma. SIM is considered to be the first morphological manifestation of gastric premalignant lesions, and is characterized by the presence of non-secretory columnar cells of intestinal epithelium which have a prominent strait border of microvilli, goblet cells and Paneth cells (Owen, 1989; Correa, 1992).

The intestinal type of gastric cancer, with which we are concerned, has a complex aetiology. It is believed that nitrates and nitrites (precursors of carcinogenic *N*-nitroso compounds), pickled foods, excess salt, bile reflux and bacterial overgrowth in atrophic mucosa play a significant role in gastric carcinogenesis (Correa, 1992; Hill, 1994; Fontham, 1997). During the last decade the attention of many investigators has been focused on *Helicobacter pylori* infection and its possible role in initiating superficial gastritis, as well as GAG and SIM (De Koster *et al.*, 1994; Crespi and Citarda, 1996; Reed, 1996; Fontham, 1997). At the onset of infection, *H. pylori* produces some inflammatory cytokines; it provokes the infiltration of mucosa with macrophages and polymorphonuclear leukocytes as a host response that is accompanied by the formation of an excess of genotoxic free radicals, namely peroxynitrite, nitrosonium ions, nitric oxide, nitrites, and *N*-nitroso mutagens and carcinogens (Hill, 1994; Correa, 1995; Mannick *et al.*, 1996; Ruiz *et al.*, 1996). It is known that *H. pylori* infection provokes the development of gastric atrophy. At this stage the production by *H. pylori* of cytotoxic proteins leads to the loss of acid-secretory parietal cells, and to an increase in pH that promotes the overgrowth of anaerobic bacteria, increased nitrite production, and the formation of an excess of *N*-nitroso mutagens and carcinogens (Mannick *et al.*, 1996; Ruiz *et al.*, 1996). A sharp decrease in the concentration of ascorbic acid in the gastric lumen during the development of atrophy (Schorah *et al.*, 1991) is another cause of an increased formation of *N*-nitroso compounds, because ascorbic acid, as well as vitamin E (Mirvish, 1996), reduces nitrites, and thereby prevents the formation of these carcinogenic substances. It should be stressed that the excess of genotoxic free radicals and carcinogens increases the risk of mutation of the p53 suppressor gene which controls apoptosis. Also, disturbances of the process of apoptosis increase the probability of survival for cells which have been initiated with a sublethal dose of carcinogen, and the start of the process of carcinogenesis (Correa, 1992). We suggested that in this situation an over-expression of proto-oncogene ornithine decarboxylase (ODC) can serve as an important driving force of gastric carcinogenesis (see below).

Numerous epidemiological observations have revealed a strong association between a low risk of gastric cancer and a relatively high intake of fresh vegetables and fruit (rich in natural antioxidants), or high plasma levels of β-carotene (Poppel and Goldbohm, 1995; Fontham, 1997). Analysis of the biochemical and pathological processes leading to the development of SIM indicates that natural antioxidants, preventing *N*-nitroso compound formation (Farinati *et al.*, 1994), and quenching and scavenging free radicals (Sies *et al.*, 1992; Sies and Stahl, 1995), help to block the process of gastric carcinogenesis at its earliest stage. Indeed, low plasma levels of β-carotene are associated with an increased risk of CAG (Tsugane *et al.*, 1995), whereas a low plasma level of ascorbic acid is associated with an increased risk of

SIM (UK Subgroup, 1992). It has also been shown that serum levels of carotene and vitamin E are significantly reduced in subjects with gastric dysplasia (Haenszel *et al.*, 1985). In light of these data, we studied the putative curative effect of natural antioxidants (β-carotene and vitamin E) in early gastric premalignant lesions (SIM), using ODC activity as a possible intermediate biochemical biomarker of antipromoter action.

ODC as a Putative Biochemical Intermediate Biomarker of Gastric Carcinogenesis

ODC catalyses the first rate-limiting step in the polyamine biosynthetic pathway, and controls cell proliferation under normal physiological stimuli (Pegg, 1988). However, being constitutively overexpressed by carcinogens, promoters or some oncogenes, ODC may play a role of oncogene (see references in Shantz and Pegg, 1994; Clifford *et al.*, 1995; Pegg *et al.*, 1995). It has been shown in cell cultures that the overexpression of ODC at the level of transcription, as well as at the level of translation of the specific mRNA for ODC, leads to the transformation of cells which display the neoplastic phenotype (Auvinen *et al.*, 1992; Moshier *et al.*, 1993; Shantz and Pegg, 1994). The neoplastic phenotype of these cells may be prevented or reversed by α-difluoromethylornithine (DFMO), an irreversible inhibitor of ODC (Höltta *et al.*, 1993; Shantz and Pegg, 1994). The variable role of ODC in cell functions is shown in Fig. 19.1. The interaction of ODC as an oncogene with other oncogenes (Pegg *et al.*, 1995) and with signalling pathways regulating proliferation and differentiation of cells (Manni *et al.*, 1997) is outside the scope of this chapter.

It should be noted that ODC overexpression plays a critical role in tumour promotion. The activity of promoters depends on their ability to induce ODC (O'Brien *et al.*, 1975). In animal models DFMO blocks ODC and thereby inhibits the production of tumours in skin, bladder, stomach, intestine, colon, oral cavity and mammary glands (Kelloff *et al.*, 1994). The specific role of ODC in tumour promotion was demonstrated recently in transgenic mice which began to express a high ODC activity in skin 12 days after birth (O'Brien *et al.*, 1997). In this multistage tumorigenesis model, the process of tumour promotion in mouse skin, after initiation with a single low dose of carcinogen, did not require the additional application of 12-*O*-tetradecanoylphorbol-13-acetate (TPA, a promoter of skin tumours), and depended solely on the time of ODC overexpression.

Clinical observations have revealed abnormally high ODC activity in patients with premalignant lesions of the oesophagus (Garewal *et al.*, 1988) and colon (Luk and Baylin, 1984; Porter *et al.*, 1987). We have shown that ODC activity increases gradually during the course of pathological processes in human gastric mucosa which lead to premalignant lesions and gastric cancer (Table 19.1). In some CAG patients ODC activity is very high; it may

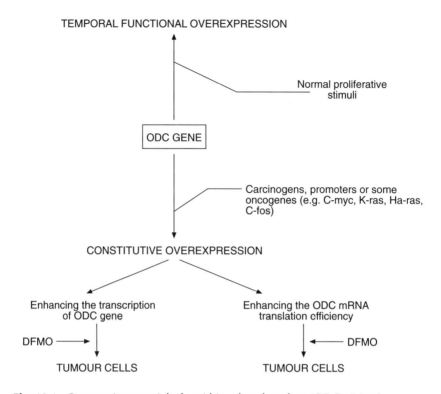

Fig. 19.1. Oncogenic potential of ornithine decarboxylase (ODC). DFMO, α-difluoromethylornithine.

be seen as an indicator of the process of tumour promotion at the biochemical level, preceding the appearance of premalignant lesions.

We have previously found that DFMO sharply inhibits ODC overexpression in rat stomach mucosa induced by the carcinogen *N*-methyl-*N'*-nitro-*N*-nitrosoguanidine (Bukin and Draudin-Krylenko, 1994). However, as the half-life of ODC in mammalian tissues is a mere 20 min (Pegg, 1988), it is therefore necessary to administer DFMO frequently during a prolonged period for it to be effective. Since this is clearly difficult, down-regulation of ODC activity by DFMO might not be a practical means to achieve antipromoter action in humans.

Antipromoter and Curative Effects of β-Carotene and Vitamin E in Early Gastric Premalignant Lesions

Our preliminary data on patients with CAG, either alone or accompanied by SIM, revealed that supplementation with β-carotene (20 mg day^{-1}) (Bukin *et al.*, 1993, 1995), or vitamin E (400 IU day^{-1}) (Bukin *et al.*, 1996, 1997) for

Table 19.1. ODC activity in human antral gastric mucosa during the course of pathological process, leading to premalignant lesions and carcinoma.

Condition of mucosa	ODC activity[a] (mean ± SD (range))
Normal	7.2 ± 1.8 (4.2–11.9)
Superficial gastritis	22.7 ± 5.9 (14.3–39.5)
Chronic atrophic gastritis (CAG)	51.4 ± 5.6 (30.4–108.0)
Small intestinal metaplasia (SIM)	56.1 ± 8.0 (39.5–90.8)
Colonic metaplasia	58.3 ± 11.4 (42.6–92.3)
Moderate or severe dysplasia	78.2 ± 14.4 (54.3–125.9)
Carcinoma	107.0 ± 16.7 (75.6–166.5)

[a] ODC activity is shown in units; one unit is the formation of 1 pmol $^{14}CO_2$ h^{-1} mg^{-1} protein.

1 or 3 months produced a substantial decrease in ODC levels in antral and fundal stomach mucosa. Taking into account the critical role of ODC overexpression at the tumour promotion stage, we suggested that this effect of β-carotene and vitamin E may be viewed as an antipromoter action. It seems that this effect *per se* may decrease the risk of gastric cancer. However, this assumption can be evaluated only in long-term large-scale intervention trials.

To date, we have focused on the possible capacity of natural antioxidants, when given for relatively long periods (6–12 months), to act as antipromoters and produce regression of early gastric premalignant lesions. In our study we used synthetic all-*trans*-β-carotene (Hoffmann-La Roche, Basel, Switzerland) and All Natural Vitamin E (Vital Life Products, Klaire Laboratories International, San Marcos, California), containing 70% D-α-tocopherol and a 30% mixture of D-β-, D-δ- and D-δ-tocopherols derived from soy oil.

So as to select patients for the intervention trial we carried out an initial gastroscopy (performed with endoscopic system Evis-100, Olympus, Japan). We usually took four biopsies for histological analysis and for determination of *H. pylori* status by the 1-min urease test (Arvind *et al.*, 1988). *H. pylori*-positive SIM patients were treated with a standard chemotherapeutic schedule (de nol colloidal bismuth subcitrate, metronidazole and tetracycline) (Bukin *et al.*, 1997); clearance of *H. pylori* was confirmed by the urease test and histological examination performed 3 or 4 weeks after the end of treatment. Only *H. pylori*-negative patients were enrolled.

Prior to treatment and at 3 or 6 months and at 12 months, six or seven biopsies were taken from the antrum at 2–4 cm from the pylorus, two or three biopsies for ODC assay, and four for histological analysis (one each from the lesser and greater curvatures, and two from the lateral walls). The standard procedure for the assay of ODC activity in human stomach mucosa using a sensitive radioisotope method was described previously (Bukin *et al.*, 1995). The levels of β-carotene and vitamin E in plasma were determined by a high performance liquid chromatography (HPLC) method (Nierenberg and Lester, 1985) using the HP 1090M chromatographic system (Hewlett-Packard, USA) equipped with Hypersil C18 columns and an ultra-violet (UV) diode array detector. For histological analysis, biopsy specimens were stained using haematoxylin and eosin. SIM was diagnosed if Paneth cells, goblet cells, as well as non-secretory columnar cells of metaplastic epithelium, having a prominent strait border of microvilli-like small intestinal epithelium, were present. In a few cases, besides the signs of SIM, sectorial colonic metaplasia was also observed. The disappearance of cells typical of SIM in all examined biopsies of a particular patient was considered to denote the regression of the premalignant lesion.

The design of the 1-year double-blind placebo-controlled trial with β-carotene was as follows. Subjects had SIM and CAG. They were matched for age and sex and received daily 20 mg of β-carotene in 10 ml of refined sunflower oil (n = 18) or a placebo (10 ml of the oil) (n = 11). Biochemical and histological examinations were carried out in both groups at 3 and 12 months after the start of intervention, as well as at 3 months after the cessation of intervention.

Initial plasma levels of β-carotene in the patients (0.11 ± 0.08 mg l^{-1}) were below normal (0.2–0.4 mg l^{-1}) (Gerster, 1993). Low initial levels of β-carotene increased to 1.02 ± 0.46 mg l^{-1} after 3 months of supplementation, and to 1.46 ± 0.62 mg l^{-1} after 12 months. No such change was seen in the placebo group. ODC activity in the placebo group did not change during the study, whereas in the β-carotene group it decreased by 46% after 3 and by 51% after 12 months of intervention.

The effect of β-carotene on SIM regression is summarized in Table 19.2. No regression was detected in the placebo group. In the β-carotene group, however, statistically significant SIM regression was observed in 50% of patients after 1 year. In Table 19.3 the β-carotene-dependent alterations of frequency in four biopsies from 16 patients (in whom all four biopsies were good enough for histological analysis) are presented. It is evident that after 1 year of treatment no signs of SIM were observed in any of the four biopsies in nine of the 16 patients. In Table 19.3 the total number of biopsies with or without SIM from 18 patients receiving β-carotene is presented. The data reveal that after 1 year of treatment, the total number of biopsies with SIM has decreased by more than half. We therefore conclude that β-carotene cured about half of SIM patients. However, this conclusion is based on the analysis of multiple biopsy specimens and does

Table 19.2. Effect of β-carotene intervention on SIM regression: ratio of patients with SIM regression to total cases.

β-carotene		Placebo	
After 3 months	After 1 year	After 3 months	After 1 year
1/18	9/18*	0/11	0/11

*Difference from placebo group is statistically significant (P<0.05); response rate is 50% (95% confidence interval 26–74%).

not rule out the possibility of residual areas of SIM at the end of treatment. For this reason the data should be interpreted with caution. Nevertheless, our results demonstrate that β-carotene at a daily dose of 20 mg can produce a partial regression of SIM after 1 year.

It should be noted that 3 months after the cessation of β-carotene supplementation, its level in plasma sharply decreased, ODC activity in some patients substantially increased, and in two patients the histological signs of SIM reappeared. This indicates that after the main treatment period, low maintenance doses of β-carotene are required.

In view of the curative effect of β-carotene on early gastric premalignant lesions, we decided to investigate the curative effect of natural vitamin E,

Table 19.3. Frequency of SIM in four biopsies from each patient before and during the 1 year of β-carotene treatment.

Time of examination	Part 1 Presence (+) or absence (−) of SIM in four biopsies					Part 2 Total number of biopsies[a]	
	(++++)	(+++−)	(++−−)	(+−−−)	(−−−−)	With SIM	Without SIM
Before treatment	8(50%)[b]	6(38%)	2(12%)	0(0%)	0(0%)	57	12
After 3 months treatment	9(56%)	5(31%)	1(6%)	0(0)%	1(6%)	55	13
After 1 year treatment	3(18%)	2(13%)	1(6%)	1(6%)	9(56%)	26[c]	44
3 months after the end of treatment	3(18%)	2(13%)	2(13%)	2(13%)	7(44%)	28[d]	42

[a] Of the 18 patients, in some only two or three biopsies out of four were suitable for histological examination.
[b] Number of patients with different SIM frequencies in biopsies; % in brackets.
[c] Decrease of SIM frequency is statistically significant (P < 0.001).
[d] Not significantly different from the previous estimation after 1 year of treatment.

which also has antioxidant properties and manifested an antipromoter action in our experiments. Selection of patients for this trial, as well as gastroscopic, biochemical and histological analyses, was performed as in the previous trial with β-carotene. Two groups of SIM patients, matched for age and sex, received daily one capsule of natural vitamin E (400 IU) or a placebo (refined soy oil). The patients were examined 6 and 12 months after the start of treatment, as well as 10 months after the cessation of treatment. There were initially 18 patients in each group but the number who completed the study was 14 in the vitamin E group and 16 in the placebo group. The initial plasma levels of vitamin E in the vitamin E and placebo groups were 6.4 ± 0.9 and 6.7 ± 1.1 mg l^{-1}, respectively. This did not change significantly in the placebo group, whereas in the vitamin E group after 6 and 12 months of supplementation, the levels reached 17.0 ± 1.8 and 21.2 ± 2.3 mg l^{-1}, respectively.

The effect of a high dose of vitamin E on ODC activity in antral gastric mucosa was as follows. The initial, abnormally high ODC activity (62.6 ± 7.8 units) progressively decreased by 53% after 6 months of vitamin E supplementation and by 65% after 12 months ($P < 0.01$). No change in ODC activity was seen in the placebo group.

The effect of vitamin E on SIM regression is shown in Table 19.4. In the placebo group no SIM regression was observed after 6 or 12 months. By contrast, in the vitamin E group, after 6 and 12 months of intervention, statistically significant regression by 57% (eight patients of 14) and by 71% (ten patients of 14), respectively, was observed. It should be noted that in some cases, only two or three of four biopsies were suitable for histological examination. The prevalence of SIM in total biopsies of the vitamin E treatment group decreased from 84 to 44 and 18% after 6 and 12 months, respectively ($P < 0.01$).

The staining procedure used at the final gastroscopy (Misumi *et al.*, 1990) revealed numerous vast patches of stained areas in all patients receiving the placebo. Similar observations were made in those patients receiving vitamin E whose biopsies demonstrated SIM histologically. Conversely, in ten of 14 patients who were histologically negative for SIM after 1 year of vitamin E supplementation, only small isolated patches of stained areas were observed. Comparison of these results with histological data revealed that although the regression of SIM produced in some patients taking vitamin E was pronounced, it was not complete.

It should be stressed that 10 months after the cessation of vitamin E supplementation, the curative effect seems to have diminished (Table 19.4). The number of patients with SIM regression reduced from ten of 14 to seven of 14, and the prevalence of biopsies with SIM among total biopsies significantly increased from 18 to 48%. It appears, therefore, that as in the case of β-carotene, treatment with large doses of vitamin E requires subsequent treatment with a relatively low maintenance dose of the antioxidant.

Table 19.4. The dynamics of SIM regression and frequency of SIM observations in multiple biopsies in SIM patients during and after supplementation with vitamin E (patients received 400 IU of vitamin E daily for 1 year).

Time of examination	SIM regression				Frequency of SIM biopsies			
	Vitamin E		Placebo		Vitamin E		Placebo	
	No. of regressions to total no. of patients	%	No. of regressions to total no. of patients	%	No. of SIM biopsies to total (%)	Differences versus initial level	No. of SIM biopsies to total (%)	Differences versus initial level
Before treatment	0/14	0	0/16	0	42/50 (84)		47/57 (82)	
After 6 months	8/14	57*	0/16	0	21/48 (44)	$X^2 = 15,6$; $P < 0.01$	50/59 (85)	$X^2 = 0.07$; $P > 0.05$
After 12 months	10/14	71**	0/16		8/44 (18)	$X^2 = 38.1$; $P < 0.01$	45/52 (87)	$X^2 = 0.11$; $P > 0.05$
10–11 months after vitamin E cessation	7/14	50***			22/46 (48)	$X^2 = 12.5$; $P < 0.01$		

* 95% confidence interval, 31–83%; ** 95% confidence interval, 47–95%; *** 95% confidence interval, 27–73%.

Discussion

Dietary antioxidants may play a significant role in the prevention of gastric cancer, especially in populations with a poor diet and low antioxidant status as a result of low consumption of fresh vegetables and fruit. Earlier, in a large intervention trial in Linxian, People's Republic of China, an area with an extremely high rate of upper stomach cancer, supplementation of patients for more than 5 years with natural antioxidants (β-carotene, vitamin E and selenium, administered together) resulted in a 21% reduction in gastric cancer mortality (Blot *et al.*, 1993). In recent studies in Russia (Tomsk, Siberia) it was shown that an antioxidant complex (vitamins A, C and E) could cause a partial regression of gastric mucosal dysplasia (Kolomiyetz, 1997). The results of our biochemical and clinical investigations demonstrate that natural antioxidants – β-carotene and vitamin E – manifest antipromoter properties and may be effective in the treatment of early gastric premalignant lesions. The curative effect in our studies was comparable with data obtained by Garewal (1994), who used β-carotene and vitamin E in the treatment of premalignant lesions of the oral cavity (leukoplakia).

The mechanism of SIM regression produced by antioxidants remains to be elucidated. We hypothesize that the curative action of β-carotene and vitamin E is related to their antioxidant action, which is closely linked to the suppression of abnormally high ODC activity. This is the simplest explanation. In addition, β-carotene and vitamin E can modify gene expression, as well as cell proliferation and differentiation, by mechanisms which do not depend on their antioxidant properties (Moser, 1995). For example, a metabolite of β-carotene, 4-retinoic acid, participating in cell differentiation, can suppress the overexpression of ODC in a mouse model of skin carcinogenesis (Verma, 1979). β-Carotene causes up-regulation expression of *connexine 43*, a gene coding for the structural unit of a gap junction; in cell culture this activity is statistically correlated with the ability to inhibit neoplastic transformation (Bertram and Bortkiewicz, 1995). The ability of β-carotene and natural or synthetic carotenoids to induce gap junction communications does not correlate with their antioxidant properties (the capacity to quench singlet oxygen) (Stahl *et al.*, 1997). In cell culture, vitamin E inhibits protein kinase C activity, the element of signal transduction pathways that leads to inhibition of cell proliferation (Azzi *et al.*, 1995; Meydani, 1995). Vitamin E (DL-α-tocopherol) induces in culture of some cancer cells the process of apoptosis, which also is not linked to its antioxidant action (Siguonas *et al.*, 1997). Clearly, many further studies need to be done to clarify the actual mechanism of SIM regression by β-carotene and vitamin E. In the meantime, the results of three large-scale intervention trials in Colombia, Venezuela and Europe will be available soon, in which antioxidants have been used in patients with gastric premalignant lesions (Buiatti and Munos, 1996). These results will permit us to better understand the practical value of these nutritional factors for gastric cancer prevention.

References

Arvind, A.S., Cook, R.S., Tabaqchali, S. and Farthing, M.J.G. (1988) One-minute endoscopy room test for *Campylobacter pylori*. *Lancet* 1, 704.

Auvinen, M., Paasinen, A., Andersson, L.C. and Höltta, F. (1992) Ornithine decarboxylase is critical for cell transformation. *Nature (London)* 360, 355–358.

Azzi, A., Boscoboinik, D., Marilley, D., Ozer, N.K., Stauble, B. and Tasinato, A. (1995) Vitamin E: a sensor and an information transducer of the cell oxidative state. *American Journal of Clinical Nutrition* 62 (Suppl.), 1337S–1346S.

Bertram, J.S. and Bortkiewicz, H. (1995) Dietary carotenoids inhibit neoplastic transformation and modulate gene expression in mouse and human cells. *American Journal of Clinical Nutrition* 62 (Suppl.), 1327S–1336S.

Blot, W.J., Taylor, P.R., Guo, W., Daysey, S., Wang, G.-Q., Yang, C.S., Zheng, S.F., Gail, M., Li, G.-Y., Yu, Y., Liu, B., Tangrea, J., Sun, Y., Liu, F., Fraumeni, J.F., Zhang, Y.-H. and Li, B. (1993) Nutrition intervention trials in Linxian, China: supplementation with specific vitamin/mineral combinations, cancer incidence, and disease-specific mortality in the general population. *Journal of the National Cancer Institute* 85, 1482–1492.

Buiatti, F. and Muñoz, N. (1996) Chemoprevention of stomach cancer. In: Hakama, M., Beral, V., Buiatti, F., Faivre, J. and Parkin, D.M. (eds) *Chemoprevention in Cancer Control*. IARC, Scientific Publications No. 136, IARC, Lyon, pp. 35–41.

Bukin, Yu.V. and Draudin-Krylenko, V.A. (1994) Approaches to regulation of ornithine decarboxylase activity in normal and premalignant stomach mucosa. In: *Abstracts of 9th Meeting on Vitamin B6 and Carbonyl Catalysis, Capri, Italy*, Second University of Naples, Naples, p. 145.

Bukin, Yu.V., Zaridze, D.G., Draudin-Krylenko, V.A., Orlov, E.N., Sigacheva, N.A., Fu Dawei, Kurtzman, M.Ya., Schlenskaya, I.N., Gorbacheva, O.N., Nechipai, A.M., Kuvshinov, Yu.P., Poddubny, B.K. and Maximovitch, D.M. (1993) Effect of beta-carotene supplementation on the activity of ornithine decarboxylase (ODC) in stomach mucosa of patients with chronic atrophic gastritis. *European Journal of Cancer Prevention* 2, 61–68.

Bukin, Yu.V., Draudin-Krylenko, V.A., Orlov, E.N., Kuvshinov, Yu.P., Poddubniy, B.K., Vorobyeva, O.V. and Shabanov, M.A. (1995) Effect of prolonged beta-carotene or DL-alpha-tocopheryl acetate supplementation on ornithine decarboxylase activity in human atrophic stomach mucosa. *Cancer Epidemiology, Biomarkers and Prevention* 4, 865–870.

Bukin, Yu.V., Poddubniy, B.K., Kuvshinov, Yu.P., Draudin-Krylenko, V.A. and Shabanov, M.A. (1996) The effects of certain vitamins and natural anti-oxidants on ornithine decarboxylase activity and on atrophic and premalignant changes in the human gastric mucosa. *Digestive Endoscopy* 8, 184–191.

Bukin, Yu.V., Draudin-Krylenko, V.A., Kuvshinov, Yu.P., Poddubniy, B.K. and Shabanov, M.A. (1997) Decrease of ornithine decarboxylase activity in premalignant gastric mucosa and regression of small intestinal metaplasia in patients supplemented with high doses of vitamin E. *Cancer Epidemiology, Biomarkers and Prevention* 6, 543–546.

Clifford, A., Morgan, D., Yuspa, S., Peralta Soler, A. and Gilmour, S. (1995) Role of ornithine decarboxylase in epidermal carcinogenesis. *Cancer Research* 55, 1680–1686.

Correa, P. (1988) A human model of gastric carcinogenesis. *Cancer Research* 48, 3854–3860.

Correa, P. (1992) Human gastric carcinogenesis: a multistep and multifactorial process. First American Cancer Society Award Lecture on Cancer Epidemiology and Prevention. *Cancer Research* 52, 6735–6740.

Crespi, M. and Citarda, F. (1996) Current opinion. *Helicobacter pylori* and gastric cancer: an overrated risk? *Scandinavian Journal of Gastroenterology* 3, 1041–1046.

De Koster, F., Buset, M., Fernandes, F. and Deltenre, M. (1994) *Helicobacter pylori*: the link with gastric cancer. *European Journal of Cancer Prevention* 3, 247–257.

Farinati, F., Cardin, R., Della Libera, G., Herszenyi, L., Marafin, C., Molari, A., Plebani, M., Rugge, M. and Naccarato, R. (1994) The role of anti-oxidants in the chemoprevention of gastric cancer. *European Journal of Cancer Prevention* 3 (Suppl. 2), 93–98.

Fontham, E.T.H. (1997) Prevention of upper gastrointestinal tract cancers. In: Bendich, A. and Deckelbaum, R.J. (eds) *Preventive Nutrition*. Humana Press, Totowa, New Jersey, pp. 33–56.

Garewal, H. (1994) Chemoprevention of oral cancer: beta-carotene and vitamin E in leukoplakia. *European Journal of Cancer Prevention* 3, 101–107.

Garewal, H.S., Gerner, E.W., Sampliner, R.E. and Roc, D. (1988) Ornithine decarboxylase and polyamine levels in columnar upper gastrointestinal mucosa in patients with Barrett's esophagus. *Cancer Research* 48, 3288–3291.

Gerster, H. (1993) Anticarcinogenic effect of common carotenoids. *International Journal of Vitamin and Nutritional Research* 63, 93–121.

Haenszel, W., Correa, P., Lopez, A., Cuello, C., Zarama, G., Zavala, D. and Fontham, E.T.H. (1985) Serum micronutrient levels in relation to gastric pathology. *International Journal of Cancer* 36, 43–48.

Hill, M.J. (1994) Mechanisms of gastric carcinogenesis. *European Journal of Cancer Prevention* 3 (Suppl. 2), 25–29.

Höltta, F., Auvinen, M. and Andersson, L.C. (1993) Polyamines are essential for cell transformation for pp60v-src: delineation of molecular events relevant for the transformed phenotype. *Journal of Cell Biology* 122, 903–914.

Kelloff, G.J., Boone, C.W., Crowell, J.A., Steel, V.F., Lubet, L. and Sigman, C.C. (1994) Chemopreventive drug development: perspectives and progress. *Cancer Epidemiology, Biomarkers and Prevention* 3, 85–89.

Kolomiyetz, L.A. (1997) Endogenous risk factors for gastric cancer. MD thesis. Cancer Research Institute of Tomsk, Russia (in Russian).

Luk, G.D. and Baylin, S.B. (1984) Ornithine decarboxylase as a biological marker in familial colonic polyposis. *New England Journal of Medicine* 331, 80–83.

Manni, A., Wechter, R., Gilmour, S., Verderame, M.F., Mauger, D. and Demers, L.M. (1997) Ornithine decarboxylase over-expression stimulates mitogen-activated protein kinase and anchorade-independent growth of human breast epithelial cells. *International Journal of Cancer* 70, 175–182.

Mannick, E.E., Bravo, L.E., Zarama, G., Reaple, J.L., Zhang, X.-I., Ruiz, B., Fontham, E.T.H., Mera, N., Miller, M.J.S. and Correa, P. (1996) Inducible nitric oxide synthase, nitrotyrosine, and apoptosis in *Helicobacter pylori* gastritis: effect of antibiotics and antioxidants. *Cancer Research* 56, 3238–3243.

Meydani, M. (1995) Vitamin E. *Lancet* 345, 170–175.

Mirvish, S.S. (1996) Inhibition by vitamins C and E of *in vivo* nitrosation and vitamin C occurrence in the stomach. *European Journal of Cancer Prevention* 5 (Suppl. 1), 131–136.

Misumi, A., Murakami, A., Harada, K. and Donahue, P.F.D. (1990) Endoscopic dye techniques in the upper gastrointestinal tract: evaluation of esophageal and gastric pathology. *Problems in General Surgery* 7, 75–86.

Moser, U. and de Min, C. (1996) Cancer prevention: role of vitamins and carotenoids. *European Journal of Cancer Prevention* 5 (Suppl. 2), 95–100.

Moshier, J.S., Dosescu, J., Skunca, M. and Luk, G.D. (1993) Transformation of NIH/3T3 cells by ornithine decarboxylase overexpression. *Cancer Research* 53, 2618–2622.

Nierenberg, D.W. and Lester, D.C. (1985) Determination of vitamin A and E in serum and plasma using a simplified clarification method and high-performance liquid chromatography. *Journal of Chromatography, Biomedical Application* 345, 275–279.

O'Brien, T.G., Simsiman, R.S. and Boutwell, R.K. (1975) Induction of polyamine-biosynthetic enzymes in mouse epidermis by tumor promoting agents. *Cancer Research* 35, 1662–1670.

O'Brien, T.G., Megosh, L.C., Gilliard, G. and Peralta Soler, A. (1997) Ornithine decarboxylase overexpression is a sufficient condition for tumor promotion in mouse skin. *Cancer Research* 57, 2630–2637.

Owen, D.A. (1989) Stomach. In: Sternberg, S.S. (ed.) *Diagnostic Surgical Pathology*, Vol. 2. Raven Press, New York, pp. 937–965.

Parkin, D.M., Pisani, P. and Ferlay, J. (1993) Estimates of the worldwide incidence of eighteen major cancers in 1985. *International Journal of Cancer* 54, 594–606.

Pegg, A. (1988) Polyamine metabolism and its importance in neoplastic growth and as a target for chemotherapy. *Cancer Research* 48, 759–774.

Pegg, A., Shantz, L.M. and Coleman, C.S. (1995) Ornithine decarboxylase as a target for chemoprevention. *Journal of Cellular Biochemistry* 22 (Suppl.), 132–138.

van Poppel, G. and Goldbohm, A. (1995) Epidemiological evidence for β-carotene and cancer prevention. *American Journal of Clinical Nutrition* 62 (Suppl.), 1393S–1402S.

Porter, C.W., Herrera-Ornelas, L., Pera, P., Petrelli, N.F. and Mittelman, A. (1987) Polyamine biosynthetic activity in normal and neoplastic human colorectal tissues. *Cancer* 60, 1275–1281.

Reed, P.I. (1996) *Helicobacter pylori* and gastric cancer. *European Journal of Cancer Prevention* 5 (Suppl. 2), 49–55.

Ruiz, B., Correa, P., Fontham, F.T.H. and Ramakrishnan, T. (1996) Antral atrophy, *Helicobacter pylori* colonization, and gastric pH. *American Journal of Clinical Pathology* 105, 96–101.

Schorah, C.J., Sobala, G.M., Sanderson, M., Collis, M. and Primrose, J.N. (1991) Gastric juice ascorbic acid: effects of disease and implication for gastric carcinogenesis. *American Journal of Clinical Nutrition* 53 (Suppl. 1), 287–293.

Shantz, L.M. and Pegg, A.E. (1994) Overproduction of ornithine decarboxylase caused by relief of translational repression is associated with neoplastic transformation. *Cancer Research* 54, 2313–2316.

Sies, H. and Stahl, W. (1995) Vitamins E and C, beta-carotene, and other carotenoids as antioxidants. *American Journal of Clinical Nutrition* 62 (Suppl.), 1315S–1321S.

Sies, H., Stahl, W. and Sundquist, A.R. (1992) Antioxidant functions of vitamins. Vitamins E and C, beta-carotene, and other carotenoids. *Annals of the New York Academy of Sciences* 669, 7–20.

Sigounas, G., Anagnostou, A. and Steiner, M. (1997) DL-alpha-Tocopherol induces apoptosis in erythroleukemia, prostate, and breast cancer cells. *Nutrition and Cancer* 28, 30–35.

Stahl, W., Nicolai, S., Briviba, K., Hanusch, M., Broszeit, G., Peters, M., Martin, H.-D. and Sies, H. (1997) Biological activities of natural and synthetic carotenoids: induction of gap junctional communication and singlet oxygen quenching. *Carcinogenesis* 18, 89–92.

Tsugane, S., Kabuto, M. and Gey, F. (1995) Precancerous lesions of the stomach. *Antioxidant Vitamins Newsletter* 11, 9.

UK Subgroup of the ECP-EURONUT-IM Study Group (1992) Plasma vitamin concentrations in patients with intestinal metaplasia and in controls. *European Journal of Cancer Prevention* 1, 177–186.

Verma, A.K., Shapas, B.G., Kice, H.M. and Boutwell, R.K. (1979) Correlation of the inhibition by retinoids of tumor promoter-induced mouse epidermal ornithine-decarboxylase activity and of skin tumor promotion. *Cancer Research* 39, 419–425.

Wanebo, H.J., Kennedy, B.J. and Chmiel, J. (1993) Cancer of the stomach. A patient care study by the American College of Surgeons. *Annals of Surgery* 218, 583–592.

Oxidative Stress, Vitamin E and Diabetes

20

SUSHIL K. JAIN

*Departments of Pediatrics, Physiology, and
Biochemistry and Molecular Biology,
Louisiana State University Medical
Center, Shreveport, Louisiana, USA*

Introduction

Diabetic patients with uncontrolled hyperglycaemia are at greater risk of development of cardiovascular disease, retinopathy, nephropathy and neuropathy. At least some of these abnormalities may be genetic, others are associated with increased glycation of membranes and proteins, and some may be associated with the activation of aldose reductase caused by hyperglycaemia and sorbitol accumulation. Risk factors such as oxidation of lipoproteins, protein glycation, platelet hyperaggregability and hyper-coagulability of blood are, at least to some extent, direct consequences of hyperglycaemia and contribute in varying degrees to the development of cardiovascular disease (CVD) in diabetes mellitus (Ruderman *et al.*, 1992). Recently, it has been proposed that some of the complications of diabetes are associated with the increased activity of reactive oxygen species (ROS) and oxidative cellular damage.

Cellular Oxidative Stress and Dysfunctions in Diabetes

Glucose can react with proteins *in vivo* to form stable covalent adducts (glycation). The aldehyde group in the glucose is condensed with amino groups on proteins via Schiff's base linkage, and this aldimine product can be rearranged to the corresponding ketoamine and amadori products which can generate oxygen radicals during autooxidation. However, generation of oxygen radicals may also be independent of the glycation. For example, oxygen radicals may be generated from the autooxidation of glucose or ketoaldehydes, or from the increased activity of the cytochrome P-450

© CAB *International* 1999. *Antioxidants in Human Health*
(eds T.K. Basu, N.J. Temple and M.L. Garg)

system, such as that caused by excess formation of NADPH from the increased glucose metabolism (Jain, 1989). Generation of different kinds of active oxygen radicals can oxidize membrane lipids or proteins and inactivate enzymes, which can impair cellular function and integrity and lead to cell injury.

Morel and Chisolm (1989) have observed oxidized lipoproteins in diabetic rats. This has implications for atherogenesis as even a minimal oxidation of lipoproteins may induce the expression and secretion of monocyte chemotactic protein-1 by smooth muscle cells, which plays a pivotal role in the arterial intimal monocyte-macrophage recruitment and atherogenesis (Cushing *et al.*, 1990). Oxidation modifies not only the fatty acids and phospholipid moieties but, probably most important, the amino acid side chains of apolipoprotein B, analogous to the modifications produced by malondialdehyde (MDA), an end product of lipid peroxidation (Cushing *et al.*, 1990). As a result, oxidized low-density lipoproteins (LDL) are no longer recognized by the LDL receptor and results in the intracellular accumulation of cholesterol (Goldstein *et al.*, 1979; Hessler *et al.*, 1983). Oxidized LDL is cytotoxic and is likely responsible for foam cell necrosis and the development of an extracellular lipid core and atherosclerotic lesions. Further, elevated plasma triglycerides (TG) in diabetic patients may also contribute to atherogenesis and thromboses (Ruderman *et al.*, 1992).

Platelets from diabetic subjects exhibit an enhanced adhesiveness, increased aggregability to various agonists, decreased survival and increased generation of thromboxane (Watanabe *et al.*, 1988; Gisinger *et al.*, 1990). Thromboxane is known to induce not only aggregation, but also vaso-constrictor activity. At least some of these functional changes may be a result of the non-enzymatic glycation of platelet proteins, particularly glycoproteins and the altered phospholipid asymmetry of platelets in diabetes (Lupu *et al.*, 1988). Glycated LDL enhances thrombin-induced aggregation, and glycated collagen increases its platelet aggregating potency. Increased platelet aggregability is conventionally associated with an enhanced thrombotic risk (Jones and Peterson, 1981). Similarly, red blood cells (RBC) of diabetic patients are known to have several abnormalities, such as excessive aggregation, reduced deformability, hyperviscosity, glycosylation of proteins, sorbitol accumulation, oxidative damage, phosphatidylserine (PS) externalization in the outer membrane bilayer and increased adhesivity to endothelial cells (Wautier *et al.*, 1981; Limpson, 1985; Wali *et al.*, 1988; Jain *et al.*, 1989a, 1990b, 1991; Watala and Jozwiak, 1989; Rajeshwari *et al.*, 1991; Jain and McVie, 1994; Jain and Levine, 1995). It has been suggested that both platelets and RBC are involved in endothelial alteration, platelet deposition, atherosclerotic processes and the impairment of diabetic microvascular flow and complications.

Numerous studies of diabetes in both humans and animals provide evidence of accelerated oxidation of lipids, proteins and other cellular components, and suggest, in at least some types of tissue, a potential relationship with hyperglycaemia. Additionally, Gallaher *et al.* (1993) have recently shown a fivefold increased excretion of urinary MDA in streptozotocin-induced diabetic rats over that in normal rats.

Oxidative damage is known to result in increased platelet aggregation. Platelets of diabetics have enhanced MDA formation. MDA can cross-link membrane components and destabilize membrane lipid asymmetry and cause the externalization of PS (Jain, 1984, 1985; Wali *et al.*, 1987), which can then activate aggregation of platelets. MDA or PS externalization is also known to promote phagocytosis, adherence, membrane permeability, and reduction in deformability and survival of RBC (Wali *et al.*, 1987; Jain *et al.*, 1989a, 1990b). RBC of diabetic patients are known to have PS externalization, increased adherence to endothelial cells, increased membrane permeability and reduced cell deformability and survival (Jain *et al.*, 1983).

Potential Role of Antioxidant Supplementation on Complications of Diabetes

Our body is continuously generating ROS, collectively called oxidative stress. If not detoxified, ROS can result in oxidative cellular damage and impaired body functions. For example, increased oxidative stress can cause oxidative modification of plasma lipoproteins, associated with an increased risk of atherosclerosis and CVD. A number of studies have provided increasing evidence that elevated glucose levels can generate ROS such as superoxide, hydroxyl and hydrogen peroxide in cell-free systems, endothelial cells and RBC (Jain, 1989; Jain *et al.*, 1989b, 1991; Rajeshwari *et al.*, 1991). Oxidative stress is increased in different tissues in both experimental diabetes and in diabetic patients. Long-term effects of diabetes include glycation of proteins, increased risk of CVD, atherosclerosis, retinopathy, nephropathy and neurological dysfunctions. A similar abnormality can be induced *in vitro* or in animal models under conditions of increased oxidative stress, which suggests that increased oxidative damage from hyperglycaemia may make some contribution to the development of diabetic complications.

Vitamin E Supplementation and CVD Risk Factors in Diabetes

Clinical trials in type II diabetic patients have shown that supplementation with pharmacological doses of vitamin E (900–2000 IU day^{-1} for 2–4 months) results in both a decrease (Ceriello *et al.*, 1991; Paolisso *et al.*, 1993; Jain *et al.*, 1996) and no effect (Reaven *et al.*, 1995; Fuller *et al.*, 1996) on blood glycosylated haemoglobin (GHb); a decrease (Bierenbaum *et al.*, 1985) and no effect on blood glucose (Ceriello *et al.*, 1991; Paolisso *et al.*, 1993; Reaven *et al.*, 1995; Jain *et al.*, 1996a); a decrease (Bierbaum *et al.*, 1985; Ceriello *et al.*, 1991; Jain *et al.*, 1996a) and no effect (Reaven *et al.*,

1995) on TG; lower plasma lipid peroxide levels (Jain *et al.*, 1996b); and reduced LDL oxidizability (Reaven *et al.*, 1995; Fuller *et al.*, 1996) compared with placebo treatments.

We have recently carried out the first trial on type I diabetic patients. We examined the effects of daily supplementation with vitamin E on blood GHb, glucose, TG and cholesterol levels. Since blood GHb can be affected by the red cell count, we also determined the effect of vitamin E on red cell indices, not previously examined in any of the clinical trials with diabetic patients. In a randomized double-blind study 35 diabetic patients visiting the clinic were assigned to a modest dose of oral vitamin E 100 IU day^{-1} or placebo capsule daily for 3 months. There was no control on the diet of these patients.

There was no difference between vitamin E and placebo patients in age (12.1 ± 1.0 vs. 12.7 ± 1.0 years), sex (7M/6F vs. 10M/6F), race (4B/9W vs. 4B/12W), duration of diabetes (4.7 ± 1.0 vs. 5.7 ± 1.1 years), duration of supplementation (13.3 ± 0.4 vs. 13.6 ± 0.4 weeks) and weight gain during 3 months (2.39 ± 0.57 vs. 2.04 ± 0.49 kg). Serum glucose apparently fell during vitamin E supplementation but this was not significant (Table 20.1). There was no significant effect of vitamin E or placebo on total, HDL or LDL cholesterol. There was also no change in mean insulin dosage by either group of patients during the study.

Vitamin E levels were significantly higher, and GHb and TG levels significantly lower in patients supplemented with vitamin E compared with respective baseline values. Placebo treatment did not affect these parameters. Vitamin E lowered the GHb level in 70% (nine out of 13) in comparison to 44% (seven out of 16) after placebo treatment (Fig. 20.1).

Table 20.1. Effect of vitamin E supplementation on type I diabetic patients.

Group	Vitamin E		Placebo	
	Baseline	Suppl.	Baseline	Suppl.
Vitamin E (μmol l^{-1})	16 ± 1	$29 \pm 2^*$	19 ± 1	18 ± 2
Glucose (mmol l^{-1})	11.6 ± 1.3	$8.8 \pm 1.2^\dagger$	9.7 ± 1.7	12.0 ± 0.9
GHb (%)	12.8 ± 0.8	$11.5 \pm 0.4^{**}$	12.3 ± 0.7	12.1 ± 0.5
TG (mmol l^{-1})	2.9 ± 0.3	$2.2 \pm 0.2^{***}$	2.8 ± 0.5	3.1 ± 0.6
Total chol. (mmol l^{-1})	3.9 ± 0.2	3.9 ± 0.2	4.2 ± 0.2	4.2 ± 0.2
LDL-chol. (mmol l^{-1})	2.1 ± 0.1	2.2 ± 0.1	2.4 ± 0.2	2.3 ± 0.2
HDL-chol. (mmol l^{-1})	1.4 ± 0.1	1.4 ± 0.1	1.4 ± 0.1	1.4 ± 0.1
Insulin use (IU kg^{-1} BW)	0.89 ± 0.1	0.86 ± 0.1	1.0 ± 0.1	0.97 ± 0.1

Values are mean $\pm$ SE. Values marked $^*(P < 0.0001)$, $^{**}(P < 0.05)$, and $^{***}(P < 0.03)$ were significantly different in comparison with respective baseline values. P value for † was <0.08. $n = 13$ (vitamin E) or 16 (placebo).
Out of 35 enrolled, six were deleted for non-compliance.

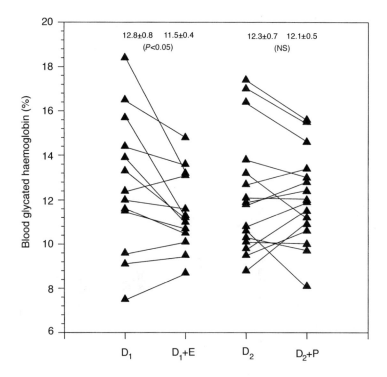

Fig. 20.1. Blood GHb level of individual diabetic patient before and after vitamin E or placebo treatment. Normal range of GHb values determined from the age-matched normal siblings of the diabetic patients is 5.86 ± 0.12 ($n = 22$). D_1 and D_2 are respective baseline values before E or P supplementation of different patients.

Figure 20.2 illustrates that vitamin E lowered the TG level in 77% (ten out of 13) in comparison to 50% (eight out of 16) of placebo-treated diabetic patients. Several red cell indices were also measured but were unaffected: RBC count, haemoglobin concentration, haematocrit and mean corpuscular volume (data not shown).

The present study reports a significant beneficial effect of even modest vitamin E supplementation (100 IU day^{-1}) on GHb and TG levels in type I diabetic patients. The mechanism of the inhibitory effect of vitamin E on glycation is not known. When GHb levels are graphed for individual patients, the beneficial effect of vitamin E appears to be mainly in patients with poor glycaemic control. The effect of vitamin E supplementation on GHb may be explained by the following possible mechanisms: improved insulin sensitivity and improved utilization of glucose; and improved circulation (Voselsang, 1948; Paolisso *et al.*, 1994); and vitamin E inhibition of free-radical production which otherwise may promote glycation (Jain and Palmer, 1997). The decrease in GHb level does not seem to be due to a

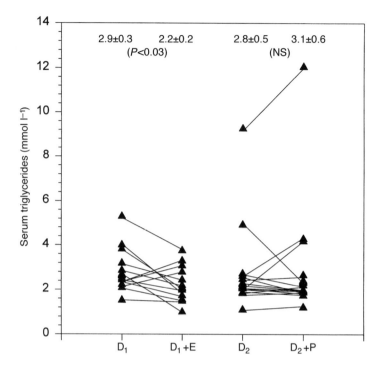

Fig. 20.2. Serum TG level of individual diabetic patient before and after the vitamin E or placebo treatment. The normal range of TG determined in age-matched normal siblings of the diabetic patients is 2.32 ± 0.21(n = 22).

decrease in red cell indices because there was no change in the RBC count, haemoglobin or haematocrit level after vitamin E treatment.

The present study also found an inhibitory effect of vitamin E on TG accumulation in type I diabetic patients. There was a significant correlation between serum glucose and TG levels in the vitamin E-supplemented group ($r = 0.63$, $P = 0.02$) but not in the placebo-treated group ($r = 0.25$, $P = 0.34$). However, the relationship between GHb and TG was not significant in either the vitamin E ($r = 0.29$, $P = 0.34$) or the placebo-supplemented ($r = 0.21$, $P = 0.44$) group. This suggests that decreased TG may be related to an improvement in the fasting blood glucose. The decrease in TG in vitamin E-supplemented patients could also be due to an increase in lipoprotein lipase activity as has been observed in vitamin E-supplemented diabetic rats (Pritchard *et al.*, 1986).

In conclusion, a large body of data supports the occurence of cellular oxidative damage in diabetic patients. A number of small clinical trials indicate that vitamin E supplementation can lower oxidative stress and some of the risk factors for CVD in diabetic patients. A large-scale clinical trial is warranted so as to determine the potential benefit of vitamin E in reducing long-term risk of CVD in diabetics.

Acknowledgements

This study was supported in part by the Research Award from the National American Diabetes Association and American Heart Association (LA Affiliate).

References

Bierenbaum, M.L., Noonan, F.J., Machlin, L.J., Machlin, S., Stier, A., Watson, P.B., Naso, A.M. and Fleischman, A.I. (1985) The effect of supplemental vitamin E on serum parameters in diabetics, postcoronary and normal subjects. *Nutrition Reports International* 31, 1171–1180.

Ceriello, A., Giugliano, D., Quatraro, A., Donzella, C., Dipalo, G. and Lefebvre, P.J. (1991) Vitamin E reduction of protein glycosylation in diabetes. *Diabetes Care* 14, 68–72.

Cushing, S.D., Berliner, J.A., Valente, A.J. and Territo, M.C. (1990) Minimally modified low density lipoprotein induces monocyte chemotactic protein 1 in human endothelial cells and smooth muscle cells. *Proceedings of the National Academy of Sciences, USA* 87, 5134–5138.

Fuller, C.J., Chandalia, M., Garg, A., Grundy, S.M. and Jialal, I. (1996) RRR-alpha-tocopherol acetate supplementation at pharmacological doses decreases low-density-lipoprotein oxidative susceptibility but not protein glycation in patients with diabetes mellitus. *American Journal of Clinical Nutrition* 63, 753–759.

Gallaher, D.D., Csallany, A.S., Shoeman, D.W. and Olson, J.M. (1993) Diabetes increases excretion of urinary malonaldehyde conjugates in rats. *Lipids* 28, 663–666.

Gisinger, C., Watanabe, J. and Colwell, J.A. (1990) Vitamin E and platelet eicosanoids in diabetes mellitus. *Prostoglandins, Leukotrienes and Essential Fatty Acids* 40, 169–176.

Goldstein, J.L., Ho, Y.K., Basu, S.K. and Brown, M.S. (1979) Binding site on macrophages that mediates uptake and degradation of acetylated low density lipoprotein, producing massive cholesterol deposition. *Proceedings of the National Academy of Sciences, USA* 76, 333–337.

Hessler, J.R., Morel, D.W., Lewis, L.J. and Chisolm, G.M. (1983) Lipoprotein oxidation and lipoprotein-induced cytotoxicity. *Atherosclerosis* 3, 215–222.

Jain, S.K. (1984) The accumulation of malonyldialdehyde, a product of fatty acid peroxidation, can disturb aminophospholipid organization in the membrane bilayer of human erythrocytes. *Journal of Biological Chemistry* 259, 3391–3394.

Jain, S.K. (1985) *In vivo* externalization of phosphatidylserine and phosphatidylethanolamine in the membrane bilayer and hypercoagulability by the lipid peroxidation of erythrocytes in rats. *Journal of Clinical Investigation* 76, 281–286.

Jain, S.K. (1989) Hyperglycemia can cause membrane lipid peroxidation and osmotic fragility in human red blood cells. *Journal of Biological Chemistry* 264, 21340–21345.

Jain, S.K. and Levine, S.N. (1995) Elevated lipid peroxidation and vitamin E quinone levels in heart ventricles of streptozotocin-treated diabetic rats. *Free Radical Biology and Medicine* 18, 337–341.

Jain, S.K. and McVie, R. (1994) Effect of glycemic control, race (white versus black), and duration of diabetes on reduced glutathione content in erythrocytes of diabetic patients. *Metabolism* 43, 306–309.

Jain, S.K. and Palmer, M. (1997) The effect of oxygen radicals metabolites and vitamin E on glycation of proteins. *Free Radical Biology and Medicine,* 22:4, 593–596.

Jain, S.K., Mohandas, N., Clark, M. and Shohet, S.B. (1983) The effect of malonydialdehyde, a product of lipid peroxidation, on the deformability, dehydration, and 51Cr-survival of erythrocytes. *British Journal of Haematology* 53, 247–255.

Jain, S.K., McVie, R., Duett, J. and Herbst, J.J. (1989a) Erythrcoyte membrane lipid peroxidation and glycosylated hemoglobin in diabetes. *Diabetes* 38, 1539–1543.

Jain, S.K., Ross, J.D., Levy, G.J., Little, R.L. and Duett, J. (1989b) The accumulation of malonyldialdehyde, an end product of membrane lipid peroxidation, can cause potassium leak in normal and sickle red blood cells. *Biochemical Medicine and Metabolic Biology* 42, 60–65.

Jain, S.K., Levine, S.N., Duett, J. and Hollier, B. (1990a) Elevated lipid peroxidation levels in red blood cells of streptozotocin-treated diabetic rats. *Metabolism* 39, 971–975.

Jain, S.K., Ross, J.D., Levy, G.J. and Duett, J. (1990b) The effect of malonyldialdehyde on viscosity of normal and sickle red blood cells. *Biochemical Medicine and Metabolic Biology* 44, 37–41.

Jain, S.K., Levine, S.N., Duett, J. and Hollier, B. (1991) Reduced vitamin E and increased lipofuscin products in erythrocytes of diabetic rats. *Diabetes* 40, 1241–1244.

Jain, S.K., McVie, R., Jaramillo, J.J., Palmer, M. and Smith, T. (1996a) Effect of modest vitamin E supplementation on blood glycated hemoglobin and triglyceride levels and red cell indices in Type-1 diabetic patients. *Journal of the American College of Nutrition* 15, 458–461.

Jain, S.K., McVie, R., Jaramillo, J.J., Palmer, M., Smith, T., Meachum, Z.D. and Little, R.L. (1996b) The effect of modest vitamin E supplementation on lipid peroxidation products and other cardiovascular risk factors in diabetic patients. *Lipids* 31, S87–S90.

Jones, R.L. and Peterson, C.M. (1981) Hematologic alterations in diabetes mellitus. *American Journal of Medicine* 70, 339–352.

Limpson, L.O. (1985) Intrinsic stiffening of red blood cells as the fundamental cause of diabetic nephropathy and microangiopathy. *Nephron* 39, 344–351.

Lupu, F., Calb, M. and Fixman, A. (1988) Alterations of phospholipid asymmetry in the membrane of spontaneously aggregated platelets in diabetes. *Thrombosis Research* 50, 605–616.

Morel, D.W. and Chisolm, G.M. (1989) Antioxidant treatment of diabetic rats inhibits lipoprotein oxidation and cytotoxicity. *Journal of Lipid Research* 30, 1827–1834.

Paolisso, G., D'Amore, A., Galzerano, D., Balbi, B., Giugliano, D., Varricchio, M. and D'Onofrio, F. (1993) Daily vitamin E supplements improve metabolic control but not insulin secretion in elderly type II diabetic patients. *Diabetes Care* 16, 1433–1437.

Paolisso, G., DiMaro, G., Galzerano, D., Cacciapuoti, F., Varricchio, G., Varricchio, M. and D'Onofrio, F. (1994) Pharmacological doses of vitamin E and insulin action in elderly subjects. *American Journal of Clinical Nutrition* 59, 1291–1296.

Pritchard, K.A. Jr, Patel, S.T., Karpen, C.W., Newman, H.A. and Panganamala, R.V. (1986) Triglyceride-lowering effect of dietary vitamin E in streptozocin-induced diabetic rats. Increased lipoprotein lipase activity in livers of diabetic rats fed high dietary vitamin E. *Diabetes* 35, 278–281.

Rajeswari, P., Natarajan, R., Nadler, J.L. and Kumar, D. (1991) Glucose induces lipid peroxidation and inactivation of membrane associated iron transport enzymes in human erythrocytes *in vivo* and *in vitro*. *Journal of Cell Physiology* 149, 100–109.

Reaven, P.D., Herold, D.A., Barnett, J. and Edelman, S. (1995) Effects of vitamin E on susceptibility of low-density lipoprotein and low-density lipoprotein subfractions to oxidation and on protein glycation in NIDDM. *Diabetes Care* 18, 807–816.

Ruderman, N.B., Williamson, J.R. and Brownlee, M. (1992) Glucose and diabetic vascular disease. *FASEB Journal* 6, 2905–2914.

Vogelsang, A. (1948) Cumulative effect of alpha tocopherol on the insulin requirements in diabetes mellitus. *Medical Record* 161, 363–365.

Wali, R.K., Jaffe, S., Kumar, D., Sorgente, N. and Kalra, V.K. (1987) Increased adherence of oxidant-treated human and bovine erythrocytes to cultured endothelial cells. *Journal of Cell Physiology* 133, 25–36.

Wali, R.K., Jaffe, S., Kumar, D. and Kalra, V.K. (1988) Alterations in organization of phospholipids in erythrocytes as factor in adherence to endothelial cells in diabetes mellitus. *Diabetes* 37, 104–111.

Watala, C. and Jówiak, Z. (1989) Phospholipid asymmetry in red blood cell membranes of type 1 diabetic children. *Medical Science Research* 17, 895–896.

Watanabe, J., Wohltmann, H.J., Klein, R.L. and Colwell, J.A. (1988) Enhancement of platelet aggregation by low-density lipoproteins from IDDM patients. *Diabetes* 37, 1652–1657.

Wautier, J.L., Paton, R.C., Wautier, M.P., Pintigny, D., Abadie, E., Passa, P. and Caen, J.P. (1981) Increased adhesion of erythrocytes to endothelial cells in diabetes mellitus and its relation to vascular complications. *New England Journal of Medicine* 305, 237–242.

An Investigation of *in Vivo* Antioxidant Status and DNA Damage in Patients With IDDM

21

MARY HANNON-FLETCHER[1], CIARA HUGHES[1], MAURICE J. O'KANE[2], KENNETH W. MOLES[2], CHRISTOPHER R. BARNETT[1] AND YVONNE A. BARNETT[1]

[1] *Cancer and Ageing Research Group, University of Ulster, Coleraine, Northern Ireland, UK;* [2] *Altnagelvin Area Hospital, Londonderry, Northern Ireland, UK*

Introduction

Free radicals, including the reactive intermediates of oxygen metabolism, have been implicated in the aetiology and pathogenesis of diabetes mellitus (Wolff, 1987; Brownlee *et al.*, 1988; Cerami *et al.*, 1988; Hunt *et al.*, 1990; Hunt and Wolff, 1991; DCCT, 1993). Free radicals may cause damage to cellular biomolecules including the nucleic acids, proteins, lipids and carbohydrates (Pryor, 1976; Aruoma *et al.*, 1989; Halliwell and Gutteridge, 1989; Dizdaroglu *et al.*, 1991; Shibutani *et al.*, 1991; Gutteridge, 1992). This damage may result in altered physiological function. Defence systems exist within organisms which: (i) reduce the excessive production of free radicals; (ii) remove excessive quantities of free radicals once they have been formed, and (iii) remove and/or repair free radical damage if it occurs. These defence systems include: enzymatic and non-enzymatic antioxidants. Examples are: superoxide dismutase (SOD), catalase (CAT) and glutathione peroxidase (GPx); transferrin, ferritin, caeruloplasmin, vitamins A, C and E; proteolytic enzymes; and DNA repair pathways (Pacifici and Davies, 1991; Barnett, 1994).

There are wide variations in the occurrence and onset of long-term complications in insulin-dependent diabetes mellitus (IDDM) patients (Raskin and Rosenstock, 1986), with some individuals displaying poor glycaemic control rarely developing overt complications, and others showing severe complications despite good glycaemic control. This suggests that factors other than glycaemic control may be involved in the development of complications. Differences in the *in vivo* defence systems against free radical damage, between individuals with IDDM, may account for the wide variations in the occurrence and onset of long-term complications. To begin to assess the validity of this hypothesis, we carried out a study of *in vivo* antioxidant status, basal levels of DNA damage in whole blood and phytohaemagglutinin (PHA)-stimulated lymphocytes, and hydrogen peroxide (H_2O_2)-induced DNA repair capacity in PHA-stimulated lymphocytes, within a group of 20 IDDM patients and 11 healthy controls.

Materials and Methods

Subjects

Twenty patients with IDDM (eight diagnosed for <12 years (mean age 28.8 ± 3.3 years; seven males and one female; three of whom were smokers) and 12 diagnosed for >17 years (mean age 51.7 ± 4.2 years; eight females and four males; two of whom were smokers)) were recruited from the Diabetes Clinic at Altnagelvin Hospital, Londonderry, Northern Ireland. Patients were assessed for the presence of diabetic complications, namely retinopathy, nephropathy, neuropathy and macrovascular disease. The control group consisted of 11 healthy individuals recruited from the University of Ulster (mean age 26.9 ± 1.0 years; six females and five males; none of whom were smokers or had a family history of diabetes). Although the controls were age-matched with the IDDM subjects diagnosed <12 years, the mean age of both these groups was considerably less than that of the other IDDM patients. The results of previous investigations within our laboratory did not show any effect of age on *in vivo* antioxidant status or any significant increase in background levels of DNA damage within PHA-stimulated lymphocytes between healthy subjects aged 20–30 years and those aged 50–54 years (King *et al.*, 1994; Barnett and King, 1995). In light of these previous findings we were confident that any differences in *in vivo* antioxidant status and/or basal levels of DNA damage between our controls and IDDM subjects (diagnosed for >17 years) would be a consequence of the pathology and not an age effect. Ethical approval for this study was obtained from the University of Ulster Ethical Committee and from the Ethical Committee at Altnagelvin Hospital.

Collection and processing of blood samples

Samples of peripheral blood (25 ml) were collected from each study subject. 20 ml was collected into lithium heparin-coated vacutainers® (Becton-Dickinson). Of this, 10 ml was transferred on to ice for subsequent processing to determine antioxidant status and basal levels of DNA damage within nucleated blood cells. A further 10 ml was used to isolate mononuclear cells (MNCs). Basal levels of DNA damage and DNA repair capacity were determined within lymphocytes separated from the MNCs. The remaining 5 ml was transferred to an ethylene diamine tetraacetic acid (EDTA)-coated tube (Monoject) for high performance liquid chromatography (HPLC) analysis of glycated haemoglobin (HbA_{1c}) levels according to the method described by John *et al.* (1992).

Assessment of *in vivo* antioxidant status

As an assessment of *in vivo* antioxidant status, we quantified the following analytes: plasma levels of vitamin C according to the method described by Heiliger *et al.* (1980); plasma levels of vitamins A, E and β-carotene according to the method described by Thurnham and Smith (1988); erythrocyte activities of CAT, GPx and SOD according to methods described by Aebi (1974), Paglia and Valentine (1967) and Jones and Suttle (1981), respectively; and plasma levels of uric acid and ceruloplasmin (CPL) were measured according to the methods of Barham and Trinder (1972) and Schosinsky *et al.* (1974), respectively.

Determination of plasma glucose and plasma iron

Plasma glucose was determined using an automated method described by Stevens (1970) and plasma iron was measured using a commercial kit supplied by Randox Ltd (Crumlin, Northern Ireland) based on the method of Stookey (1970).

Quantification of DNA damage and repair in whole blood and PHA-stimulated lymphocytes

MNCs were isolated from whole blood using a method described by Bôyum (1980) and were stored frozen at $-20°C$. Thawing, PHA stimulation (5 µg ml^{-1}; HA15, Wellcome Diagnostics) and subsequent culture of lymphocytes (in RPMI 1640 with 10% fetal calf serum, 4% sodium pyruvate (200 µg ml^{-1}), 100 U ml^{-1} and 100 µg ml^{-1} streptomycin) was carried out using the method described by Barnett and King (1995).

Quantification of basal levels of DNA damage (expressed as percentage single-stranded DNA; %SS-DNA) in 30 µl of whole blood or in 2×10^5 PHA-stimulated lymphocytes was performed using a sandwich enzyme-linked immunosorbent assay (ELISA), described by van Loon *et al.* (1992). The ELISA is based on the action of the monoclonal antibody, D1B, directed against single-stranded DNA (SS-DNA). Lymphocyte samples were subjected to controlled, partial alkaline unwinding, to convert single-strand breaks and alkali labile sites into stretches of SS-DNA to which the antibody molecules could subsequently bind. The extent of binding was then assayed by the addition of an alkaline phosphatase-labelled D1B in a sandwich ELISA. The chromogenic substrate, *p*-nitrophenyl phosphate, was then added and the optical density, proportional to the degree of SS-DNA, was determined using a microtitre plate reader.

Assessment of 200 μmol l^{-1} H_2O_2-induced DNA damage and repair in PHA-stimulated lymphocytes was performed according to the method described by Barnett and King (1995). Essentially, lymphocytes were treated on ice (to minimize DNA repair) for 1 h with H_2O_2. Untreated lymphocyte cultures (controls) were prepared in parallel. Following treatment, an aliquot of lymphocyte suspension was removed and processed for the quantification of DNA damage. The remainder of the H_2O_2-treated lymphocytes were placed in an incubator at 37°C (to facilitate DNA repair) and aliquots of lymphocytes were removed at 45, 90 and 120 min and processed for the quantification of DNA damage. By monitoring the rate of decrease of the H_2O_2-induced DNA damage within the lymphocyte cultures it was possible to assess the DNA repair capacity of the lymphocytes from each study subject.

Results

Of the eight IDDM patients diagnosed for less than 12 years, only one presented with a complication (retinopathy), whereas five of the subjects in the diagnosed for more than 17 years group presented with at least one complication (retinopathy, neuropathy, nephropathy or ischaemic heart disease). Because of small numbers it was not possible to determine by statistical analysis whether the values obtained for the various endpoints were different in IDDM patients who had complications compared with those who did not, but this did not appear to be the case. A similar examination did not reveal any striking differences in the endpoints measured between smokers and non-smokers.

%HbA$_{1c}$ levels (Table 21.1) were significantly increased in both IDDM groups in comparison with controls ($P < 0.0001$). The range of %HbA$_{1c}$ levels indicated that all patients were under acceptable clinical control.

There were no significant differences in mean levels of plasma glucose, plasma iron, haemoglobin concentration, plasma vitamins C, E and β-carotene, erythrocyte SOD or CAT levels, for both groups of IDDM patients when compared to controls and also when the levels of these analytes within the two groups of IDDM patients were compared (Table

Table 21.1. Biochemical measurements from blood samples.

Analyte	Control	Subjects	
		IDDM <12 year	IDDM >17 years
Glucose (mmol l^{-1})	4.01 ± 0.25	6.46 ± 1.66	6.92 ± 1.51
%HbA1c	4.55 ± 0.07	*7.49 ± 0.62	*7.67 ± 0.35
Iron (μmol l^{-1})	16.70 ± 2.86	18.13 ± 3.66	14.58 ± 1.82
Haemoglobin (g dl^{-1})	12.97 ± 0.16	12.83 ± 0.56	12.50 ± 3.64
β-Carotene (μmol l^{-1})	0.01 ± 0.002	0.01 ± 0.003	0.02 ± 0.001
Vitamin C (μmol l^{-1})	49.22 ± 5.74	36.20 ± 5.16	44.02 ± 7.04
Vitamin E (μmol l^{-1})	12.11 ± 1.76	10.50 ± 1.13	11.20 ± 0.59
Vitamin A (μmol l^{-1})	0.75 ± 0.07	0.61 ± 0.05	**0.55 ± 0.05
GPx (U gHb^{-1})	31.62 ± 2.35	****14.05 ± 4.37	*15.09 ± 1.72
SOD (U gHb^{-1})	880.8 ± 38.5	776.9 ± 34.1	814.9 ± 28.4
CAT (k gHb^{-1})	29.28 ± 8.85	46.53 ± 1.47	27.78 ± 4.70
CPL (U l^{-1})	587.0 ± 28.7	***782.4 ± 65.7	***770.1 ± 42.7
Uric acid (mg dl^{-1})	4.63 ± 0.35	4.00 ± 0.49	****3.00 ± 0.29

Values are mean ± SEM for all groups.
*$P < 0.0001$, **$P < 0.05$, ***$P < 0.01$ and ****$P < 0.002$ compared to control.

21.1). The mean level of vitamin A was decreased in all IDDM patients (to a significant extent in those diagnosed for >17 years; $P < 0.05$; Table 21.1). Similarly, erythrocyte GPx activity was significantly reduced in all IDDM patients (<12 years, $P < 0.002$; >17 years, $P < 0.001$) and uric acid levels were significantly decreased in IDDM patients diagnosed >17 years ($P < 0.002$; Table 21.1), when compared to controls. In contrast, CPL activity was significantly increased in all IDDM patients ($P < 0.01$; Table 21.1) compared to the control group.

Basal levels of DNA damage (expressed as %SS-DNA) in whole blood from both IDDM groups were significantly increased when compared to controls (<12 years, $P < 0.02$; >17 years, $P < 0.002$; Table 21.2). However, there were no significant differences in the basal levels of DNA damage in PHA-stimulated lymphocytes from IDDM patients, when compared to controls (Table 21.2). In addition, there were no significant differences in the capacity of lymphocytes from the diabetic patients to repair H_2O_2-induced DNA damage over a 120 min time course (Fig. 21.1).

Discussion

It has been reported that IDDM represents a condition of oxidative stress (Wolff, 1987; Brownlee *et al.*, 1988; Cerami *et al.*, 1988; Hunt *et al.*, 1990; Hunt and Wolff, 1991; DCCT, 1993). In support of this, the results for the

Table 21.2. Basal levels of DNA damage (%SS-DNA).

		Subjects	
Sample	Controls	IDDM <12 years	IDDM >17 years
Whole blood	2.57 ± 0.49	*4.47 ± 0.65	5.23 ± 0.51
Lymphocytes	26.09 ± 1.63	27.79 ± 1.89	**30.73 ± 1.55

Values are mean ± SEM for all groups.
*$P < 0.02$, and **$P < 0.002$ when compared to control.

levels of the various antioxidants within IDDM patients in this study have revealed alterations which suggest a state of oxidative stress. We do not believe that the altered antioxidant status was due to an age-related effect since we have previously shown that there are no age-related changes in antioxidant status in healthy humans (aged 18–69 years; Barnett and King, 1995).

A number of studies of IDDM patients have reported changes in the levels of the antioxidant enzymes SOD, CAT and GPx, but reports have

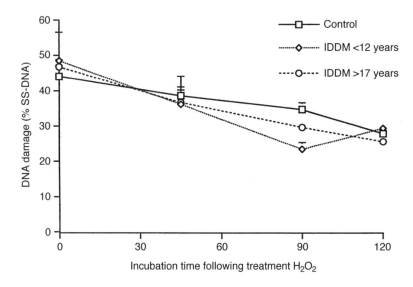

Fig. 21.1. Graph illustrating the repair of H_2O_2-induced DNA damage within cultured lymphocytes from IDDM patients and controls over a 120 min time course. Lymphocyte cultures were treated for 1 h on ice with 200 μM H_2O_2. Lymphocytes were then incubated at 37°C. Aliquots of lymphocytes were removed at 0, 45, 90 and 120 min and processed for the determination of DNA damage (% SS-DNA).

been inconsistent (Matkovics *et al.*, 1982; Hagglof *et al.*, 1983; Godin and Wohaieb, 1987; Uzel *et al.*, 1987; Thompson and Godin, 1995). In our study we did not find any differences in SOD or CAT activities within IDDM patients, compared to controls, though we did find decreased levels of GPx activity in both groups of IDDM patients. Our results did not reveal any significant differences in plasma levels of vitamins C, E and β-carotene within IDDM patients. This supports work by Oberly (1986) who was not able to show reduced antioxidant vitamin levels in diabetes. However, Seghieri and colleagues (1993) reported reduced serum levels of vitamin C in diabetic patients.

We did, however, find decreases in vitamin A and uric acid levels within IDDM patients (significant in those subjects diagnosed for >17 years). In animal studies, vitamin A has been shown to be an effective anticarcinogen. One of the anticarcinogenic mechanisms of action of vitamin A may be via scavenging reactive intermediates formed and/or by direct interaction with DNA and so directly protecting against reactive intermediates (Ioannides *et al.*, 1991). In light of the possible protective action against reactive intermediates, a reduced level of vitamin A in the IDDM patients might result in an increased level of potentially biomolecule-damaging radicals.

Uric acid comprises 30–65% of the peroxyl radical-scavenging capacity of blood plasma (Becker, 1993) and the reduced level of this important antioxidant in the IDDM patients may contribute to a situation of oxidative stress *in vivo*. The increased levels of CPL activity found within IDDM patients, and which has also been found by others (Mooradian and Morley, 1987) possibly reflects the greater inflammatory conditions in IDDM, since CPL is an acute phase reactant (DiSilvestro, 1990).

In this study we were interested in whether changes in the levels of the various antioxidants in the IDDM patients contributed to increased background levels of DNA damage. Other studies have demonstrated increased levels of lipid peroxidation in the leukocytes, plasma or erythrocytes of diabetic patients, in conjunction with alterations to certain antioxidants (Parthiban *et al.*, 1995; Reaven, 1995; Akkus *et al.*, 1996). We found a significant increase in basal levels of DNA damage in the whole blood of IDDM patients, the increase being greatest in those subjects diagnosed for >17 years. Since the subjects in the >17 years diagnosed group were considerably older (mean age 51.7 ± 4.2 years) compared with those in the <12 years diagnosed group (mean age 28.8 ± 3.3 years), the greater levels of DNA damage may simply reflect the fact that certain nucleated blood cells would have been around for longer *in vivo* and so would be more likely to suffer biomolecule damage from exogenous and endogenous entities. Subsequent quantification of DNA damage levels in PHA-stimulated lymphocytes from the IDDM patients did not show any significant difference when compared to the control group. The background levels of DNA damage in PHA-stimulated lymphocytes were found to be six- to eightfold higher than the levels in whole blood. The increased damage within the lymphocytes is probably the consequence of their exposure to conditions of oxidative stress *in vitro*, from the increased oxygen tension in the medium compared to the blood (Collins *et al.*, 1997), and thus any difference existing *in vivo* in background levels of DNA damage within lymphocytes from IDDM patients and controls would very likely be masked. There is evidence from the studies of Dandona *et al.* (1996) for a state of oxidative stress within diabetic patients sufficient to lead to DNA damage. They measured levels of oxidative DNA damage in freshly isolated, unstimulated mononuclear cells from IDDM and non-insulin-dependent diabetes mellitus patients and found significantly higher levels of the oxidised purine base 8-hydroxy-deoxyguanosine, a recognized biomarker of oxidant-induced DNA damage. We did not find any difference in the repair of H_2O_2-induced DNA damage within PHA-stimulated lymphocytes between controls and IDDM patients. Unstimulated lymphocytes (like many found *in vivo*) are less proficient at DNA repair than PHA-stimulated lymphocytes (*in vitro*) (Collins *et al.*, 1995) and so individual differences in the repair of DNA damage *in vivo* may contribute to the observed variation in onset of diabetic complications. We are currently investigating this possibility.

Conclusion

In conclusion, the results from this preliminary study suggest that IDDM is associated with alterations to *in vivo* antioxidant status which may contribute to increased whole blood levels of DNA damage.

References

Aebi, H. (1974) Catalase *in vitro*. *Methods in Enzymatic Analysis* 2, 121–126.

Akkus, I., Kalak, S., Vural, H., Caglayan, O., Menekse, E., Can, G. and Durmus, B. (1996) Leukocyte lipid peroxidation, superoxide dismutase, glutathione peroxidase and serum and leukocyte vitamin C levels of patients with type II diabetes mellitus. *Clinica Chimica Acta* 244, 221–227.

Aruoma, O.I., Halliwell, B., Gajewski, E. and Dizdaroglu, M. (1989) Damage to the bases in DNA induced by hydrogen peroxide and ferric ion chelates. *Journal of Biological Chemistry* 264, 20509–20512.

Barham, D. and Trinder, P. (1972) Improved colour reagent for determination of blood glucose by oxidase system. *Analyst* 97, 142–145.

Barnett, Y.A. (1994) Nutrition and the ageing process. *British Journal of Biomedical Science* 52, 278–287.

Barnett, Y.A. and King, C.M. (1995) An investigation of antioxidant status, DNA repair capacity and mutation as a function of age in humans. *Mutation Research* 338, 115–128.

Becker, B.F. (1993) Towards the physiological function of uric acid. *Free Radical Biology and Medicine* 14, 615–631.

Bôyum, A. (1980) *Isolation of Mononuclear Cells and Granulocytes from Human Blood*. Norwegian Defence Research Establishment, Division for Toxicology, Kjeller, Norway. Paper iv, pp. 77–89.

Brownlee, M., Cerami, A. and Vlassara, H. (1988) Advanced glycosylation end-products in tissue and the biochemical basis of diabetic complications. *New England Journal of Medicine* 318, 1315–1321.

Cerami, A., Vlassara, H. and Brownlee, M. (1988) Role of advanced glycosylation products in complications of diabetes. *Diabetes Care* 11 (Suppl. 1), 73–79.

Collins, A.R., Ai-guo, M. and Duthie, S. (1995) The kinetics of repair of oxidative DNA damage (strand breaks and oxidised pyrimidines) in human cells. *Mutation Research* 336, 69–77.

Collins, A.R., Duthie, S.J., Fillion, L., Gedik, C.M., Vaughan, N. and Wood, S.G. (1997) Oxidative DNA damage in human cells: the influence of antioxidants and DNA repair. *Biochemical Society Transactions* 25, 326–331.

Dandona, P., Thusu, K., Cook, S., Snyder B., Makowski, J., Armstrong, D. and Nicotera, T. (1996) Oxidative damage to DNA in diabetes mellitus. *Lancet* 347, 444–445.

The Diabetes Control and Complications Trial (DCCT) (1993) *New England Journal of Medicine* 329, 977–986.

DiSilvestro, R.A. (1990) Influence of dietary copper, copper injections and inflammations on rat serum caeruloplasmin activity levels. *Nutrition Research* 10, 355–358.

Dizdaroglu, M., Nackerdien, Z., Chao, B.C., Gajewski, E. and Rao, G. (1991) Chemical nature of *in vivo* DNA base damage in hydrogen peroxide-treated mammalian cells. *Archives in Biochemistry and Biophysics* 286, 388–390.

Godin, D.V. and Wohaieb, S.A. (1987) Reactive oxygen radical processes in Diabetes. In: Signal, P.K. (ed.) *Free Radicals in the Pathophysiology of Heart Disease*. Martinus Nijhoff Publishing, Boston, Massachusetts, pp. 302–322.

Gutteridge, J.M.C. (1992) Ageing and free radicals. *Medical Laboratory Sciences* 49, 313–318.

Hagglof, B., Marklund, S.L. and Holmgren, G. (1983) CuZn-superoxide dismutase, catalase and glutathione peroxidase in lymphocytes and erythrocytes in insulin-dependent diabetic children. *Acta Endocrinology* 102, 235–239.

Halliwell, B. and Gutteridge, J.M.C. (1989) Protection against oxidants in biological systems; the superoxide theory of toxicity. In: Halliwell, B. and Gutteridge, J.M.C. (eds) *Free Radicals in Biology*, 2nd edn. Clarendon Press, Oxford, pp. 152–156.

Heiliger, F. (1980) Ascorbic acid analysis by HPLC. *Current Methods in Separation* 2, 4–5.

Hunt, J.V. and Wolff, S.P. (1991) Oxidative glycation and free radical production: a causal mechanism of diabetic complications. *Free Radical Research Communication* 12–13, 115–123.

Hunt, J.V., Smith, C.C.T. and Wolff, S.P. (1990) Autoxidative glycosylation and possible involvement of peroxides and free radicals in LDL modification by glucose. *Diabetes* 39, 1420–1424.

Ioannides, C., Ayrton, A.D., Keele, A., Lewis, D.F.V., Flatt, P.R. and Walker, R. (1991) Mechanism of the *in vitro* antimutagenic action of retinol. *Mutagenesis* 5, 257–262.

John, W.G., Bullock, D.G. and MacKenzie, F. (1992) Methods for analysis of glycated haemoglobins: what is being measured? *Diabetic Medicine* 9, 15–19.

Jones, D.G. and Suttle, N.F. (1981) Some effects of copper deficiency on leucocyte function in sheep and cattle. *Research in Veterinary Science* 31, 151–156.

King, C.M., Gillespie, E.S., McKenna, P.G. and Barnett, Y.A. (1994) An investigation of mutation as a function of age in humans. *Mutation Research* 316, 79–90.

van Loon, A.A.W.M., Groenendijk, R.H., Timmerman, A.J., van der Schans, G.P., Lohman, P.H.M. and Baan, R.A. (1992) Quantitative detection of DNA damage in cells after exposure to ionizing radiation by means of an improved immunochemical assay. *Mutation Research* 274, 19–27.

Matkovics, B., Varga, Sz.I., Szabo, L. and Witas, H. (1982) The effect of diabetes on the activities of the peroxide metabolism enzymes. *Hormone and Metabolism Research* 14, 77–79.

Mooradian, A.D. and Morley, J.E. (1987) Micronutrient status in diabetes mellitus. *American Journal of Clinical Nutrition* 45, 877–895.

Oberly, L.W. (1986) Free radicals and diabetes. *Free Radical Biology and Medicine* 5, 113–124.

Pacifici, R.E. and Davies, K.J.A. (1991) Protein, lipid and DNA repair systems in oxidative stress: the free radical theory revised. *Journal of Gerontology* 37, 166–180.

Paglia, D.E. and Valentine, W.N. (1967) Characteristics of erythrocyte glutathione peroxidase. *Journal of Laboratory and Clinical Medicine* 70, 158–159.

Parthiban, A., Vijayalingam, S., Shanmugasundaram, K.R. and Mohan, R. (1995) Oxidative stress and the development of diabetic complications – antioxidants and lipid peroxidation in erythrocytes and cell membrane. *Cell Biology International* 19, 987–993.

Pryor, W.A. (1976) The role of free radical reactions in biological systems. In: Pryor, W.A. (ed.) *Free Radicals in Biology*, Vol. IV. Academic Press, London, pp. 1–49.

Raskin, P. and Rosenstock, J. (1986) Blood glucose control and diabetic complications. *Annals of Internal Medicine* 105, 254–263.

Reaven, P. (1995) Dietary and pharmacologic regimens to reduce lipid peroxidation in non-insulin-dependent diabetes mellitus. *American Journal of Clinical Nutrition* 62 (Suppl. 6), 1483S–1489S.

Schosinsky, K.H., Lehmann, H.P. and Beller, M.F. (1974) Measurement of caeruloplasmin activity in serum by use of *O*-dianesidinedihydrochloride. *Clinical Chemistry* 20, 1556–1563.

Seghieri, G., Martinoli, L., Micelli, M., Ciuti, M., D'Alessandri, G., Gironi, A., Palmieri, L., Anichini, R., Bartolomei, G. and Franconi, F. (1993) Renal excretion of ascorbic acid in insulin-dependent diabetes mellitus. *International Journal of Vitamin and Nutrition Research* 64, 119–124.

Shibutani, S., Takeshita, M. and Grollman, A.P. (1991). Insertion of specific bases during DNA synthesis past the oxidation damaged 8-oxodG. *Nature* (London) 394, 431–434.

Stevens, J. (1970) Determination of glucose by an automatic analyser. *Clinica Chimica Acta* 32, 199–201.

Stookey, L. (1970) Ferrozine – a new spectrophotometric reagent for iron. *Analytical Chemistry* 42, 779–781.

Thompson, K.H. and Godin, D.V. (1995) Micronutrients and antioxidants in the progression of diabetes. *Nutrition Research* 15, 1377–1410.

Thurnham, D.I. and Smith, E.F. (1988) Concurrent liquid-chromatographic assay of retinol, α-tocopherol, β-carotene, α-carotene, lycopene and β-cryptoxanthine in plasma, with tocopherol acetate as an internal standard. *Clinical Chemistry* 34, 377–381.

Uzel, N., Sivas, A., Uysal, M. and Oz, H. (1987) Erythrocyte lipid peroxidation and glutathione peroxidase activities in patients with diabetes mellitus. *Hormone and Metabolism Research* 287, 89–90.

Wolff, S.P. (1987) The potential role of oxidative stress in diabetes and its complications: novel implications for theory and therapy. In: Crabbe, M.J.C. (ed.) *Diabetic Complications: Scientific and Clinical Aspects.* Churchill Livingstone, New York, pp. 167–220.

Nutrition and the Risk for Cataract 22

ALLEN TAYLOR, PAUL JACQUES AND ESTHER EPSTEIN

Jean Mayer USDA Human Nutrition Research Center on Aging, Tufts University, Boston, Massachusetts, USA

Introduction

Although the number of associations between nutriture and age-related eye diseases have burgeoned in the last decade, early studies regarding antioxidant properties of nutrients were performed virtually immediately after the discovery of ascorbate in the early part of the century.

Studies regarding the aetiology of cataract now include laboratory and epidemiological investigations. This chapter briefly reviews available data regarding associations between antioxidant nutrients and eye lens cataract in humans. Readers can refer to other recent reviews (Taylor, 1992, 1999; Taylor *et al.*, 1993; Jacques *et al.*, 1994) for more thorough treatments, particularly with respect to animal studies. Due to editorial concerns with brevity, much of the rich body of pioneering work is, of necessity, given limited coverage here.

The primary function of the eye lens is to collect and focus light on the retina. To do so it must remain clear throughout life. The lens is located posterior to the cornea and iris and receives nutriture from the aqueous humor. Although the lens appears to be free of structure it is exquisitely designed. A single layer of epithelial cells is found directly under the anterior surface of the collagenous membrane in which it is encapsulated. The epithelial cells at the germinative region divide, migrate posteriorly and differentiate into lens fibres. The fibres elaborate crystallins as their primary gene products; these are the predominant proteins of the lens. The fibres also lose their organelles. New cells are formed throughout life but older cells are usually not lost. Instead, they are compressed into the centre or nucleus of the lens. There is a coincident dehydration of the proteins and the lens itself. Together with modifications of the protein (noted below) and other constituents, these changes result in a less flexible lens upon ageing.

As the lens ages, the proteins are photooxidatively damaged, aggregate and accumulate in lens opacities. Dysfunction of the lens due to opacification is called cataract. The term 'age-related cataract' is used to distinguish lens opacification associated with old age from opacification associated with other causes, such as congenital and metabolic disorders (Taylor, 1999).

The solid mass of the lens is about 98% protein. Because these proteins undergo minimal turnover as the lens ages, they are subject to the chronic stresses of exposure to light and oxygen. Consequently, it is not surprising that these proteins are extensively damaged in the aged lens. Lens opacities develop as the damaged proteins aggregate and precipitate (Taylor *et al.*, 1993). Fibre cell membrane lipid damage is also associated with lens opacities (Berman, 1991; Jacques and Chylack, 1991; Jacques *et al.*, 1994). Smoking and ultraviolet light, which appear to induce oxidative stress, are also associated with elevated cataract risk, as well as with depletion of plasma ascorbate and carotenoid levels (reviewed in Taylor *et al.*, 1988; West *et al.*, 1989, 1992).

In young lenses, damaged proteins are usually maintained at harmless levels by defence systems. Primary defences that directly protect the lens against the initial oxidative insult include small molecule antioxidants (e.g. vitamins C and E, and carotenoids) and antioxidant enzyme systems (e.g. superoxide dismutase, catalase and the glutathione redox cycle) (Fridovich, 1984; Zigler and Goosey, 1984; Rathbun *et al.*, 1990; Giblin *et al.*, 1992; Varma *et al.*, 1999). The lens also has secondary defence systems, which include proteolytic enzymes that selectively identify and remove damaged or obsolete proteins (Taylor and Davies, 1987; Berger *et al.*, 1988; Jahngen-Hodge *et al.*, 1991; Huang *et al.*, 1993; Obin *et al.*, 1994; Shang and Taylor, 1995; Taylor, 1999). Accumulation of (photo-)oxidized (and/or otherwise modified) proteins in older lenses indicates that protective systems are not keeping pace with the insults that damage lens proteins. This occurs in part because, like bulk proteins, enzymes that comprise some of the protective systems are damaged by photo-oxidation (Blondin and Taylor, 1987; Taylor and Davies, 1987).

Many cell-free, *in vitro* and animal studies have addressed putative roles for antioxidants in maintenance of lens and retina function. These were reviewed recently and inspired the epidemiological work described below (Taylor, 1999). In order to fully appreciate the data presented below, readers should be aware that the various studies used different lens classification schemes, different definitions of high and low levels of nutrients and different age groups of subjects.

More than ten epidemiological studies have examined the associations between cataract and antioxidant nutrients (Mohan *et al.*, 1989; Robertson *et al.*, 1989; The Italian–American Cataract Study Group, 1991; Jacques and Chylack, 1991; Leske *et al.*, 1991; Hankinson *et al.*, 1992b; Knekt *et al.*, 1992;

Mares-Perlman *et al.*, 1994; Seddon *et al.*, 1994; Vitale *et al.*, 1994; Jacques *et al.*, 1997). Seven of the studies were retrospective case–control studies comparing the nutrient levels of cataract patients with that of similarly aged individuals with clear lenses (Mohan *et al.*, 1989; Robertson *et al.*, 1989; The Italian–American Cataract Study Group, 1991; Jacques and Chylack, 1991; Leske *et al.*, 1991; Mares-Perlman *et al.*, 1994; Vitale *et al.*, 1994). Our ability to interpret data from retrospective studies, such as these, is limited by the concurrent assessment of lens status and nutrient levels. Prior diagnosis of cataract might influence behaviour of cases including diet and might also bias reporting of usual diet. Three other studies assessed nutrient levels and/or supplement use, and then followed individuals with intact lenses for 8 (Hankinson *et al.*, 1992b; Knekt *et al.*, 1992), and 5 years (Seddon *et al.*, 1994), respectively. Prospective studies, such as these, are less prone to bias because assessment of exposure is performed before the outcome is present. These latter studies did not directly assess lens status, but used cataract extraction, or reported diagnosis of cataract as a measure of cataract risk. Extraction may not be a good measure of cataract incidence (development of new cataract), because it incorporates components of both incidence and progression in severity of existing cataract. However, extraction is the result of visually disabling cataract and is the endpoint that we wish to prevent. Although Hankinson *et al.* (1992b) measured nutrient intake over a 4-year period, Knekt *et al.* (1992) used only one measure of serum antioxidant status, and Seddon *et al.* (1994) used only one measure of supplement use. One measure may not provide an accurate assessment of usual, long-term nutrient levels. Multiple measures may be the best nutritional correlate of cataract (Jacques *et al.*, 1997). In the Vitamin C and Cataract Study and the Nutrition and Vision Project, nutrient intake was determined several times prior to enrolment in the study and examination of lens status.

Vitamin C

Vitamin C is probably the most effective, least toxic water-soluble antioxidant identified in mammalian systems (Levine, 1986; Frei *et al.*, 1988). Lens concentrations of vitamin C (mmol l^{-1}) are many times higher than in plasma or other tissues and are related to dietary intake in humans (Taylor *et al.*, 1991, 1997). The concentration of vitamin C in the lens is increased with dietary supplements beyond levels achieved in persons who already consume more than two times the recommended daily allowance (RDA) (60 mg day^{-1}) for vitamin C (Taylor *et al.*, 1991). However, lens and vitamin C levels may be compromised upon ageing and/or cataractogenesis (Berger *et al.*, 1988, 1989). Although biochemically plausible, there are no data to demonstrate that vitamin C shortage induces damage in the lens *in vitro* or *in vivo* (Blondin and Taylor, 1987; Garland, 1991; Naraj and Monnier, 1992).

Vitamin C has been considered in ten published studies (Mohan *et al.*, 1989; Robertson *et al.*, 1989; Jacques and Chylack, 1991; The Italian–American Cataract Study Group, 1991; Leske *et al.*, 1991, 1998; Hankinson *et al.*, 1992b; Mares-Perlman *et al.*, 1994; Vitale *et al.*, 1994; Jacques *et al.*, 1997) and observed to be inversely associated with at least one type of cataract in eight of these studies (Fig. 22.1). In an early study, Jacques and Chylack (1991) observed that among persons with higher vitamin C intakes (>490 mg day^{-1}), the prevalence of cataract was 25% of the prevalence among persons with lower intakes (<125 mg day^{-1}) (RR, 0.25; CI, 0.06–1.09).

Several studies found correlations between vitamin C supplement use and risk for cataract. In our Nutrition and Vision Project (Jacques *et al.*, 1997), age-adjusted analyses based on 165 women with high vitamin C intake (mean = 294 mg day^{-1}) and 136 women with low vitamin C intake (mean = 77 mg day^{-1}) indicated that the women who took vitamin C supplements for ≥10 years had >70% lower prevalence of early opacities (RR, 0.23; CI, 0.09–0.60) (Fig. 22.1A) and > 80% lower risk of moderate opacities (RR, 0.17; CI, 0.03–0.87) at any site compared with women who did not use vitamin C supplements (Fig. 22.1B) (Jacques *et al.*, 1997). Recent re-examination of 600 of the members of the same cohort indicates that comparable data can be anticipated. This corroborated work by Hankinson *et al.* (1992b) who noted that women who had consumed vitamin C supplements for >10 years had a 45% reduction in rate of cataract surgery (RR, 0.55; CI, 0.32–0.96) (Fig. 22.1G). In comparison with the data noted above, Mares-Perlman and co-workers (1994) report that past use of supplements containing vitamin C was associated with a reduced prevalence of nuclear cataract (RR, 0.7; CI, 0.5–1.0), but an increased prevalence of cortical cataract (adjusted RR, 1.8; CI, 1.2–2.9) after controlling for age, sex, smoking and history of heavy alcohol consumption. Mohan *et al.* (1989) also noted an 87% (RR, 1.87; CI, 1.29–2.69) increased prevalence of mixed cataract with posterior subcapsular and nuclear involvement for each standard deviation increase in plasma vitamin C levels. Vitale and co-workers (1994) observed that persons with plasma levels greater than 80 μmol l^{-1} and below 60 μmol l^{-1} had similar prevalences of both nuclear (RR, 1.31; CI, 0.61–2.39) and cortical (RR, 1.01; CI, 0.45–2.26) cataract after controlling for age, sex and diabetes. Similarly, no differences in cataract prevalence were observed between persons with high (>261 mg day^{-1}) and low (<115 mg day^{-1}) vitamin C intakes. One other study (The Italian–American Cataract Study Group, 1991) failed to observe any association between prevalence of cataract and vitamin C intake.

Vitamin E

Vitamin E, a natural lipid-soluble antioxidant, can inhibit lipid peroxidation (Machlin and Bendich, 1987) and appears to stabilize lens cell membranes (Libondi *et al.*, 1985). Vitamin E may be affected by ascorbate (see legend

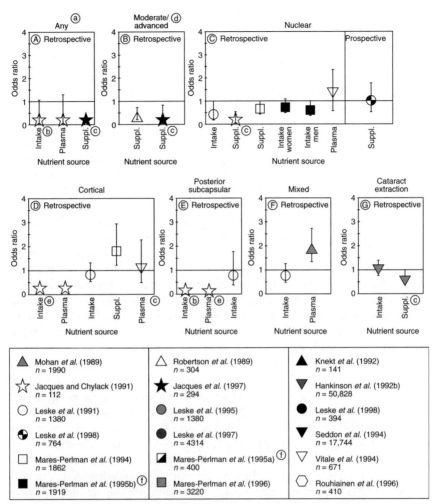

Fig. 22.1. Cataract risk ratio, high versus low intake (with or without supplements) or plasma levels of vitamin C. Types of cataract are: any, moderate/advanced, nuclear, cortical, posterior subcapsular, mixed or cataract extraction. Data for retrospective and prospective studies are presented independently. Adapted from Taylor *et al.* (1997).

to Fig. 22.1) and may enhance glutathione recycling, helping to maintain reduced glutathione levels in the lens and aqueous humor (Costagliola *et al.*, 1986).

Four studies assessing plasma vitamin E levels also reported significant inverse associations with cataract (Fig. 22.2). Some of these reached statistically significant observations. Vitale and co-workers (1994) observed the age-, sex- and diabetes-adjusted prevalence of nuclear cataract to be about 50% less (RR, 0.52; CI, 0.27–0.99) (Fig. 22.2C) among persons with plasma vitamin E concentrations greater than 29.7 μmol l^{-1} compared to persons with levels below 18.6 μmol l^{-1}. A similar comparison showed that the prevalence of cortical cataract did not differ between those with high and low plasma vitamin E levels (RR, 0.96; CI, 0.52–1.78) (Fig. 22.2D). Jacques and Chylack (1991) also observed the prevalence of posterior subcapsular cataract to be 67% lower (RR, 0.33; CI, 0.03–4.13) (Fig. 22.2E) lower among persons with plasma vitamin E levels above 35 μmol l^{-1} relative to persons with levels below 21 μmol l^{-1} after adjustment for age, sex, race and diabetes; however, the effect was not statistically significant. Prevalence of any early cataract (RR, 0.83; CI, 0.20–3.40) (Fig. 22.2A) or cortical cataract (RR, 0.84; CI, 0.20–3.60) (Fig. 22.2D) did not differ between those with high and low plasma levels. Plasma vitamin E was also inversely associated with prevalence of cataract in a large Italian study after adjusting for age and sex, but the relationship was no longer statistically significant after adjusting for other factors such as education, sunlight exposure and family history of cataract (The Italian–American Cataract Study Group, 1991). Leske *et al.* (1995) also demonstrated that individuals with high plasma vitamin E levels had significantly lower prevalence of nuclear cataract (RR, 0.44; CI, 0.21–0.90), but vitamin E was not associated with cataracts at other lens sites. Mares-Perlman *et al.* (1995a) completed a recent study in which they observed an inverse (non-significant) relationship (RR, 0.61; CI, 0.32–1.19) between serum γ-tocopherol (which has lower biological vitamin E activity than α-tocopherol) and severity of nuclear sclerosis but a positive, significant relationship between elevated serum α-tocopherol levels and severity of nuclear cataract (RR, 2.13; CI, 1.05–4.34).

In contrast with the studies noted above, Mares-Perlman and co-workers (1994) observed only weak, non-significant associations between vitamin E supplement use and nuclear (RR, 0.9; CI, 0.6–1.5) and cortical (RR, 1.2; CI, 0.6–2.3) cataract. Hankinson *et al.* (1992b) found no association between vitamin E intake and cataract surgery. Women with high vitamin E intakes (median = 210 mg day^{-1}) had a similar rate of cataract surgery (RR, 0.96; CI, 0.72–1.29) to women with low intakes (median = 3.3 mg day^{-1}). In partial contrast with their positive correlations between serum α-tocopherol levels and cataract, Mares-Perlman *et al.* (1995a) found that dietary vitamin E was associated with diminished risk for nuclear cataract in men, but not in women (Mares-Perlman *et al.*, 1995b).

Two prospective studies demonstrated a reduced risk for cataract progress among individuals with higher plasma vitamin E. Rouhiainen *et al.* (1996) found a 73% reduction in risk for cortical cataract progression (RR, 0.27; CI, 0.08–0.83) (Fig. 22.2D), whereas Leske *et al.* (1998) reported a 42% reduction in risk for nuclear cataract progression (RR, 0.58; CI, 0.36–0.94)

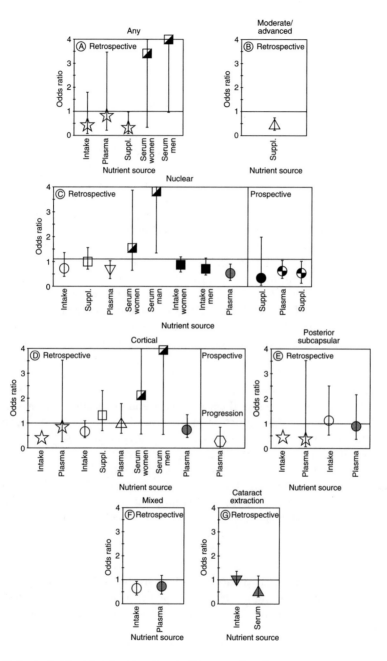

Fig. 22.2. As in Fig. 22.1, but for vitamin E (α-tocopherol).

(Fig. 22.2C). Vitamin E supplementation was related to a lower risk for progress of nuclear opacity (RR, 0.43; CI, 0.19–0.99) (Leske *et al.*, 1998).

Carotenoids

The carotenoids, like vitamin E, are natural lipid-soluble antioxidants (Machlin and Bendich, 1987). β-Carotene is the best known carotenoid because of its importance as a vitamin A precursor. It exhibits particularly strong antioxidant activity at low partial pressures of oxygen (15 torr) (Burton and Ingold, 1984). Partial pressure of oxygen in the core of the lens is approximately 20 torr (Kwan et al., 1972). However, it is only one of approximately 400 naturally occurring carotenoids (Erdman, 1988), and other carotenoids may have similar or greater antioxidant potential (Krinsky and Deneke, 1982; DiMascio et al., 1991). In addition to β-carotene, α-carotene, lutein and lycopene are important carotenoid components of the human diet (Micozzi et al., 1990). Carotenoids have been identified in the lens in approximately 10 ng g^{-1} wet weight concentrations (Daicker, 1987; Yeum et al., 1995), but there are no laboratory data relating carotenoids to cataract formation.

Jacques and Chylack (1991) observed that persons with high-plasma total carotenoid concentrations (>3.3 μmol l^{-1}) had less than one-fifth the prevalence of cataract compared to persons with low plasma carotenoid levels (<1.7 μmol l^{-1}) (RR, 0.18; CI, 0.03 1.03) after adjustment for age, sex, race and diabetes. However, they were unable to observe an association between carotene intake and cataract prevalence. Persons with carotene intakes above 18,700 IU day^{-1} had the same prevalence of cataract as those with intakes below 5677 IU day^{-1} (RR, 0.91; CI, 0.23–3.78). Knekt and co-workers (1992) reported that among age- and sex-matched cases and controls, persons with serum β-carotene concentrations above approximately 0.1 μmol l^{-1} had a 40% reduction in the rate of cataract surgery compared with persons with concentrations below this level (RR, 0.59; CI, 0.26–1.25). Hankinson and co-workers (1992b) reported that the multivariate-adjusted rate of cataract surgery was about 30% lower (RR, 0.73; CI, 0.55–0.97) for women with high carotene intakes (median = 14,558 IU day^{-1}) compared with women with low intakes of this nutrient (median = 2935 IU day^{-1}). However, while cataract surgery was inversely associated with total carotene intake, it was not strongly associated with consumption of carotene-rich foods, such as carrots. Rather, cataract surgery was associated with lower intakes of foods such as spinach that are rich in lutein and xanthin carotenoids, rather than β-carotene. The study by Mares-Perlman et al. (1995b) indicates that higher levels of individual or total carotenoids in the serum are not associated with less severe nuclear or cortical cataract overall. However, associations differed between men and women. A significant trend for lower risk ratio for either opacity with serum levels of β-carotene was observed in men. A marginally significant trend for lower risk of cortical opacities with higher levels of β-carotene was also noted for men. Higher serum levels of α-carotene, β-cryptoxanthin, and lutein were significantly related to lower risk for nuclear sclerosis only in men who smoked. In contrast, higher levels of some carotenoids were often directly associated with elevated nuclear sclerosis and cortical cataract, particularly in women. Vitale and colleagues (1994) also examined the relationships between plasma β-carotene levels and age-, sex- and diabetes-adjusted prevalence of cortical and nuclear cataract. Although the data suggested a weak inverse association between plasma β-carotene and cortical cataract and a weak positive association between this nutrient and nuclear cataract, neither association was statistically significant.

Antioxidant Nutrient Combinations

We were the first research group to report relationships between the risk for cataracts and various indices of antioxidants (for review, see Taylor and Jacques, 1997). However, it is not clear whether the nutrients are acting additively or synergistically. Thus, until this question is resolved (in progress), there may be only limited use to such discussion.

Nevertheless, the following are considered to be important data. The first, and perhaps most important, study in terms of revealing the utility of diet indicates a significant fivefold decrease in risk ratio for cataract between persons consuming ≥1.5 servings of fruits and/or vegetables daily (Jacques and Chylack, 1991) (Fig. 22.3). Relationships between multiple antioxidant nutrients and cataract risk are further supported by multivitamin use data. Leske and co-workers (1991) found that use of multivitamin supplements was associated with decreased prevalence for each type of cataract: 60%, 48%, 45% and 30%, respectively, for posterior subcapsular (RR, 0.40; CI, 0.21–0.77), cortical (RR, 0.52; CI, 0.36–0.72), nuclear (RR, 0.55; CI, 0.33–0.92), and mixed (RR, 0.70; CI, 0.51–0.97) cataracts. Seddon and co-workers (1994) also observed a reduced risk for incident cataract for users of multivitamins (RR, 0.73; CI, 0.54–0.99). Preliminary analyses from the Nutrition and Vision Project also indicate diminished risk for early stages of cataract for persons who took multivitamin supplements for more than 10 years.

Conclusions

Age-related eye diseases can be devastating in terms of quality of life of our most frail and with respect to national public health and economics. While it is too early to declare that increased consumption or intake of specific levels of nutrients is associated with diminished risk of cataract at any one location in the eye, the impression one gets from examining results from the work carried out to date is that nutrient intake can be optimized to delay cataract. Optimization of nutriture can be achieved through better diets and, perhaps, with the aid of supplements once appropriate levels of specifically beneficial nutrients are defined. Appropriate contemporary questions with respect to decreased risk for cataract might be: (i) how much of a nutrient is the

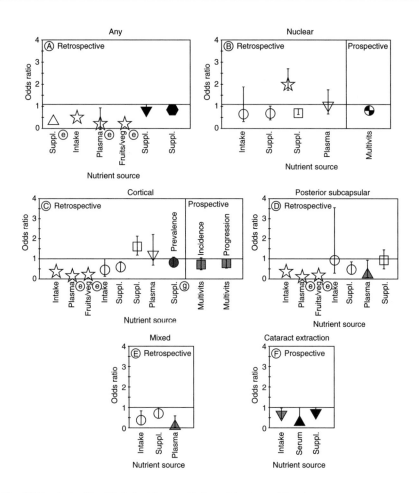

Fig. 22.3. As in Fig. 22.1, but for multiple nutrients and foods.

optimal intake? (ii) for how long or when would intake of the nutrient be useful? and (iii) is nutrient intake related to slowed progress or delayed onset of cataract? The answer to these questions is almost at hand. Two studies indicated that persons who consumed supplements of ascorbate for over 10 years have decreased risk for cataract or cataract extraction. However, these results should be corroborated by other research, including quantitative information regarding the quantity and the term of intake of other nutrients as well. The epidemiological data also indicate that it is imperative to execute longitudinal studies and possibly intervention trials.

Acknowledgements

This work was supported in part by grants EY08566, USDA contract 53-3K06-0-1 and Hoffmann-La Roche Inc.

References

Berger, J., Shepard, D., Morrow, F., Sadowski, J., Haire, T. and Taylor, A. (1988) Reduced and total ascorbate in guinea pig eye tissues in response to dietary intake. *Current Eye Research* 7, 681–686.

Berger, J., Shepard, D., Morrow, F. and Taylor, A. (1989) Relationship between dietary intake and tissue levels of reduced and total vitamin C in the guinea pig. *Journal of Nutrition* 119, 1–7.

Berman, E.R. (1991) *Biochemistry of the Eye*. Plenum Press, New York.

Blondin, J. and Taylor, A. (1987) Measures of leucine aminopeptidase can be used to anticipate UV-induced age-related damage to lens proteins: ascorbate can delay this damage. *Mechanisms of Ageing and Development* 41, 39–46.

Blondin, J., Baragi, V.J., Schwartz, E., Sadowski, J. and Taylor, A. (1986) Delay of UV-induced eye lens protein damage in guinea pigs by dietary ascorbate. *Free Radical Biology and Medicine* 2, 275–281.

Burton, W. and Ingold, K.U. (1984) Beta-carotene: an unusual type of lipid antioxidant. *Science* 224, 569–573.

Costagliola, C., Iuliano, G., Menzione, M., Rinaldi, E., Vito, P. and Auricchio, G. (1986) Effect of vitamin E on glutathione content in red blood cells, aqueous humor and lens of humans and other species. *Experimental Eye Research* 43, 905–914.

Daicker, B., Schiedt, K., Adnet, J.J. and Bermond, P. (1987) Canthaxamin retinopathy. An investigation by light and electron microscopy and physiochemical analyses. *Graef's Archives of Clinical and Experimental Ophthalmology* 225, 189–197.

Di Mascio, P., Murphy, M.E. and Sies, H. (1991) Antioxidant defense systems: the role of carotenoids, tocopherols and thiols. *American Journal of Clinical Nutrition* 53, 194S–200S.

Erdman, J. (1988) The physiologic chemistry of carotenes in man. *Clinical Nutrition* 7, 101–106.

Frei, B., Stocker, R. and Ames, B.N. (1988) Antioxidant defenses and lipid peroxidation in human blood plasma. *Proceedings of the National Academy of Sciences, USA* 85, 9748–9752.

Fridovich, I. (1984) Oxygen: aspects of its toxicity and elements of defense. *Current Eye Research* 3, 1–2.

Garland, D.D. (1991) Ascorbic acid and the eye. *American Journal of Clinical Nutrition* 54, 1198S–1202S.

Giblin, F.J., McReady, J.P. and Reddy, V.N. (1992) The role of glutathione metabolism in detoxification of H_2O_2 in rabbit lens. *Investigative Ophthalmology and Visual Science* 22, 330–335.

Hankinson, S.E., Willett, W.C., Colditz, G.A., Seddon, J.M., Rosner, B., Speizer, F.E. and Stamper M.J. (1992a) A prospective study of cigarette smoking and risk of cataract surgery in women. *Journal of the American Medical Association* 268, 994–998.

Hankinson, S.E., Stampfer, M.J., Seddon, J.M., Colditz, G.A., Rosner, B., Speizer, F.E. and Willett, W.C. (1992b) Nutrient intake and cataract extraction in women: a prospective study. *British Medical Journal* 305, 335–339.

Huang, L.L., Jahngen-Hodge, J. and Taylor, A. (1993) Bovine lens epithelial cells have a ubiquitin-dependent proteolysis system. *Biochimica Biophysica Acta* 1175, 181–187.

The Italian–American Cataract Study Group (1991) Risk factors for age-related cortical, nuclear, and posterior subcapsular cataracts. *American Journal of Epidemiology* 133, 541–553.

Jacques, P.F. and Chylack, L.T. Jr (1991) Epidemiologic evidence of a role for the antioxidant vitamins and carotenoids in cataract prevention. *American Journal of Clinical Nutrition* 53, 352S–355S.

Jacques, P.F. and Taylor, A. (1991) Micronutrients and age-related cataracts. In: Bendich, A. and Butterworth, C.E. (eds) *Micronutrients in Health and in Disease Prevention*. Marcel Dekker, New York, pp. 359–379.

Jacques, P.F., Chylack, L.T. Jr and Taylor, A. (1994) Relationships between natural antioxidants and cataract formation. In: Frei, B. (ed.) *Natural Antioxidants in Human Health and Disease*. Academic Press, Orlando, Florida, pp. 513–533.

Jacques, P.F., Taylor, A., Hankinson, S.E., Willett, W.C., Mahnken, B., Lee, Y., Vaid, K. and Lahav, M. (1997) Long-term vitamin C supplement use and prevalence of early age-related lens opacities. *American Journal of Clinical Nutrition* 66, 911–916.

Jahngen-Hodge, J., Laxman, E., Zuliani, A. and Taylor, A. (1991) Evidence for ATP ubiquitin-dependent degradation of proteins in cultured bovine lens epithelial cells. *Experimental Eye Research* 52, 341–347.

Jahngen-Hodge, J., Cyr, D., Laxman, E. and Taylor, A. (1992) Ubiquitin and ubiquitin conjugates in human lens. *Experimental Eye Research* 55, 897–902.

Knekt, P., Heliovaara, M., Rissanen, A., Aromaa, A. and Aaran, R. (1992) Serum antioxidant vitamins and risk of cataract. *British Medical Journal* 305, 1392–1394.

Krinsky, N.I. and Deneke, S.S. (1982) Interaction of oxygen and oxy-radicals with carotenoids. *Journal of the National Cancer Institute* 69, 205–210.

Kwan, M., Niinikoski, J. and Hunt, T.K. (1972) *In vivo* measurement of oxygen tension in the cornea, aqueous humor, and the anterior lens of the open eye. *Investigative Ophthalmology and Visual Science* 11, 108–114.

Leske, M.C., Chylack, L.T. Jr and Wu, S. (1991) The lens opacities case–control study risk factors for cataract. *Archives of Ophthalmology* 109, 244–251.

Leske, M.C., Wu, S.Y., Hyman, L., Sperduto, R., Underwood, B., Chylack, L.T., Milton, R.C., Srivastava, S. and Ansari, N. (1995) Biochemical factors in the lens opacities. Case–control study. The Lens Opacities Case–Control Study Group. *Archives of Ophthalmology* 113, 1113–1119.

Leske, M.C., Wu, S.Y., Connell, A.M.S. and Hyman, I. (1997) Lens opacities, demographic factors and nutritional supplements in the Barbados Eye Study. *International Journal of Epidemiology* 26, 1314–1322.

Leske, M.C, Chylack, L.T. Jr, He, Q., Wu, S.Y., Schoenfeld, E., Friend, J., Wolfe, J. and The LSC Group. (1998) Antioxidant vitamins and nuclear opacities—The Longitudinal Study of Cataract. *Ophthalmology* 105, 831–836.

Levine, M. (1986) New concepts in the biology and biochemistry of ascorbic acid. *New England Journal of Medicine* 314, 892–902.

Libondi, T., Menzione, M. and Auricchio, G. (1985) *In vitro* effect of alpha-tocopherol on lysophosphatidylcholine-induced lens damage. *Experimental Eye Research* 40, 661–666.

Luthra, R., Wa, S.-Y., Leske, M.C., Nemesure, B., He, Q. and BES Group (1997) Lens opacities and use of nutritional supplements: the Barbados Study. *Investigative Ophthalmology and Visual Science* 8, S450.

Machlin, L.J. and Bendich, A. (1987) Free radical tissue damage: protective role of antioxidant nutrients. *FASEB J.* 1, 441–445.

Mares-Perlman, J.A., Klein, B.E.K., Klein, R. and Ritter, L.L. (1994) Relationship between lens opacities and vitamin and mineral supplement use. *Ophthalmology* 101, 315–325.

Mares-Perlman, J.A., Brady, W.E., Klein, B.E.K., Klein, R., Palta, M., Bowen, P. and Stacewicz-Sapuntzakis, M. (1995a) Serum carotenoids and tocopherols and severity of nuclear and cortical opacities. *Investigative Ophthalmology and Visual Science* 141, 276–288.

Mares-Perlman, J.A., Brady, W.E., Klein, B.E.K., Klein, R., Haus, G.J., Palta, M., Ritter, L.L. and Shoff, S.M. (1995b) Diet and nuclear lens opacities. *American Journal of Epidemiology* 141, 322–334.

Mares-Perlman, J.A., Brady, W.E., Klein, B.E.K., Klein, R. and Palta, M. (1996) Supplement use and 5-year progression of cortical opacities. *Investigative Ophthalmology and Visual Science* 37, 137.

Micozzi, M.S., Beecher, G.R., Taylor, P.R. and Khachik, F. (1990) Carotenoid analyses of selected raw and cooked foods associated with a lower risk for cancer. *Journal of the National Cancer Institute* 82, 282–285.

Mohan, M., Sperduto, R.D., Angra, S.K., Milton, R.C., Mathur, R.L., Underwood, B., Jafery, N. and Pandya, C.B. (1989) India–US case–control study of age-related cataract. *Archives of Ophthalmology* 107, 670–676.

Naraj, R.M. and Monnier, V.M. (1992) Isolation and characterization of a blue fluorophore from human eye lens crystallins: *in vitro* formation from Maillard reaction with ascorbate and ribose. *Biochimica Biophysica Acta* 1116, 34–42.

Obin, M.S., Nowell, T. and Taylor, A. (1994) The photoreceptor G-protein transducin (G_t) is a substrate for ubiquitin-dependent proteolysis. *Biochemical and Biophysical Research Communications* 200, 1169–1176.

Rathbun, W.B., Holleschau, A.M., Murray, D.L., Buchanan, A., Sawaguchi, S. and Tao, R.V. (1990) Glutathione synthesis and glutathione redox pathways in naphthalene cataract in the rat. *Current Eye Research* 9, 45–53.

Robertson, J.McD., Donner, A.P. and Trevithick, J.R. (1989) Vitamin E intake and risk for cataracts in humans. *Annals of the New York Academy of Science* 570, 372–382.

Rouhianen, P., Rouhiainen, H. and Salonen, T.J. (1996) Association between low plasma vitamin E concentration and progression of early cortical lens opacities. *American Journal of Epidemiology* 144, 496–500.

Schwab, L. (1990) Cataract blindness in developing nations. *International Ophthalmology Clinics* 30, 16–18.

Seddon, J.M., Christen, W.G., Manson, J.E., LaMotte, F.S., Glynn, R.J., Buring, J.E. and Hennekens C.H. (1994) The use of vitamin supplements and the risk of cataract among US male physicians. *American Journal of Public Health* 84, 788–792.

Shang, F. and Taylor, A. (1995) Oxidative stress and recovery from oxidative stress are associated with altered ubiquitin conjugating and proteolytic activities in bovine lens epithelial cells. *Biochemistry Journal* 307, 297–303.

Taylor, A. (1992) Vitamin C. In: Hartz, S.C., Russell, M. and Rosenberg, I.H. (eds) *Nutrition in the Elderly: The Boston Nutritional Status Survey*. Smith Gordon Ltd, London, pp. 147–150.

Taylor, A. (1993) Cataract: relationships between nutrition and oxidation. *Journal of the American College of Nutritionists* 12, 138–146.

Taylor, A. (1999) Nutritional and environmental influences on risk for cataract. In: Taylor, A. (ed.) *Nutritional and Environmental Influences on Vision*. CRC Press, Boca Raton, Florida (in press).

Taylor, A. and Davies, K.J.A. (1987) Protein oxidation and loss of protease activity may lead to cataract formation in the aged lens. *Free Radical Biology of Medicine* 3, 371–377.

Taylor, A. and Jacques, P.F. (1997) Antioxidant status and risk for cataract. In: Bendich, A. and Deckelbaum, R.J. (eds) *Preventive Nutrition*. Humana Press, Totowa, New Jersey, pp. 267–283.

Taylor, A., Jacques, P.F., Nadler, D., Morrow, F., Sulsky, S.I. and Shepard, D. (1991) Relationship in humans between ascorbic acid consumption and levels of total and reduced ascorbic acid in lens, aqueous humor, and plasma. *Current Eye Research* 10, 751–759.

Taylor, A., Jacques, P.F. and Dorey, C.K. (1993) Oxidation and aging: impact on vision. *Journal of Toxicology and Industrial Health* 9, 349–371.

Taylor, A., Jacques, P., Nowell, T., Perrone, G., Blumberg, J., Handelman, G., Jozwiak, B. and Nadler, D. (1997) Vitamin C in human and guinea pig aqueous, lens and plasma in relation to intake. *Current Eye Research* 16, 857–864.

Taylor, H.R, West, S.K., Rosenthal, F.S., Newland, H.S., Abbey, H. and Emmett, E.A. (1988) Effect of ultraviolet radiation on cataract formation. *New England Journal of Medicine* 319, 1429–1433.

Varma, S.D., Devamanoharan, P.S. and Ali, A.H. (1999) Oxygen radicals in the pathogenesis of cataract – possibilities for therapeutic intervention. In: Taylor, A. (ed.) *Nutritional and Environmental Influences on Vision*. CRC Press, Boca Raton, Florida (in press).

Vitale, S., West, S., Hallfrisch, J., Alston, C., Wang, F., Moorman, C., Muller, D., Singh, V. and Taylor, H.R. (1994) Plasma antioxidants and risk of cortical and nuclear cataract. *Epidemiology* 4, 195–203.

West, S. (1992) Does smoke get in your eyes? *Journal of the American Medical Association* 268, 1025–1026.

West, S.K., Munoz, B., Emmett, E.A. and Taylor, H.R. (1989) Cigarette smoking and risk of nuclear cataracts. *Archives of Ophthalmology* 107, 1166–1169.

Yeum, K.-J., Taylor, A., Tang, G. and Russell, R. (1995) Measurement of carotenoids, retinoids, and tocopherols in human lenses. *Investigative Ophthalmology and Visual Science* 36, 2756–2761.

Zigler, J.S. and Goosey, J.D. (1984) Singlet oxygen as a possible factor in human senile nuclear cataract development. *Current Eye Research* 3, 59–65.

Reactive Oxygen Species and Age-related Macular Degeneration

23

RAVINDRA NATH[1], AMOD GUPTA[2], RAJENDRA PRASAD[3], SURINDER S. PANDAV[2] AND RAJINDER KUMAR[3]

Departments of [1] Experimental Medicine and Biotechnology, [2] Ophthalmology and [3] Biochemistry, Postgraduate Institute of Medical Education and Research, Chandigarh, India

Introduction

Age-related macular degeneration (AMD) is the second most common eye disease after cataract causing blindness in developed countries. It is a major cause of loss of vision in an ageing population (Young, 1987; Klein *et al.*, 1992; Seddon *et al.*, 1997). The clinical manifestations of AMD vary greatly, ranging from drusen and minimal disturbance of retinal pigment to massive subretinal exudation. There are two types of AMD. Dry AMD is the most common, and is associated with slow degeneration of the macula. The other type of AMD is wet, caused by an abnormal growth of blood vessels behind the retina. The specific changes that trigger the disease process whereby the retina becomes damaged are unknown. Oxidative stress is often cited as a leading mechanism causing ageing and degenerative disorders. This likely includes age-related ocular disorders (Prashar *et al.*, 1993). In view of the above findings, in the present chapter we have focused on the oxidative free radical status, which could be one of the most prominent factors in the pathogenesis of AMD, and the potential role of antioxidants in protection against eye diseases.

© CAB *International* 1999. *Antioxidants in Human Health*
(eds T.K. Basu, N.J. Temple and M.L. Garg)

Age-related Macular Degeneration

Loss of vision due to AMD may be slow or progressive due to geographic atrophy of retinal pigment epithelium (RPE) or may be due to sudden haemorrhage or exudation under the retina from the choroid neovascular membranes. In either case, visual handicap is severe and no satisfactory treatment is available. The incidence of AMD rises with age and is unusual below age 55. Once damage occurs, it cannot be reversed. Laser therapy has been used increasingly to halt the progression of choroidal neovascular membranes which commonly cause severe loss of vision.

Disturbances of RPE pigmentation and drusen formation are the classical signs of AMD (Green *et al.*, 1985). Loss of vision is due to increased neovascular invasion when drusen are large and confluent (Gregor *et al.*, 1977; Sarks, 1980). Histologically AMD is characterized by abnormalities in the Bruch's membrane which becomes thicker, hyalinized and more basophilic. Aberrant forms of collagen, densification and calcification of the Bruch's membrane may be seen.

A basal lamina deposit (BLD) of amorphous or granular eosinophilic material is seen between the RPE and its basal lamina in AMD. Continuous thick BLD are associated with severe degenerative changes in the RPE (Hoshino *et al.*, 1984). Formation of these deposits is closely correlated with the histological and clinical development of AMD.

Pigmentary changes, drusens and thickening of Bruch's membrane are common findings in the elderly eye (Feeney-Burns *et al.*, 1985). Accumulation of BLD and penetration of Bruch's membrane by neovessels have also been documented in ageing eyes. Thus, all major changes that occur in AMD are also seen in ageing eyes. But normally they do not progress to cell death and loss of function. Therefore, AMD can be considered to be an exaggerated form of normal ageing where loss of visual function occurs because senescent changes progress to degenerative disease.

Retinal Pigment Epithelium and the Antioxidant Defence System

The functional integrity of the retina depends on the maintenance activities of the RPE (Handelman and Dratz, 1986). The RPE cells ingest and degrade numerous rod outer segments every day, a process that renews the photoreceptors (Bok, 1985). However, phagocytosis initiates the production of superoxide anions $O_2 \cdot$, a reactive form of oxygen that can cause cellular damage directly or by conversion to the more reactive and damaging hydroxyl radical ($\cdot OH$).

Exposure of the RPE to these reactive oxygen species can also result from the photic reaction (Newsome *et al.*, 1986; Young, 1988). Another cause is high pO_2 values due to the diffusion of oxygen through the RPE from the adjacent choroidal circulation. By these means oxygen radical damage may accelerate the age-related changes (Sohal, 1987). The accumulation of ageing pigment, lipofuscin, is probably accelerated as a result of lipid degradation and lipid peroxidation (Dorey *et al.*, 1989; Bazan *et al.*, 1990). Retinal metabolism results in the production of several highly reactive species of oxygen, a process which might be speeded up by exposure to light (Pacifici and Davies, 1991; Halliwell *et al.*, 1992). These radicals are deleterious to the cellular components such as proteins, nucleic acids, lipids and carbohydrates. The high content of polyunsaturated fatty acids (PUFA) in the photoreceptor outer segment membranes makes photoreceptors more susceptible to free radical damage.

Antioxidant enzymes such as catalase, glutathione peroxidase, glutathione reductase and superoxide dismutase (SOD) protect against oxidative damage by catalysing decomposition of reactive oxygen species. The role of these enzymes in protecting the RPE from oxygen radical damage is critically important (Handelman and Dratz, 1986; Liles *et al.*, 1991). The two species of SOD (copper–zinc and manganese) break down superoxide anions forming H_2O_2 as a product (Equation 23.1). As previously mentioned, H_2O_2 can, in turn, give rise to reactive hydroxyl radicals (Equation 23.2).

$$2\,O_2\!\cdot\, + 2H^+ \xrightarrow[\text{Cu}^{2+}/\text{Zn}^{2+} \text{ or } \text{Mn}^{2+}]{\text{SOD}} H_2O_2 + O_2 \tag{23.1}$$

$$H_2O_2 \xrightarrow[\text{Fe}^{2+}]{\text{Cu}^{2+}} OH^- + \cdot OH \tag{23.2}$$

Thus SOD acts in concert with two other antioxidant enzymes, catalase and glutathione peroxidase, both of which convert H_2O_2 to H_2O and O_2, which are non-toxic. The combined action of these enzymes forms one metabolic pathway for protection against oxidative assault (Slater, 1979; Hayden *et al.*, 1990).

The activity of catalase is closely linked to the mechanism of rod outer segment (ROS) degradation. Catalase is localized within the peroxisomes of the RPE (Robinson *et al.*, 1977; Beard *et al.*, 1988) and after the fusion of the peroxisome with the phagosome, catalase is also present within secondary lysosomes, which contain ROS in various stages of degradation (Cohen *et al.*, 1970). Phagocytosis of ROS has been reported to cause a mobilization of peroxisomes *in vivo* and to increase catalase activity in cultured human RPE cells (Beard *et al.*, 1988; Boulton *et al.*, 1990). As a result, the most important role of catalase activity in the RPE may be the prevention of lipid peroxidation and lysosomal enzyme inhibition by removing H_2O_2 from the phagosomes. SOD activity has no significant correlation with ageing or macular degeneration, while catalase activity has been reported to be decreased with age and macular degeneration in both macular and peripheral RPE (Liles *et al.*, 1991).

The data from our laboratory on the activities of SOD and glutathione peroxidase in the RBCs suggest that there is a significant reduction in the activities of these enzymes in patients with AMD compared with age-matched controls. A strong correlation ($r = -0.99$) was observed between age of the patients and decreased activity of antioxidant enzymes (Prashar *et al.*, 1993). We can conclude, therefore, that oxidative stress is more pronounced in subjects with AMD as there is a decrease in levels of antioxidant enzymes. Moreover, oxidative stress could be one of the factors responsible for the development of AMD.

Protective Role of Antioxidants in Eye Health

As with our general health, good nutrition is essential for maintaining healthy vision. As with other diseases discussed in this book, it is the antioxidant nutrients which play a crucial role.

Vitamins A, E and C

For over 60 years, vitamin A has been associated with good eyesight. It is essential for forming the retinal photoreceptor pigments which are the basis of vision. Vitamin A deficiency causes eye tissue to shrink and harden, leading to over-sensitivity to bright light, dry and inflamed eyes and eyelids, and finally to night blindness. Vitamin A deficiency is still the prime cause of child blindness in developing countries. It is also associated with advanced AMD (Seddon *et al.*, 1994).

Seddon *et al.* (1994) studied the effect of antioxidant supplementation in patients with an advanced form of AMD. In those subjects given a multivitamin–mineral antioxidant supplement containing vitamin E (400 mg day^{-1}), vitamin C (500 mg day^{-1}), selenium (250 μg day^{-1}) and β-carotene (9 mg day^{-1}), distance visual acuity stabilized over a 18 month period whereas in those given placebo it declined. The supplements successfully halted or reversed the degenerative macular changes in 60% of subjects. This study suggests that vitamins A, C, E and β-carotene have a protective effect in preventing or slowing down the degenerative changes in the macula in early or late stages of AMD.

Carotenoids

Carotenoids have been shown to have a protective role against damaging ultraviolet (UV) light and free radicals. Two carotenoids, lutein and zeaxanthin, are present in relatively high concentrations in the eye and it is thought that they act both as a blue light filter and as antioxidants protecting against free radicals. The best dietary sources of lutein and zeaxanthin are spinach, red peppers, kale, broccoli, peas and celery.

In animals, the formation of drusen in the retina occurs faster in those deprived of carotenoids (Seddon *et al.*, 1994). Similarly, population studies show that people who eat more carotenoid-rich vegetables, particularly those containing lutein and zeaxanthin, have a significantly lower risk of developing AMD (Seddon *et al.*, 1994). Khachik *et al.* (1997) have concluded from their studies that the proposed oxidative reductive pathways for lutein and zeaxanthin in human retina may therefore play an important role in the prevention of AMD and cataracts. Thus, from these studies it can be concluded that nutritional status plays a vital role in maintaining the functional integrity of the eye.

Zinc

Zinc supplementation has been shown to enhance activity of antioxidant enzymes, notably catalase and SOD (Newsome and Swartz, 1988; Pacifici and Davies, 1991). By this means, zinc inhibits the free radical chain reaction and is known to possess antioxidant properties (Hidalgo *et al.*, 1988; Ophir and Chevian, 1992). Oral administration of zinc induces production of metallothionein to which it binds to form zinc-metallothionein, which is stored in the Ehrlich cells (Krezoski *et al.*, 1988). High concentrations of zinc have been reported in the ocular tissue, especially choroid, retina and RPE (Echert, 1979; Karcioglu, 1982).

Newsome and co-workers (1988) published the results of a double-blind, randomized, placebo-controlled study that investigated the effect of oral zinc supplementation on the natural course of AMD. They reported a significantly lower incidence of visual loss in the treatment group, which also had a lower frequency of exudative lesions during the follow-up period. Stur *et al.* (1996) reported a 2-year double-blind randomized placebo-controlled study including 112 patients with AMD and choroidal neovascularization, pigment epithelium detachment or both, in one eye, and visual acuity of better than 20/40 and macular degeneration without any exudative lesion in the second eye. It was concluded that oral zinc substitution has no short-term effect on the course of AMD in patients who have an exudative form of the disease in one eye. In our study, 60 patients with AMD and exudative lesions were recruited randomly into two groups (30 patients in each group) (unpublished observations). One group was given 89.5 mg daily of elemental zinc as $ZnSO_4$ and the other group was given placebo. The patients were kept under treatment for 18 months, with follow-up every 3 months and antioxidant status was assessed. It was found that levels of antioxidant enzymes (catalase, SOD and glutathione peroxidase) were increased and lipid peroxidation was decreased significantly. Further studies are being done to correlate the biochemical findings with the clinical outcome of oral zinc supplementation.

Conclusion

Oxidative stress, as assessed by antioxidant enzymes, is more pronounced in subjects with AMD as compared to age-matched controls. Our observations of decreased enzyme activities in RBCs of AMD subjects compared with controls suggest that RBCs can be used as an indicator of tissue oxidant status in studying the progress of the disease. Such studies may support the theory which proposes that abnormalities in RPE function are involved in AMD. In the absence of a definite cause-and-effect relationship, various agents are being investigated for their possible association with AMD. Recently, attention has been focused on the possible involvement of various trace elements. Zinc has received particular attention. Administration of oral zinc has been shown to be useful in patients with AMD which is explained, at least in part, by its enhancement of antioxidant status. Several epidemiological studies have questioned the role of zinc and emphasized the importance of the long-term dietary intake of other antioxidants such as β-carotene, α-tocopherol and vitamin C. Clearly, further epidemiological and intervention studies are required to determine the relationship between changes in nutritional status and clinical outcome in patients with AMD.

References

Bazan, H.E., Bazan, N.G., Feeney-Burns, L. and Berman, E.R. (1990) Lipids in human lipofuscin-enriched subcellular fractions of two age populations. *Investigative Ophthalmology and Visual Science* 31, 1433–1443.

Beard, M.E., Davies, T., Holloway, M. and Holtzman, E. (1988) Peroxisomes in pigment epithelium and Muller cells of amphibian retina possess D-amino acid oxidase as well as catalase. *Experimental Eye Research* 47, 795–806.

Bok, D. (1985) Retinal photoreceptors–pigment epithelium interactions: Friedenwald lecture. *Investigative Ophthalmology and Visual Science* 26, 1659–1695.

Boulton, M., Moriarty, P. and Unger, W. (1990) Human retinal pigment epithelial cell in culture: a means of studying aging and disease process? In: *Program and Abstracts of the Ninth International Congress for Eye Research*, July 29–August 4. Helsinki, Finland, Abstract 581.

Cohen, G., Dembiec, D. and Marcus, J. (1970) Measurement of catalase activity in tissue extracts. *Analytical Biochemistry* 34, 30–38.

Dorey, C.K., Khouri, G.G., Syniuta, L.A., Curran, S.A. and Weiter, J.J. (1989) Superoxide production by porcine retinal pigment epithelium *in vitro*. *Investigative Ophthalmology and Visual Science* 30, 1047–1054.

Echert, C.D. (1979) A comparative study of the concentrations of Ca, Fe, Zn and Mn in ocular tissues. *Federation Proceedings* 38, 872 (Abstract 3396).

Feeney-Burns, L. and Eldred, G.E. (1983) The fate of the phagosome: Conversion to age pigment and impact in human RPE. *Transactions of the Ophthalmological Society of the UK* 103, 416–421.

Feeney-Burns, L., Hilderbrand, E.S. and Eldridge, S. (1985) Age-related changes in the ultrastructure of Bruch's membrane. *American Journal of Ophthalmology* 100, 686–697.

Green, W.R., McDonnell, P.J. and Yeo, J.H. (1985) Pathologic features of senile macular degeneration. *Ophthalmology* 92, 615–627.

Gregor, Z., Bird, A.C. and Chisholm, I.H. (1977) Senile disciforn macular degeneration in the second eye. *British Journal of Ophthalmology* 61, 141–147.

Halliwell, B., Gutteridge, J.M.C. and Cross, C.E. (1992) Free radicals, antioxidants in human disease: where are we now. *Journal of Laboratory Clinical Medicine* 110, 599–620.

Handelman, G.J. and Dratz, E.A. (1986) The role of antioxidants in the retina and retinal pigment epithelium and the nature of pro-oxidant-induced damage. *Advances in Free Radical in Biology and Medicine* 2, 1–89.

Hayden, B.J., Zihu, L., Sens, D., Tapert, M. and Croueh, R.K. (1990) Cytolysis of corneal epithelial cells by hydrogen peroxide. *Experimental Eye Research* 50, 11–16.

Hidalgo, J., Compmany, L., Borras, M., Garvey, J.S. and Armario, A. (1988) Metallothionein in response to stress in rats: role in free radical scavenging. *American Journal of Physiology* E255, 518–524.

Hoshino, M., Mizano, K. and Ichikawa, H. (1984) Aging alterations of retina and choroid of Japanese: light microscopic study of macular region of 176 eyes. *Japanese Journal of Ophthalmology* 28, 89–102.

Kabayashi, M., Tanaka, T. and Usui, T. (1982) Inactivation of lysosomal enzymes by the respiratory burst of polymorphonuclear leukocytes. *Journal of Laboratory Clinical Medicine* 100, 896–907.

Karcioglu, Z.A. (1982) Zinc in the eye. *Survey of Ophthalmology* 27, 114–122.

Khachik, F., Berustein, P.S. and Garland, D.L. (1997) Identification of lutein and zeaxanthin oxidation products in human and monkey retinas. *Investigative Ophthalmology and Visual Science* 38, 1802–1811.

Klein, R., Klein, B. and Linton, K.L.P. (1992) Prevalence of age-related maculopathy: the Beaver Dam study. *Ophthalmology* 99, 933–943.

Krezoski, S.K., Villalobos, J., Shaw, C.F. and Petering, D.H. (1988) Kinetic lability of zinc bound to metallothionein in Ehrlich cells. *Biochemical Journal* 255, 483–491.

Liles, M.R., Newsome, D.A. and Oliver, P.D. (1991) Measurement of catalase activity in tissue extracts. *Analytical Biochemistry* 34, 30–38.

Newsome, D.A. and Swartz, M. (1988) Oral zinc in macular degeneration. *Archives of Ophthalmology* 106, 192–197.

Newsome, D.A., Berson, E. and Bonner, R. (1986) Possible role of optical radiation in retinal degenerations. In: Waxler, M. and Kilchins, V. (eds) *Optical Radiation and Visual Health*. CRC Press, Boca Raton, Florida, pp. 89–102.

Niwa, Y., Sakare, T., Yokoyama, M., Skosey, J.L. and Miyachi, Y. (1985) Reverse relationship between lysosomal enzyme release and active oxygen generation in stimulated human neutrophils. *Molecular Immunology* 22, 973–980.

Ophir, A. and Chevion, M. (1992) A possible role of free radical in the transplantation of retinal pigment epithelial cells. *Ophthalmology Surgery* 23, 284–287.

Pacifici, R.E. and Davies, K.J.A. (1991) Protein, lipid and DNA repair systems in oxidative stress: the free radical theory of aging revisited. *Gerontology* 37, 166–180.

Prashar, S., Pandav, S.S., Gupta, A. and Nath, R. (1993) Antioxidant enzymes in RBCs as a biological index of age related macular degeneration. *Acta Ophthalmologica* 171, 214–218.

Robinson, W.G. and Kuwabara, T. (1977) Vitamin A storage and peroxisome in retinal pigment epithelium and liver. *Investigative Ophthalmology and Visual Science* 16, 1110–1117.

Sarks, S.H. (1980) New vessel formation beneath the retinal pigment epithelium in senile eyes. *British Journal of Ophthalmology* 57, 951–965.

Seddon, J.M., Ajani, U.A., Sperduto, R.D., Hiller, R., Blair, N., Burton, T.C., Farber, M.D., Gragoudes, E.S., Hiller, J., Miller, D.T., Yannuzzi, L.A. and Willet, W. (1994) Dietary carotenoids, vitamins A, C and E and advanced age related macular degeneration: Eye Disease Case Control Study Group. *Journal of the American Medical Association* 272, 1413–1420.

Seddon, J.M., Anjali, U.A., Sperduto, R.D., Hiller, R., Blair, N., Burton, T.C., Farber, M.D., Gragoudas, E.S., Hallor, J., Miller, D.T., Yannuzzi, L.A. and Willet, W. (1997). Multi-center ophthalmic and nutritional age-related macular degeneration study – Part 2. Antioxidant intervention and conclusions. *Journal of the American Optometrist Association* 67, 30–49.

Slater, T.F. (1979) Mechanisms of protection against the damage produced in biological systems by oxygen-derived radicals. *Ciba Foundation Symposium* 65, 143–162.

Small, M.L., Green, W.R. and Alpar, J.J. (1976) Senile macular degeneration. *Archives of Ophthalmology* 94, 601–607.

Sohal, R.S. (1987) The free radical theory of aging: a critique. In: Rothstein, M. (ed.) *Review of Biological Research in Aging*. Alan R. Liss, New York, pp. 385–415.

Stur, M., Tittl, M., Reitner, A. and Meisinger, V. (1996) Oral zinc and the second eye in age-related macular degeneration. *Investigative Ophthalmology and Visual Science* 37, 1225–1235.

Young, R. (1988) Solar radiations and age related macular degeneration. *Survey of Ophthalmology* 32, 252–269.

Young, W.R. (1987) Pathophysiology of age related macular degeneration. *Survey of Ophthalmology* 31, 291–307.

Antioxidants and Respiratory Disease 24

IAN S. YOUNG[1],
HEATHER E. ROXBOROUGH[2]
AND JAYNE V. WOODSIDE[3]

[1] Department of Clinical Biochemistry,
Institute of Clinical Science, Belfast,
UK; [2] Cardiovascular Research,
The Rayne Institute, London, UK;
[3] Department of Surgery, University
College London Medical School, London, UK

Introduction

Oxygen is essential to life, yet is also potentially toxic as a result of its capacity to participate in the formation of oxygen free radicals and reactive oxygen species. This is a particular problem for the lung, which, as a consequence of its large surface area and direct exposure to inhaled gases and atmospheric pollutants, is at high risk of oxidant injury. Of special concern in this regard are ozone (O_3) and nitrogen dioxide (NO_2) (Putman et al., 1997). The antioxidant defences of pulmonary epithelial lining fluid (ELF) and lung tissue therefore play an important role in protecting the respiratory system against oxidant damage (Fig. 24.1).

Antioxidants in Respiratory Tract Lining Fluids

The fluids which line the respiratory tract form a first line of defence against the potential adverse effects of inhaled oxidants (Cross et al., 1994). Various antioxidants are present in ELF, including low-molecular-weight chain-breaking antioxidants, antioxidant enzymes and transition metal-binding proteins (Fig. 24.2). In particular, several small chain-breaking antioxidants are present in substantial concentrations.

Uric acid is the major low-molecular-weight antioxidant in upper respiratory tract fluids (Peden et al., 1993). It is co-secreted with lactoferrin

Ozone formation from smog and UV radiation

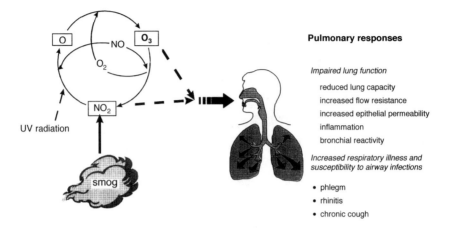

Fig. 24.1. Effects of inhaled air pollutants on respiratory function.

into the upper airways, and is closely associated with mucin. In plasma, urate is the most potent scavenger of ozone, and it probably has the same action in the respiratory tract (Cross *et al.*, 1992). Urate can also chelate transition metals and this may contribute to its antioxidant activity.

Ascorbate is the most important aqueous phase chain-breaking antioxidant in plasma (Frei *et al.*, 1989), and makes a major contribution to antioxidant protection in the lung, particularly the lower respiratory tract. This is likely to be due mainly to the direct radical-scavenging properties of ascorbate, but its capacity to recycle vitamin E may also be important. In animals, ascorbate is secreted in the reduced form by lower respiratory tract cells (Slade *et al.*, 1993), but it is uncertain whether this happens in humans. Ascorbate protects against the bronchoconstriction induced by exposure to both ozone (Chatham *et al.*, 1987) and NO_2 (Mohsenin, 1987) in healthy subjects, as well as against the increased bronchial responsiveness observed during upper respiratory tract infections (Bucca *et al.*, 1989).

Glutathione is the third low-molecular-weight antioxidant present in significant amounts in ELF, again mostly in the lower respiratory tract. Normal levels are more than 50 times those found in plasma. Glutathione is synthesized within cells lining the respiratory tract and subsequently released into the ELF, sometimes in response to inhaled pollutants (Boehme *et al.*, 1992a). Glutathione may directly scavenge free radicals, in the process being converted into the oxidized form. In addition, it acts as an essential cofactor for the antioxidant enzyme glutathione peroxidase which is present in ELF (Boehme *et al.*, 1992b). Oxidized glutathione can then be recycled by glutathione reductase, which is also known to be present (Buhl *et al.*, 1996).

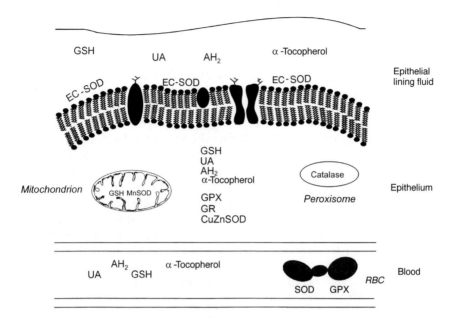

Fig. 24.2. Distribution of antioxidants in the respiratory tract. GSH, glutathione; UA, uric acid; AH_2, ascorbate; EC-SOD, extracellular superoxide dismutase; Mn SOD, manganese superoxide dismutase; GPX, glutathione peroxidase; GR, glutathione reductase; CuZnSOD, copper zinc superoxide dismutase; RBC, red blood cells.

α-Tocopherol has been measured in only low concentrations in ELF in comparison with the above antioxidants (Cross *et al.*, 1994). This is unsurprising given that the respiratory lining is essentially an aqueous environment with very little lipid present. Nonetheless, vitamin E depletion has been shown in animal models to increase the susceptibility of the lung to oxidant injury (Pryor, 1991). Most of the α-tocopherol is likely to be associated with components of surfactant, which constitutes the main lipid components present in ELF. However, significant amounts of α-tocopherol along with other lipid-phase chain-breaking antioxidants, including ubiquinol and the carotenoids, are likely to be present in the membranes of respiratory tract-lining cells, and these will play an important role in protecting cells from oxidant damage. The relatively high concentrations of the aqueous phase antioxidants in the ELF, as described above, will ensure that the membrane antioxidants can be efficiently recycled.

As well as the low-molecular-weight antioxidants, a variety of metal-binding proteins and antioxidant enzymes have been identified in ELF, as well as the enzymes involved in glutathione metabolism. These include lactoferrin, transferrin, albumin, ceruloplasmin (ferroxidase activity), catalase and superoxide dismutase (SOD) (Cantin *et al.*, 1990; Halliwell and Gutteridge, 1990). Under normal conditions ELF contain very little in the way of transition metals, but in the presence of lung inflammation, metals may be released from damaged cells, and transition metal binding proteins will then serve an important antioxidant function. Albumin has copper-binding activity, but will also serve as a sacrificial antioxidant by virtue of its rich content of sulphydryl groups (Neuzil and Stocker, 1994).

In addition to fluid, mucin is present in the upper respiratory tract and surfactant in the lower respiratory tract (in particular the bronchoalveolar regions). Mucin consists of a core glycoprotein rich in threonine and serine with a number of cysteine-rich domains which are involved in disulphide formation (Girod *et al.*, 1992). These disulphide bridges are important in giving mucin its characteristic consistency. The abundant thiol groups also provide mucin with the capacity to directly scavenge many oxidants. Moreover, mucins are known to have transition metal-binding properties (Cooper *et al.*, 1985). Mucins are excreted in increased amounts following exposure of airways to pollutants and other irritants and are likely to provide a substantial contribution to the antioxidant protection of upper airways.

Effect of Pollution

A number of epidemiological studies have investigated the proposed association between ozone and airways disease. These have shown asthma to be prevalent in areas with higher levels of ambient ozone, with outdoor ozone pollution exacerbating symptoms (Bates *et al.*, 1990). A significant association has also been demonstrated between incidence of upper and lower respiratory tract symptoms and high ambient ozone levels. As the ELF and bronchial epithelium are the first to come into contact with gaseous pollutants, antioxidant defences of ELF and lung tissue play an important role in protecting the respiratory system against oxidant damage. Once these antioxidants are depleted, the bronchial epithelium will undergo oxidative injury, resulting in enhancement of eicosanoid metabolism and subsequent generation of products of the arachidonic acid pathway which contribute to the development of early symptoms and decrement in lung function. Damage to the bronchial epithelium will also result in generation of tachykinins (e.g. substance P). Tachykinins contribute to the early symptomatic responses and changes in lung function. The simultaneous depletion in epithelial lining fluid of the enzyme neutral endopeptidase will exaggerate their local effects. These biochemical changes elicit a broad spectrum of pathophysiological responses including airway inflammation, alterations in airway epithelial permeability and increased airway reactivity to bronchoconstrictor agents.

Gaseous pollutants have been shown to cause airway injury in the normal population as well as potentiating allergen sensitization in asthmatics.

Therefore, the need for an adequate lung antioxidant barrier in the general population is clear. Differential utilization of water-soluble antioxidants in ELF upon contact with ozone and nitric oxide has been noted with uric acid proving the most potent, followed by ascorbic acid and finally glutathione. Exposure to ozone therefore leads to rapid depletion of urate in ELF; however, little information is available with regard to the reactivity or metabolic fate of urate oxidation products and it is possible that these are harmful. Inter-subject variations in the concentrations of these antioxidants could present one possible explanation for the observed variation in symptomatic responsiveness to air pollutants (Kelly and Mudway, 1997). Antioxidant composition of ELF is therefore thought to be crucial in determining an individual's sensitivity to gaseous pollutants and therefore susceptibility to respiratory disease (Fig. 24.3).

Cigarette Smoking and Pulmonary Antioxidants

Cigarette smoking is a major risk factor for the development of pulmonary disease, including emphysema, chronic bronchitis and lung cancer. Amongst its many toxic components, cigarette smoke contains substantial quantities of free radicals in both gas and particulate/tar phases (Churg and Cherukupalli, 1993). These include superoxide and nitric oxide, which may combine to produce peroxynitrites, the highly damaging hydroxyl radical (Zang *et al.*, 1995), tar semiquinone-free radicals and various xenobiotic electrophiles (Pryor, 1992). In addition, cigarette smokers have increased numbers of pulmonary inflammatory cells which will provide a secondary source of increased free radical production (MacNee *et al.*, 1989), and circulating leukocytes have an increased oxidative burst (Ludwig and Hoidal, 1982), which will make a significant contribution to oxidative damage in the airways (Fig. 24.3). Smoking is associated with increased levels of lipid peroxidation products in plasma, exhaled breath and lung tissue (Petruzzelli *et al.*, 1990; Duthie *et al.*, 1991, 1993; Morrow *et al.*, 1995). Elevated levels of DNA and protein damage products can also be detected (Reznick *et al.*, 1992), which may contribute to smoking-induced cancer and emphysema. In the latter case, it is likely to be of importance that exposure to tobacco smoke inactivates the anti-protease α_1-antitrypsin which opposes the action of neutrophil elastase (Hubbard *et al.*, 1987). Hereditary α_1-antitrypsin deficiency leads to the development of severe and premature emphysema, while inactivation of the enzyme by radical components of tobacco smoke is likely to play a role in the development of emphysema in smokers.

Smoking is associated with reduced antioxidant levels in various body fluids. This is due to a combination of reduced dietary intake of fruit and vegetables and repetitive sessions of oxidative stress (Rahman and MacNee, 1996). Smokers, however, also show evidence of increased turnover of

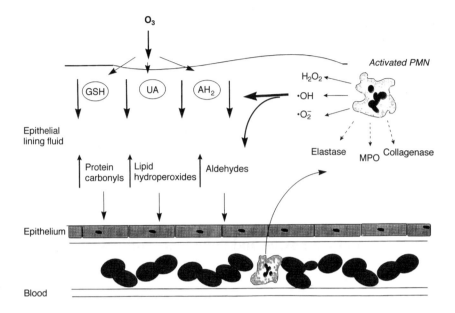

Fig. 24.3. The role of ozone and activated leukocytes (PMN, polymorphonuclear leukocyte) in oxidative damage in the lung. GSH, glutathione; UA, uric acid; AH_2, ascorbate; MPO, myeloperoxidase.

many chain-breaking antioxidants with low plasma vitamin E status recently attributed to both a reduction in the ability to absorb α-tocopherol and increased clearance of the freshly absorbed vitamin E. Smokers are hence likely to have an increased vitamin E requirement to maintain normal plasma levels. Studies suggest a depletion of ascorbate, α-tocopherol, β-carotene and selenium in serum of chronic smokers (Chow *et al.*, 1986; Bridges *et al.*, 1993; Mezzetti *et al.*, 1995), and decreased ascorbate and α-tocopherol have also been described in leukocytes from smokers (Barton and Roath, 1976; Theron *et al.*, 1990). However, there is some evidence of a compensatory increase in red blood cell antioxidant enzymes, including SOD and catalase (Toth *et al.*, 1986).

Several studies have reported an increase in gluatathione in ELF of smokers (Linden *et al.*, 1989; Morrison *et al.*, 1994). This may be as a consequence of increased cell turnover due to chronic airways inflammation. Ascorbate may also be somewhat increased in ELF from smokers (Bui *et al.*, 1992), while α-tocopherol is decreased (Pacht *et al.*, 1986). Results relating to antioxidant enzymes in macrophages from human lungs have been variable, with both increased activity of SOD and catalase (McCusker and Hoidal, 1990) and decreased activity (Kondo *et al.*, 1994) having been reported.

Chronic Obstructive Pulmonary Disease

Chronic obstructive pulmonary disease (COPD) is an obstructive airway disorder characterized by a gradually progressive and irreversible decrease in forced expiratory volume (FEV_1) (Siafakas et al., 1995). The condition usually arises due to chronic bronchitis or emphysema and the airflow obstruction may be accompanied by airway hyperreactivity. Asthma is generally differentiated from COPD, although distinguishing the two in a patient who smokes and has allergies can be difficult. This decrease is due to narrowing of the airway lumen and occurs as a direct result of disturbances in airway and interstitial lung tissue. There are a number of known risk factors for COPD, including air pollution, recurrent bronchopulmonary infection, socio-economic status and childhood history of respiratory infection. A strong relationship between age and COPD is also noted, with occurrence rare before 40 years and incidence increasing rapidly until 60–70 years of age when it becomes more stable, which is due in part to increased mortality in this age group. The most marked association observed, however, is between smoking and COPD, with nearly 90% of all COPD patients being smokers.

Considerable evidence now links COPD with oxidative stress (Crystal, 1990; Rahman et al., 1996), with iron apparently playing a key role. Iron concentrations of smokers are known to be increased in alveolar macrophages, ELF and upper lobes (Thompson et al., 1991; Nelson et al., 1996). This is due to a combination of iron present in the cigarette and to the increased release of iron from its binding proteins, which occurs as a result of biochemical disturbances induced by cigarette smoke (Lapenna et al., 1995). As superoxide and hydrogen peroxide will react in the presence of iron to produce the more potent oxidizing agent, the hydroxyl radical, the resultant increase in oxidative stress is clear. Cigarette smoke has also been estimated to contain 500 mg kg^{-1} nitric oxide and 10^{15} radicals per puff and so will provide a rich source of oxidants which will again contribute to the increase in oxidative stress (Pryor and Stone, 1993; Eiserich et al., 1994).

Increased airway and parenchymal inflammation is a frequent feature of COPD, with numbers of neutrophils, alveolar macrophages (AM) and eosinophils reported to be increased in COPD lung biopsies (Bosken et al., 1992; Costabel and Guyman, 1992; Saetta et al., 1993). This effect is further compounded by the finding that polymorphonuclear leukocytes (PMN) and AM from smokers release more superoxide than those from non-smoking controls (Ludwig and Hoidal, 1982; Schaberg et al. 1992). Infections may also contribute to oxidative stress in patients with COPD, as the resultant phagocyte recruitment and activation in the lung will lead to an increase in oxidative stress. This is exacerbated by the disturbance in antioxidant defence noted in smokers, as described previously. The overall increase in free radical production and decreased antioxidant status is reflected in the increase in oxidative stress biomarkers: lipid peroxidation, protein carbonyl formation and DNA damage (Schwalb and Anderson, 1989; Lapenna *et al.*, 1995; Lenz *et al.*, 1996).

Although the imbalance in lung oxidant–antioxidant status is clear both in COPD and in smokers, it is still unknown why only 20% of smokers develop the disease. Smoking may combine/interact with other risk factors in the disease aetiology (Snider, 1989). As exposure to inhaled oxidants from cigarette smoke appears consistent among those with comparable smoking histories, the answer to this question could lie in the involvement of genetic, dietary and environmental factors that help to control the antioxidant–oxidant balance. Greater understanding of the determinants which both coarse- and fine-tune this balance is therefore required. Further evidence of the role of antioxidants in COPD is also discussed in Chapter 25.

Asthma

Asthma is a major health problem worldwide, with a prevalence of at least 10% among children and 5% among adults in Western countries (Burney *et al.*, 1990). It is characterized by airway lability, with spontaneously variable or reversible airflow obstruction, a bronchoconstrictor response to methacholine or histamine, or daily or diurnal variability in peak expiratory flow (Sears, 1993). There is strong evidence that the prevalence of asthma has increased substantially in the last 25 years in a number of populations (Burr *et al.*, 1989; Ninan and Russel, 1992). This has been accompanied by an increase in allergy, and it is generally accepted that only part of the increase is attributable to improved diagnosis (Gergen and Weiss, 1992). Over the same period the genetic background has obviously remained constant, and there is no evidence of a significant rise in any pollutants. Attention must therefore focus on other environmental or lifestyle changes which may have increased susceptibility to asthma. One potential candidate is dietary change associated with reduced consumption of fresh fruit and vegetables and hence nutritional antioxidants.

Whatever the underlying factor precipitating asthma, airways inflammation is a key feature (Holgate, 1997), characterized by the presence of eosinophils, T lymphocytes and mast cells in the airways. These cells produce a wide range of inflammatory mediators, including free radicals. Reduced antioxidant intake in the diet would decrease the availability of key antioxidants in respiratory tract lining fluids and hence increase the susceptibility of airways to free radical damage. In the UK, data from the National Food Surveys show a 26% fall in fresh fruit consumption and a 51% fall in green vegetable consumption between 1961 and 1991, although these data are open to criticism as they do not include restaurant meals (MAFF, 1989). Epidemiological data suggest that greater antioxidant consumption is associated with reduced bronchial reactivity and wheeze in both adults and children (Schwartz and Weiss, 1990; Strachan *et al.*, 1991; Britton *et al.*, 1995; Cook *et al.*, 1997; Soutar *et al.*, 1997). The evidence appears to be greatest for vitamin C, which is in keeping with the well-established role of ascorbate as an antioxidant in respiratory tract lining fluids as discussed above. The only study to compare the effects of different nutrients on lung function found that both vitamin E and vitamin C were related to forced expiratory volume in 1 s (FEV$_1$). However, in a mulitivariate analysis only the association with vitamin C persisted (Britton *et al.*, 1995). Two studies have reported a beneficial role for vitamin C preventing decreases in FEV$_1$ following exercise or methacholine challenge (Schacter and Schlessinger, 1982; Mohsenin *et al.*, 1983), and vitamin C has also been shown to attenuate bronchoconstriction induced by inhaling ozone or NO$_2$ (Chatham *et al.*, 1987; Mohsenin, 1987). Results with regard to the ability of vitamin C to reduce the response to histamine challenge are less clear cut, with studies giving both positive (Zuskin *et al.*, 1975) and negative (Malo *et al.*, 1986) results. It may be that the beneficial effects of increased vitamin C are restricted to subjects who are genetically predisposed to increased bronchial reactivity, as suggested by some recent studies (Cook *et al.*, 1997; Soutar *et al.*, 1997).

While the evidence is strongest for a role of vitamin C in protecting against bronchoconstriction, other micronutrients could be important. Reduced selenium levels have been reported in patients with asthma (Stone *et al.*, 1989; Flatt *et al.*, 1990), and reduced serum retinol has also been associated with bronchoconstriction (Morabia *et al.*, 1990). The apparent inverse association between vitamin C intake and asthma could be confounded by other nutrients which tend to be present in the same dietary sources. One possible candidate is magnesium, which influences muscle contraction and has been related to wheezing and airway hyperreactivity (Britton *et al.*, 1994).

Neonatal Lung Disease

Chronic lung disease of prematurity (CLD) is a major cause of morbidity and mortality in premature babies due to a combination of underdeveloped lungs and a requirement for mechanical ventilation with high concentrations of oxygen. Acute lung disease in preterm infants is accompanied by a marked influx of inflammatory cells into the lungs (Arnon *et al.*, 1993). The combination of this with high concentrations of inspired oxygen, the relative immaturity of antioxidant defence systems and ischaemia–reperfusion injury as collapsed lung segments re-expand may lead to significant free radical-induced lung damage (Saugstad, 1990). The administration of surfactant with a resultant marked transitory increase in oxygenation may also augment reperfusion injury (Halahakoon *et al.*, 1995). A poor clinical outcome in very low birthweight infants is associated with increased levels of lipid peroxidation products in exhaled breath, although these may originate in sites other than the lung (Pitkanen *et al.*, 1990). The factors which lead some infants to recover from acute respiratory insufficiency while others go on to develop CLD are poorly understood, but it is possible that poor antioxidant defences are involved.

Little information is available with regard to the development of antioxidant enzymes in premature infants, although in one study the administration of bovine superoxide dismutase to 45 premature infants was associated with reduced oxygen dependency in the treated group (Rosenfeld *et al.*, 1984). Selenium deficiency has been recognized in premature infants (Lockitch *et al.*, 1989) and is associated with glutathione peroxidase deficiency (Sluis *et al.*, 1992). In animal models (rat, rabbit, hamster and guinea pig), antioxidant enzyme availability is markedly reduced in those born prematurely (<85% gestation time), and this is associated with increased susceptibility to lung damage (Frank and Sosenko, 1987). Treatment with corticosteroids in human mothers prior to delivery leads to induction of antioxidant enzymes in babies and protection against lung damage (Frank *et al.*, 1985). Treatment of human mothers with steroids is also associated with a reduction in lung disease in infants, and an increase in antioxidant enzymes may be one of several mechanisms involved.

So far as low-molecular-weight antioxidants are concerned, several studies reported reduced levels of glutathione in ELF in premature infants (Grigg *et al.*, 1993; Reise *et al.*, 1997). In plasma, ascorbate levels are relatively high, which reflects the several-fold increase in ascorbate in cord blood compared with maternal plasma (Silvers *et al.*, 1994). This is likely to result in normal or increased availability of ascorbate in ELF. However, premature babies have reduced serum transferrin, which tends to be abnormally saturated, resulting in circulating non-protein-bound redox reactive iron (Lindeman *et al.*, 1992). Leakage of this fluid into alveolar fluid relatively well supplied with ascorbate might result in a pro-oxidant reaction leading to the generation of hydroxyl radicals. This would normally be inhibited by the ferroxidase activity of ceruloplasmin, but ceruloplasmin levels are also reduced in premature infants (Rosenfeld *et al.*, 1986), and the ferroxidase activity of ceruloplasmin can be inhibited by the high concentrations of ascorbate found in neonates (Powers *et al.*, 1995). In the case of vitamin E, no data are available regarding concentrations in ELF in neonates. However, a meta-analysis of eight randomized controlled trials of vitamin E supplementation did not indicate any protective effect against chronic lung disease (Heffner and Repine, 1989), suggesting that vitamin E deficiency is not a major factor predisposing to oxidant injury in this setting.

Cystic Fibrosis

Recently, there have been major advances in the understanding of the underlying genetic defect in cystic fibrosis (CF). However, the causes of lung damage and pulmonary fibrosis which are responsible for the majority of deaths from CF remains unclear. Lung dysfunction in CF consists of progressive airflow obstruction caused by accumulation of thick, viscous secretions and the gradual destruction of the bronchiolar and larger airways (Brown *et al.*, 1996). In addition, CF patients suffer from diminished pancreatic function, resulting in the inadequate breakdown and absorption of fat-soluble nutrients. This leads to deficiencies in α-tocopherol and β-carotene, and therefore a reduction in overall antioxidant defence. In addition, CF patients have a 1000-fold increase in lung neutrophil numbers; this is due to a heightened immune response as a result of repetitive pulmonary infections. Once activated, these neutrophils are a major source of free radicals. CF patients are therefore placed under increased oxidative stress. As a result, patients with normal antioxidant status show increased oxidant damage. As CF patients have insufficient antioxidant defences to cope with this increase in oxidative stress, oxidative lung damage will result, which is likely to exacerbate the progressive decrease in pulmonary function noted. Antioxidant supplementation might therefore prove beneficial in reducing the rate of deterioration in pulmonary function in CF.

Other Respiratory Diseases

Idiopathic pulmonary fibrosis is characterized by pulmonary inflammation of unknown aetiology leading to alveolar epithelial injury and progressive fibrosis. Release of oxidant species by inflammatory cells is thought to play a significant role in the progression of the condition (Cantin *et al.*, 1987). Reduced glutathione concentrations in ELF seem to be a characteristic feature (Cantin and Begin, 1991). An imbalance between oxidants and antioxidants in the lung may also play a role in the respiratory manifestations of acquired immune deficiency syndrome (Buhl, 1994). Adult respiratory distress syndrome (ARDS) is characterized by severe hypoxaemia, pulmonary infiltration and decreased respiratory compliance, occurring in a variety of clinical settings and with a uniformly poor prognosis. Massive infiltration of the lungs by neutrophils with consequent oxidant injury occurs. A prominent deficit of glutathione in ELF is again a prominent feature (Bunnell *et al.*, 1991; Lykens *et al.*, 1992) with systemic evidence of increased antioxidant turnover (Cross *et al.*, 1990).

Antioxidant Therapy and Respiratory Disease

As discussed above, depletion of antioxidants will increase tissue sensitivity to oxidant injury in a variety of respiratory diseases. This therefore raises the possibility that augmenting lung antioxidant levels will be effective in preventing or treating respiratory disease. The aim of such treatment would be to increase antioxidant levels in ELF or in epithelial cells lining the airways and alveoli. There are two potential routes for the administration: either systemically or via inhalation of an aerosol. So far as antioxidant enzymes are concerned, options for increasing levels are at present very limited. Liposome-encapsulated enzymes could be administered by inhalation and might be taken up by epithelial cells (Tanswell and Freeman, 1987). Superoxide dismutase bound to a heparin-like molecule can attach to the surface of vascular endothelial cells and help to protect them against oxidant injury (Inoue *et al.*, 1990). In the longer term, it may be possible to selectively increase the transcription of antioxidant enzyme genes in lung cells. At present, these forms of treatment are only at the experimental stage.

It is much more feasible to increase concentrations of low-molecular-weight antioxidants in ELF. The administration of ascorbate, glutathione, α-tocopherol or urate by nebulized aerosol would be technically straight-forward. The use of glutathione aerosol therapy has been investigated in idiopathic pulmonary fibrosis and human immunodeficiency virus infection, where ELF glutathione levels were increased and there seemed to be some reduction in oxidant injury at the epithelial surface (Borok *et al.*, 1991; Holroyd *et al.*, 1993). In mice exposed to oxygen, reduced glutathione protected lungs against injury when administered via the trachea in liposomes, but not when given intraperitoneally to mice exposed to air (Smith and Anderson, 1992), so the mode of administration might be important. The effects of the administration of other antioxidants by this route has so far not been reported.

Glutathione cannot be administered orally, due to lack of bioavailability. However, oral or intravenous administration of *N*-acetylcysteine (NAC) is an effective means of increasing glutathione in plasma, red blood cells and ELF (Bridgeman *et al.*, 1994), and observational studies suggest a possible beneficial effect in adult respiratory distress syndrome (Bernard, 1990). Administration of ascorbate or α-tocopherol by the oral route effectively increases antioxidant concentrations in many body fluids, but no data are available with regard to effects on lung lining fluids. Perhaps of more relevance to public health, recent evidence has shown that a switch to a diet rich in fruit and vegetables will result in a significant increase in plasma levels of ascorbate and carotenoids. However, further studies are required to show whether this type of intervention will translate into improved respiratory function in subjects with asthma or other respiratory disease.

Conclusions

A variety of antioxidants are present in ELF and play an important role in protecting the lung against oxidant injury which occurs as a consequence of neutrophil activation during inflammatory processes or following inhalation of cigarette smoke or pollutants. Epidemiological and experimental evidence suggests that reduced levels of nutritional antioxidants, particularly vitamin C, may predispose to the development of asthma and other respiratory diseases. The assessment of strategies to augment lung antioxidant levels is at an early stage. This could be achieved by increased consumption of fruit and vegetables or by pharmacological administration of antioxidants by oral or intravenous routes or by inhalation.

References

Arnon, S., Grigg, J. and Silverman, M. (1993) Pulmonary inflammatory cells in ventilated preterm infants – effect of surfactant treatment. *Archives of Disease in Childhood* 69, 44–48.

Barton, G.M. and Roath, O.S. (1976) Leukocyte ascorbic acid in abnormal leukocyte states. *International Journal for Vitamin and Nutrition Research* 46, 271–274.

Bates, D.V., Baker-Anderson, M. and Sizto, R. (1990) Asthma attack periodicity: a study of hospital emergency visits in Vancouver. *Environmental Research* 51, 51–70.

Bernard, G.R. (1990) Potential of *N*-acetylcysteine as treatment for the adult respiratory-distress syndrome. *European Respiratory Journal* 3, 496–498.

Boehme, D.S., Maples, K.R. and Henderson, R.F. (1992a) Glutathione release by pulmonary alveolar macrophages in response to particles *in vitro*. *Toxicology Letters* 60, 53–60.

Boehme, D.S., Hotchkiss, J.A. and Henderson, R.F. (1992b) Glutathione and GSH-dependent enzymes in bronchoalveolar lavage fluid cells in response to ozone. *Experimental and Molecular Pathology* 56, 37–48.

Borok, Z., Buhl, R., Grimes, G.J., Bokser, A.D., Hubbard, R.C., Holroyd, K.J., Roum, J.H., Czerski, D.B., Cantin, A.M. and Crystal, R.G. (1991) Effect of glutathione aerosol on oxidant–antioxidant imbalance in idiopathic pulmonary fibrosis. *Lancet* 338, 215–216.

Bosken, C.H., Hards, J., Gatter, K. and Hogg, J.C. (1992) Characterization of the inflammatory reaction in the peripheral airways of cigarette smokers using immunocytochemistry. *American Review of Respiratory Disease* 145, 911–917.

Bridgeman, M.E., Marsden, M., Selby, C., Morrison, D. and MacNee, W. (1994) Effect of *N*-acetylcysteine on the concentrations of thiols in plasma, bronchoalveolar lavage fluid, and lung-tissue. *Thorax* 49, 670–675.

Bridges, A.B., Scott, N.A., Parry, G.J. and Belch, J.J. (1993) Age, sex, cigarette smoking and indices of free radical activity in healthy humans. *European Journal of Medicine* 2, 205–208.

Britton, J., Pavord, I., Richards, K., Wisniewski, A., Knox, A., Lewis, S., Tattersfield, A. and Weiss, S. (1994) Dietary magnesium, lung-function, wheezing, and airway hyperreactivity in a random adult-population sample. *Lancet* 344, 357–362.

Britton, J.R., Pavord, I.D., Richards, K.A., Knox, A.J., Wisniewski, A.F., Lewis, S.A., Tattersfield, A.E. and Weiss, S.T. (1995) Dietary antioxidant vitamin intake and lung-function in the general population. *American Journal of Respiratory and Critical Care Medicine* 151, 1383–1387.

Brown, R.K., Wyatt, H., Price, J.F. and Kelly, F.J. (1996) Pulmonary dysfunction in cystic fibrosis is associated with oxidative stress. *European Respiratory Journal* 9, 334–339.

Bucca, C., Rolla, G., Arossa, W., Caria, E., Elia, C., Nebiolo, F. and Baldi, S. (1989) Effect of ascorbic-acid on increased bronchial responsiveness during upper airway infection. *Respiration* 55, 214–219.

Buhl, R. (1994) Imbalance between oxidants and antioxidants in the lungs of HIV-seropositive individuals. *Chemical and Biological Interactions* 91, 147–158.

Buhl, R., Meyer, A. and Vogelmeier, C. (1996) Oxidant–protease interaction in the lung. Prospects for antioxidant therapy. *Chest* 110, 267–272.

Bui, M.H., Sauty, A., Collet, F. and Leuenberger, P. (1992) Dietary vitamin-C intake and concentrations in the body-fluids and cells of male smokers and non-smokers. *Journal of Nutrition* 122, 312–316.

Bunnell, E., Merola, A.J. and Pacht, E.R. (1991) Oxidized glutathione (GSSG) is increased in the epithelial lining fluid (ELF) of patients with the adult respiratory-distress syndrome (ARDS). *Clinical Research* 39, 754.

Burney, P.J., Chinn, S. and Rona, R.J. (1990) Has the prevalence of asthma increased in children – evidence from the national study of health and growth 1973–86. *British Medical Journal* 300, 1306–1310.

Burr, M.L., Butland, B.K., King, S. and Vaughan-Williams, E. (1989) Changes in asthma prevalence: two surveys 15 years apart. *Archives of Disease in Childhood* 64, 1452–1456.

Cantin, A.M. and Begin, R. (1991) Glutathione and inflammatory disorders of the lung. *Lung* 169, 123–138.

Cantin, A.M., North, S.L., Fells, G.A., Hubbard, R.C. and Crystal, R.G. (1987) Oxidant-mediated epithelial cell injury in idiopathic pulmonary fibrosis. *Journal of Clinical Investigation* 79, 1665–1673.

Cantin, A.M., Fells, G.A., Hubbard, R.C. and Crystal, R.G. (1990) Antioxidant macromolecules in the epithelial lining fluid of the normal human lower respiratory tract. *Journal of Clinical Investigation* 86, 962–971.

Chatham, M.D., Eppler, J.H., Sauder, L.R., Green, D. and Kulle, T.J. (1987) Evaluation of the effects of vitamin-C on ozone-induced bronchoconstriction in normal subjects. *Annals of the New York Academy of Sciences* 498, 269–279.

Chow, C.K., Thacker, R.R., Changchit, C., Bridges, R.B., Rehm, S.R., Humble, J. and Turbek, J. (1986) Lower levels of vitamin-C and carotenes in plasma of cigarette smokers. *Journal of the American College of Nutrition* 5, 305–312.

Churg, A. and Cherukupalli, K. (1993) Cigarette-smoke causes rapid lipid-peroxidation of rat tracheal epithelium. *International Journal of Experimental Pathology* 74, 127–132.

Cook, D.G., Carey, I.M., Whincup, P.H., Papacosta, O., Chirico, S., Bruckdorfer, K.R. and Walker, M. (1997) Effect of fresh fruit consumption on lung function and wheeze in children. *Thorax* 52, 628–633.

Cooper, B., Creeth, J.M. and Donald, A.S. (1985) Studies of the limited degradation of mucus glycoproteins. The mechanism of the peroxide reaction. *Biochemical Journal* 228, 615–626.

Costabel, U. and Guyman, J. (1992) Effect of smoking on bronchoalveolar lavage constituents. *European Respiratory Journal* 5, 776–779.

Cross, C.E., Forte, T., Stocker, R., Louie, S., Yamamoto, Y., Ames, B.N. and Frei, B. (1990) Oxidative stress and abnormal cholesterol-metabolism in patients with adult respiratory-distress syndrome. *Journal of Laboratory and Clinical Medicine* 115, 396–404.

Cross, C.E., Reznick, A.Z., Packer, L., Davis, P.A., Suzuki, Y.J. and Halliwell, B. (1992) Oxidative damage to human plasma proteins by ozone. *Free Radical Research Communications* 15, 347–352.

Cross, C.E., van der Vliet, A., O'Neill, C.A., Louie, S. and Halliwell, B. (1994) Oxidants, antioxidants, and respiratory tract lining fluids. *Environmental Health Perspectives* 102, S185–S191.

Crystal, R.G. (1990) Alpha-1-antitrypsin deficiency, emphysema, and liver-disease – genetic-basis and strategies for therapy. *Journal of Clinical Investigation* 85, 1343–1352.

Duthie, G.G., Arthur, J.R. and James, W.T. (1991) Effects of smoking and vitamin E on blood antioxidant status. *American Journal of Clinical Nutrition* 53, S1061–S1063.

Duthie, G.G., Arthur, J.R., Beattie, J.G., Brown, K.M., Morrice, P.C., Robertson, J.D., Shortt, C.T., Walker, K.A., James, W.T. and Rimm, E. (1993) Cigarette-smoking, antioxidants, lipid-peroxidation, and coronary heart-disease. *Annals of the New York Academy of Sciences* 686, 120–129.

Eiserich, J.P., Vossen, V., O'Neill, C.A., Halliwell, B., Cross, C.E. and van der Vliet, A. (1994) Molecular mechanisms of damage by excess nitrogen oxides: nitration of tyrosine by gas-phase cigarette smoke. *FEBS Letters* 353, 53–56.

Flatt, A., Pearce, N., Thomson, C.D., Sears, M.R., Robinson, M.F. and Beasley, R. (1990) Reduced selenium in asthmatic subjects in New-Zealand. *Thorax* 45, 95–99.

Frank, L. and Sosenko, I.S. (1987) Prenatal development of lung antioxidant enzymes in four species. *Journal of Pediatrics* 110, 106–10.

Frank, L., Lewis, P.L. and Sosenko, I.S. (1985) Dexamethasone stimulation of fetal-rat lung antioxidant enzyme-activity in parallel with surfactant stimulation. *Paediatrics* 75, 569–574.

Frei, B., England, L. and Ames, B.N. (1989) Ascorbate is an outstanding antioxidant in human blood plasma. *Proceedings of the National Academy of Sciences, USA* 86, 6377–6381.

Gergen, P.J. and Weiss, K.B. (1992) The increasing problem of asthma in the United-States. *American Review of Respiratory Disease* 146, 823–824.

Girod, S., Zahm, J.M., Plotkowski, C., Beck, G. and Puchelle, E. (1992) Role of the physicochemical properties of mucus in the protection of the respiratory epithelium. *European Respiratory Journal* 5, 477–487.

Grigg, J., Barber, A. and Silverman, M. (1993) Bronchoalveolar lavage fluid glutathione in intubated premature-infants. *Archives of Disease in Childhood* 69, 49–51.

Halahakoon, C., Bell, A.H., Young, I.S., Halliday, H.L. and McClure, B.G. (1995) EEG activity and antioxidant status after exosurf administration. *Paediatric Research Communications* 8, 218.

Halliwell, B. and Gutteridge, J.C. (1990) The antioxidants of human extracellular fluids. *Archives of Biochemistry and Biophysics* 280, 1–8.

Heffner, J.E. and Repine, J.E. (1989) Pulmonary strategies of antioxidant defense. *American Review of Respiratory Disease* 140, 531–554.

Holgate, S.T. (1997) The cellular and mediator basis of asthma in relation to natural history. *Lancet* 350, 5–9.

Holroyd, K.J., Buhl, R., Borok, Z., Roum, J.H., Bokser, A.D., Grimes, G.J., Czerski, D., Cantin, A.M. and Crystal, R.G. (1993) Correction of glutathione deficiency in the lower respiratory-tract of HIV-seropositive individuals by glutathione aerosol treatment. *Thorax* 48, 985–989.

Hubbard, R.C., Ogushi, F., Fells, G.A., Cantin, A.M., Jallat, S., Courtney, M. and Crystal, R.G. (1987) Oxidants spontaneously released by alveolar macrophages of cigarette smokers can inactivate the active-site of alpha1-antitrypsin, rendering it ineffective as an inhibitor of neutrophil elastase. *Journal of Clinical Investigation* 80, 1289–1295.

Inoue, M., Watanabe, N., Morino, Y., Tanaka, Y., Amachi, T. and Sasaki, J. (1990) Inhibition of oxygen-toxicity by targeting superoxide-dismutase to endothelial-cell surface. *FEBS Letters* 269, 89–92.

Kelly, F.J. and Mudway, I.S. (1997) Sensitivity to ozone: could it be related to an individual's complement of antioxidants in lung epithelium lining fluid? *Redox Report* 3,199–206.

Kondo, T., Tagami, S., Yoshioka, A., Nishimura, M. and Kawakami, Y. (1994) Current smoking of elderly men reduces antioxidants in alveolar macrophages. *American Journal of Respiratory and Critical Care Medicine* 149, 178–182.

Lapenna, D., De Gioia, S., Mezzetii, A., Ciofani, G., Consoli, A., Marzio, L. and Cuccurullo, F. (1995) Cigarette smoke, ferritin and lipid peroxidation. *American Journal of Respiratory and Critical Care Medicine* 151, 431–435.

Lenz, A.G., Costabel, U. and Maier, K.L. (1996) Oxidized BAL fluid proteins in patients with interstitial lung diseases. *European Respiratory Journal* 9, 307–312.

Lindeman, J.H.N., Houdkamp, E., Lentjes, E.G.W.M., Poothuis, B.J.H.M. and Berger, H.M. (1992) Limited protection against iron-induced lipid peroxidation by cord blood plasma. *Free Radical Research Communications* 16, 285–294.

Linden, M., Hakansson, L., Ohlsson, K., Sjodin, K., Tegner, H., Tunek, A. and Venge, P. (1989) Glutathione in bronchoalveolar lavage fluid from smokers is related to humoral markers of inflammatory cell activity. *Inflammation* 13, 651–658.

Lockitch, G., Jacobson, B., Quigley, G., Dison, P. and Pendray, M. (1989) Selenium deficiency in low birth weight neonates: an unrecognised problem. *Journal of Paediatrics* 114, 865–870.

Ludwig, P.W. and Hoidal, J.R. (1982) Alterations in leukocyte oxidative-metabolism in cigarette smokers. *American Review of Respiratory Disease* 126, 977–980.

Lykens, M.G., Davis, W.B. and Pacht, E.R. (1992) Antioxidant activity of bronchoalveolar lavage fluid in the adult respiratory-distress syndrome. *American Journal of Physiology* 262, L169–L175.

MacNee, W., Wiggs, B., Belzberg, A.S. and Hogg, J.C. (1989) The effect of cigarette-smoking on neutrophil kinetics in human lungs. *New England Journal of Medicine* 321, 924–928.

Malo, J.L., Cartier, A., Pineau, L., Larcheveque, J., Ghezzo, H. and Martin, R.R. (1986) Lack of acute effects of ascorbic-acid on spirometry and airway responsiveness to histamine in subjects with asthma. *Journal of Allergy and Clinical Immunology* 78, 1153–1158.

McCusker, K. and Hoidal, J. (1990) Selective increase of antioxidant enzyme-activity in the alveolar macrophages from cigarette smokers and smoke-exposed hamsters. *American Review of Respiratory Disease* 141, 678–682.

Mezzetti, A., Lapenna, D., Pierdomenico, S.D., Calafiore, A.M., Costantini, F., Riariosforza, G., Imbastaro, T., Neri, M. and Cuccurullo, F. (1995) Vitamin-E, vitamin-C and lipid-peroxidation in plasma and arterial tissue of smokers and nonsmokers. *Atherosclerosis* 112, 91–99.

Ministry of Agriculture, Fisheries and Food (1989) Household food consumption and expenditure 1987. In: *Annual Report of the National Food Survey Committee.* HMSO, London.

Mohsenin, V. (1987) Effect of vitamin-C on NO_2-induced airway hyperresponsiveness in normal subjects – a randomized double-blind experiment. *American Review of Respiratory Disease* 136, 1408–1411.

Mohsenin, V., Dubois, A.B. and Douglas, J.S. (1983) Effect of ascorbic-acid on response to methacholine challenge in asthmatic subjects. *American Review of Respiratory Disease* 127, 143–147.

Morabia, A., Menkes, M.S., Comstock, G.W. and Tockman, M.S. (1990) Serum retinol and airway-obstruction. *American Journal of Epidemiology* 132, 77–82.

Morrison, D., Lannan, S., Langridge, A., Rahman, I. and MacNee, W. (1994) Effect of acute cigarette smoking on epithelial permeability, inflammation and oxidant status in the airspaces of chronic smokers. *Thorax* 49, 1077.

Morrow, J.D., Frei, B., Longmire, A.W., Gaziano, J.M., Lynch, S.M., Shyr, Y., Strauss, W.E., Oates, J.A. and Roberts, L.J. (1995) Increase in circulating products of lipid-peroxidation (F-2- isoprostanes) in smokers – smoking as a cause of oxidative damage. *New England Journal of Medicine* 332, 1198–1203.

Nelson, M.E., Obrienladner, A.R. and Wesselius, L.J. (1996) Regional variation in iron and iron-binding proteins within the lungs of smokers. *American Journal of Respiratory and Critical Care Medicine* 153, 1353–1358.

Neuzil, J. and Stocker, R. (1994) Free and albumin-bound bilirubin are efficient co-antioxidants for α-tocopherol inhibiting plasma and low density lipoprotein lipid peroxidation. *Journal of Biological Chemistry* 269, 16712–16719.

Ninan, T.K. and Russell, G. (1992) Respiratory symptoms and atopy in Aberdeen schoolchildren – evidence from 2 surveys 25 years apart. *British Medical Journal* 304, 873–875.

Pacht, E.R., Kaseki, H., Mohammed, J.R., Cornwell, D.G. and Davis, W.B. (1986) Deficiency of vitamin-E in the alveolar fluid of cigarette smokers – influence on alveolar macrophage cyto-toxicity. *Journal of Clinical Investigation* 77, 789–796.

Peden, D.B., Swiersz, M., Ohkubo, K., Hahn, B., Emery, B. and Kaliner, M.A. (1993) Nasal secretion of the ozone scavenger uric acid. *American Review of Respiratory Disease* 148, 455–461.

Petruzzelli, S., Hietanen, E., Bartsch, H., Camus, A.M., Mussi, A., Angeletti, C.A., Saracci, R. and Giuntini, C. (1990) Pulmonary lipid-peroxidation in cigarette smokers and lung-cancer patients. *Chest* 98, 930–935.

Pitkanen, O.M., Hallman, M. and Andersson, S.M. (1990) Correlation of free oxygen radical induced lipid-peroxidation with outcome in very-low-birth-weight infants. *Journal of Paediatrics* 116, 760–764.

Powers, H.J., Loban, A., Silvers, K. and Gibson, A.T. (1995) Vitamin-C at concentrations observed in premature babies inhibits the ferroxidase activity of ceruloplasmin. *Free Radical Research* 22, 57–65.

Pryor, W.A. (1991) Can vitamin-E protect humans against the pathological effects of ozone in smog. *American Journal of Clinical Nutrition* 53, 702–722.

Pryor, W.A. (1992) Biological effects of cigarette-smoke, wood smoke, and the smoke from plastics – the use of electron-spin-resonance. *Free Radical Biology and Medicine* 13, 659–676.

Pryor, W.A. and Stone, K. (1993) Oxidants in cigarette smoke: radicals, hydrogen peroxides, peroxynitrate, and peroxynitrite. *Annals of the New York Academy of Sciences* 686, 12–28.

Putman, E., van Golde, L.M. and Haagsman, H.P. (1997) Toxic oxidant species and their impact on the pulmonary surfactant system. *Lung* 175, 75–103.

Rahman, I. and MacNee, W. (1996) Role of oxidants/antioxidants in smoking-induced lung diseases. *Free Radical Biology and Medicine* 21, 669–681.

Rahman, I., Morrison, D., Donaldson, K. and MacNee, W. (1996) Systemic oxidative stress in asthma, COPD, and smokers. *American Journal of Respiratory and Critical Care Medicine* 154, 1055–1060.

Reise, J.A., Taylor, G.W., Fardy, C.H. and Silverman, M. (1997) Glutathione and neonatal lung disease. *Clinica Chimica Acta* 265, 113–119.

Reznick, A.Z., Cross, C.E., Hu, M.L., Suzuki, Y.J., Khwaja, S., Safadi, A., Motchnik, P.A., Packer, L. and Halliwell, B. (1992) Modification of plasma proteins by cigarette smoke as measured by protein carbonyl formation. *Biochemical Journal* 286, 607–611.

Rosenfeld, W., Evans, H., Concepcion, L., Jhaveri, R., Schaeffer, H. and Friedman, A. (1984) Prevention of bronchopulmonary dysplasia by administration of bovine superoxide-dismutase in preterm infants with respiratory-distress syndrome. *Journal of Paediatrics* 105, 781–785.

Rosenfeld, W., Concepcion, L., Evans, H., Jhaveri, R., Sahdev, S. and Zabaleta, I. (1986) Serial trypsin inhibitory capacity and ceruloplasmin levels in prematures at risk for bronchopulmonary dysplasia. *American Review of Respiratory Disease* 134, 1229–1232.

Saetta, M., Stefano, A., Maestrelli, P., Ferraresso, A., Drigo, R., Potena, A., Ciaccia, A. and Fabbri, L.M. (1993) Activated T-lymphocytes and macrophages in bronchial mucosa of subjects with chronic bronchitis. *American Review of Respiratory Disease* 147, 301–306.

Saugstad, O.D. (1990) Oxygen-toxicity in the neonatal-period. *Acta Paediatrica Scandinavica* 79, 881–892.

Schaberg, T., Haller, H., Rau, M., Kaiser, D., Fassbender, M. and Lode, H. (1992) Superoxide anion release induced by platelet-activating factor is increased in human alveolar macrophages from smokers. *European Respiratory Journal* 5, 3877–3893.

Schacter, E.N. and Schlessinger, A. (1982) The attenuation of exercise induced bronchospasm by ascorbic acid. *Annals of Allergy* 49, 146–151.

Schwalb, G. and Anderson, R. (1989) Increased frequency of oxidant-mediated DNA strand breaks in mononuclear leukocytes exposed to activated neutrophils from cigarette smokers. *Mutation Research* 228, 95–99.

Schwartz, J. and Weiss, S.T. (1990) Dietary factors and their relation to respiratory symptoms – The Second National Health and Nutrition Examination Survey. *American Journal of Epidemiology* 132, 67–76.

Sears, M.R. (1993) The definition and diagnosis of asthma. *Allergy* 48, 12–16.

Siafakas, N.M., Vermeire, P., Pride, N.B., Paoletti, P., Gibson, J., Howard, P., Yernault, J.C., DeCramer, M., Higgenbottom, T., Postma, D.S. and Rees, J. (1995) Optimal assessment and management of chronic obstructive pulmonary disease (COPD): a consensus statement of the European Respiratory Society (ERS). *European Respiratory Journal* 8, 1398–1420.

Silvers, K.M., Gibson, A.T. and Powers, H.J. (1994) High plasma vitamin-C concentrations at birth associated with low antioxidant status and poor outcome in premature-infants. *Archives of Disease in Childhood* 71, F40–F44.

Slade, R., Crissman, K., Norwood, J. and Hatch, G. (1993) Comparison of antioxidant substances in bronchoalveolar lavage cells and fluid from humans, guinea pigs, and rats. *Experimental Lung Research* 19, 469–484.

Sluis, K.B., Darlow, B.A., George, P.M., Mogridge, N., Dolamore, B.A. and Winterbourn, C.C. (1992) Selenium and glutathione-peroxidase levels in premature-infants in a low selenium community (Christchurch, New-Zealand). *Paediatric Research* 32, 189–194.

Smith, L.J. and Anderson, J. (1992) Oxygen-induced lung damage – relationship to lung mitochondrial glutathione levels. *American Review of Respiratory Disease* 146, 1452–1457.

Snider, G.L. (1989) Chronic obstructive pulmonary disease: risk factors, pathophysiology, and pathogenesis. *Annual Review of Medicine* 40, 411–429.

Soutar, A., Seaton, A. and Brown, K. (1997) Bronchial reactivity and dietary antioxidants. *Thorax* 52, 166–170.

Stone, J., Hinks, L.J., Beasley, R., Holgate, S.T. and Clayton, B.A. (1989) Reduced selenium status of patients with asthma. *Clinical Science* 77, 495–500.

Strachan, D.P., Cox, B.D., Erzinclioglu, S.W., Walters, D.E. and Whichelow, M.J. (1991) Ventilatory function and winter fresh fruit consumption in a random sample of British adults. *Thorax* 46, 624–629.

Tanswell, A.K. and Freeman, B.A. (1987) Liposome-entrapped antioxidant enzymes prevent lethal O_2 toxicity in the newborn rat. *Journal of Applied Physiology* 63, 347–352.

Theron, A.J., Richards, G.A., Vanrensburg, A.J., Vandermerwe, C.A. and Anderson, R. (1990) Investigation of the role of phagocytes and antioxidant nutrients in oxidant stress mediated by cigarette-smoke. *International Journal for Vitamin and Nutrition Research* 45, 261–266.

Thompson, A.B., Bohling, T., Heires, A., Linder, J. and Rennard, S.I. (1991) Lower respiratory tract iron burden is increased in association with cigarette smoking. *Journal of Laboratory and Clinical Medicine* 117, 494–499.

Toth, K.M., Berger, E.M., Beehler, C.J. and Repine, J.E. (1986) Erythrocytes from cigarette smokers contain more glutathione and catalase and protect endothelial-cells from hydrogen-peroxide better than do erythrocytes from non-smokers. *American Review of Respiratory Disease* 134, 281–284.

Zang, L.Y., Stone, K. and Pryor, W.A. (1995) Detection of free-radicals in aqueous extracts of cigarette tar by electron-spin-resonance. *Free Radical Biology and Medicine* 19, 161–167.

Zuskin, E., Lewis, A.J. and Bouhuys, A. (1975) Inhibition of histamine induced airways constriction by ascorbic acid. *Journal of Allergy and Clinical Immunology* 51, 218–226.

Oxidative Stress and Antioxidants in Cystic Fibrosis

25

LISA WOOD, CLARE COLLINS AND MANOHAR GARG

Discipline of Nutrition and Dietetics,
Faculty of Medicine and Health Sciences,
University of Newcastle, Callaghan, Australia

Introduction

Cystic fibrosis (CF) is the most commonly occurring lethal autosomal recessive disorder. Disease frequency varies considerably among ethnic groups, being highest among Caucasians, where approximately one in 2500 newborns are affected. CF is rarely seen in people of mongoloid or negroid origin (Pencharz and Durie, 1993). CF is carried by mutations in a single gene on the long arm of chromosome 7 that encodes the CF transmembrane conductance regulator (CFTR) (Collins, 1992). CFTR has multiple functions involving fluid balance across epithelial cells. It acts as a chloride channel activated by cyclic adenosine monophosphate (cAMP) and may stimulate other chloride channels. It also inhibits sodium absorption by epithelial sodium channels. Mutations in the CFTR gene result in defective chloride transport in the epithelial cells of the respiratory, hepatobiliary, gastro-intestinal and reproductive tracts, and the pancreas. The ineffective transport of chloride, sodium and water, causes secretions to be extremely viscous, leading to obstruction, destruction and scarring of various exocrine ducts (Ramsey and Boat, 1994; Ramsey, 1996).

The primary cause of morbidity and mortality in CF patients is respiratory failure (FitzSimmons, 1993). Obstruction of airways by thick mucus gives rise to infection, especially due to *Pseudomonas* spp. bacteria (Boat *et al.*, 1989; Pencharz and Durie, 1993; Brown *et al.*, 1996). This bacteria causes repeated lower respiratory tract infections, eliciting intense inflammatory response ('respiratory burst') by neutrophils. This damages the airway, as excess free radical production is not efficiently neutralized by the body's antioxidant defences. The resulting oxidative damage to cells is referred to as 'oxidative stress'. The stimulated neutrophils also produce excess quantities of neutrophil elastase that damages cells, reducing the host's ability to resist bacterial infection (Birrer *et al.*, 1994; Allen, 1996; Buhl *et al.*, 1996). A vicious cycle develops in the respiratory tract that results in progressive bronchiectasis and ultimately respiratory failure and early death (Balfour-Lynn and Dinwiddie, 1996). Median survival age of up to 30 years has been reported for CF patients in Canada and USA. British children born with CF in 1990 were given a median life expectancy of 40 years (Elborn *et al.*, 1991; FitzSimmons, 1993). Essentially, the patient's length of survival is directly linked to the preservation of lung function. As well as respiratory problems, there are many other clinical manifestations of CF, the most serious being gastrointestinal complications leading to malabsorption, as well as impaired fertility, nasal polyps and sinus disease.

Important Antioxidants in CF

As much of the oxidative stress in CF occurs in the respiratory tract, the antioxidants present in the respiratory epithelial cells and the respiratory tract lining fluid (RTLF), are critically important. Of particular significance is glutathione (GSH), as it is the dominant antioxidant in epithelial lining fluid (ELF) (Buhl *et al.*, 1996). By virtue of its thiol group, GSH can react directly with key reactive oxygen species (ROS), including the hydroxyl radical ($\cdot$OH), superoxide ($O_2\cdot^-$) and hydrogen peroxide (H_2O_2). GSH is also important intracellularly in the protection of membrane lipids, through its ability to regenerate vitamin E and C. GSH is also an important component in the detoxification of H_2O_2 by GSH peroxidase (GSH-Px). Mucus may play an important antioxidant role in CF, due to its presence in RTLF. Several components in mucus, such as carbohydrates, are powerful scavengers of ROS, including $\cdot$OH. There are also many protein thiols and disulphide bonds, which scavenge $\cdot$OH and $HOCl/OCl^-$ (van der Vliet *et al.*, 1997). The other major antioxidants, such as vitamin E, vitamin C, β-carotene and the GSH-Px and superoxide dismutase (SOD) enzymes, are also believed to play a role in CF, as the antioxidants found in plasma, erythrocytes and platelets, form the antioxidant defence system of peripheral blood.

Factors Contributing to Oxidative Stress in CF

There is much evidence to suggest that the deleterious effects of oxidative stress on cell function play an important role in the pathogenesis of many degenerative diseases. The lungs and airway tissue are particularly prone to oxidative attack and damage, being the interface between the atmosphere and the body, continuously exposed to oxidants in inhaled air and to blood-borne toxins (van der Vliet *et al.*, 1997). They are exposed to the highest O_2 tension of any body tissue. In addition, oxidant products are generated by the action of phagocytic cells, ensuring a constant pressure of free radicals in the lung environment. Oxidants not only damage lipids, proteins and DNA but also mediate a variety of specific effects that could diminish lung function and/or lung repair mechanisms. These include increased mucus production, impaired cilia function, stimulation of thromboxane (vasoconstrictor), injury of fibroblasts and reduced surfactant activity (Shelhamer *et al.*, 1995). It is not surprising that there are many respiratory tract diseases in which oxidative stress is believed to play a role.

Oxidative stress is of particular importance in CF, as the disease combines an infectious pathology with a syndrome of malabsorption, both potentially capable of favouring the deleterious effects of ROS. While the body's immune response to infection increases production of ROS, malabsorption of food reduces protection by dietary antioxidants. The key factors believed to contribute to the overall excess of oxygen free radicals in CF are summarized in Box 25.1.

Free radical production due to inflammation in CF

In CF, the bacteria colonized in the mucus accumulated in the lungs leads to chronic infection and inflammation. The large numbers of bacteria present (especially *Pseudomonas* spp.) attract neutrophils (Konstan and

Box 25.1. Factors contributing to oxidative stress in CF.

Factors increasing production of oxidants

- Increased immune response due to chronic infection and inflammation (i.e. activated neutrophils)
- Cytokines causing priming of leukocytes and phagocytes
- Increased levels of TNFα, IL-1, -6 and -8 and LTB$_4$
- Disordered iron metabolism, resulting in excess free iron for catalysis of free radical reactions
- *P. aeruginosa* secreting pyochelin/pyocyanin
- Increased production of nitric oxide
- Formation of xanthine oxidase
- Increased metabolic rate, thus increasing oxygen consumption and leakage of electrons from the mitochondrial electron transport chain
- Heightened activity of cytochrome P450 oxidative enzyme

Factors reducing antioxidant protection

- Fat malabsorption leading to deficiency of fat-soluble vitamins
- Increased turnover of antioxidant vitamins and enzymes

Berger, 1993). As neutrophils (phagocytic cells) come into contact with bacteria, they internalize the bacteria in a vacuole called a phagolysosome. As the bacterium is being internalized, an NADPH-dependent superoxide-generating system is activated and begins to secrete superoxide into the phagolysosome (Equation 25.1).

$$2O_2 + NADPH \rightarrow 2O_2^- \cdot + NADP^+ + H^+ \qquad (25.1)$$

A dismutation reaction follows (catalysed by SOD), resulting in production of H_2O_2 (Equation 25.2). This combines with chlorine ions to generate hypochlorous acid, HOCl, in a reaction that is catalysed by neutrophil myeloperoxidase (Davies, 1995; Sen, 1995) (Equation 25.3).

$$2O_2^- \cdot + 2H^+ \xrightarrow{\text{SOD}} H_2O_2 + O_2 \qquad (25.2)$$

$$H_2O_2 + Cl^- + H^+ \rightarrow HOCl + H_2O \qquad (25.3)$$

HOCl then reacts to produce another strong oxidant, probably ·OH. This may be by one of the following mechanisms (Equation 25.4 or 25.5):

$$HOCl + O_2^- \cdot \rightarrow \cdot OH + Cl^- + O_2 \qquad (25.4)$$

$$HOCl + Fe^{2+} \rightarrow \cdot OH + Cl^- + Fe^{3+} \qquad (25.5)$$

Thus, during this 'respiratory burst', the neutrophils have released high concentrations of the ROS, superoxide ($O_2^- \cdot$), the hydroxyl radical (·OH), hydrogen peroxide (H_2O_2) and hypochlorous acid (HOCl). The bacterium ingested by the phagolysosome has been exposed to this high concentration of free radicals, leading to its destruction. Some of these free radicals, however, leak into the cell (Crystal, 1991).

At the same time, alveolar macrophages release the cytokine interleukin-8 (IL-8), which is also a neutrophil chemoattractant (Khan *et al.*, 1995). Other neutrophil chemoattractants found in CF include the complement component C5a, the lipoxygenase products leukotriene B_4 (LTB$_4$), and other cytokines including interleukin-1 and -6 and tumour necrosis factor-α (TNFα) (Konstan and Berger, 1993; Bonfield *et al.*, 1995; Ward, 1997). As a result, 1000-fold increases in the number of neutrophils can be observed in CF (Holsclaw, 1993). Neutrophils typically represent less than 5% of the cells recovered by bronchoalveolar lavage in normal adults. However, in CF adults, neutrophils may comprise more than 95% of the cell population (Allen, 1996).

Also, during periods of inflammation or infection, neutrophil elastase (NE) is released by neutrophils (Birrer *et al.*, 1994). NE is a highly destructive protease, capable of hydrolysing all the major connective tissue proteins that form the lung matrix. In the healthy lung, a system of antiproteases exists to inactivate excesses of NE and other proteases. One important protease is α_1-antitrypsin (α_1-AT). However, the enormous numbers of neutrophils, and hence the excessive concentration of NE in CF overwhelms the antiproteases, allowing active neutrophil elastase to remain unbound and chronically injure the epithelium (Birrer *et al.*, 1994; Buhl *et al.*, 1996). The excess of NE also adversely affects the CF airways by enhancing mucus secretion, modifying ciliary motion and mucociliary clearance, exacerbating release of IL-8 secretion from epithelia, thereby attracting more neutrophils and by reducing the host's ability to resist bacterial infection by interfering with neutrophil phagocytosis (Birrer *et al.*, 1994; Bilton and Mahadeva, 1997). Neutrophils are thus responsible for much of the lung damage in CF. The oxygen free radicals they generate cause oxidative damage and the proteolytic enzymes (e.g. neutrophil elastase, NE) cause breakdown of the epithelium.

Another proposed aspect of the inflammatory response causing oxidative stress, particularly in the respiratory tract, is the production of increased levels of nitric oxide (NO·) due to exposure of cells to the various cytokines that are released by activated macrophages and neutrophils (van der Vliet *et al.*, 1997; Ward, 1997). Significant quantities of NO· are continuously produced in human airway epithelium by the inducible nitric oxide synthetase (NOS) isoform. This has been evidenced by its detection in expired air of healthy animals and humans. While NO· has many helpful physiological properties, such as regulation of blood pressure, excesses are thought to be harmful, and have been implicated in such conditions as chronic inflammation, stroke and septic shock. Although direct reactions of NO· with most biological molecules are slow, its reaction with other free radicals is very rapid. In particular, NO· reacts with O_2^-· at near diffusion-limited rates, to form the cytotoxic species peroxynitrite ($ONOO^-$). $ONOO^-$ has many potentially deleterious effects, including oxidation of lipids. Nitration of phenolic compounds, including the amino acid tyrosine, has also been observed, although the biological significance of this is still unknown (van der Vliet *et al.*, 1997). There is some suggestion that excess NO· may actually inhibit lipid peroxidation if the supply of O_2^-· is limited. NO· reacts fast with the lipophilic peroxyl radicals, important propagating species in the chain reaction of lipid peroxidation, to generate alkyl peroxynitrates (ROONO). These are far more stable than $ONOO^-$. In the presence of high concentrations of NO· relative to O_2^-·, production of ROONO is favoured, as there is limited O_2^-· available for formation of $ONOO^-$. This inhibits lipid peroxidation, as the excess NO· scavenges the peroxyl radicals to form the non-toxic ROONO (Halliwell, 1996).

Following inflammation, the xanthine dehydrogenase enzyme is converted to the oxidase form xanthine oxidase. This can catalyse the formation of uric acid, O_2^-· and H_2O_2 from xanthine (or hypoxanthine), thus providing another source of ROS (Sen, 1995; Nakazawa et al., 1996).

It is known that the bacteria *Pseudomonas aeruginosa*, which colonizes the lungs in CF, is itself a source of ROS. It secretes pyochelin and pyocyanin, which can damage pulmonary artery endothelial cells *in vitro* by affecting the endothelial cell-mediated redox cycling of pyocyanin, leading to the production of $O_2^-\cdot/\ H_2O_2$. This is then converted to the $\cdot OH$ radical through the catalytic activity of ferripyochelin (Britigan *et al.*, 1992).

Free-radical production due to increased metabolic rate in CF

In conjunction with the increased oxidative burden resulting from the immune response to pulmonary infection in CF, free radical generation is heightened by the increase in metabolic rate (Brown and Kelly, 1994a). In a normal, healthy host, small amounts of ROS are continuously generated as unwanted by-products of normal respiration, as the chemical heat energy necessary for life is obtained. More than 95% of the oxygen we breathe is reduced by four electrons to produce water, catalysed by the cytochrome oxidase enzyme in the mitochondrial electron transport chain. Thus, oxygen becomes a sink for electrons (Reilly *et al.*, 1991; Davies, 1995; Nakazawa *et al.*, 1996). Although this system is efficient, at each step in the chain, the electron carrier is predisposed to side reactions with molecular oxygen, instead of passing the electron on to the next electron carrier in the chain. Thus, electrons leak from the chain and ROS are produced. About 1.5% of the consumed oxygen is not reduced to water, but produces ROS which are liberated into the ambient medium (Davies, 1995). In CF patients, an elevated resting metabolic rate is observed. This is directly related to the severity of lung infection, the increased work of breathing, enteral feeding and certain drugs. As a result, energy requirements and oxygen uptake are 120–150% of normal (MacDonald, 1996). This increases the quantity of unwanted by-products of respiration that are produced in CF patients (Brown *et al.*, 1994a).

Free-radical production due to exogenous oxidants in CF

Exogenous oxidants such as cigarette smoke (containing NO, NO_2, $ONOO^-$) and air pollution (containing NO_2, O_3, SO_2, CCl_4) are metabolized by cytochrome P450 enzymes. These enzymes are responsible for protecting cells from environmental poisons, by metabolizing non-nutrient lipochemicals that are taken up from the environment. Metabolism by P450 enzymes, which is heightened in CF, causes generation and release of free radicals, in particular superoxide (Brown *et al.*, 1994a; Sen, 1995).

Reduced antioxidant protection due to malabsorption in CF

Exocrine pancreatic insufficiency is a common problem in CF (Gaskin *et al.*, 1982). The pancreas produces thick secretions that often block the pancreatic ducts, preventing the digestive enzymes from reaching the intestines. Attempts are made to correct malabsorption by oral administration of pancreatic enzyme replacements given with food. However, residual steatorrhea and azotorrhea are still usual (Pencharz and Durie, 1993). This amplifies oxidative injury due to severe deficiencies in fat-soluble antioxidants, such as vitamin E and carotenoids, resulting in impaired antioxidant protection. These deficiencies commonly develop by the age of 3 months (Sokol *et al.*, 1989). Some examples of these dietary deficiencies are described in Table 25.1.

Evidence Linking Oxidative Stress to CF

There is much evidence to support the increase of oxidative stress in CF (Table 25.1). A range of indices of oxidative stress in CF are listed, including increases in the concentration of lipid peroxides (e.g. TBARS, breath pentane), increased levels of protein and DNA damage and decreases in the plasma levels of antioxidants (e.g. selenium, ascorbic acid, α-tocopherol, β-carotene, GSH and GSH-Px).

In 1994, Brown examined several markers of oxidative damage to proteins and lipids. Increased lipid peroxidation was observed, as indicated by higher plasma levels of TBARS and free fatty acid hydroperoxides. Elevated protein peroxidation however, was not observed, suggesting that CF patients are more susceptible to lipid oxidative damage. It appears that different mechanisms of damage are in operation or that the susceptibility to damage and breakdown of the subsequent metabolites differs between proteins and lipids. Concentrations of antioxidants including vitamin E, vitamin C and protein sulphydryls were within normal ranges, although a wide range was observed, particularly for vitamin E. This suggests that CF patients are more susceptible to oxidative damage, even in the presence of normal concentrations of plasma antioxidants. Thus, increased antioxidant levels above normal may be required (Brown *et al.*, 1994b).

Another study by Brown and colleagues (1996) of patients whose plasma concentrations of vitamins E and C had been normalized with supplements, indicated that although antioxidant levels were within the normal range, they were found to correlate with pulmonary function. Patients showing antioxidant levels at the higher end of the normal range were observed to have better pulmonary function. This information suggests that patients with severe disease have a higher requirement for antioxidants, which caused levels in these patients to be depleted. Supplementation should aim to increase plasma antioxidant levels *above* the levels found in healthy controls, to help to alleviate the increased oxidative burden of the disease. The study also reported that decreased lung function correlates with elevated plasma malondialdehyde, a product of lipid peroxidation. Patients with severe lung dysfunction were also shown to have significantly higher levels of lipid hydroperoxides than patients with mild pulmonary symptoms, while protein carbonyls were not significantly affected. These data support the suggestion that lipid peroxidation rather than protein peroxidation is closely associated with CF pulmonary dysfunction.

Table 25.1. Markers of oxidative stress in CF.

Biochemical marker	Effect observed	Reference
Plasma α-tocopherol levels	Decreased	Willison *et al.*, 1985
		Winklhofer-Roob *et al.*, 1990a, 1995a, 1996
		Biggemann *et al.*, 1988
		Congden *et al.*, 1981
		Farrell *et al.*, 1977
Plasma β-carotene levels	Decreased	Homnick *et al.*, 1993
		Winklhofer-Roob *et al.*, 1991, 1994, 1995a,b,c, 1996b
		Portal *et al.*, 1995
		Rust *et al.*, 1998
		Lepage *et al.*, 1996
Plasma lutein levels	Decreased	Homnick *et al.*, 1993
		Winklhofer-Roob *et al.*, 1995c
Plasma/LDL lycopene levels	Decreased	Winklhofer-Roob *et al.*, 1995a,b,c, 1996b
		Homnick *et al.*, 1993
Plasma α-carotene levels	Decreased	Winklhofer-Roob *et al.*, 1995a,b
		Homnick *et al.*, 1993
Plasma vitamin A (retinol) level	Decreased	Homnick *et al.*, 1993
ELF GSH levels	Decreased	Roum *et al.*, 1990, 1993
Plasma GSH levels	Decreased	Roum *et al.*, 1993
GSH-Px activity	Decreased	Winklhofer-Roob *et al.*, 1990b
		Portal *et al.*, 1995
Whole blood Se levels	Decreased	Lloyd-Still *et al.*, 1980
Plasma TBARS levels	Elevated	Portal *et al.*, 1995
		Brown *et al.*, 1994b
		Winklhofer-Roob *et al.*, 1995c, 1996b
		Lepage *et al.*, 1996
Plasma malondialdehyde (MDA) levels	Increased levels correlate with decreased lung function	Brown *et al.*, 1996
Breath pentane and ethane levels	Elevated	Kneepkens *et al.*, 1992
Prooxidant cytokines (TNFα, IL-1β, -6, -8)	Increased	Bonfield *et al.*, 1995
		Elborn *et al.*, 1993
Regulatory cytokines (IL-10)	Decreased	Bonfield *et al.*, 1995
Plasma organic hydroperoxides levels	Elevated	Portal *et al.*, 1995
		Brown *et al.*, 1994b
Major lipoperoxidation substrates (e.g. linoleic and arachidonic acid)	Decreased	Portal *et al.*, 1995
Oxidative damage to DNA	Increased	Brown *et al.*, 1995
Ascorbic acid, α-tocopherol and sulphydryls levels	Decreased levels correlate with decreased lung function	Brown *et al.*, 1996
Urinary 8-hydroxydeoxyguanosine (oh8dG)	Increased	Brown *et al.*, 1995
Susceptibility of LDL to oxidation	Increased	Winklhofer-Roob *et al.*, 1995a,c
TRAP levels	Decreased	Langley *et al.*, 1993
Free iron in sputum	Increased	Britigan *et al.*, 1991
Sputum chloramine concentration	Increased	Witko-Sarsat *et al.*, 1995
Sputum myeloperoxidase concentration	Increased	Witko-Sarsat *et al.*, 1995
Serum myeloperoxidase concentration	Increased	Niggemann *et al.*, 1995
Monocyte oxidase activity	Increased	Regelmann *et al.*, 1991
8-iso-PGF$_{2\alpha}$	Increased	Collins *et al.*, 1998

LDL, low-density lipoprotein; TBARS, thiobarbiturate-reactive substance; TRAP, total radical trapping potential.

Vitamin deficiencies have been reported in many studies of CF patients. Portal *et al.* (1995) studied a group who were taking varying levels of α-tocopherol (0–43.7 mg kg^{-1} day^{-1}) and retinol (0–1000 IU kg^{-1} day^{-1}) supplements. None of the patients in the group were taking β-carotene supplements. The group showed very low plasma levels of β-carotene and vitamin A compared with normal controls. Portal reported lower levels of linoleic and arachidonic acid, the major substrates for lipid peroxidation, and a corresponding increase in TBARS and organic hydroperoxides, which all supports the suggestion that these patients are experiencing increased oxidative stress. Homnick *et al.* (1993) showed that carotenoid levels (β-carotene, lutein, lycopene and α-carotene) were lower in CF patients, as were retinol levels. This significant difference remained when carotenoid levels were adjusted for serum cholesterol, to account for the carotenoids being carried by the blood in association with cholesterol. These data also indicate that carotenoid levels were lower in CF patients who have increased inflammation. Vitamin E deficiencies were also observed in unsupplemented patients by Biggemann *et al.* (1988), while vitamin A levels were normal (supplemented with 5000 IU day^{-1}). With pancreatic insufficiency being such a common problem in CF, vitamin E deficiency in unsupplemented patients has been commonly reported (Farrell *et al.*, 1977; Congden *et al.*, 1981).

According to other researchers, pancreatic insufficiency in CF, combined with increased oxidant status, frequently leads to deficiencies of the fat-soluble vitamins despite routine supplementation. One study found that 45% of supplemented patients were deficient in plasma vitamin E and 87% of unsupplemented patients were deficient. Similarly, 17% of supplemented patients were deficient in erythrocyte vitamin E, while 50% of unsupplemented patients were deficient (Winklhofer-Roob *et al.*, 1990a).

Winklhofer-Roob *et al.* (1995b,c, 1996b) also report that severe carotenoid deficiency is commonly observed in CF patients compared to controls. Low levels of β-carotene were shown to be associated with increased lipid peroxidation as measured by reduced LDL resistance to oxidation. Other groups have found similar deficiencies in β-carotene and other carotenoids, such as α-carotene and lycopene (Lepage *et al.*, 1996; Rust *et al.*, 1998).

Reduced levels of antioxidant enzymes and enzyme components have also been reported. GSH levels in epithelial lining fluid and plasma in CF patients have been found to be reduced to about one-third of normal, suggesting increased utilization due to increased oxidant levels (Roum *et al.*, 1990, 1993). GSH-Px activities have also been found to be low in erythrocytes of CF patients (Winklhofer-Roob *et al.*, 1990b). Lower Se concentrations in CF patients have also been observed, suggesting increased utilization of the GSH-Px enzyme; however GSH-Px levels were normal (Lloyd-Still and Ganther, 1980). Lower activity of plasma GSH-Px was observed by Portal *et al.* (1995), suggesting disturbed antioxidant status. Reported levels of Se, Zn and SOD enzyme however were normal.

Brown *et al.* (1995) studied the extent of oxidative damage to DNA in CF patients by measuring a urinary marker, 8-hydroxydeoxyguanosine (OH^{8}dG), which is specifically produced during hydroxyl radical attack on DNA. Compared with controls, the concentration of urinary OH^{8}dG was found to be significantly higher in CF patients, despite plasma levels of vitamin E having been normalized with supplements. No correlation with clinical status was observed, however. One possible explanation is that the DNA damage observed is not being caused by oxygen free radicals produced by the inflammatory process, but rather by the free radicals formed by elevated oxidative metabolism in the mitochondria.

The myeloperoxidase (MPO) enzyme is a key component in the phagocytosis of bacteria, catalysing production of hypochlorous acid and chlorinated amine compounds. These are reduced to powerful oxidants, including ·OH, which cause oxidative damage to cells. Thus an increase in MPO leads to increased oxidative stress. A paper by Niggemann *et al.* (1995) reported that serum levels of the MPO enzyme were elevated in CF patients. Another study (Witko-Sarsat *et al.*, 1995) showed elevated MPO levels in the sputum of CF patients.

The proinflammatory cytokines tumour necrosis factor-α (TNFα) and interleukins 1β, 6 and 8 (IL-1β, IL-6 and IL-8), which are produced by alveolar macrophages in response to bacteria, promote the destruction of lung tissue by encouraging production of ROS. High levels of these have been observed in CF patients (Elborn *et al.*, 1993; Bonfield *et al.*, 1995). Decreased production of the regulatory molecule interleukin 10 (IL-10) has also been observed, diminishing the body's ability to correct excesses of the proinflammatory cytokines (Bonfield *et al.*, 1995).

Increased levels of chloramines, long-lived oxidants produced by neutrophils, have also been observed to accumulate in sputum of CF patients. Chloramine may contribute to oxidative stress in CF by scavenging GSH, mediating immunodepressive effects, or interacting with other inflammatory mediators such as TNFα and NO (Witko-Sarsat *et al.*, 1995).

Other indicators of increased oxidant production have been observed in CF. Increased levels of free iron have been reported in sputum from CF patients. This free iron catalyses free radical production (Britigan *et al.*, 1991). An *in vitro* study found monocytes from CF patients display increased oxidase activity, resulting in increased oxygen uptake and superoxide formation (Regelmann *et al.*, 1991).

TRAP (total radical trapping potential) is an assay designed to describe the relative contribution from each antioxidant in a system, giving an indication of the strength of the antioxidant screen. Langley *et al.* (1993) reported a decrease in TRAP in CF patients compared with normal controls, suggesting decreased ability to protect against oxidative stress. This was despite increased levels of urate (probably due to the high purine content of pancreatic enzymes), sulphydryl and vitamin C. This suggests that the vitamin C may have been acting as a prooxidant in this system. Other authors have also reported increased plasma uric acid concentrations (Nousia-Arvanitakis *et al.*, 1977).

More recently, plasma isoprostane (8-iso-PGF$_{2\alpha}$) levels of CF patients were also found to be elevated compared to normal controls (Collins *et al.*, in press). Isoprostanes are a recently discovered series of bioactive prostaglandin F$_2$-like compounds (termed F$_2$ isoprostanes). They are produced independently of the cyclooxygenase enzyme by the peroxidation of arachidonic acid, catalysed by free radicals (see Chapter 29). In models of oxidant injury, levels of F$_2$ isoprostanes are dramatically increased, and have thus emerged as a reliable, non-invasive index of oxidative stress *in vivo* (Awad *et al.*, 1993, 1994, 1996; Morrow *et al.*, 1993, 1995; Nanji *et al.*, 1994; Awad and Morrow, 1995; Bachi *et al.*, 1996). Most other methods previously used to assess *in vivo* oxidative stress suffer from a lack of specificity and/or sensitivity and are unreliable. The increased plasma 8-iso-PGF$_{2\alpha}$ levels of CF patients also correlated with a reduction in plasma β-carotene concentration despite antioxidant supplementation.

These are just some of the many examples of biochemical data which indicate that CF patients experience increased oxidative stress and have increased requirements for antioxidants.

Antioxidant Therapy in CF

Antioxidant therapy must inhibit the production of oxidizing species, without compromising the host's response to infection. Oxidants play an important role in the body's defences against microorganisms. Thus, the introduction of high levels of antioxidants may interfere with this mechanism. As an example, mucoid *Pseudomonas* phenotypes secrete an antioxidant, slimy alginate, to protect them against neutrophil-derived antioxidants. It should be considered that introducing high levels of antioxidants may enhance the bacteria's protection system even further (van der Vliet *et al.*, 1997). Particular caution must be taken with vitamin C, which can act as a pro-oxidant in the presence of free iron. However, in CF, this should not be a problem because the bacterial siderophores which colonize the lungs bind most of the free iron available (Terry *et al.*, 1992).

In a study by Winklhofer-Roob *et al.* (1995a), a group of CF patients were observed to be vitamin E-deficient and to have lower LDL resistance to oxidation than controls. These patients' diets were supplemented with 400–800 IU day^{-1} vitamin E. Plasma vitamin E levels and LDL resistance to oxidation (as measured by the lag time preceding onset of conjugated diene formation during exposure to copper (II) ions), was normalized within 2 months. β-Carotene, lycopene and cryptoxanthin levels were low prior to the study and remained low throughout the trial. Winkhofer-Roob *et al.*

(1996a) tested three forms of vitamin E supplements (RRR-α-tocopherol, all-rac-α-tocopherol-acetate (fat soluble), and all-rac-α-tocopherol-acetate (water soluble)), and determined that each of these treatments is effective in normalizing vitamin E status in CF patients at a dosage of 400 IU day^{-1}.

Another study by Winklhofer-Roob *et al.* (1995b, 1996b), involved β-carotene supplementation over 16 months to clinically stable CF patients. Plasma α-tocopherol concentrations had already been normalized (supplementation with 330 ± 120 IU day^{-1} of RRR-α-tocopherol or all-rac-α-tocopherol acetate). β-Carotene supplementation of 0.5 mg kg^{-1} body weight day^{-1} normalized plasma β-carotene levels within 3 weeks of supplementation. Plasma α-tocopherol concentrations were also increased during the study, probably due to the sparing effect of β-carotene or improved compliance during the study. Plasma retinol concentration also increased, while still remaining below normal, probably due to conversion of β-carotene to retinol. A decrease in plasma MDA concentrations accompanied these increases in antioxidant levels, suggesting the antioxidants were effective in preventing lipid peroxidation. Plasma neutrophil elastase/α$_1$-proteinase inhibitor (NE/α$_1$-PI) complex levels also decreased, suggesting the antioxidant levels prevented oxidative inactivation of α$_1$-PI, which protects cells from the damaging effects of excess NE.

Another study by Winklhofer-Roob *et al.* (1995c) involved supplementation of clinically stable CF patients with β-carotene (0.5 mg kg^{-1} body weight day^{-1}) for 3 months. Patients already had normal plasma levels of vitamin E (receiving long-term supplementation of 330 ± 120 IU day^{-1}). Within 3 months, β-carotene levels had normalized and two measures of lipid peroxidation were also observed to have normalized. These included the resistance to oxidation of LDL and plasma MDA concentrations. A protective effect of β-carotene and α-tocopherol was suggested by the data, with the greatest increase in lag times being observed in patients with an increase in plasma levels of both antioxidants during the supplementation. If this is the case, the excellent vitamin E status of the CF patients in the study may have contributed or even been essential for the positive effect of β-carotene.

Winklhofer-Roob *et al.* (1997) recently examined the potential for vitamin C supplementation in CF patients. Plasma vitamin C concentrations in CF patients taking no or low-dose (median 40 mg day^{-1}) vitamin C from multivitamin supplements did not differ from control subjects. However, vitamin C did decrease with age in CF. Thus it cannot be determined if this is due to an increased demand for vitamin C, due to the oxidative stress brought on by the disease, or decreased intake, or if this vitamin facilitates the progression of the disease. The decrease in vitamin C with age was accompanied by an increase in plasma MDA, TNFα, white blood cell count, IL-6, NE/α$_1$-PI complexes and α-acid glycoprotein (markers of inflammation). Also, patients with vitamin C concentrations less than 40 μM l^{-1} showed relatively high indices of inflammation, with patients having concentrations >80 µM l^{-1} clearly showing lower values. This suggests that plasma vitamin C levels >80 µM l^{-1} may indeed provide a protective effect for CF patients. This is possibly due to the scavenging effect of oxygen free radicals, which prevent activation of alveolar macrophages and neutrophils, release of proinflammatory cytokines and inactivation of antiproteases. Optimum levels of supplementation need to be determined before high dose supplementation is recommended for CF patients, particularly in light of the recent evidence suggesting that vitamin C acts as a prooxidant when present in high concentrations.

A study of β-carotene supplementation in CF children has shown that lipid peroxidation may have been corrected by the introduction of this antioxidant (Lepage *et al.*, 1996). Plasma levels of MDA were elevated in CF patients, despite normal vitamin E and A status (due to regular supplementation with 200 mg day^{-1} all-rac-α-tocopherol acetate and 4000 IU day^{-1} vitamin A). Supplementation with 15 mg day^{-1} β-carotene for 2 months normalized β-carotene levels and MDA levels, with plasma concentrations of these being inversely correlated. Thus it appears that normal levels of vitamin A and E do not provide adequate protection from oxidants, and β-carotene is an essential component of the body's antioxidant defences.

Another study by Rust *et al.* (1998), demonstrated that β-carotene levels in CF patients were significantly lower than age-matched controls, as were α-carotene and lycopene. Supplementation with high doses of β-carotene (1 mg kg^{-1} body weight day^{-1}), was able to increase β-carotene levels into the normal range. Plasma concentrations of α-tocopherol, retinol and ascorbate were normal at the commencement of the study and remained unchanged (levels had been normalized by supplementation with 1–2 mg day^{-1} retinol, 50–200 mg day^{-1} ascorbate and 110–380 mg day^{-1} α-tocopherol-acetate). The normalized levels of β-carotene appeared to reduce the extent of lipid peroxidation, as indicated by plasma MDA which significantly decreased to values found in healthy individuals.

No clinical symptoms were measured in any of the above supplementation trials. Thus the ability of the supplements to improve overall patient outcome is unknown. In conclusion, the studies undertaken to date indicate that CF patients experience oxidative stress and commonly have low levels of plasma antioxidants. Supplementation which normalizes plasma antioxidant levels can reduce oxidative damage in CF. In fact, the existing evidence suggests that antioxidant levels *above* normal may be required in CF to minimize oxidative stress. The interaction that occurs between antioxidants themselves means that the balance is critical. Table 25.2 summarizes the results from several antioxidant supplementation trials, all leading to an improvement in one or more biochemical markers. However, the optimal doses of antioxidants have not been determined and further work is required to determine both optimal dose and resulting clinical improvement. A recent review of antioxidant supplementation across a range of conditions, suggested that considering the synergistic effect of the major antioxidants, vitamin E, vitamin C and β-carotene proportions of supplementation should be 1:2:0.1 (Furst, 1996). Another review suggests that the optimal proportion of supplementation of these vitamins to prevent cardiovascular disease is 1:5:0.1 (Blumberg, 1995). The optimal ratio needs to be determined for CF patients, due to the common deficiencies in fat soluble vitamins that are associated with the disease, and which lead to an increased demand for vitamin A, vitamin E and the carotenoids.

Isoprostanes have emerged as the most accurate and reliable marker of *in vivo* oxidative stress, and will be an important method of monitoring the oxidant burden in CF patients. This will be critically important in any supplementation studies using high levels of antioxidants, particularly considering the recent concerns regarding the prooxidant properties of some vitamins, particularly vitamin C.

Other Respiratory Diseases

Antioxidant supplementation trials in respiratory diseases (other than CF) are discussed below.

Chronic obstructive pulmonary disease (COPD)

COPD is an obstructive airway disorder characterized by a slowly progressive and irreversible decrease in lung function. A review by Repine *et al.* (1997) discusses several clinical trials of *N*-acetylcysteine (NAC), a synthetic antioxidant, that have all led to relief of symptoms such as decreased sputum viscosity and purulence and improved sputum expectoration. NAC treatment has also been observed to decrease the number of viral infections and the airway bacterial colonization in COPD patients, as well as reducing the rate of decline in forced expiratory volume in 1 s (FEV_1) compared with controls (Repine *et al.*, 1997). A recent supplementation study in 29,133 male COPD patients used a combination of vitamin E (50 mg day^{-1}) and β-carotene (20 mg day^{-1}). No reduction in the recurrence of symptoms was observed, including chronic cough, phlegm or dyspnea. However, a baseline diet high in these antioxidants had a preventative effect (Rautalahti *et al.*, 1997). This negative result may be due to dose levels being insufficient to achieve a substantial increase in blood levels of antioxidants. This effect is compounded by the fact that all the subjects were smokers and had been smoking for a median of 36 years, which increases the demand for antioxidants. (In fact, it is suggested that smokers should ingest at least 200 mg day^{-1} vitamin C to provide the same protection as that provided by 60 mg day^{-1} in non-smokers (Schectman *et al.*, 1991).) There may have also been a shortage of dietary vitamin C among participants, thus preventing reduction of the α-tocopherol radical formed in the α-tocopherol radical reaction back to functional α-tocopherol. Thus the imbalance in serum

Table 25.2. Antioxidant supplementation in CF patients.

Vit. A	Vit. E	Vit. C	β-Carotene (mg day^{-1})	Biochemical marker changed	Study duration (months)	Reference
	400–800 IU day^{-1}			LDL resistance to oxidation norm	2	Winklhofer-Roob et al., 1995a
	330 ± 120 IU day^{-1}		0.5 mg kg^{-1} BW day^{-1}	Plasma MDA ↓ NE/α_1-PI ↓	16	Winklhofer-Roob et al., 1996b
	330 ± 120 IU day^{-1}		0.5 mg kg^{-1} BW day^{-1}	LDL resistance to oxidation norm Plasma MDA norm	3	Winklhofer-Roob et al., 1995c
4000 IU day^{-1}	200 mg day^{-1}		15 mg day^{-1}	Plasma MDA norm	2	Lepage et al., 1996
1–2 mg day^{-1}	110–380 mg day^{-1}	50–200 mg day^{-1}	1 mg kg^{-1} BW day^{-1}	Plasma MDA norm	3	Rust et al., 1998

BW, body weight; norm, normalized; ↑, increased; ↓, decreased.

concentrations of vitamin E, C and β-carotene may have invalidated the protective effects of increased vitamin E and β-carotene levels.

Adult respiratory distress syndrome (ARDS)

ARDS is another respiratory disease involving serious lung dysfunction in which oxidative stress has been implicated. NAC was administered to patients with established ARDS. Concentrations of cysteine and GSH were increased and patients experienced a significant improvement in pulmonary function as measured by chest radiographs. Cardiac output was also improved, translating to an increase in both oxygen delivery and oxygen consumption (Bernard, 1991).

Idiopathic pulmonary fibrosis (IPF)

IPF is a destructive lung disease, characterized by pulmonary inflammation, alveolar epithelial injury and progressive fibrosis. Several studies have implicated increased oxidant burden in the pathophysiology of the disease (Strausz *et al.*, 1990; Borok *et al.*, 1991). GSH deficiency has been observed in IPF patients. A study was undertaken to attempt to normalize GSH levels in epithelial lining fluid (ELF). GSH (600 mg) was administered via aerosol twice daily for 3 days to individuals with IPF (Borok *et al.*, 1991). Significant increases in GSH levels were observed in ELF, with a corresponding decrease in spontaneous lung inflammatory cell superoxide anion release, suggesting that the aerosolized GSH was relieving oxidant burden. Similar results were achieved in IPF patients following oral therapy with 600 mg NAC, three times daily for 5 days. GSH levels in bronchoalveolar lavage-obtained fluid increased significantly.

Asthma

Asthma is another respiratory disease involving increased concentrations of ROS (Greene, 1995). Vitamin C has been suggested to reduce the severity of asthma symptoms. Data from NHANES suggested that vitamin C intake positively correlates with lung function in asthmatics, as measured by FEV_1. Other intervention trials have indicated that vitamin C improves symptoms in asthmatics (Schachter and Schlesinger, 1982; Mohsenin and DuBois, 1987). Troisi *et al.* (1995) studied the relationship between several dietary antioxidants and the incidence of asthma in a group of 760 females over a 10 year period. Vitamin E from diet, but not from supplements, was inversely related to asthma risk. Positive associations were found for vitamins C and E from supplements. These results may be explained by the women at high risk of asthma, or displaying asthmatic symptoms, initiating use of vitamin supplements prior to diagnosis of asthma. Also, dose levels were inconsistent, thus the level of supplementation may not have been sufficient to induce an adequate increase in blood levels of antioxidants. A previous study has suggested that a significant decrease in frequency and severity of asthma attacks was achieved using 1 g of ascorbic acid daily for 14 weeks (Anah, 1980). Such high doses were not involved in the study by Troisi *et al.* (1995).

References

Allen, E.D. (1996) Opportunities for the use of aerosolized α_1-antitrypsin for the treatment of cystic fibrosis. *Chest* 110, 256S–260S.

Anah, C.O. (1980) High dose ascorbic acid in Nigerian asthmatics. *Tropical and Geographical Medicine* 32, 132–137.

Awad, J.A. and Morrow, J.D. (1995) Excretion of F_2-isoprostanes in bile: a novel index of hepatic lipid peroxidation. *Hepatology* 22, 962–968.

Awad, J.A., Morrow, J.D., Kihito, T. and Roberts, L.J. (1993) Identification of non-cyclooxygenase-derived prostanoid (F_2-isoprostane) metabolites in human urine and plasma. *Journal of Biological Chemistry* 268, 4161–4169.

Awad, J.A., Burk, R.F. and Roberts, L.J. (1994) Effect of selenium deficiency and glutathione-modulating agents on diquat toxicity and lipid peroxidation in rats. *Journal of Pharmacology and Experimental Therapeutics* 270, 858–864.

Awad, J.A., Horn, J.-L., Roberts, L.J. and Franks, J.J. (1996) Demonstration of halothane-induced hepatic lipid peroxidation in rats by quantification of F_2-isoprostanes. *Anesthesiology* 84, 910–916.

Bachi, A., Zuccato, E., Baraldi, M., Fanelli, R. and Chiabrando, C. (1996) Measurement of urinary 8-epi-prostaglandin $F_{2\alpha}$, a novel index of lipid peroxidation *in vivo*, by immunoaffinity extraction/gas chromatography-mass spectrometry. Basal levels in smokers and nonsmokers. *Free Radical Biology and Medicine* 20, 619–624.

Balfour-Lynn, I.M. and Dinwiddie, R. (1996) Role of corticosteroids in cystic fibrosis lung disease. *Journal of the Royal Society of Medicine* 89, 8–13.

Bernard, G.R. (1991) *N*-acetylcysteine in experimental and clinical acute lung injury. *American Journal of Medicine* 91, 54–59.

Biggemann, B., Laryea, M.D., Schuster, A., Griese, M., Reinhardt, D. and Bremer, H.J. (1988) Status of plasma and erythrocyte fatty acids and vitamin A and E in young children with cystic fibrosis. *Scandinavian Journal of Gastroenterology* 23, 134–141.

Bilton, D. and Mahadeva, R. (1997) New treatments in adult cystic fibrosis. *Journal of the Royal Society of Medicine* 90, 2–5.

Birrer, P., McElvaney, G., Rudeberg, A., Wirz Sommer, C., Liechti-Gallati, S., Kraemer, R., Hubbard, R. and Crystal, R.G. (1994) Protease–antiprotease imbalance in the lungs of children with cystic fibrosis. *American Journal of Respiratory and Critical Care Medicine* 150, 207–213.

Blumberg, J.B. (1995) Considerations of the scientific substantiation for antioxidant vitamins and β-carotene in disease prevention. *American Journal of Clinical Nutrition* 62, 1521S-1526S.

Boat, T.F., Welsh, M.J. and Beaudet, A.L. (1989) *The Metabolic Basis of Inherited Disease.* McGraw-Hill, New York, pp. 2649–2680.

Bonfield, T.L., Panuska, J.R., Konstan, M.W., Hilliard, K.A., Hilliard, J.B., Ghnaim, H. and Berger, M. (1995) Inflammatory cytokines in cystic fibrosis lungs. *American Journal of Respiratory and Critical Care Medicine* 152, 2111–2118.

Borok, Z., Buhl, R., Grimes, G.J., Bokser, A.D., Hubbard, R.C., Holroyd, K.J., Roum, J.H., Czerski, D.B., Cantin, A.M. and Crystal, R.G. (1991) Effect of glutathione aerosol on oxidant–antioxidant imbalance in idiopathic pulmonary fibrosis. *The Lancet* 338, 215–216.

Britigan, B.E., Roeder, T.L., Rasmussen, G.T., Shasby, D.M., McCormick, M.L. and Cox, C.D. (1992) Interaction of the *Pseudomonas aeruginosa* secretory products pyocyanin and pyochelin generates hydroxyl radical and causes synergistic damage to endothelial cells. *Journal of Clinical Investigation* 90, 2187–2196.

Brown, R.K. and Kelly, F.J. (1994a) Role of free radicals in the pathogenesis of cystic fibrosis [editorial]. *Thorax* 49, 738–742.

Brown, R.K. and Kelly, F.J. (1994b) Evidence for increased oxidative damage in patients with cystic fibrosis. *Pediatric Research* 36, 487–493.

Brown, R.K., McBurney, A., Lunec, J. and Kelly, F.J. (1995) Oxidative damage to DNA in patients with cystic fibrosis. *Free Radical Biology and Medicine* 18, 801–806.

Brown, R.K., Wyatt, H., Price, J.F. and Kelly, F.J. (1996) Pulmonary dysfunction in cystic fibrosis is associated with oxidative stress. *European Respiratory Journal* 9, 334–339.

Buhl, R., Meyer, A. and Vogelmeier, C. (1996) Oxidant–protease interaction in the lung. Prospects for antioxidant therapy. *Chest* 110, 267S–272S.

Collins, C.E., Quaggiotto, P., O'Loughlin, E.V., Henry, R.L. and Garg, M.L. (1998) Elevated plasma levels of F2alpha-isoprostane in cystic fibrosis. *Lipids* (submitted in June, 1998).

Collins, F.C. (1992) Cystic fibrosis: molecular biology and therapeutic implications. *Science* 256, 774–779.

Congden, P.J., Bruce, G. and Rothburn, M.M. (1981) Vitamin status in treated patients with cystic fibrosis. *Archives of Disease in Childhood* 56, 708–714.

Crystal, R.G. (1991) Oxidants and respiratory tract epithelial injury: pathogenesis and strategies for therapeutic intervention. *American Journal of Medicine* 91, 39S–44S.

Davies, K.J. (1995) Oxidative stress: the paradox of aerobic life. *Biochemical Society Symposia* 61, 1–31.

Elborn, J.S., Shale, D.J. and Britton, J.R. (1991) Cystic fibrosis: current survival and population estimates to the year 2000. *Thorax* 46, 881–885.

Elborn, J.S., Cordon, S.M., Western, P.J., Macdonald, I.A. and Shale, D.J. (1993) Tumour necrosis factor-alpha, resting energy expenditure and cachexia in cystic fibrosis. *Clinical Science* 85, 563–568.

Farrell, P.M., Bieri, J.G., Fratantoni, J.F., Wood, R.E. and Di Sant'Agnese, P.A. (1977) The occurrence and effects of human vitamin E deficiency. A Study of patients with cystic fibrosis. *Journal of Clinical Investigation* 60, 233–241.

FitzSimmons, S. (1993) The changing epidemiology of cystic fibrosis. *Journal of Pediatrics* 122, 1–9.

Furst, P. (1996) The role of antioxidants in nutritional support. *Proceedings of the Nutrition Society* 55, 945–961.

Gaskin, K., Gurwitz, D., Durie, P., Corey, M. and Livison, H. (1982) Improved respiratory prognosis in patients with cystic fibrosis with normal fat absorption. *Journal of Pediatrics* 100, 857–862.

Greene, L.S. (1995) Asthma and oxidant stress: nutritional, environmental and genetic risk factors. *Journal of the American College of Nutrition* 14, 317–324.

Halliwell, B. (1996) Oxidative stress, nutrition and health. Experimental strategies for optimization of nutritional antioxidant intake in humans. *Free Radical Research* 25, 57–74.

Holsclaw, D.S. (1993) Cystic fibrosis and pulmonary involvement from multiple perspectives. *Seminars in Respiratory Infections* 7, 141–150.

Homnick, D.N., Cox, J.H., DeLoof, M.J. and Ringer, T.V. (1993) Carotenoid levels in normal children and in children with cystic fibrosis. *Journal of Pediatrics* 122, 703–707.

Khan, T.Z., Wagener, J.S., Bost, T., Martinez, J., Accurso, F.J. and Riches, D.W.H. (1995) Early pulmonary inflammation in infants with cystic fibrosis. *American Journal of Respiratory and Critical Care Medicine* 151, 1075–1082.

Konstan, M.W. and Berger, M. (1993) *Infection and Inflammation of the Lung in Cystic Fibrosis.* Marcel Dekker, New York.

Langley, S.C., Brown, R.K. and Kelly, F.J. (1993) Reduced free-radical-trapping capacity and altered plasma antioxidant status in cystic fibrosis. *Pediatric Research* 33, 247–250.

Lepage, G., Champagne, J., Ronco, N., Lamarre, A., Osberg, I., Sokol, R.J. and Roy, C.C. (1996) Supplementation with carotenoids corrects increased lipid peroxidation in children with cystic fibrosis. *American Journal of Clinical Nutrition* 64, 87–93.

Lloyd-Still, J.D. and Ganther, H.E. (1980) Selenium and glutathione peroxidase levels in cystic fibrosis. *Pediatrics* 65, 1010–1012.

MacDonald, A. (1996) Nutritional management of cystic fibrosis. *Archives of Disease in Childhood* 74, 81–7.

Mohsenin, V. and DuBois, A.B. (1987) Vitamin C and airways. *Annals of the New York Academy of Science* 498, 259–268.

Morrow, J.D., Moore, K.P., Awad, J.A., Ravenscraft, M.D., Marini, G., Badr, K.F., Williams, R. and Roberts, L.J. (1995) Marked overproduction of non-cyclooxygenase derived prostanoids (F_2-isoprostanes) in the hepatorenal syndrome. *Journal of Lipid Mediators* 6, 417–420.

Nakazawa, H., Genka, C. and Fujishima, M. (1996) Pathological aspects of active oxygens/free radicals. *Japanese Journal of Physiology* 46, 15–32.

Nanji, A.A., Khwaja, S. and Sadrzadeh, S.M.H. (1994) Eicosanoid production in experimental alcoholic liver disease is related to vitamin E levels and lipid peroxidation. *Molecular and Cellular Biochemistry* 140, 85–89.

Niggemann, B.T.S., Magdorf, K. and Wahn, U. (1995) Myeloperoxidase and eosinophil cationic protein in serum and sputum during antibiotic treatment in cystic fibrosis patients with *Pseudomonas aeruginosa* infection. *Mediators of Inflammation* 4, 282–288.

Nousia-Arvanitakis, S., Stapleton, F.B., Linshaw, I.Y.A. and Kennedy, J. (1977) Therapeutic approach to pancreatic extract-induced hyperuricosuria in cystic fibrosis. *Journal of Pediatrics* 90, 302–305.

Pencharz, P.B. and Durie, P.R. (1993) Nutritional management of cystic fibrosis. *Annual Review of Nutrition*, 111–136.

Portal, B.C., Richard, M.-J., Faure, H.S., Hadjian, A.J. and Favier, A.E. (1995) Altered antioxidant status and increased lipid peroxidation in children with cystic fibrosis. *American Journal of Clinical Nutrition*, 843–847.

Ramsey, B.W. and Boat, T.F. (1994) Outcome measures for clinical trials in cystic fibrosis. Summary of a Cystic Fibrosis Foundation consensus conference. *Journal of Pediatrics* 124, 177–192.

Ramsey, B.W. (1996) Management of pulmonary disease in patients with cystic fibrosis. *New England Journal of Medicine* 335, 179–188.

Rautalahti, M., Virtamo, J., Haukka, J., Heinonen, O.P., Sundvall, J., Albanes, D. and Huttunen, J.K. (1997) The effect of α-tocopherol and β-carotene supplementation on COPD symptoms. *American Journal of Respiratory and Critical Care Medicine* 156, 1447–1452.

Regelmann, W.E., Skubitz, K.M. and Herron, J.M. (1991) Increased monocyte oxidase activity in cystic fibrosis heterozygotes and homozygotes. *American Journal of Respiratory Cell Molecular Biology* 5, 27–33.

Reilly, P.M., Schiller, H.J. and Bulkley, G.B. (1991) Pharmacologic approach to tissue injury mediated by free radicals and other reactive oxygen metabolites. *American Journal of Surgery* 161, 488–503.

Repine, J.E., Bast, A. and Lankhorst, I. (1997) Oxidative stress in chronic obstructive pulmonary disease. Oxidative Stress Study Group. *American Journal of Respiratory and Critical Care Medicine* 156, 341–357.

Roum, J.H., Ruhl, R., McElvaney, N.G., Borok, Z., Hubbard, R.C., Chernick, M., Cantin, A.M. and Crystal, R.G. (1990) Cystic fibrosis is characterised by a marked reduction in glutathione levels in pulmonary epithelial lining fluid. *American Review of Respiratory Disease* 141, A87.

Roum, J.H., Buhl, R., McElvaney, N.G., Borok, Z. and Crystal, R.G. (1993) Systemic deficiency of glutathione in cystic fibrosis. *Journal of Applied Physiology* 75, 2419–2424.

Rust, P., Eichler, I., Renner, S. and Elmadfa, I. (1998) Effects of long term oral β-carotene supplementation on lipid peroxidation in patients with cystic fibrosis. *International Journal of Vitaminology and Nutritional Research* 68, 83–87.

Schachter, E.N. and Schlesinger, A. (1982) The attenuation of exercise induced bronchospasm by ascorbic acid. *Annals of Allergy* 49, 146–151.

Schectman, G., Byrd, J.C. and Hoffman, R. (1991) Ascorbic acid requirements for smokers: analysis of a population survey. *American Journal of Clinical Nutrition* 53, 1466–1470.

Sen, C.K. (1995) Oxygen toxicity and antioxidants: state of the art. *Indian Journal of Physiology and Pharmacology* 39, 177–196.

Shelhamer, J.H., Levine, S.J., Wu, T., Jacoby, D.B., Kaliner, M.A. and Rennard, S.I. (1995) NIH conference, airway inflammation. *Annals of Internal Medicine* 123, 288–304.

Sokol, R.J., Reardon, M.C., Accurso, F.J., Stall, C., Narkewicz, M., Abman, S.H. and Hammond, K.B. (1989) Fat-soluble-vitamin status during the first year of life in infants with cystic fibrosis identified by screening of newborns. *American Journal of Clinical Nutrition* 50, 1064–1071.

Strausz, J., Muller-Quernheim, J. and Steppling, H. (1990) Oxygen radical production by alveolar inflammatory cells in idiopathic pulmonary fibrosis. *American Review of Respiratory Disease* 141, 124–128.

Terry, J.M., Pina, S.E. and Mattingly, S.J. (1992) Role of energy metabolism in conversion of nonmucoidal *Pseudomonas aeruginosa* to the mucoid type. *Infection and Immunity* 60, 1329–1335.

Troisi, R.J., Willett, W.C., Weiss, S.T., Trichopoulos, D., Rosner, B. and Speizer, F.E. (1995) A prospective study of diet and adult-onset asthma. *American Journal of Respiratory and Critical Care Medicine* 151, 1401–1408.

van der Vliet, A., Eiserich, J.P., Marelich, G.P., Halliwell, B. and Cross, C.E. (1997) Oxidative stress in cystic fibrosis: does it occur and does it matter? *Advances in Pharmacology* 38, 491–513.

Ward, P.A. (1997) Recruitment of inflammatory cells into lung: roles of cytokines, adhesion molecules and complement. *Journal of Laboratory and Clinical Medicine* 129, 400–404.

Willison, H.J., Muller, D.P.R., Matthews, S., Jones, S., Kriss, A., Stead, R.J., Hodson, M.E. and Harding, A.E. (1985) A study of the relationship between neurological function and serum vitamin E concentrations in patients with cystic fibrosis. *Journal of Neurology, Neurosurgery and Psychiatry* 48, 1097–1102.

Winklhofer-Roob, B., Shmerling, D.H., Schimek, M.G. and Tuchschmid, P. (1990a) Significance of DL-α-tocopherol acetate supplementation in patients with cystic fibrosis (abstr.). *Pediatric Research* 28, 283.

Winklhofer-Roob, B.M., Schmerling, D.H. and Tuchschmid, P.E. (1990b) Parameters of the antioxidant protective system in patients with cystic fibrosis (abstr.). *Pediatric Research* 27, 533.

Winklhofer-Roob, B.M., Ziouzenkova, O., Puhl, H., Ellemunter, H., Greiner, P., Muller, G., van't Hof, M.A., Esterbauer, H. and Schmerling, D.H. (1995a) Impaired resistance to oxidation of low density lipoprotein in cystic fibrosis: improvement during vitamin E supplementation. *Free Radical Biology and Medicine* 19, 725–733.

Winklhofer-Roob, B.M., van't Hof, M.A. and Shmerling, D.H. (1995b) Response to oral β-carotene supplementation in patients with cystic fibrosis: a 16-month follow-up study. *Acta Paediatrica* 84, 1132–1136.

Winklhofer-Roob, B.M., Puhl, H., Khoschsorur, G., van't Hof, M.A., Esterbauer, H. and Shmerling, D.H. (1995c) Enhanced resistance to oxidation of low density lipoproteins and decreased lipid peroxide formation during β-carotene supplementation in cystic fibrosis. *Free Radical Biology and Medicine* 18, 849–859.

Winklhofer-Roob, B.M., van't Hof, M.A. and Schmerling, D.H. (1996a) Long-term oral vitamin E supplementation in cystic fibrosis patients: RRR-α-tocopherol compared with all-rac-α-tocopheryl acetate preparations. *American Journal of Clinical Nutrition* 63, 722–728.

Winklhofer-Roob, B.M., Schlegel-Haueter, S.E., Khoschsorur, G., van't Hof, M.A., Suter, S. and Schmerling, D.H. (1996b) Neutrophil elastase/α_1-proteinase inhibitor complex levels decrease in plasma of cystic fibrosis patients during long-term oral β-carotene supplementation. *Pediatric Research* 40, 130–134.

Winklhofer-Roob, B.M., Ellemunter, H., Fruhwirth, M., Schlegel-Haueter, S.E., Khoschsorur, G., van't Hof, M.A. and Schmerling, D.H. (1997) Plasma vitamin C concentrations in patients with cystic fibrosis: evidence of associations with lung inflammation. *American Journal of Clinical Nutrition* 65, 1858–1866.

Witko-Sarsat, V., Delacourt, C., Rabier, D., Bardet, J., Nguyen, A.T. and Descamps-Latscha, B. (1995) Neutrophil-derived long-lived oxidants in cystic fibrosis sputum. *American Journal of Respiratory and Critical Care Medicine* 152, 1910–1916.

The Influence of Antioxidants on Cognitive Decline in the Elderly

26

WALTER J. PERRIG, PASQUALINA PERRIG AND HANNES B. STÄHELIN

Institute of Psychology,
University of Bern, Bern, Switzerland

Introduction

The importance of vitamin supplementation on cognitive functioning in general and on memory competence in particular is a subject of great practical relevance. The question as to what extent the biochemical status of vitamins is related to an optimal cognitive functioning and how it could be employed against memory decrease in age is a vital scientific challenge. Since age-related memory decrease is subject to vast individual variation which has not yet been explained in a satisfactory manner, the quest for possible causes or predictors becomes a crucial one.

There are two promising main research approaches to address the question of what is responsible for age-related cognitive decline. These include: (i) the information processing approach with analyses of cognitive activities in terms of changes in elementary components; and (ii) the health status approach focusing on the influence of health or disease factors on cognitive performance (Salthouse, 1992; Rabbitt, 1993). Ideally, these two approaches should be integrated. Thus, the cognitive approach can point to appropriate studies on theoretically distinctive cognitive functions and their age-correlated changes in a normal population. This knowledge can then be used to differentiate the influence of health-related factors on cognitive performance.

There is no doubt that declining cognitive function can be the result of age-associated chronic diseases such as Alzheimer's disease, vascular degenerative changes and many other related disorders. There appears to be a substantial amount of evidence demonstrating common causes and controls of ageing and disease processes (Halliwell, 1994). From this we can plausibly infer that each factor influencing biological cell functioning could have an impact on cognitive processes. Concerning the effects of vitamins, there is empirical evidence for the cell-protective effects of antioxidants on brain metabolism (Bell *et al.*, 1990; Tucker *et al.*, 1990). Moreover, inverse correlations between dietary antioxidant intake or plasma levels and subsequent disease have been demonstrated (Volicer and Crino, 1990; Kozlowski, 1992; Evans, 1993). From these facts one might assume that increased oxidative stress is responsible for disturbances in memory functions.

In a prospective epidemiological study (Inter Disciplinary Study on Ageing, IDA), we addressed this hypothesis and searched for relationships between antioxidants, prooxidants and mental functioning. We found significant correlationships between the antioxidants α-tocopherol, β-carotene, ascorbic acid and different measures of memory (Perrig *et al.*, 1997).

From these findings we can assume that vitamins do play an important role in brain ageing and cognitive functioning. However, because of the quasi-experimental nature of the study we cannot satisfactorily explain the exact mechanisms that are responsible for the relationships which were observed. Biological dispositions (lipoprotein concentrations as transport vehicles for fat-soluble vitamins) or nutritional habits are the two most plausible explanations for our findings. The biological hypothesis suggests that higher levels of plasma vitamins in our subjects directly cause improved cognitive performance through their antioxidative and cell-protective effects. According to the nutritional habits perspective, the intellectually more competent or better educated subjects are more concerned with health-related nutritional behaviour. In this case, higher plasma vitamin levels are not necessarily the cause but rather the consequence of higher cognitive competence. From the practical perspective the first explanation would put a much higher demand on people to increase their vitamin intake. In either case, the relationship we found in our study delivers an important message. Even making the assumption that antioxidative vitamins do not have a direct impact on cognitive performance through biochemical means in the cell, our data show that a higher level of plasma vitamins is associated with better cognitive performance. Bearing in mind the well-established cell-protective effects of antioxidants we would be in any case well advised to be concerned about vitamin intake.

Clearly, further research is needed so as to better understand the effects of vitamins on cognitive processes. The present contribution is devoted to this goal. In particular, we are looking for evidence that could help to clarify the mechanisms underlying the relationship between antioxidants and cognitive performance that we found in our study. We will first present a review of the literature and report on new data from our IDA study. In these analyses we will include additional vitamins or provitamins. In the final section we report our conclusions, which integrate the results of the two lines of analyses presented here with the findings we reported previously (Perrig *et al.*, 1997).

Antioxidants and Memory Performance: a Review

Concerning the question of the relationship between vitamins and cognitive performance, there have been two types of study: (i) epidemiological and quasi-experimental studies that report correlational results, and (ii) experimental studies that report the effects of vitamin treatment.

Of course, the second type of study is of special importance because the experimental approach should lead us more directly to causal relationships between vitamins and memory performance. Unfortunately, there are very few such studies available at present. In the present review we focus on research on human subjects and on cognitive performance.

In a cross-sectional study involving 260 non-institutionalized men and women, aged over 60 years, Goodwin *et al.* (1983) found that subjects with low blood levels of vitamins C and B_{12} scored worse on tests for abstract thinking ability and memory, while subjects with low levels of riboflavin or folic acid scored worse on categories tests. The nutritional analysis was based on diet history. Similarly, in a cross-sectional study involving 28 healthy persons aged over 60, Tucker *et al.* (1990) observed several significant correlations (e.g. for plasma carotene and vitamin C) but in somewhat contradictory ways. Demanding tasks correlated preferentially with nutrition status. The authors suggested that task performance and brain physiology are sensitive to changes in nutrition but this viewpoint has not been proven. La Rue *et al.* (1997) examined the association between nutritional status (measured in 1980 and 1986) and cognitive performance (1986) in 137 normal elderly community residents aged 66–90 years. Although associations were relatively weak in this well-nourished and cognitively intact sample, the pattern of results suggests some important directions for further research (e.g. higher past intake of vitamins E, A, B_6, and B_{12} were related to better performance on visuospatial recall and abstraction tests). The Rotterdam Study examined the cross-sectional relationship between cognitive function and dietary intake of antioxidants (β-carotene and vitamins C and E) in 5182 persons aged 55–95 years. Results show that a lower intake of β-carotene was associated with impaired cognitive function (measured with the MMSE, a screening method of cognitive function to detect dementing disorders), whereas there was no association between cognitive function and the intakes of vitamins C and E (Jama *et al.*, 1996). In the SENECA-EURONUT Investigation, subjects from European towns born between 1911 and 1914 were analysed. In this study plasma carotene, ascorbic acid and α-tocopherol concentrations correlated with the MMSE (Haller *et al.*, 1996).

Sram *et al.* (1993) examined the effects of long-term supplementation (24 months) with vitamin C (1000 mg day^{-1}) and vitamin E (300 mg day^{-1}) in two homes for people with considerable morbidity and a high incidence of malnutrition. Eight subjects were selected from each home for psychological tests and biochemical analysis. The results from different measurements during the treatment phase provided only suggestive evidence for positive effects on cognitive functioning. The preliminary finding of a favourable effect of very high thiamin dosages (3–8 g day^{-1}) in Alzheimer's disease were not followed further (Maedor *et al.*, 1993). In a recent study involving patients with mild to moderate Alzheimer's disease treated with 1800 IU α-tocopherol daily, this led to a significant slowing in the deterioration of mental function, leading to a delay in institutionalization compared with untreated controls (Sano *et al.*, 1997). The therapeutic effect was comparable to the effect of selegilin therapy alone. Interestingly, the combination of selegilin and α-tocopherol did not increase treatment efficacy.

This review of the literature reveals only a very limited number of relevant studies. The research field actually presents a variety of approaches that have produced suggestive evidence that vitamins might have an impact on cognitive functioning. However, we cannot state with any certainty which vitamin(s) will affect what kind of cognitive processes. Much more systematic research is clearly needed. The large diversity in methodology, study populations and measure of cognitive performance are factors probably responsible for the inconsistent findings. For instance, in a study where the MMSE is used for a population at risk for dementia there might be enough variation in this measure to allow correlations with plasma vitamins. With a healthy elderly population this measure will produce little variation, thereby preventing correlations with vitamins. This shows that it will be difficult to relate findings from one study to another, given large differences in populations and methods.

Vitamins and Memory Function: New Results from the Basel Longitudinal Project (IDA)

In this section we present research that was done with a sample that can be considered representative of a healthy elderly population. The Basel longitudinal project (IDA) with status measurements in 1993 and 1995 is part of a medical study (the Basel Prospective Study) that collected mostly biomedical data from a large sample of initially 6400 healthy people in 1960, 1965 and 1971 (Widmer *et al.*, 1981).

In a previous study (Perrig *et al.*, 1997) we investigated the relationship between present (1993) and long-term (1971) serum antioxidant status, and different memory functions in a healthy, elderly population. The memory criterion is not as easy to evaluate as it might appear at first glance. Almost every human performance is related to memory in one way or another.

Therefore, we have to classify different cognitive performance tasks based on actual knowledge about structures and functions of memory. We were interested in the unique predictive power of plasma antioxidant levels (ascorbic acid, β-carotene and α-tocopherol) collected in 1971 (Stahelin *et al.*, 1991) and 1993 on different memory performances (priming, working-memory, free recall, recognition and vocabulary) measured in 1993. In multivariate regression analyses we corrected for potentially confounding factors such as systolic blood pressure, serum cholesterol and ferritin as well as age, gender and level of education.

High systolic blood pressure is one of the major risk factors for stroke and vascular dementia (Binswanger disease). High cholesterol is also related to stroke, TIA, and indirectly reflects apoEe4 status. Thus, both are to some extent risk-related to cognitive function and dementia. They therefore have to be allowed for in evaluating the effect of antioxidants on cognitive functioning. Ferritin is an indicator of tissue iron stores and thus of the pro-oxidative potential in the presence of free radicals (Volicer and Crino, 1990; Evans, 1993). In addition, ascorbic acid may have pro-oxidative activity in the presence of high endogenous ferritin content (Sram *et al.*, 1993). Thus, since these measurements were available for 1971 and 1993, it was important to include them in the analyses.

In the present study we expanded the array of examined antioxidants by including three additional bioactive compounds: α-carotene, cryptoxanthin and lycopene, which were determined only in 1993. We also computed the correlation of plasma levels of vitamin A (measured in 1971 and 1993). We expect that this will help to clarify the question of whether correlations found between plasma antioxidant levels and memory performance are based on a causal relationship or not. The hypothesis is based on the assumption that free radicals influence the rate of ageing and neurodegeneration and hence affect memory performance. Since in our previous evaluation only β-carotene of the vitamin A complex was analysed, the observed effect could be attributable to a pro-vitamin A property. In comparison with the effects of the antioxidants analysed in our previous study we can expect that α-carotene, cryptoxanthin and lycopene investigated here invalidates or corroborates the antioxidant hypothesis on memory function, since lycopene has no pro-vitamin A action and the other carotenes only a rather weak effect.

Methods

Participants

Of 848 persons invited, 442 agreed to participate. They were healthy and were aged 65–94 (mean age: 75; 312 males and 132 females) (Perrig-Chiello *et al.*, 1996). The investigation took place at the Geriatric University Clinic of Basel between April and September 1993. Participants arrived in the morning in the fasting state. After the anthropometric and clinical data collection, blood samples were drawn. Participants received a breakfast, followed by a psychometric testing.

Antioxidants: assessment and description

In this analysis we included the carotenoids α-carotene, cryptoxanthin and lycopene, which were determined in 1993. The plasma vitamin analyses were performed by Hoffman-La Roche, Basel, Switzerland, according to the methods described by Heinimann *et al.* (1996).

Memory functions: assessment and description

Different memory parameters (priming, working memory, free recall and recognition) were assessed for this study. The WAIS-R Vocabulary Test was administered in this standardized subtest of the Wechsler Adult Intelligence Scale, subjects have to give definitions of words, assessing aspects of:

- semantic long-term memory.

For the other memory variables a computerized test was used (Perrig *et al.*, 1995). This 20 min procedure assesses memory resources in terms of:

- explicit memory (free recall, recognition),
- implicit memory (priming in a perceptual identification task, clarification),
- working-memory (dual task procedure).

This memory test is based on the theoretical insights of experimental psychology into the modular structures and functions of memory known to be influenced by age in differential ways (Perrig and Perrig, 1993; Perrig *et al.*, 1993). Also, in terms of psychometrical standards, the test is a reliable and valid instrument with norms for 5-year cohorts aged between 65 and 95. German, French and English versions of the test now exist, with norms for the German version.

Test procedure

In the initial (learning) phase, participants were presented with a picture containing two identical scenes on a computer screen (one on the left side, the other on the right). The scenes consisted of easy-to-name objects, animals, digits, words and distinctive textures. Participants had to scan for missing parts in the left-hand side image, and they were informed that they would be questioned later on the content of the scenes. No further hint was given on what kind of memory test would be administered later.

Memory assessment was performed as follows:

- *Implicit memory*: 15 old pictures presented in the original scene and 15 new pictures of easy-to-name objects were shown in a fixed random order and had to be identified and named as quickly as possible. In this procedure, each picture on the computer scene was generated by a recursive function. This function randomly selects a coordinate on the screen and from there on draws a line of 10 pixels of the picture to be presented. From the phenomenological perspective, the subjects see small, black horizontal lines appear somewhere on the screen. These lines continuously construct a picture which becomes clearer and clearer until it is complete. Priming was calculated as percent gain in naming speed of old pictures compared to new pictures: ((new − old)/new)*100.

- *Working memory capacity*: To test working-memory capacity, a dual task procedure was used. The picture naming task described above was repeated, using the old pictures and a set of new pictures. The subjects had to identify and name these pictures as quickly as possible. The secondary task consisted of simultaneously responding as quickly as possible to little suns flashing either on the left or the right side of the computer screen, by pressing a key on a button box with the left- or right-hand index finger. To account for possible trade-offs between the two tasks, we calculated the rate of correct responses to the flashing suns and the response time in the naming task. These two measures were standardized (z values) and summed to produce a compound measure of working memory capacity.

- *Explicit memory*: About 20 min after the acquisition phase, a free-recall and a recognition task were administered. The subjects were asked to freely recall all the elements they could remember having seen in the initial scene, where they did the error scanning. The number of correctly remembered items was counted. Finally the subjects were presented with a picture containing elements (objects and animals) from the initial scene in the learning phase and elements that were used in the picture-naming task later on in the test procedure. The subject's task was to identify the elements of the initial scene. In the data analyses, the recognition performance is represented by the discrimination indexed from the signal detection theory, which integrates hit and false-alarm rates.

Results

Table 26.1 presents the intercorrelations between retinol, and the carotenoids analysed in this study (α-carotene, cryptoxanthin and lycopene), and the antioxidants (β-carotene, ascorbic acid and α-tocopherol) analysed in the Perrig *et al.* (1997) study. It can be seen that retinol does not correlate with the other carotenoids and antioxidants. While β-carotene shows substantial correlations with the other carotenoids, this is not the case for the two antioxidants, α-tocopherol and ascorbic acid, used in our previous study.

Table 26.1. Intercorrelations of the vitamin A complex and the antioxidants, α-tocopherol and ascorbic acid.

	Retinol	α-Carotene	Cryptoxanthin	Lycopene	β-Carotene	Ascorbic acid	α-Tocopherol
Retinol	1	0.01	0.00	−0.08	0.06	−0.11**	0.25*
α-Carotene		1	0.33*	0.21*	0.74*	0.19*	0.18*
Cryptoxanthin			1	0.24*	0.48*	0.23*	0.18*
Lycopene				1	0.34*	0.09	0.19*
β-Carotene					1	0.24*	0.25*
Ascorbic acid						1	0.02*
α-Tocopherol							1

* $P < 0.0005$; ** $P < 0.01$.

Table 26.2 presents the correlations between the vitamin A complex (retinol, the carotenoids α-carotene, cryptoxanthin and lycopene) and the memory measures. In order to look for differential effects we added the data of α-tocopherol, and ascorbic acid analysed earlier. When available, we used data from both times of investigations (1971 and 1993). The data from Table 26.2 show that retinol, α-carotene and α-tocopherol have no or weak correlation with memory performance. Beside the effects of β-carotene on cognitives measures, established in our previous study, we also find significant correlations for cryptoxanthin and lycopene.

All memory measures except priming correlate significantly with different antioxidants, showing that higher serum vitamin levels are associated with better performance. Although we find correlations between different vitamins and the measures for working memory capacity, free recall and recognition, the most substantial and reliable effects seem to be related to WAIS-Vocabulary. Ascorbic acid and cryptoxanthin correlate only with this performance measure.

In a further analysis we used analysis of variance (ANOVAs) to measure the effect of serum vitamins on memory performances beside the effects of age and education, two important variables known to strongly influence cognitive performances. The median of the serum vitamin was used to split our subjects into low-level and high-level vitamin groups. In the age variable, a median of 73 years was used to separate the young-old from the old-old. Concerning education, we distinguished three groups of study

Table 26.2. Correlations of the vitamin A complex, α-tocopherol and ascorbic acid with memory performances (1993).

	Priming	Working memory	Free recall	Recognition	WAIS-Vocabulary
Retinol 1971	−0.03	−0.05	−0.14[**]	−0.05	0.08
Retinol 1993	−0.03	−0.03	−0.02	0.03	0.12
Vitamin A Pro-vitamins:					
α-Carotene 1993	−0.05	0.04	0.12	0.11	0.13
β-Carotene 1971	0.04	0.14[**]	0.10	0.18[*]	0.17[*]
β-Carotene 1993	0.02	0.08	0.17[*]	0.19[*]	0.16[**]
Cryptoxanthin 1993	0.01	0.07	0.10	0.09	0.17[*]
Vitamin A Pre-stage component:					
Lycopene 1993	0.01	0.14[**]	0.14[**]	0.15[**]	0.14[**]
Ascorbic acid 1993	−0.05	0.03	0.10	0.06	0.16[**]
α-Tocopherol 1993	0.07	0.05	0.05	0.08	0.04

[*] $P < 0.0005$; [**] $P < 0.01$.

participants. Thus we had a 2 × 2 × 3 quasi-experimental factorial design with the between-subjects factors vitamin (low level and high level), age (young-old and old-old), and education (1, primary level = 9 years of education; 2, secondary level = 12 years of education; and 3, university level). We tested the influence of these three factors on the five dependent memory variables: priming, working-memory capacity, free recall, recognition and the WAIS-R Vocabulary Test. We analysed the effects of α-carotene, cryptoxanthin and lycopene. Because of the modest correlation between retinol and the memory parameters, retinol was not included in this analysis. In this three-factorial design the serum vitamin showed no effect in the analyses of α-carotene and lycopene. Cryptoxanthin, on the other hand, had a clear effect on performance in the WAIS-R Vocabulary Test, beside age and education. These results are presented in Fig. 26.1.

General Discussion and Conclusions

The influence of vitamin supplementation on cognitive functioning in general and on memory competence in particular, especially in the elderly, is a subject of great theoretical and practical relevance. Nutrients may affect cognitive functions in several ways. The integrity of the nutrient and energy supply to the brain is critically dependent on the vascular system; thus stroke and related disorders contribute significantly to disability in old age. Because the risk factors for stroke can be reduced by the intake of protective

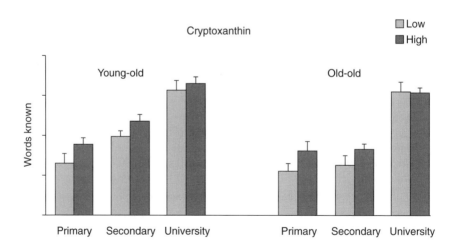

Fig. 26.1. Effects of cryptoxanthin (high, low), age (young-old, old-old) and education (primary, secondary, university) on performance in the WAIS-R Vocabulary Test (means and standard errors).

micronutrients, cognitive impairment can be partially avoided, at least indirectly, by this means. In addition to these influences of nutrition on energy supply, there might be other ways in which nutrition affects brain function. The efficiency of biochemical mechanisms in neurotransmitter synthesis, in intermediary metabolism, in protecting cells from oxidative stress, in the cytokines and other signalling molecules, has been related to level of nutrition. This is obvious in situations of malnutrition. In this study we have concentrated on the question of whether such nutrition effects can be shown to affect cognitive functions in study samples which are more or less representative of a normal, healthy population. Thus, we concentrated on relationships between vitamins and cognitive functions in a non-risk population. When free radicals contribute significantly to brain ageing, it is a plausible assumption that mechanisms protecting against free radical action will also maintain better cognitive functioning.

From a review of the literature we learned that only a very limited number of studies could be of help in answering our question. The research field dealing with the effects of vitamins on cognitive function actually presents a variety of approaches that are presented here and that give suggestive evidence for the conjecture that antioxidants might have an impact on cognitive functioning. However, we cannot come to any firm conclusions about which vitamins will affect what kind of cognitive processes in what kind of population. Much more systematic research is clearly needed. The large diversity of methodological approaches, selected populations and measures of cognitive performance create many problems in the interpretation of the data.

In the empirical part of this chapter we presented data that we collected from more than 400 elderly participants, aged 65–95 years. In the present study we examined the relationship of the bioactive compounds, α-carotene, cryptoxanthin and lycopene, together with vitamin A, to different cognitive performances. These results, taken together with the findings published earlier (Perrig *et al.*, 1997), clearly show differential effects of various vitamins and pro-vitamins on specific cognitive measures.

First of all we did not find any relationship between vitamin A and the cognitive measures. α-Carotene has small or no correlations; cryptoxanthin and lycopene, on the other hand, show substantial and highly significant correlations with different measures of memory performance. As in our previous study, the data in the priming measure cannot be predicted by any vitamin, while there are significant correlations between working memory capacity, free recall and recognition, and vitamins. As before, the performance in the WAIS-R Vocabulary Test was predicted best by vitamin status. The highest correlations being with cryptoxanthin and lycopene. It was for this measure that we found in the ANOVA a significant main effect for cryptoxanthin, besides age and education. And it was this measure again that had shown significant effects of β-carotene and ascorbic acid in the ANOVA of our previous study.

These are important similarities that suggest a high degree of reliability in our data. In fact the question of reliability is an important one in these kind of quasi-experimental studies. Reliability of the cognitive measures can influence the correlations with other variables. Therefore, it is important to note that the vocabulary and explicit memory measures generally show much higher reliability than implicit memory measures such as priming (Meier and Perrig, 1999). Although these methodological questions are important, we want to concentrate now on the question of how far our data can supply evidence for the two hypotheses, namely biological causal relation versus nutritional habit indication. The biological hypothesis suggests that higher levels of plasma vitamins directly cause improved cognitive performance through their antioxidative and cell-protective effects. The nutritional habits hypothesis assumes that the intellectually more competent or better-educated subjects are more concerned with health-related nutritional behaviour. In this case, higher plasma vitamin levels are not necessarily the cause but rather the consequence of higher cognitive competence.

We believe that our data give quite strong evidence against the hypothesis that the eating behaviour of more competent or better educated subjects is responsible for a higher vitamin intake. If this were the case then we would not expect differential effects between vitamins and cognitive performance. In other words, we should have the same correlations between vitamin A, α-carotene and α-tocopherol and the cognitive measures that we found among β-carotene, ascorbic acid, lycopene and cryptoxantin and cognitive performance. Furthermore, we do not find higher plasma levels of vitamins in more highly educated people. Finally the effects of antioxidants on memory performances, found in our study, do not appear to be based on the intake of vitamin supplements. In our study cohorts, only about 6% of the subjects mentioned vitamin supplementation. These subjects did not show higher levels of plasma vitamins nor better performance in the cognitive tasks. In addition, the study was carried out during spring and summer seasons, when the intake of vitamin supplements is rather low.

Explaining the biological mechanisms, the underlying relationship, between vitamins and cognitive performance seems to be a difficult and complex challenge. Because of the reliable effects of β-carotene on cognitive performance we might assume a pro-vitamin A property to be responsible. Consistent with this assumption we find correlations between cryptoxanthin and cognitive performance. However, inconsistent with this fact, we do not find effects of α-carotene, but on the other hand we do find significant correlations between cognitive performance and lycopene, which has no pro-vitamin A action. When we consider the antioxidants in our study, α-tocopherol has smaller effects on cognition than ascorbic acid or β-carotene. Here again we have to consider the possibility that different reliabilities in the measures could be responsible. But we also have arguments against such statistical artefacts. In our previous study (Perrig *et al.*, 1997) we found remarkable correlations between the 1971 and 1993 values for all three antioxidants (for α-tocopherol, $r = 0.47$; β-carotene, $r = 0.43$; and ascorbic acid, $r = 0.22$). These correlations over such a long time indicate stability in the measured parameters. Such high stability could not be measured with instruments of low reliability. In the same way, the lack of correlation between vitamin A and the cognitive parameters is not the result of lower reliability since the correlation between both vitamin A measures (1971 and 1993) is high ($r = 0.45$).

Unfortunately, at present it is impossible to relate a consistent pattern of results to a theoretical view of how plasma vitamins influence different forms of cognitive function. There are simply not enough data available that can be compared to the same tasks and the same plasma vitamins. It is noteworthy that Tucker *et al.* (1990) observed a significant positive correlation of plasma carotene with word fluency but negative correlations with tonal memory span. Goodwin *et al.* (1983), who did not measure carotene, found a significant correlation between ascorbic acid and recall of paragraphs from the Wechsler Verbal Memory Test. Neither study measured α-tocopherol. In the SENECA investigation, Haller *et al.* (1996) reported that α-tocopherol concentrations correlated with the MMSE. The lack of effect of α-tocopherol in our study might be due to the especially high α-tocopherol status in our population. While there is a reasonable ascorbic acid and β-carotene plasma concentration in our sample, the α-tocopherol level is particularly high. Thus in other populations with a poor α-tocopherol status, the latter may become a more important predictor.

With respect to the relationship between vitamins and cognition, we may be able to explain the differential effects of vitamins on cognitive measures by considering differences and similarities in the transport vehicles and dietary sources of vitamins and their metabolism. It is noteworthy that in our sample cholesterol has positive correlations with α-tocopherol and, to a lesser degree, with β-carotene, but not with ascorbic acid. This finding might be explained by the fact that α-tocopherol and β-carotene are transported with plasma lipoproteins, which, if determined in the fasting state, remain rather constant in a given person with stable eating habits and lifestyle, and thus show less fluctuation in their plasma levels. Ascorbic acid, by contrast, is water-soluble and not protein bound and thus subject to more rapid changes. This suggests that a single plasma ascorbic acid determination will misclassify a number of individuals and the actual long-term correlation might be higher than indicated by the observed correlation coefficient. Furthermore, ascorbic acid and β-carotene reflect similar eating habits since both are important constituents of fruit and vegetables, whereas the main sources for α-tocopherol are fat and oils. Consistent with this is our finding that ascorbic acid and β-carotene correlate significantly with each other. Summarizing the differential effects of vitamins on the different memory parameters used in our study, performance in the WAIS-R Vocabulary Test is the one predicted best by antioxidants. After including possible confounding variables such as age, education and gender in multiple regression analyses, ascorbic acid, β-carotene and cryptoxanthin remained significant predictors. Performances in dual task performance, free recall and recognition also correlate significantly with different vitamins, especially with β-carotene and lycopene. But these effects do not hold up in the multiple regression analyses. For the moment we have two possible explanations for this data pattern. First, it appears that the vitamin effects are manifested in activities that represent long-term states. The reason for this could well be in the special biochemical representation of information in the cells. Second, it could also be that the methods with which we measure semantic long-term memory are more reliable. More systematic research will lead us to clearer insights in this very complex matter.

Acknowledgements

We thank the Swiss National Science Foundation for the support of the study (Nr. 4032 – 035642) and Hoffmann-La Roche, Basel, Switzerland, for performing and sponsoring the analyses of the serum vitamin.

References

Bell, J.R., Edman, J.S., Marty, D.W. and Sathin, A. (1990) Vitamin β-su β-1-su β-2 and folate status in acute geropsychiatric inpatients: affective and cognitive characteristics of a vitamin nondeficient population. *Biological Psychiatry* 27, 125–137.

Evans, P.H. (1993) Free radicals in brain metabolism and pathology. *British Medical Bulletin* 19, 577–587.

Goodwin, J.S., Goodwin, J.M. and Garry, P.J. (1983) Association between nutritional status and cognitive functioning in a healthy elderly population. *Journal of the American Medical Association* 249, 2917–2921.

Haller, J., Weggemans, R.M., Ferry, M. and Guigoz, Y. (1996) Mental health: mini-mental state examination and geriatric depression score of elderly Europeans in the SENECA study of 1993. *European Journal of Clinical Nutrition* 50 (Suppl. 2), 112–116.

Halliwell, B. (1994) Free radicals, antioxidants, and human disease: curiosity, cause, or consequence? *Lancet* 344, 721–724.

Heinimann, K., Staehelin, H.B., Perrig-Chiello, P. and Perrig, W.J. (1996) Lipoprotein und Plasma-Lipide bei 429 Betagten und Hochbetagten: Bedeutung als Risikofaktor, Einfluss von Ernährung und Lebensstil. *Schweizerische Medizinische Wochenschrift* 126, 1487–1494.

Jama, J.W., Launer, L.J., Witteman, J.C., den Breeijen, J.H., Breteler, M.M.B., Grobbee, D.E. and Hofman, A. (1996) Dietary antioxidants and cognitive function in a population-based sample of older persons. The Rotterdam Study. *American Journal of Epidemiology* 144, 175–280.

Kozlowski, B.W. (1992) Megavitamin treatment of mental retardation in children: a review of effects on behaviour and cognition. *Journal of Child and Adolescence Psychoparmacology* 2, 307–320.

La Rue, A., Koehler, K.M., Wayne, S.J., Chiulli, S.J., Haaland, K.Y. and Garry, P.J. (1997) Nutritional status and cognitive functioning in a normally aging sample: a 6-y reassessment. *American Journal of Clinical Nutrition* 65, 20–29.

Maedor, K.J., Nichols, M.E., Franke, P., Durkin, M.W., Oberzan, R.L., Moore, E.E. and Loring, D.W. (1993) Evidence for a central cholinergic effect of high-dose thiamine. *Annals of Neurology* 34, 724–726.

Meier, B. and Perrig, W.J. (1999) Low reliability of perceptual priming: consequences for the interpretation of functional dissociations between explicit and implicit memory. *Quarterly Journal of Experimental Psychology*, in press.

Perrig, W.J. and Perrig, P. (1993) Life-span aspects in explicit and implicit memory. *German Journal of Psychology* 17, 307–309.

Perrig, W.J., Wippich, W. and Perrig, P. (1993) *Unbewusste Informationsverarbeitung.* Huber, Bern.

Perrig, W.J., Hofer, D., Kling, V., Meier, B., Perrig-Chiello, P., Ruch, M. and Serafin, D. (1995) Computerunterstützer Gedächtnis-Funktions-Test (C-GFT) Version 1. Manual und Disketten für IBM. Institut für Psychologie, Universität Basel, Switzerland.

Perrig, W., Perrig, P. and Stähelin, H.B. (1997) The relation between antioxidants and memory performance in the old and very old. *Journal of the American Geriatric Society* 45, 718–724.

Perrig-Chiello, P., Perrig, W.J., Stähelin, H.B., Krebs, E. and Ehrsam, R. (1996) Autonomie, Wohlbefinden und Gesundheit im Alter: eine interdisziplinäre Altersstudie (IDA). *Zeitschrift für Gerontologie und Geriatrie* 29, 95–109.

Rabbitt, P. (1993) Does it all go together when it goes? *Quarterly Journal of Experimental Psychology Human Experimental Psychology* 46A, 385–434.

Salthouse, T.A. (1992) *Mechanisms of Age–Cognition Relations in Adulthood.* Lawrence Erlbaum, Hillsdale, New Jersey.

Sano, M., Ernesto, C., Thomas, R.G., Klauber, M.R., Schafer, K., Grundman, M., Woodbury, P., Growdon, J., Cotman, C.W., Pfeiffer, E., Schneider, L.S. and Thal, L.J. (1997) A controlled trial of selegiline, alpha-tocopherol, or both as treatment of Alzheimer's disease. The Alzheimer's Disease Cooperative Study. *New England Journal of Medicine* 336, 1216–1222.

Sram, R.J., Binkova, B., Topinka, J., Kotesovec, F., Fojtikova, I., Hanel, I., Klaschka, J., Kocisova, J., Prosek, M. and Machelek, J. (1993) Effect of antioxidant supplementation in an elderly population. In: Bronzetti *et al.* (eds) *Antimutagenesis and Anticarcinogenesis Mechanisms III.* Plenum Press, New York.

Stähelin, H.B., Gey, K.F., Eichholzer, M., Lüdin, E., Bernasconi, F., Thurneysen, J. and Brubacher, G. (1991) Plasma antioxidant vitamins and subsequent cancer mortality in the 12-year follow-up of the prospective Basel Study. *American Journal of Epidemiology* 133, 766–775.

Tucker, D.M., Penland, J.G., Sandstead, H.H., Milne, D.B., Heck, D.G. and Klevay, L.M. (1990) Nutrition status and brain function in aging. *American Journal of Clinical Nutrition* 52, 93–102.

Volicer, L. and Crino, P.B. (1990) Involvement of free radicals in dementia of the Alzheimer type: a hypothesis. *Neurobiology and Aging* 11, 567–571.

Widmer, L.K., Stähelin, H.B., Nissen, C. and da Silva, A. (1981) (eds) *Venen-Arterien-Krankheiten koronare Herzkrankheiten- bei Berufstätigen*. Huber, Bern.

Schizophrenia: Role of Oxidative Stress and Essential Fatty Acids

27

RAVINDER REDDY[1] AND JEFFREY K. YAO[1,2]

[1]*University of Pittsburgh Medical Center, Western Psychiatric Institute and Clinic, Pittsburgh, Pennsylvania, USA;* [2]*Pittsburgh VA Healthcare System, Pittsburgh, Pennsylvania, USA*

Introduction

Schizophrenia is a devastating psychiatric disorder that has yet to reveal its pathophysiology. It is a complex disorder with a broad range of behavioural and biological manifestations. One of its most distressing aspects is the relatively high proportion of patients who do not respond well to treatment. It is estimated that the annual economic burden of this illness to the USA is $40–60 billion. It is probable that a significant portion of that cost is expended in taking care of patients with a poor outcome. While much of the research in the past 100 years has focused on elucidating the aetiology of the disorder, less attention has been paid to understanding the biological mechanisms that mediate poor outcome. There is evidence that membrane deficits, primarily concentrations of membrane phospholipid and essential fatty acids (EFA), may be associated with clinical features of the illness associated with poor outcome. Further, there is also evidence that oxidative stress, well known as a cause of membrane abnormalities, occurs in schizophrenia. These findings, which we review below, converge to suggest a meaningful relationship between oxidative stress, membrane deficits and poor outcome in schizophrenia.

Schizophrenia and Clinical Outcome

Schizophrenia is a brain disorder with protean manifestations. It has a lifetime prevalence of 1%, with a relatively early age of onset – late adolescence and early adulthood. It is characterized by psychotic symptoms ('positive' symptoms such as hallucinations and delusions), impaired thinking and bizarre behaviour sometime during the course of the illness. Many patients have 'negative' symptoms that are just as, if not more, troublesome as positive symptoms, and include decreased emotional arousal and social drive, paucity of mental activity, motor retardation and decreased ability to experience pleasure. While positive symptoms are often episodic in nature, and generally responsive to treatment, negative symptoms tend to be persistent and treatment-resistant. Treatment of this disorder includes long-term administration of antipsychotic agents, rehabilitation, family and community support, and education. However, in spite of current best treatment efforts, the clinical outcome of schizophrenia remains highly variable. While long-term follow-up studies indicate that 50–68% of schizophrenic patients have a favourable outcome (Hegarty *et al.*, 1994), a substantial proportion still have a long-term poor outcome that is devastating to themselves, their families and society.

There are several clinical characteristics of the illness that have been consistently associated with poor outcome, including poor premorbid adjustment, long duration of psychosis prior to treatment or delayed intervention, prominent negative symptoms early in illness, persistence of positive symptoms even with optimal treatment, and medication discontinuation (reviewed in Ram *et al.*, 1992; Wyatt, 1995). Biological factors, such as structural brain abnormalities, neurological 'soft' signs, being male and possibly genetic loading for schizophrenia are associated with poor outcome.

Whether these mediators of poor outcome are independent biological factors or reflect a more fundamental, possibly a unitary, pathology has yet to be determined. A multiplicity of theories have been proposed over the years that aim to conceptualize the pathophysiology of schizophrenia, including neuronal maldevelopment, impaired neurotransmission, a role for viral infections, autoimmune dysfunction, and many others. While most theoretical constructs are aimed at aetiological explication, and not predicting outcome, it is likely that pathological processes active at the onset of illness are involved in determining outcome, or at least interact with other factors that modify it. A further consideration is the large variety of apparently disparate biological findings reported in schizophrenia (Lieberman and Koreen, 1993). Also, very likely there is aetiological heterogeneity, in which case there probably exists a final common pathogenetic pathway (or very few). The issue at hand, therefore, is to identify candidate pathological process(es) that account for the constellation of clinical and biological features in schizophrenic patients which are associated with poor outcome.

A point of convergence for the above-mentioned theoretical models occurs at the level of the neuronal membrane, which is the structural and functional site of neurotransmitter receptors, ion channels, signal transduction and drug effects. The membrane is also a point where there is a natural intersection between genetic and environmental factors (Horrobin *et al.*, 1995). Membrane defects, such as those induced by decreased arachidonic acid (AA) in phospholipids, can significantly alter a broad range of membrane functions, and *ipso facto* behaviour through multiple 'down-stream' effects. Previous results from our laboratory and those of other investigators show alterations in EFA metabolism and membrane dynamics, and are associated with indices of poor outcome.

Importance of Membrane EFA in Schizophrenia

EFA are attached to cell membrane lipids, primarily phospholipids such as phosphatidylcholine, phosphatidylethanolamine, phosphatidylserine and phosphatidylinositol that make up 80% of total phospholipids. The two types of EFA, defined on the basis of the first double-bond position, are the omega-6 (*n*-6) and omega-3 (*n*-3) series. Neuronal membrane phospholipids contain high proportions of essential polyunsaturated fatty acids (PUFA), primarily AA (*n*-6) and docosahexaenoic acid (DHA; *n*-3). In addition to helping to maintain normal membrane structure and function, EFA also are critical in all aspects of normal brain development (Tacconi *et al.*, 1997).

Since the dynamic functional state of all membranes, including neuronal, is dependent on their composition, even small changes in key EFA that make up phospholipids, such as AA and DHA, can lead to a broad range of membrane dysfunction involving receptor binding, neurotransmission, signal transduction and prostaglandin synthesis. Further, AA is itself a second messenger. Thus, deficits in membrane EFA may explain many biological, physiological and clinical consequences observed in schizophrenia (see review by Horrobin, 1996).

Alterations in Phospholipids and PUFA in Schizophrenia

Early studies, reviewed by Rotrosen and Wolkin (1987), reported a variety of alterations in plasma or red blood cell (RBC) membrane phospholipid concentrations in psychotic patients. These findings included variable alterations in levels of phosphatidylcholine, phosphatidylserine and phosphatidylinositol, but consistent reductions in phosphatidylethanolamine levels. The variability in the findings may be due to differences in diagnostic methods and laboratory methodology. Further, the previous results may have been confounded by the recent finding of a bimodal distribution of RBC AA and DHA in chronic schizophrenic patients, in contrast with the unimodal distribution seen in normal controls (Glen *et al.*, 1994; Peet *et al.*, 1994). While a majority of previous studies were done in chronic schizophrenic patients, studies of patients with recent-onset schizophrenia also show decreased RBC phosphatidylethanolamine (Keshavan *et al.*,

1993a), and decreases in the four key membrane phospholipids were found in fibroblasts from similar patients (Mahadik *et al.*, 1994).

EFA concentrations have been investigated only recently. Significant reductions in RBC AA concentration have been reported in hospitalized neuroleptic-treated schizophrenic patients (Peet *et al.*, 1994). Similarly, significant decreases of both plasma AA and linoleic acid (18:2, *n*-6), a precursor of AA, but an increase in total omega-3 fatty acids, was reported in three schizophrenic patient groups from England, Scotland and Ireland (Horrobin *et al.*, 1989). A decrease in plasma linoleic acid, but not in AA, was reported in Japanese schizophrenic patients (Kaiya *et al.*, 1991). Decreases in PUFA were also demonstrated in RBC membranes of schizophrenic patients (Vaddadi *et al.*, 1989; Glen *et al.*, 1994; Laugharne *et al.*, 1996; Peet *et al.*, 1996). More recently, Yao *et al.* (1994b) reported a significant decrease of PUFA, particularly linoleic acid and AA, in the RBC ghost membranes of schizophrenic patients on and off treatment with the antipsychotic haloperidol. Thus, reductions in blood linoleic acid levels in schizophrenia appear to be a consistent finding. Decreases in membrane AA concentration have been found in fibroblasts of first-episode schizophrenic patients (Mahadik *et al.*, 1996). This finding suggests that these EFA abnormalities are present early in the course of illness and not necessarily a consequence of neuroleptic treatment. Since membrane defects in schizophrenia have been found in a variety of peripheral cell types (platelets, RBC and fibroblasts), Horrobin (1996) proposed that these membrane compositional defects may occur in all cell membranes in the body, thus detectable in both extra-neural tissues as well as the CNS.

Alterations of Brain Membrane Lipids

A particularly vexing problem has been the inability to examine phospholipid metabolism *in vivo* so as to determine whether peripheral findings of membrane deficits in schizophrenia also occur in the brain. With the advent of ^{31}P magnetic resonance spectroscopy (MRS) methods, it has become possible to non-invasively study *in vivo* phosphorus metabolism in humans. In the earliest reports using ^{31}P MRS, Pettegrew *et al.* (1991, 1993) demonstrated significant reductions of phosphomonoesters (phospholipid precursors) and significantly increased levels of phosphodiesters (phospholipid breakdown products) in the frontal cortices of neuroleptic-naive first-episode schizophrenic patients as compared to healthy controls. In addition, increased ATP levels and decreased inorganic orthophosphate were also found. It was suggested that changes in membrane phospholipids may be related to molecular changes that precede onset of clinical symptoms and brain structural changes in schizophrenia, while changes in high-energy phosphate metabolism may be state-dependent (Pettegrew *et al.*, 1993). Subsequently, several other investigators have reported similar findings of membrane phospholipid perturbations in both acutely and chronically ill patients (reviewed in Keshavan and Pettegrew, 1997). Keshavan *et al.* (1993b) suggested a possible familial basis for membrane phospholipid changes in schizophrenia, based on ^{31}P MRS findings.

Direct evidence of decreased fatty acid levels comes from a post-mortem study of the frontal cortex of schizophrenic patients and normal controls (Horrobin *et al.,* 1991). We recently conducted a preliminary post-mortem study of the caudate in 11 schizophrenic patients, five psychiatric controls and ten normal control subjects, and found in schizophrenic patients significant reductions of membrane phosphatidylethanolamine, phosphatidylcholine, AA and linoleic acid (unpublished data). These findings, taken together with evidence from peripheral tissues and ^{31}P MRS, lend further support to the notion of membrane pathology in schizophrenia.

Free Radicals and the Antioxidant Defence System

To better comprehend the relationship between changes in brain membrane lipids and schizophrenia, we must look at the question of free radical biochemistry and oxidative stress. A consequence of aerobic metabolism is the generation of potentially toxic free radicals, which are chemical species with unpaired electrons (primarily the reactive oxygen species, superoxide and hydroxyl radicals). They are generated *in vivo* during many normal biochemical reactions involving oxygen, including the mitochondrial electron transfer chain, NADPH-dependent oxidases, and oxidation of PUFA and catecholamines (Kalyanaraman, 1989; Cohen, 1994; Rice-Evans, 1994). The superoxide radicals produced during these reactions are dismutated to hydrogen peroxide. Hydrogen peroxide is itself not a free radical, but is susceptible to autoxidation to yield the hydroxyl radical, one of the most reactive free radical species. Complex protective strategies have evolved against free radical toxicity. Under normal physiological conditions, free radical-mediated damage is kept under control by the antioxidant defence system, comprising a series of enzymatic and non-enzymatic components. The most important antioxidant enzymes include superoxide dismutases (SOD), catalase (CAT) and glutathione peroxidase (GSH-Px). These enzymes act cooperatively at different sites in the metabolic cascade of free radicals (Fig. 27.1).

Hydrogen peroxide produced by SOD is decomposed to water and oxygen by the haem protein, CAT and selenium-dependent GSH-Px, thereby preventing the formation of hydroxyl radicals. Failure of this first-line antioxidant defence can lead to an initiation of lipid peroxidation, and subsequent loss of membrane lipids. Since SOD, CAT and GSH-Px are critical at different stages of free radical metabolism, altered activity of one enzyme without compensatory changes in other antioxidant systems may leave membranes vulnerable to damage.

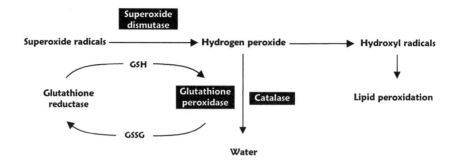

Fig. 27.1. Key enzymes in the antioxidant defence system.

The non-enzymatic antioxidant components – which may be equally important in the overall antioxidant defence system – consist of molecules that react with reactive oxygen species, preventing the propagation of lipid peroxidation. The most common non-enzymatic antioxidant molecules are glutathione, α-tocopherol (vitamin E), ascorbic acid (vitamin C), β-carotene, albumin, bilirubin and uric acid.

What is Oxidative Stress?

Oxidative stress is a state when there is a disequilibrium between pro-oxidant processes and the antioxidant defence system in favour of the former, and occurs as a consequence of increased production of free radicals, or when the antioxidant defence system is inefficient, or a combination of both events. Oxidative stress, regardless of the specific cause, can result in the initiation of any number of pathophysiological processes leading to cellular toxicity.

Free radicals target cellular components including lipids, proteins, DNA and carbohydrates. Protein oxidation can lead to loss of sulphydryl groups, in addition to modifications of amino acids, leading to the formation of carbonyl moieties. Accumulation of oxidized proteins may be involved in loss of various biochemical and physiological functions. DNA can also be damaged. These alterations can affect the viability of DNA and modify gene expression. Lipids, by virtue of their location in cell membranes, are particularly vulnerable to peroxidation.

Evidence for Free Radical-mediated Pathology in Schizophrenia

It was proposed over 40 years ago that toxic radicals had a role in the aetiology of schizophrenia (Hoffer *et al.*, 1954). Only in the last two decades has there been accumulating evidence that supports Hoffer's proposition. Studies generally have examined indirect measures of free radical activity, as direct measures of free radicals *in vivo* are difficult and cumbersome. Most studies have examined the activities of key antioxidant enzymes in plasma and RBC, based on the assumption that alterations in enzyme activities, which are tightly coupled with free radical production, reflect oxidative stress. A few recent studies have examined levels of non-enzymatic antioxidants, and levels of peroxidation products that provide a more direct indicator of oxidative damage.

Increased RBC SOD activity has been reported in schizophrenic patients in some studies (Michelson *et al.*, 1977; Golse *et al.*, 1978; Abdalla *et al.*, 1986; Reddy *et al.*, 1991; Wang, 1992; Vaiva *et al.*, 1994) but not in others (Sinet *et al.*, 1983; Yao *et al.*, 1998a). By contrast, decreased SOD activity has been reported in neuroleptic-naive first-episode schizophrenic patients (Mukherjee *et al.*, 1996). On the other hand, GSH-Px activity in schizophrenic patients, relative to normal controls, has been found to be low in some studies (Golse *et al.*, 1977; Abdalla *et al.*, 1986; Stoklasova *et al.*, 1986) but not in others (Yao *et al.*, 1998b). In one study, GSH-Px was found to be increased (Zhang *et al.*, 1998). Similarly, CAT activity has been reported to be decreased in some studies (Glazov and Mamzev, 1976; Reddy *et al.*, 1991, 1993), but not others (Mukherjee *et al.*, 1996; Yao *et al.*, 1998a). Some of the variability in the findings is likely due to differences in patient samples, particularly differences in the duration of illness (acute vs. chronic illness) and laboratory methodology.

A significant contribution to the total antioxidant capacity comes from antioxidant molecules in plasma, such as vitamins E and C, albumin and uric acid. Lower vitamin E:cholesterol ratios have been found in chronic schizophrenic patients (McCreadie *et al.*, 1995) as well decreased lipid-corrected vitamin E levels in schizophrenic patients with tardive dyskinesia (Brown *et al.*, 1998). Lower plasma and urinary vitamin C levels were found decreased, relative to normal controls, even after controlling for diet (Suboticanec *et al.*, 1990). We recently found significantly lower plasma total antioxidant capacity (TAS) in male schizophrenic patients compared to matched normal controls (Yao *et al.*, 1998c). Further, we found reductions in bilirubin and albumin levels (Yao *et al.*, 1998c) as well as reductions in plasma uric acid in schizophrenic patients (Yao *et al.*, 1998d).

Alterations in the antioxidant defence system do not necessarily indicate the presence of oxidative stress and possible membrane lipid damage. Evidence of peroxidative damage, such as measures of lipid peroxidation by-products, is required. This type of evidence in schizophrenia, while limited, has been consistent. There is substantial evidence that oxidative stress *can directly lead* to the type of specific membrane defects described earlier, and that AA is particularly susceptible to oxidative damage (Katsuki and Okuda, 1995). One intriguing finding in schizophrenic patients of an inverse relation between RBC AA concentration and thiobarbituric acid-reactive substances (an index of lipid peroxidation) supports the proposed relations between oxidative stress and membrane pathology (Peet *et al.*, 1994). There is abundant evidence that free radicals are involved in membrane pathology in the CNS (Halliwell, 1992), and may play a role in neuropsychiatric disorders, including schizophrenia (Lohr, 1991). Several independent lines of evidence indicate the presence of oxidative stress in schizophrenia, including measures of oxidative membrane damage products, elevations of which have been reported in first-episode and chronic schizophrenic patients (reviewed in Reddy and Yao, 1996).

Increased blood malondialdehyde levels have been reported in schizophrenic patients relative to normal controls (Prilipko, 1984, 1992; Guliaeva *et al.*, 1988; Sram and Binkova, 1992; McCreadie *et al.*, 1995). More critically, there is evidence of plasma lipid peroxidation at the onset of psychosis in never-medicated, first-episode schizophrenic patients (Scheffer *et al.*, 1995; Mahadik *et al.*, 1998). Increased concentrations of pentane, a marker of lipid peroxidation, have been reported in schizophrenic patients (Kovaleva *et al.*, 1989; Phillips *et al.*, 1993).

The findings discussed above all indicate oxidative stress in *peripheral* tissues. Given that schizophrenia is a brain disorder, what evidence exists for any similar abnormalities in the brain? There have been two reports of post-mortem SOD activity in schizophrenia. A recent study found increased manganese-SOD activity in the temporal and frontal cortices (Loven *et al.*, 1996). An earlier study, that examined only the diencephalon, found no differences between schizophrenic patients and control subjects (Wise *et al.*, 1974). While only suggestive of oxidative stress, electron microscopic studies of brains from schizophrenics have reported large amounts of lipofuscin-like material in oligodendrocytes (Miyakawa *et al.*, 1972), abnormal pigment-laden neurons (Averback, 1981), and axonal deposits of lipofuscin-like bodies (Senitz and Winkelman, 1981). Lipofuscin is a by-product of lipid peroxidation. Most post-mortem brain studies of schizophrenic patients have not reported gliosis, a potential response to neuronal loss (Roberts, 1991). A general, but possibly misleading, assumption is that cell death is a necessary consequence of oxidative stress. If oxidative stress does play a pathophysiological role in schizophrenia, then it is more likely that the membrane abnormalities are sublethal and lead to neuronal dysfunction.

Clinical Implications of Membrane Deficits and Oxidative Stress in Schizophrenia

Of what significance are the alterations in membrane and oxidative stress? The constraint on understanding the clinical implications of these alterations are that the specific pathophysiology in schizophrenia remains unknown. However, there are several intriguing associations between clinical features of schizophrenia and the biochemical measures at issue. For example, in the prefrontal cortex, a key area implicated in schizophrenia, there is evidence for both phospholipid abnormality (e.g. Pettegrew *et al.*, 1993) and impaired free radical metabolism (Levon *et al.*, 1996). Since PUFA are preferentially vulnerable to free radical insult, it is conceivable that decreased membrane EFA levels also exist in these areas. Prominent negative symptoms have been associated with low levels of RBC AA levels (Glen *et al.*, 1994) and low levels of GSH-Px (Buckman *et al.*, 1990). Positive symptoms have been associated with low RBC AA levels (Peet *et al.*, 1995) and correlated with SOD activity (Khan and Das, 1997). We have observed a significant correlation between positive symptoms and plasma GSH-Px (Yao *et al.*, 1998b), and an inverse correlation between negative symptoms and SOD activity in drug-free chronic schizophrenic patients (Yao *et al.*, 1998a). Taken together, these findings suggest that membrane deficits and oxidative stress may mediate illness expression, and further suggest the possibility of therapeutic approaches using currently available treatments (Mahadik and Evans, 1997; Reddy and Yao, 1999).

EFA Supplementation in Schizophrenia

Early studies of EFA supplementation, based on its efficacy in animal models (Costall *et al.*, 1984), were aimed at treating tardive dyskinesia (TD), a motor abnormality associated with chronic antipsychotic treatment. Several studies reported decreased TD severity in open clinical and blind placebo-controlled trials (Nohria and Vaddadi, 1982; Kaiya, 1984). However, in a double-blind placebo-controlled study of EFA supplementation, Vaddadi *et al.* (1989) showed that EFA alone did not improve TD, though it did produce a significant improvement in Weschler memory scale scores and psychopathology scores in a group of psychiatric (primarily schizophrenic) patients. Similar results were obtained by other investigators (Soulairac *et al.*, 1983; Bourguignon, 1984; Wolkin *et al.*, 1986). The failure of these EFA trials to improve movement disorder could be due to using a low dosage, inadequate length of the trial, small number of patients, as well as chronicity and irreversibility of TD (Vaddadi, 1996). However, the improvement in cognitive functioning may be the more important finding of these studies. These few studies suggest that the potential exists for adjunctive treatment with EFA supplementation and possibly antioxidants. However, before embarking on expensive controlled treatment trials, studies are first needed that convincingly demonstrate that oxidative stress and decreased membrane EFA have a role in modifying outcomes in schizophrenia. These studies are underway in our and other laboratories.

Future Directions

We have provided a brief overview of studies that demonstrate the presence of membrane deficits and oxidative stress in schizophrenia, and have suggested that membrane deficits are a consequence of oxidative stress. The obvious implication of these findings is the possibility of therapeutic interventions. However, any rational approach to using adjunctive EFA supplementation and antioxidants will require a series of studies to establish the parameters within which treatment recommendations can be made. For example, it would be important to determine whether these treatments are effective at all stages of illness or only during 'windows' of maximal efficacy (such as at the onset of illness). Vitamin E treatment of tardive dyskinesia has been shown to be most effective when the duration of the dyskinesia is less than 5 years (Lohr and Lavori, 1998; Reddy and Yao, 1998). Further, it would be advantageous to identify whether there are any specific symptom complexes or outcome variables which would be targets for such treatment. It is possible that EFA supplementation and/or antioxidants will be most beneficial as non-specific modifiers of clinical course of the illness, increasing the likelihood of a favourable outcome.

There are a number of known demographic and environmental factors, independent of schizophrenia, that are associated with oxidative stress (Bridges *et al.*, 1993) and need to be taken into account. These include diet, cigarette smoking (Halliwell, 1993), alcohol consumption (Nordmann *et al.*, 1992), environmental pollutants (Papas, 1996) and co-morbid medical conditions. These factors could be additive to the already existing oxidative stress and membrane deficits in schizophrenia.

Finally, it needs to be determined whether the membrane deficits and oxidative stress observed in schizophrenia also have any aetiological relevance. Horrobin (1998) argues for such a possibility. Since phospholipids are key to normal brain development (Clandinin and Jumpsen, 1997), any deviation in fatty acid metabolism during the early critical brain developmental phases and later brain structural modulation can lead to the type of structural abnormalities seen in schizophrenia (Horrobin, 1998). There is also a suggestion that free radicals have a role in cellular development and differentiation (Allen and Ballin, 1989). It is conceivable that there exists a cascade of events leading from impaired antioxidant status to oxidative stress, leading then to membrane deficits, finally resulting in abnormal brain development. This may be one risk factor for the later development of schizophrenia. If this model is shown to be true, then the possibility also exists of developing preventive strategies against schizophrenia.

Acknowledgements

This work was supported in part by the National Alliance for Research in Schizophrenia and Affective Disorders (NARSAD) Young Investigator Award (RR) and a Veterans Administration Merit Review grant (JKY).

References

Abdalla, D.S.P., Manteiro, H.P., Olivera, J.A.C. and Bechara, C.H. (1986) Activities of superoxide dismutase and glutathione peroxidase in schizophrenic and manic depressive patients. *Clinical Chemistry* 32, 805–807.

Allen, R.G. and Ballin, A.K. (1989) Oxidative influence on development and differentiation: an overview of free radical theory of development. *Free Radical Biology and Medicine* 6, 631–661.

Averback, P. (1981) Structural lesions of the brain of young schizophrenics. *Canadian Journal of Neurological Sciences* 8, 73–76.

Bourguignon, A. (1984) Trial of evening primrose oil in the treatment of schizophrenia. *L'Encephale* 10, 241–250.

Bridges, A.B., Scott, N.A., Parry, G.J. and Belch, J.J. (1993) Age, sex, cigarette smoking and indices of free radical activity in health humans. *European Journal of Medicine* 2, 205–208.

Brown, K., Reid, A., White, T., Henderson, T., Hukin, S., Johnstone, C. and Glen, A. (1998) Vitamin E, lipids, lipid peroxidation products and tardive dyskinesia. *Biological Psychiatry* 43, 863–867.

Buckman, T.D., Kling, A.S., Eiduson, S., Sutphin, M.S., Steinberg, A. and Eiduson, S. (1990) Platelet glutathione peroxidase and monoamine oxidase activity in schizophrenics with CT scan abnormalities: relation to psychosocial variables. *Psychiatry Research* 31, 1–14.

Clandinin, M.T. and Jumpsen, J. (1997) Fatty acid metabolism in brain in relation to development, membrane structure, and signaling. In: Yehuda, S. and Mostofsky, D.I. (eds) *Handbook of Essential Fatty Acid Biology: Biochemistry, Physiology, and Behavioral Neurobiology.* Humana Press, Totowa, New Jersey, pp. 15–65.

Cohen, G. (1994) Enzymatic/nonenzymatic sources of oxyradicals and regulation of antioxidant defenses. *Annals of the New York Academy of Science* 738, 8–14.

Costall, B., Kelly, M. and Naylor, R.J. (1984) The antidyskinetic action of dihomo-gamma-linolenic acid in the rodent. *British Journal of Pharmacology* 83, 733–740.

Deicken, R.F., Merrin, E., Calabrese, G., Dillon, W., Weiner, M.W. and Fein, G. (1993) [31]Phosphorus MRSI in the frontal and parietal lobes in schizophrenia. *Biological Psychiatry* 33, 46A.

Glazov, V.A. and Mamzev, V.P. (1976) Catalase in the blood and leucocytes in patients with nuclear schizophrenia. *Zhurnal Nevropatologia Psikhiatrii* 4, 549–552.

Glen, A.I.M., Glen, E.M.T., Horrobin, D.F., Vaddadi, K.S., Speliman, M., Morse-Fisher, N. and Skinner, E.K. (1994) A red cell membrane abnormality in a sub-group of schizophrenic patients: evidence for two disease. *Schizophrenia Research* 12, 53–61.

Golse, B., Debray-Ritzen, P., Puget, K. and Michelson, A.M. (1977) Dosages de la superoxyde dismutases 1 plaquettaire dans les pychoses infantiles de développement. *Nouvelle Presse Medicale* 6, 2449.

Golse, B., Debray, Q., Puget, K. and Michelson, A.M. (1978) Dosages érythrocytaires de la superoxyde dismutases 1 et de la glutathion peroxydase dans les schizophrénies de l'adulte. *Nouvelle Presse Medicale* 7, 2070–2071.

Guliaeva, N.V., Levshina, I.P. and Obidin, A.M. (1988) Indices of lipid free-radical oxidation and the antiradical protection of the brain – the neurochemical correlates of the development of the general adaptation syndrome. *Zhurnal Vysshei Nervnoi Deiatelnosti Imeni I.P. Pavlova (Moscow)* 38, 731–737.

Halliwell, B. (1992) Reactive oxygen species and the central nervous system. *Journal of Neurochemistry* 59, 1609–1623.

Hegarty, J.D., Baldessarini, R.J., Tohen, M., Waternaux, C. and Oepen, G. (1994) One hundred years of schizophrenia: a meta-analysis of the outcome literature. *American Journal of Psychiatry* 151, 1409–1416.

Hoffer, A., Osmand, H. and Smythies, J. (1954) Schizophrenia: new approach. *Journal of Mental Science* 100, 29–45.

Horrobin, D.F. (1996) Schizophrenia as a membrane lipid disorder which is expressed throughout the body. *Prostaglandins, Leukotrienes and Essential Fatty Acids* 55, 3–8.

Horrobin, D.F. (1998) The membrane phospholipid hypothesis as a biochemical basis for the neurodevelopmental concept of schizophrenia. *Schizophrenia Research* 30(3), 193–208.

Horrobin, D.F., Manku, M.S., Morse-Fisher, N., Vaddadi, K.S., Courtney, P., Glen, A.I.M., Glen, E., Spellman, M. and Bates, C. (1989) Essential fatty acid in plasma phospholipids in schizophrenics. *Biological Psychiatry* 25, 562–568.

Horrobin, D.F., Manku, M.S., Hillman, S. and Glen A.I.M. (1991) Fatty acid levels in brains of schizophrenics and normal controls. *Biological Psychiatry* 30, 795–805.

Horrobin, D.F., Glen, A.I.M. and Vaddadi, K. (1994) The membrane hypothesis of schizophrenia. *Schizophrenia Research* 13, 195–207.

Horrobin, D.F., Glen, A.I.M. and Hudson, C.J. (1995) Possible relevance of phospho-lipid abnormalities and genetic interactions in psychiatric disorders: the relationship between dyslexia and schizophrenia. *Medical Hypotheses* 45, 605–613.

Kaiya, H. (1984) Prostaglandin E treatment of schizophrenia. *Biological Psychiatry* 19, 457–462.

Kaiya, H., Horrobin, D.F., Manku, M.S. and Fisher, N.M. (1991) Essential and other fatty acids in plasma in schizophrenics and normal individuals from Japan. *Biological Psychiatry* 30, 357–362.

Kalyanaraman, B. (1989) Free radicals from catecholamine hormones, neuromelanins, and neurotoxins. In: Miquel, J., Quintanilha, A.T. and Weber, H. (eds) *Handbook of Free Radicals and Antioxidants in Biomedicine*, Vol. I. CRC Press, Boca Raton, Florida, pp. 147–159.

Katsuki, H. and Okuda, S. (1995) Arachidonic acid as a neurotoxic and neurotrophic substance. *Progress in Neurobiology* 46, 607–636.

Keshavan, M.S. and Pettegrew, J.W. (1997) Magnetic resonance spectroscopy in schizophrenia and psychotic disorders. In: Krishnan, K.R.R. (ed.) *Brain Imaging in Psychiatry*. Marcel Dekker, New York, pp. 381–400.

Keshavan, M.S., Pettegrew, J.W., Panchalingam, K., Kaplan, D. and Bozik, E. (1991) ^{31}P NMR spectroscopy detects altered brain metabolism before onset of schizophrenia. *Archives of General Psychiatry* 48, 1112–1113.

Keshavan, M.S., Mallinger, A.G., Pettegrew, J.W. and Dippold, C. (1993a) Erythrocyte membrane phospholipids in psychotic patients. *Psychiatry Research* 49, 89–95.

Keshavan, M.S., Pettegrew, J.W. and Ward, R. (1993b) Are membrane phospholipid changes in schizophrenia familial? *Biological Psychiatry* 33, 37A–162A.

Khan, N.S. and Das, I. (1997) Oxidative stress and superoxide dismutase in schizophrenia. *Biochemical Society Transactions* 25, 418S.

Kovaleva, E.S., Orlov, O.N., Tsutsul'kovskia, M.I.A., Vladimirova, T.V. and Beliaev, T.S. (1989) Lipid peroxidation processes in patients with schizophrenia. *Zhurnal Nevropatologi Psikiatrii* 89, 108–110.

Laugharne, J.D., Mellor, J.E. and Peet, M. (1996) Fatty acids and schizophrenia. *Lipids* 31 (Suppl.), 163–165.

Lieberman, J.A. and Koreen, A.R. (1993) Neurochemistry and neuroendocrinology of schizophrenia: a selective review. *Schizophrenia Bulletin* 19, 371–429.

Lohr, J.B. (1991) Oxygen radicals and neuropsychiatric illness: some speculations. *Archives of General Psychiatry* 48, 1097–1106.

Lohr, J.B. and Lavori, P. (1998) Whither vitamin E and tardive dyskinesia? *Biological Psychiatry* 43, 861–862.

Loven, D.P., James, J.F., Biggs, L. and Little, K.Y. (1996) Increased manganese-superoxide dismutase activity in postmortem brain from neuroleptic-treated psychotic patients. *Biological Psychiatry* 40, 230–232.

Mahadik, S.P. and Evans, D.R. (1997) Essential fatty acids in the treatment of schizophrenia. *Drugs of Today* 33, 5–17.

Mahadik, S.P., Mukherjee, S., Correnti, E., Kelkar, H.S., Wakade, C.G., Costa, R.M. and Scheffer, R. (1994) Distribution of plasma membrane phospholipids and cholesterol in skin fibroblasts from drug-naive patients at the onset of psychosis. *Schizophrenia Research* 13, 239–247.

Mahadik, S.P., Mukherjee, S., Correnti, E.E., Kelkar, H.S., Wakade, C.G., Costa, R.M. and Scheffer, R. (1996) Plasma membrane phospholipid fatty acid composition of cultured skin fibroblasts from schizophrenic patients: comparison with bipolar and normal controls. *Psychiatry Research* 63, 133–142.

Mahadik, S.P., Mukherjee, S., Scheffer, R., Correnti, E.E. and Mahadik, J.S. (1998) Elevated plasma lipid peroxides at the onset of nonaffective psychosis. *Biological Psychiatry* 43, 674–679.

McCreadie, R.G., MacDonald, E., Wiles, D., Campbell, G. and Paterson, J.R. (1995) The Nithsdale Schizophrenia Surveys. XIV: Plasma lipid peroxide and serum vitamin E levels in patients with and without tardive dyskinesia, and normal subjects. *British Journal of Psychiatry* 167, 610–617.

Michelson, A.M., Puget, K., Durosay, P. and Bouneau, J.C. (1977) Clinical aspects of the dosage of erythrocuprein. In: Michelson, A.M., McCord, J.M. and Fridovich, I. (eds) *Superoxide and Superoxide Dismutase*. Academic Press, London, pp. 467–499.

Miyakawa, T., Sumiyoshi, S. and Deshimaru, M. (1972) Electron microscopic study on schizophrenia. Mechanism of pathological changes. *Acta Neuropathologica (Berlin)* 20, 67–77.

Mukherjee, S., Mahadik, S.P., Correnti, E.E. and Scheffer, R. (1996) The antioxidant defense system at the onset of psychosis. *Schizophrenia Research* 19, 19–26.

Nohria, V. and Vaddadi, K.S. (1982) Tardive dyskinesia and essential fatty acids: an animal model study. In: Horrobin, D.F. (ed.) *Clinical Uses of Essential Fatty Acids*, pp. 199–204.

Nordmann, R., Ribiere, C. and Rouach, H. (1992) Implication of free radical mechanisms in ethanol-induced cellular injury. *Free Radical Biology and Medicine* 12, 219–240.

Papas, A.M. (1996) Determinants of antioxidant status in humans. *Lipids* 31, S77–82.

Peet, M., Laugharne, J.D.E., Horrobin, D.F. and Reynolds, G.P. (1994) Arachidonic acid: a common link in the biology of schizophrenia. *Archives of General Psychiatry* 51, 665–666.

Peet, M., Laugharne, J.D.E., Rangarajan, N., Horrobin, D.F. and Reynolds, G. (1995) Depleted red cell membrane essential fatty acids in drug-treated schizophrenic patients. *Journal of Psychiatric Research* 29, 227–232.

Peet, M., Laugharne, J.D.E., Mellor, J. and Ramchand, C.N. (1996) Essential fatty acid deficiency in eyrthrocyte membranes from chronic schizophrenic patients, and the clinical effects of dietary supplementation. *Prostaglandins, Leukotrines and Essential Fatty Acids* 55, 71–75.

Pettegrew, J.W., Keshavan, M.S., Panchalingam, K., Strychor, S., Kaplan, D.B., Tretta, M.G. and Allen, M. (1991) Alterations in brain high energy phosphate and membrane phospholipid metabolism in first episode drug naive schizophrenics. *Archives of General Psychiatry* 48, 563–568.

Pettegrew, J.W., Keshavan, M.S. and Minshew, N.J. (1993) ^{31}P nuclear magnetic resonance spectroscopy: neurodevelopment and schizophrenia. *Schizophrenia Bulletin* 19, 335–353.

Phillips, M., Sabas, M. and Greenberg, J. (1993) Increased pentane and carbon disulfide in the breath of patients with schizophrenia. *Journal of Clinical Pathology* 46, 861–864.

Prilipko, L.L. (1984) Activation of lipid peroxidation under stress and in schizophrenia. In: Kemali, D., Morozov, P.V. and Toffano, G. (eds) *New Research Strategies in Biological Psychiatry*. Biological Psychiatry-New Perspectives, no. 3. John Libbey, London.

Prilipko, L.L. (1992) The possible role of lipid peroxidation in the pathophysiology of mental disorders. In: Packer, L., Prilipko, L. and Christen, Y. (eds) *Free Radicals in the Brain*. Springer-Verlag, Berlin, pp.146–152.

Ram, R., Bromet, E.J., Eaton, W.W., Pato, C. and Schwartz, J.E. (1992) The natural course of schizophrenia: a review of first-admission studies. *Schizophrenia Bulletin* 18, 185–207.

Reddy, R. and Yao, J.K. (1996) Free radical pathology in schizophrenia: a review. *Prostaglandins, Leukotrines and Essential Fatty Acids* 55, 33–43.

Reddy, R. and Yao, J.K. (1999) Membrane protective strategies in schizophrenia: conceptual and treatment issue. In: Glen, A.I.M., Peet, M. and Horrobin, D.F. (eds) *Phospholipid Spectrum Disorder in Psychiatry*. Marius Press, Lancashire.

Reddy, R., Mahadik, S.P., Mukherjee, M. and Murthy, J.N. (1991) Enzymes of the antioxidant system in chronic schizophrenic patients. *Biological Psychiatry* 30, 409–412.

Reddy, R., Kelkar, H., Mahadik, S.P. and Mukherjee, S. (1993) Abnormal erythrocyte catalase activity in schizophrenic patients. *Schizophrenia Research* 9, 227.

Rice-Evans, C.A. (1994) Formation of free radicals and mechanisms of action in normal biochemical processes and pathological states. In: Rice-Evans, C.A. and Burdon, R.H. (eds) *Free Radical Damage and its Control*. Elsevier, Amsterdam, pp. 131–153.

Roberts, G.W. (1991) Schizophrenia: a neuropathological perspective. *British Journal of Psychiatry* 158, 8–17.

Rotrosen, J. and Wolkin, A. (1987) Phospholipid and prostraglandin hypotheses of schizophrenia. In: Meltzer, H.Y. (ed.) *Psychopharmacology: the Third Generation of Progress.* Raven Press, New York, pp. 759–764.

Scheffer, R., Diamond, B.I., Correnti, E.E., Borison, R.L., Mahadik, S.P. and Mukherjee, S. (1995) Plasma lipid peroxidation and HVA in first episode psychosis. *Biological Psychiatry* 37, 681.

Senitz, D. and Winkelmann, E. (1981) Über morphologische Befunde in der orbitofrontalen Rinde bei Menschen mit schizophrenen Psychosen. Eine Golgi- und eine elektonenoptische Studie. *Psychiatrie, Neurologie und Medizinische Psychologie* 33, 1–9.

Sinet, P.M., Debray, Q., Carmagnol, F., Pelicier, Y., Nicole, A. and Jerome, H. (1983) Normal erythrocyte SOD values in two human diseases: schizophrenia and cystic fibrosis. In: Greenwald, R.A. and Cohen, G. (eds) *Oxy Radicals and their Scavenger Systems.* Vol. II, *Cellular and Medical Aspects.* Elsevier, New York, pp. 302–304.

Soulairac, A., Lambinet, H. and Neuman, J.C. (1983) Schizophrenia and PGs: therapeutic effects of PG precursors in the form of evening primrose oil. *Annals of Medical Psychology* 8, 883–890.

Sram, R.J. and Binkova, B. (1992) Side-effects of psychotropic therapy. In: Packer, L., Prilipko, L. and Christen, Y. (eds) *Free Radicals in the Brain.* Springer-Verlag, Berlin, pp. 153–166.

Stoklasova, A., Zapletalek, M., Kudrnova, K. and Randova, Z. (1986) Glutathione peroxidase activity of blood in chronic schizophrenics. *Sbornik Vedeckych Praci Lekarske Fakulty UK v Hradci Kralove* (Suppl.) 29(1–2), 103–108.

Suboticanec, K., Folnegovic-Smalc, V., Korbar, M., Mestrovic, B. and Buzina, R. (1990) Vitamin C status in chronic schizophrenia. *Biological Psychiatry* 28, 959–966.

Tacconi, M.T., Calzi, F. and Salmona, M. (1997) Brain lipids and diet. In: Hillbrand, M. and Spitz, R.T. (eds) *Lipids, Health, and Behavior.* American Psychological Association, Washington, DC, pp. 197–226.

Vaddadi, K.S. (1996) Dyskinesias and their treatment with essential fatty acids: a review. *Prostaglandins, Leukotrines and Essential Fatty Acids* 55, 89–94.

Vaddadi, K.S., Courtney, P., Gilleard, C.S., Manku, M.S. and Horrobin, D.F. (1989) A double blind trial of essential fatty acid supplementation in patients with tardive dyskinesia. *Psychiatry Research* 27, 313–323.

Vaiva, G., Thomas, P., Leroux, J.M., Cottencin, O., Dutoit, D. and Erb, F. (1994) Erythrocyte superoxide dismutase (eSOD) determination in positive moments of psychosis. *Therapie* 49, 343–348.

Wang, H. (1992) An investigation on changes in blood CuZn-superoxide dismutase contents in type I, II schizophrenics. *Chung Hua Shen Ching Ching Shen Ko Tsa Chih* 25, 6–8.

Wise, C.D., Baden, M.M. and Stein, L. (1974) Post-mortem measurement of enzymes in human brain: evidence of a central noradrenergic deficit in schizophrenia. *Journal of Psychiatric Research* 11, 185–198.

Wolkin, A., Jordan, B., Peselow, E., Rubinstein, M. and Rotrosen, J. (1986) Essential fatty acid supplementation in tardive dyskinesia. *American Journal of Psychiatry* 143, 912–914.

Wyatt, R.J. (1995) Antipsychotic medication and the long-term course of schizophrenia. In: Shriqui, C.L. and Nasrallah, H.A. (eds) *Contemporary Issue in the Treatment of Schizophrenia.* American Psychiatric Press, Washington, DC, pp. 385–410.

Yao, J.K., van Kammen, D.P., Gurklis, J. and Peters, J.L. (1994a) Platelet aggregation and secretion in schizophrenia. *Psychiatry Research* 54, 3–24.

Yao, J.K., van Kammen, D.P. and Welker, J.A. (1994b) Red blood cell membrane dynamics in schizophrenia. II. Fatty acid composition. *Schizophrenia Research* 13, 217–226.

Yao, J.K., Reddy, R., van Kammen, D.P. and Kelley, M.E. (1998) Superoxide dismutase and negative symptoms in schizophrenia. *Biological Psychiatry* 43, 123S–124S.

Yao, J.K., Reddy, R., McElhinny, L.G. and van Kammen, D.P. (1998a) Effect of haloperidol on antioxidant defense system enzymes in schizophrenia. *Journal of Psychiatric Research*, in press.

Yao, J.K., Reddy, R., McElhinny, L.G. and van Kammen, D.P. (1998b) Reduced status of plasma total antioxidant capacity in schizophrenia. *Schizophrenia Research* 32, 1–8.

Yao, J.K., Reddy, R. and van Kammen, D.P. (1998c) Reduced level of plasma antioxidant uric acid in schizophrenia. *Psychiatry Research* 80, 29–39.

Yao, J.K., Reddy, R. and van Kammen, D.P. (1998d) Plasma specific glutathione peroxidase and symptom severity in schizophrenia. *Biological Psychiatry*, in press.

Zhang, Z.J., Ramchand, C.N., Ramchand, R., Milner, E., Telang, S.D. and Peet, M. (1998) Glutathione peroxidase (GSHPx) activity in plasma and fibroblasts from schizophrenics and control. *Schizophrenia Research* 29, 103–104.

β-Amyloid and Oxidative Stress in the Pathogenesis of Alzheimer's Disease

28

RALPH N. MARTINS[1], CHIN WERN CHAN[1], EMMA WADDINGTON[1], GERALD VEURINK[1], SIMON LAWS[1], KEVIN CROFT[2] AND A.M. DHARMARAJAN[3]

[1]*Department of Surgery, University of Western Australia, Hollywood Private Hospital, Nedlands, Australia;* [2]*Department of Medicine, The University of Western Australia, Royal Perth Hospital, Perth, Australia;* [3]*Department of Anatomy and Human Biology, The University of Western Australia, Nedlands, Australia*

Introduction

Alzheimer's disease (AD) is a progressive neurodegenerative disorder characterized by loss of memory and cognition. AD accounts for two-thirds of all dementia cases (Ott *et al.*, 1995; Hardy, 1996). This statistic is particularly significant in the Western world where surveys have uniformly shown that more than 70% of nursing home residents suffer from dementia. Furthermore, AD, a severe form of dementia, represents the most common neurological disorder in old age and ranks as the third leading cause of natural death in the elderly in the developed world after cardiovascular disease and cancer (Hardy and Allsop, 1991). The prevalence increases exponentially with advancing age to reach one in five by 80 years of age (Evans *et al.*, 1989).

Furthermore, with successful cures for infectious diseases, rapid advances in medical technology and improved health standards many more of us will be living longer and will thus reach the age at which neurodegenerative diseases (especially AD) are common. Epidemiologists have predicted that if the average life expectancy ever reaches 100 years, one-third of the population will be affected by AD (Katzman, 1986).

Despite rapid progression in our knowledge of AD there remains no effective treatment or prevention for it. Hence, AD represents a potential crisis for the health care system. Already, the estimated cost to American society for the diagnosis and management of AD is estimated to be $60–120 billion annually (Hendrie, 1997). The majority of this is for custodial care. However, a more distressing aspect of this form of dementia is the severe burden placed upon health carers and patients' families. Consequently, AD has given rise to major medical, social and economic problems in the Western world.

The aetiology and pathogenesis of AD remains an area of great interest and debate. Progress in AD research in the last 15–20 years has been rapid, with the identification of several genes, proteins and toxins associated with the development of AD. These recent advances have provided a better understanding of the pathogenesis of AD. A key molecule central to the pathogenesis of AD is a 4 kDa peptide known as β-amyloid (Aβ). The neuronal loss seen in the AD brain is thought to result from a state of oxidative stress induced by Aβ. Oxidative stress causes metabolic and functional disruption in neurons and other cells of the central nervous system (CNS), culminating in cell death via an apoptotic mechanism.

Neuropathology of Alzheimer's Disease

Morphological characteristics of AD

The original definition of AD was based upon characteristic morphology associated with the AD brain. To this day, the histological features of the AD brain remain as hallmarks of this form of dementia.

Macroscopically, the AD brain is smaller than average. The atrophy is usually symmetrical between the hemispheres, though the degree of atrophy between lobes sometimes varies. Typically, the temporal lobes and temporal poles are more severely affected, with marked involvement of the medial temporal lobe and the associated areas. These changes in the medial temporal lobe are visible on computer tomography (CT) and magnetic resonance imaging (MRI) scans. Conversely, the primary motor and sensory regions of the brain are relatively spared.

Histopathological features of AD

Histologically, AD is characterized by the presence of neurofibrillary tangles within neurons and senile plaques located outside neurons (Alzheimer,

1907). Another common pathological feature of the AD brain is the presence of amyloid deposits in and around blood vessels known as congophilic amyloid angiopathy. A common feature of these lesions is the presence of amyloid deposits which have similar secondary structures and thus take up the dye Congo red which characteristically stains amyloid proteins having β-pleated sheets.

Neurofibrillary tangles

Neurofibrillary tangles (NFT) are found within the nerve cells. They are found in greater numbers in AD patients, primarily in regions associated with memory and other intellectual functions. A major component of the tangles is a protein called tau. Tau is responsible for directing assembly and disassembly of microtubules. In the NFT the tau protein is abnormally phosphorylated. It is thought that excessive phosphorylation of the tau protein may prevent it from stabilizing microtubules, which accumulate to form amyloid fibrils within the nerve cell, thereby causing breakdown in the structural framework. The NFT is formed later than the senile plaque and is thought to result from the toxic action of the extracellular amyloid.

Amyloid plaques

There is extensive variation in amyloid plaque morphology. However, comprehensive histological analysis has identified two categories of plaques: diffuse and neuritic (Yamaguchi *et al.*, 1988; Wisniewski *et al.*, 1989; Schmidt *et al.*, 1994). Diffuse plaques, which reflect newly formed deposits, do not elicit gliosis and are thought to be benign. They are abundant in the brains of some non-demented elderly individuals as well as in the brains of AD patients (Yamaguchi *et al.*, 1988; Wisniewski *et al.*, 1989; Schmidt *et al.*, 1994).

Neuritic plaques are focal, spherical collections of dilated, tortuous, silver-staining neuritic processes (dystrophic neurites) surrounding a central amyloid core. They are very common in AD patients. These plaques contain abundant amyloid fibrils and are intensely stained by Thioflavin S, Congo red as well as several different types of silver stains (Trojanowski *et al.*, 1993). Neuritic plaques are not common in normal ageing. Hence, this form of amyloid plaque is a better indicator of AD than the diffuse plaque. The major protein component of both the diffuse and neuritic plaque is a 4 kDa peptide termed β-amyloid.

β-Amyloid and Amyloid Precursor Protein

β-Amyloid (Aβ)

Aβ is a 4 kDa hydrophobic protein, composed of 39–43 amino acids. Aβ was discovered when it was isolated from the meningeal blood vessels (Glenner and Wong, 1984) and the cores of the amyloid plaques (Masters *et al.*, 1985) of AD patients.

There are two major types of Aβ, which differ according to the amino acid length of the peptide: Aβ1–40 and Aβ1–42. Aβ1–40 is the major form of Aβ deposited in sporadic AD (Masters et al., 1985), whereas amyloid deposits associated with early onset familial AD have been shown to contain increased amounts of Aβ1–42 (Roher et al., 1993; Suzuki et al., 1994; Yan et al., 1994; Younkin, 1995).

A number of groups have demonstrated that selected regions of Aβ have certain characteristics that may be important in understanding its behaviour and hence toxicity. The first 28 residues constitute an extra-cellular domain whereas residues 29–40/42 are involved with anchoring the peptide in the lipid membrane (Fraser et al., 1991). Pillot et al. (1996) have suggested that the fusogenic properties of the peptide's C-terminal domain destabilizes cellular membranes. The hydrophobic region of Aβ also directs folding of the peptide and aggregation. The importance of the hydrophobic region is reflected by the difference in behaviour of the two forms of Aβ. The longer peptide (Aβ1–42) aggregates more easily than Aβ1–40 and becomes a seed for the formation of insoluble amyloid fibrils, leading to the neurotoxicity seen in AD (Jarret and Lansbury, 1993). This has led some investigators to suggest that Aβ1–42 is the real culprit in the pathological development of AD. The neurotoxic action has been localized to amino acid residues 25–35 of Aβ. This region by itself has been shown to induce cell death at a much faster rate than the long forms of Aβ (Mattson, 1995).

The amyloid precursor protein

Following the discovery of Aβ, oligonucleotides based on the Aβ sequence were used to isolate complementary DNA clones encoding a precursor protein to Aβ (Goldgaber et al., 1987; Kang et al., 1987; Robakis et al., 1987; Tanzi et al., 1987). This protein was named the amyloid precursor protein (APP). The APP gene is a single copy gene that is widely conserved in evolution and is expressed in virtually all cells and tissue types of the human body.

Structure of APP

The APP gene is located on chromosome 21q21.2 (Kang et al., 1987) and consists of 18 exons which encode APP. Exons 16 and 17 together encode Aβ (Yoshikai et al., 1990). APP belongs to a family of eight transmembrane glycoproteins (Sandbrink et al., 1994). The APP gene is known to produce six different species of messenger RNAs, all sharing the same amino-terminal sequence. The three major Aβ-containing proteins are 695, 751 and 770 amino acids long. APP 695 is the major isoform found in the brain. APP751 and APP770 contain exon 7 which encodes a domain homologous to a Kunitz protease inhibitor.

Distribution of APP in the brain

APP is found in several cell types of the brain. However, the only cell type that constitutively expresses large amounts of APP are neurons. In neurons, newly synthesized APP is first delivered from the cell body to the axon but later appears in the dendrites (Simons *et al.*, 1995). APP is most commonly found in the pre- and post-synaptic membranes (Schubert *et al.*, 1991; Simons *et al.*, 1995). Microglia and astrocytes can express high levels of APP but only upon activation (Beyreuther *et al.*, 1996).

Processing of APP

Two major competing pathways exist that are capable of processing APP (Fig. 28.1). Each pathway involves the actions of proteases that cleave the protein at certain sites to produce fragments that may be either non-amyloidogenic (do not contain the full Aβ sequence) or amyloidogenic (contains the complete Aβ sequence) (Hardy and Higgins, 1992; Haass and Selkoe, 1993; Citron *et al.*, 1995).

The non-amyloidogenic pathway, which is the constitutive secretory pathway, processes the majority of APP. In this setting an α-secretase (Fig. 28.1) cleaves APP within the Aβ sequence and consequently intact Aβ is not produced (Esch *et al.*, 1990). Therefore this pathway is non-amyloidogenic and does not contribute to the pathological lesions of AD. The non-amyloidogenic products are soluble APP (APPs) and a 10 kDa APP fragment, termed p10, which only contains the first 16 amino acid residues of the Aβ sequence.

Alternatively, APP may be proteolytically cleaved by the competing amyloidogenic pathway that results in the release of fragments which include intact Aβ. An endosomal/lysosomal pathway capable of processing APP to produce Aβ-containing 11 kDa C-terminal fragments has been identified. In this route the membrane-bound APP is reinternalized from the cell surface and is then degraded into potentially amyloidogenic fragments accumulating in the lysosomes. Intact Aβ is released by the proteolytic action of two enzymes (Fig. 28.1). One protease, β-secretase, cleaves at the N terminus of Aβ producing C-terminal fragments containing the entire Aβ domain (Seubert *et al.*, 1993). A second enzyme, γ-secretase, then cleaves at the C terminus to release intact Aβ (Haass and Selkoe, 1993).

Neurotoxicity of Aβ

Research from a number of studies indicates that Aβ plays a central role in the development of AD pathology. One line of evidence stems from examination of the histological lesions where dystrophic neurites are found to surround the amyloid plaques. Furthermore, the density of astrocytes and microglia in plaques is higher than that of surrounding tissue (Braak and Braak, 1996). Experimental studies in rat hippocampal cultures have provided further support for Aβ as a causative factor in AD. Exposure to Aβ

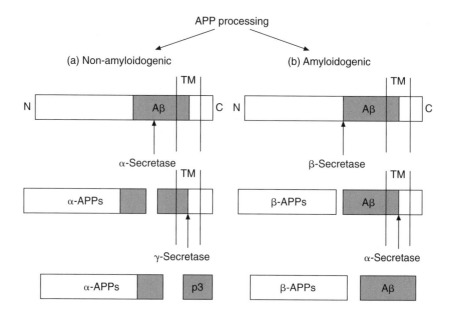

Fig. 28.1. Competing pathways of APP processing. The non-amyloidogenic pathway (a) is characterized by the activity of α-secretase, which cleaves within the Aβ domain, preventing the formation of the Aβ fragment. The amyloidogenic pathway (b) is characterized by the cleaving of the Aβ domain at the N terminus by β-secretase. After cleavage by these enzymes another postulated enzyme, γ-secretase, cleaves within the TM region at the C terminus of the Aβ domain. This allows the formation of the non-amyloidogenic p3 fragment and the amyloidogenic Aβ fragment, depending on the initial pathway. Arrows from enzymes indicate site of action; α-APPs, soluble APP resulting from α-secretase action; β-APPs, soluble APP resulting from β-secretase action; p3, non-amyloidogenic fragment; TM, transmembrane domain.

resulted in neurites displaying pathology resembling that seen in AD (dystrophic neurites) (Games *et al.*, 1995; Higgins and Cordell, 1995; Hsiao *et al.*, 1995; LaFerla *et al.*, 1995). Strong evidence in support of a primary role for Aβ in the pathogenesis of AD comes from a number of genetic studies. A few families with early-onset AD are associated with mutations in the APP gene. These pathogenic mutations are clustered within or around the Aβ sequence and result in either increased total Aβ production or else preferential production of the longer and more neurotoxic Aβ1–42 (Citron *et al.*, 1992, 1994; Cai *et al.*, 1993; Haass *et al.*, 1994; Suzuki *et al.*, 1994). Furthermore, these mutations were demonstrated to be pathogenic in transgenic animal models of AD where the inclusion of APP mutation resulted in neuropathology consistent with having AD. Additional genetic evidence is provided by individuals affected with Down's syndrome who invariably develop the neuropathology of AD. These individuals possess three copies of chromosome 21 and therefore have an increased Aβ load (Wisniewski et al., 1985; Tanzi et al., 1987; Teller et al., 1996). In addition, mutations in the presenilin genes, located on chromosomes 1 and 14, have been demonstrated to increase APP mRNA and Aβ levels (Levy-Lahad et al., 1995; Querfurt et al., 1995; Sherrington et al., 1995; Selkoe, 1996; Sheuner et al., 1996). Finally, the ε4 allele of the apolipoprotein E gene, which is a major risk factor for late-onset AD (Strittmatter et al., 1993a; Martins et al., 1995), is associated with increased density of Aβ plaques in AD brains with this ε4 genotype (Strittmatter et al., 1993b). Taken together, these numerous findings demonstrate that the various genetic causes of AD all result in a final common biochemical pathway, namely the enhanced deposition of Aβ which forms the toxic neuritic plaques and congophilic angiopathy (Table 28.1; Mattson et al., 1998).

The mechanism(s) by which Aβ exerts its toxicity is currently under intense investigation though substantial evidence already exists to suggest that its toxic effects are mediated via the production of oxygen free radicals.

Observations made by Butterfield (1997) suggest that Aβ interacts with and causes membrane lipid peroxidation damage in a selective manner and that the structure of the peptide radical is important in its ability to cause membrane damage, such that soluble non-toxic Aβ does not promote synaptosomal membrane lipid peroxidation.

One consequence of lipid peroxidation is the production of 4-hydroxy-nonenal, an aldehyde that covalently binds to membrane proteins involved in the regulation of ion homeostasis and impairs their function. These proteins include the Na^+/K^+-ATPase, the Ca^{2+}-ATPase, and the glutamate and glucose transporters (Mattson, 1998). Therefore, lipid peroxidation is an early event in the pathogenesis of AD.

In addition to AD, lipid peroxidation has been implicated in a growing list of pathological conditions which include atherosclerosis and cancer (Lawson and Maxey, 1996). Accurate and efficient assays to measure the degree of lipid peroxidation is imperative for clinical and scientific applications.

Previously, measurements of lipid peroxidation have been based on the formation of aldehydes, peroxides, conjugated dienes or malondialdehyde (MDA). The most commonly used technique involved the reaction of aldehydes, produced during the decomposition of lipid peroxides, with thiobarbituric acid. However, this method has recently been found to be both ambiguous and inaccurate (Lawson and Maxey, 1996). The measurement of MDA by the thiobarbituric acid assay was found to over-estimate the actual MDA levels by more than tenfold and hence produced an inaccurate representation of the level of lipid peroxidation (Patrono and FitzGerald, 1997). Several assays were then developed to measure peroxides, but further analysis revealed that peroxides were a very unstable class of compounds and many errors are produced (Lawson and Maxey,

Table 28.1. Genetics of Alzheimer's disease. (From Mattson, 1998.)

	Gene	Chromosome	Prevalence (%)	Onset age	Pathogenetic mechanism
Causal	APP	21	1	45–65	Increased Aβ1–42 production, decreased sAPPα
	Presenilin 1	14	8	28–50	Increased Aβ1–42 production, perturbed Ca^{2+} regulation, apoptosis
	Presenilin 2	1	1	40–55	Increased Aβ1–42 production, Apoptosis
	????	12	5	40–55	?????
Risk	Apolipoprotein E	19		60–85	Vascular damage, increased Aβ1–40 deposition
	Mitochondrial DNA	–	????	60–85	Impaired metabolism, oxidative stress

1996). Assays designed to measure conjugated dienes were found to suffer from interference at the lower end of the ultraviolet (UV) spectrum and hence lack sensitivity (Lawson and Maxey, 1996).

Currently, measurement of isoprostanes is considered the most reliable measure of lipid peroxidation due to their chemical stability and their excellent chromatographic characteristics (Lawson and Maxey, 1996). Isoprostanes are prostaglandin-like compounds generated by the free radical-induced oxidation of unsaturated fatty acids in membrane. These compounds are thought to be the best indicators of the oxidative status of an organism (also see Chapter 30).

Protein oxidation

All amino acids of proteins are susceptible to attack by oxidants and free radicals. As the free radicals attack the amino acids they cause structural modifications in both secondary and tertiary structure. Consequently, aggregation or crosslinking of proteins and protein degradation or fragmentation results in impaired activity of the affected proteins, leading to modified membrane and cellular function (Rice-Evans and Burdon, 1994). An important group of proteins that are often subject to modification by reactive oxygen species (ROS) are the cellular membrane ion transport proteins. Transport proteins, such as the Na^+/K^+-ATPases and Ca^{2+}-ATPases, if attacked, can result in ion imbalances which lead to cell death (Butterfield, 1997; Keller *et al.*, 1997).

DNA damage

Free radical damage to DNA can be observed in a wide range of cells; however, the mitochondrial DNA is particularly susceptible to oxidative stress due to a high O_2 consumption (hence they are a continuous source of oxygen radicals), and an unprotected position close to the inner membrane where free radicals are produced. Studies have shown that there is an age-related increase in oxidative damage not only to mitochondrial DNA but also to other DNA (Benzi and Moretti, 1995). A threefold enhancement of oxidative damage to DNA has also been reported in the AD brain (Benzi and Moretti, 1995). Nuclear DNA damage in the cortex of AD patients is double that of normal controls, indicating that free radicals may damage DNA in this disorder (Benzi and Moretti, 1995).

Evidence for Oxidative Stress in Alzheimer's Disease

Our group provided the first evidence in support of the role of oxidative stress in the pathogenesis of AD (Martins *et al.*, 1986). In this study, increased activities of glucose-6-phosphate dehydrogenase (G6PD) and

6-phosphogluconate dehydrogenase (6PGD) were detected in AD brains (Martins *et al.*, 1986). G6PD and 6PGD are enzymes of the hexose monophosphate shunt. We postulated that the increased activities of G6PD and 6PGD were a response to an increased demand for NADPH by the glutathione-dependent peroxide-detoxifying system (Martins *et al.*, 1986). Therefore, the increased activities of these enzymes indicate increased free radical production, specifically H_2O_2 in the AD brain. Since increased activity of G6PD and 6PGD are associated with decreased glucose utilization by the glycolytic pathway, it is tempting to speculate that the decreased glucose utilization observed in the AD brain (Balzacs and Leon, 1994) is, in part, a result of oxidative stress promoting increased G6PD and 6PGD activities and thus increased flux of glucose utilization by the hexose monophosphate pathway at the expense of the glycolytic pathway.

Another indicator of oxidative stress in AD is glutamine synthetase, an enzyme which is highly sensitive to oxidative stress. Reduced activity of glutamine synthetase has been reported in the AD brain (Smith *et al.*, 1991). Direct evidence of enhanced lipid peroxidation in the brains of AD patients has also been reported (Subbaro *et al.*, 1990). More recent evidence comes in the form of antioxidant protection against the development of AD lesions (e.g. EUK8, melatonin and vitamin E) (Behl *et al.*, 1992; Bruce *et al.*, 1996; Pappolla *et al.*, 1997) and the decreased levels of endogenous antioxidants in AD (reviewed by Shinobu and Beal, 1997).

Support for the oxidative stress hypothesis in AD has been strengthened further with research directly demonstrating the generation of free radicals by Aβ. Using sensitive assays and detection methods such as the dichlorofluorescein diacetate assay (DCFDA) and electron paramagnetic spectroscopy (EPR), several groups have identified H_2O_2 as the major ROS generated by Aβ (Behl *et al.*, 1994b; Butterfield *et al.*, 1994; Harris *et al.*, 1995; Café *et al.*, 1996).

The Central Nervous System: an Increased Susceptibility to Free Radical Damage

Free radical-induced damage is not unique to AD. It has also been implicated as the major pathogenic process underlying the other neuro-degenerative disorders: amyotrophic lateral sclerosis, Down's syndrome and Parkinson's disease.

A host of unique anatomical, physiological and biochemical charac-teristics makes the CNS more vulnerable to the effects of free radicals: in particular, the level of oxidative metabolic activity is disproportionate to the size of the brain. This is reflected by normal cerebral oxygen consumption in conscious young men which amounts to 3.5 ml O_2 100 g^{-1} brain min^{-1} (Sokoloff, 1960). Thus, in the brain, 2% of body weight accounts for 20% of the resting total body oxygen consumption.

The protection in the CNS to oxidation is low relative to other systems. Specifically there are lower levels of antioxidants (e.g. glutathione) and protective enzyme activity (e.g. glutathione peroxidase, catalase and super-oxide dismutase). Conversely, the CNS contains abundant polyunsaturated fatty membranes. Lipid membranes are extremely susceptible to free radical-mediated destruction. The cells in the CNS are non-replicating. Once they have been damaged they may be dysfunctional for life. The CNS neural network is readily disrupted.

The Relation of ROS Generation to Aβ Effects

Free radical-mediated toxicity can account for the multiple metabolic and functional impairments demonstrated when cells are exposed to Aβ. An increased vulnerability to excitotoxicity, disruption of calcium homeostasis and an impaired glucose uptake have been reported in cells treated with Aβ. Due to their destructive effects on lipid membranes and proteins, ROS can induce these cellular dysfunctions. A proposed scheme of Aβ toxicity incorporating the oxidative stress hypothesis and the major impairments in cellular function are illustrated in Fig. 28.2.

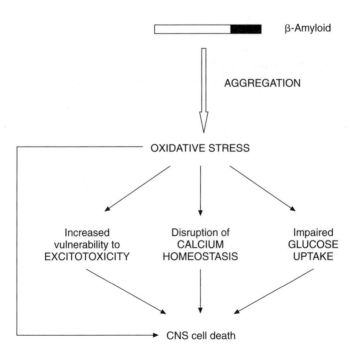

Fig. 28.2. Proposed scheme of Aβ-induced neurotoxicity resulting in cell death.

Disruption of calcium homeostasis

Administration of Aβ to neuronal cultures disrupts calcium homeostasis with a significantly increased intracellular free calcium concentration. The increased intracellular calcium levels result from the flow of calcium ions from the extracellular compartment (Joseph and Han, 1992; Zhou *et al.*, 1996). Zhou *et al.* (1996) further demonstrated that the entry of calcium was not mediated by voltage-dependent calcium channels (VDCC) by showing that Aβ still caused an increased $[Ca^{2+}]_I$ in the presence of VDCC blockers. The study also demonstrated that U83836E and vitamin E (potent antioxidants) blocked the increase in $[Ca^{2+}]_I$ and the Aβ25–35 cytotoxicity, consistent with a free radical hypothesis explaining Aβ toxicity. ROS would target the proteins important in transporting calcium to the extracellular space and disrupt lipid membranes making cells more permeable to calcium (Fig. 28.3).

Apart from free radical-mediated increases in intracellular calcium, several studies have demonstrated an ability of Aβ to form channels in planar lipid bilayer membranes (Pike *et al.*, 1991; Arispe *et al.*, 1993). The Aβ-induced channels are able to conduct calcium current (Arispe *et al.*, 1993; Mirzabckov *et al.*, 1994). However, these channels are formed at levels which are five times the physiological concentration of Aβ. It would seem more logical that the ROS-induced intracellular calcium increase is the first and primary means by which disruption of calcium homeostasis develops. Aβ aggregation to form calcium ion channels may occur but this would come at a time when ROS have induced an already substantial increase in intracellular calcium levels.

This increased intracellular calcium further potentiates oxidative stress in a number of ways. Firstly, a calcium-induced increase in phospholipase

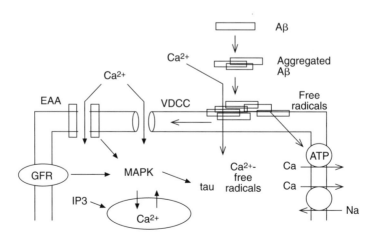

Fig. 28.3. Disruption of calcium homeostasis.

activity leads to increased arachidonic acid levels and production of oxygen radicals via fatty acid metabolism (Kontos, 1989). The mitochondria, in response to excessive calcium, develop problems with electron transport, leading to mitochondrial leakage of electrons generating superoxide anions (Beal, 1992). Thus, a cycle of ROS-induced calcium influx with further ROS generation can ensue.

Increased vulnerability to excitotoxicity

Synaptic communication in the CNS is carried out by neurotransmitters. These chemicals diffuse across the synaptic space and induce either an excitatory or inhibitory effect on postsynaptic neurons. The most common excitatory neurotransmitter is glutamate, an amino acid. Excitotoxicity is the concept by which excitatory stimulation is so intense it becomes neurotoxic and induces neuronal death.

Reports to date have implicated Aβ as increasing neuronal vulnerability to excitotoxic-mediated death (Koh *et al.*, 1990; Mattson *et al.*, 1992). One cellular process that is important for preventing excitotoxicity is the uptake of glutamate from the extracellular space via cellular protein transport systems. This leaves less glutamate to stimulate the NMDA receptor and so reduces the chance of excitotoxicity. Although neurons can take up glutamate, a more important cell is the astrocyte. These cells are abundant around synapses. Astrocytes are much more efficient than neurons at taking up glutamate (V_{max} is several-fold higher than the neurons) (McLennan, 1976; Hertz and Schousboe, 1986; Holsie *et al.*, 1986). Therefore, Aβ-induced free radical damage to astrocytic membrane proteins would hinder this important protective mechanism (Fig. 28.4).

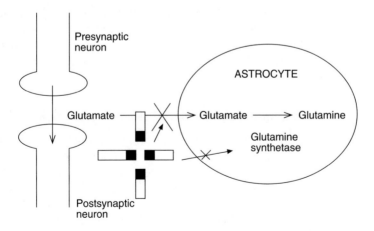

Fig. 28.4. Increased vulnerability to excitotoxicity.

Toxic glutamate is converted into the inactive metabolite glutamine by glutamine synthetase (GS). This enzyme is mainly present in astrocytes. This enzyme is inhibited under conditions of significant oxidative stress (Harris *et al.*, 1995). It is hypothesized that the reduction in GS activity may result in excessive glutamate accumulation and exacerbation of excitotoxicity. Apart from GS activity, astrocytes also secrete growth factors, which have been shown to protect hippocampal neurons in culture from Aβ-induced oxidative stress, disturbances of calcium homeostasis and neuronal death (Mattson *et al.*, 1993).

Impairment of glucose transport

The brain is a highly metabolic organ and its primary substrate is glucose which provides energy for cognitive function. Neurons themselves are incapable of glucose storage or synthesis. Glucose is obtained from the systemic circulation and the supply to the brain is one of the most highly regulated functions in the body. Hence the cognitive areas in the brain are extremely vulnerable to alterations in glucose regulation and utilization.

The results of oral glucose tolerance tests and *in vitro* studies of skin fibroblast response to glucose in AD patients have revealed systemic abnormalities in glucose regulation and availability (Craft *et al.*, 1992). Furthermore, the manipulation of glycaemic states in AD patients (increasing glucose utilization) has resulted in significant improvements in memory. Craft *et al.* (1996) induced hyperinsulinaemia, following a glucose load, and observed a corresponding improvement in memory. They hypothesized that this effect was due to improving glucose utilization in the hippocampus and surrounding medial temporal cortex. Glucose utilization is also related to the levels of the acetylcholine neurotransmitter.

In AD there are significant deficiencies of glucose uptake in neurons and vascular endothelial cells (Blanc *et al.*, 1997). In these cells a reduced number of glucose transporter proteins (GLUT1) has been reported (Horwood and Davies, 1994; Simpson *et al.*, 1994). These findings may be a consequence of Aβ-induced membrane lipid peroxidation (Fig. 28.5) (Mark *et al.*, 1997).

Interrelationship of Aβ-induced cellular dysfunction

It must be pointed out that the three forms of cellular dysfunction, excitotoxicity, disruption of calcium homeostasis and impairment of glucose uptake, are interrelated. Excitotoxicity causes an increase in intracellular calcium; likewise the disruption of calcium homeostasis increases the susceptibility of neurons to excitotoxicity. Hypoglycaemia also sensitizes cells to excitotoxic damage. Furthermore, both excitotoxicity and increased intracellular calcium can lead to the generation of more free radicals and perpetuation of Aβ-initiated oxidative stress.

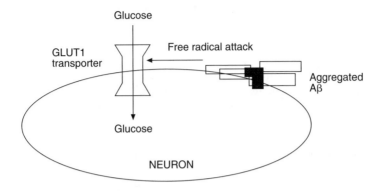

Fig. 28.5. Impaired glucose uptake.

The above discussion has mainly concentrated on the generation of ROS by Aβ. However, it is important to also be aware that there are other sources of oxidative stress in AD. The presence of advanced glycation end products (AGEs) (Smith *et al.*, 1994; Smith and Perry, 1995), redox active metals (Markesberry *et al.*, 1996; Multhaup *et al.*, 1996), leaky mitochondria (Parker *et al.*, 1994), reactive microglia (Colton *et al.*, 1994), glutamate activation of NMDA receptors (Mattson, 1995), and nitric oxide (Estevez *et al.*, 1995) in AD brains are immediate sites of ROS generation and therefore complementary to Aβ's ROS-induced damage.

β-Amyloid-induced Cell Death: Apoptosis

Apoptosis is a form of cell death morphologically distinct from necrosis. It is distinguished from necrosis by morphological, biochemical and genetic characteristics. Morphologically, cells undergoing apoptosis display chromatin condensation, cell shrinkage, membrane blebbing and the release of apoptotic bodies from the cell (Tilly and Hsueh, 1993). A distinguishing feature of apoptosis is the activation of a calcium/magnesium-dependent endonuclease, which cleaves cellular DNA at regularly spaced nucleosomal units to produce fragments in multiples of 185–200 bp (Zeleznick *et al.*, 1989; Gaido and Cidlowski, 1991; Giannakis *et al.*, 1991). The fragments are displayed as a characteristic ladder pattern after ethidium bromide staining (Wyllie, 1980).

Although the process of cell death in AD is not fully resolved, recent evidence suggests that apoptosis is the primary means of cell death (Loo *et al.*, 1993; Cotman and Anderson, 1995; Lassman *et al.*, 1995; Nagy and Eserij, 1997). This would be consistent with the oxidative stress hypothesis, as many substances that induce apoptosis also generate ROS (Buttke and Sandstrom, 1994). H_2O_2, the primary mediator of Aβ toxicity, has been shown to induce apoptosis in a variety of cell types (Lennon *et al.*, 1991).

Antioxidant Therapy in AD

Vitamin E taken at 1000 IU twice daily has recently been shown to delay the advent of a poor outcome (death, institutionalization or significant functional decline) in patients with moderate AD (reviewed by Brodaty and Sachdev, 1997). Vitamin E taken together with vitamin C may prove to be more beneficial to AD patients as vitamin C recycles vitamin E to its active form (also see Chapter 2).

Pycnogenol, which represents a group of flavonoids called proantho-cyanidins, may be a prime candidate in the treatment of disorders associated with oxidative damage (Rong *et al.*, 1994). It was shown to be a more potent scavenger of free radicals than vitamin E and ascorbic acid (Bagchi, 1997). One component of pycnogenol, procyanidin C-1 3,3',3''-tri-O-gallate, has been reported to be 50 times more potent than vitamin E under *in vitro* conditions (Uchida *et al.*, 1987). The high potency of this antioxidant certainly warrants investigation for comparison with vitamin E in animal models of AD.

Sex hormones have been shown to protect against the effects of oxidative stress. Oestrogen was found to protect cultured hippocampal neurons against $A\beta$ toxicity (Goodman *et al.*, 1996). Lipid peroxidation induced by $FeSO_4$ and $A\beta$ was also significantly attenuated in neurons and isolated membranes pretreated with oestrogens and progesterone, suggesting that these hormones may possess antioxidant capacities (Goodman *et al.*, 1996). In a recent clinical trial Tang *et al.* (1996) reported that oestrogen decreased the relative risk of developing AD and delays the age of onset of this disorder. Taken together with the *in vitro* data, oestrogen appears to protect against AD by combating oxidative stress.

Conclusions

There is now overwhelming evidence to demonstrate that in both early- and late-onset AD the 4 kDa peptide $A\beta$ is the major culprit. The literature strongly supports the hypothesis that $A\beta$ exerts its toxicity by free radical-mediated processes. The beneficial effects observed in AD patients treated with antioxidants further indicate that oxidative damage is central to the pathogenesis of AD. The most effective treatment for AD would ultimately involve drugs that inhibit or retard the production of $A\beta$. However, recent work with antioxidant therapy suggests another promising avenue. Further work with more potent antioxidants, taken in combination, and given at an earlier stage of the disease may eventually prove to be more effective in treating this devastating disease.

References

Alzheimer, A. (1907) Uber eine eigenartige. Erkrankung der Himrinde. *Allg. Z. Psychiatrie (Berlin)* 64, 164–168.

Arispe, N., Rojas, E. and Pollard, H.B. (1993) Alzheimer disease amyloid beta protein forms calcium channels in bilayer membranes: blockade by tromethamine and aluminum. *Proceedings of the National Academy of Sciences, USA* 90, 567–571.

Bagchi, D., Garg A., Krohn, R.L., Bagchi, M., Tran, M.X. and Stoh, S.J. (1997) Oxygen free radical scavenging abilities of vitamins C and E, and a grape seed proanthocyanidin extract *in vitro*. *Research Communications in Molecular Pathology and Pharmacology* 95, 179–189.

Balzacs, L. and Leon, M. (1994) Evidence of an oxidative challenge in the Alzheimer's brain. *Neurochemical Research* 19, 1131–1137.

Beal, M.F. (1992) Mechanisms of excitotoxicity in neurologic diseases. *FASEB Journal* 6(15), 3338–3344.

Behl, C., Davis, J., Cole, G.M. and Schubert, D. (1992) Vitamin E protects nerve cells from amyloid beta protein toxicity. *Biochemical and Biophysical Research Communications* 186, 944–950.

Behl, C., Davis, J.B., Klier, F. and Schubert, D. (1994a) Amyloid β peptide induces necrosis rather than apoptosis. *Brain Research* 645, 253–264.

Behl, C., Davis, J.B., Lesley, R. and Schubert, D. (1994b) Hydrogen peroxide mediates amyloid β protein toxicity. *Cell* 77, 1–20.

Benzi, G. and Moretti, A. (1995) Age- and peroxidative stress-related modifications of the cerebral enzymatic activities linked to mitochondria and the glutathione system. *Free Radical Biology and Medicine* 19, 77–101.

Beyreuther, K., Multhaup, G. and Masters, C.L. (1996) Alzheimer's disease: genesis of amyloid. In: Bock, G.R. and Goode, J.A. (eds) *The Nature and Origin of Amyloid Fibrils*. John Wiley & Sons, Chichester, pp. 119–131.

Blanc, E.M., Toborek, M., Mark, R.J., Hennig, B. and Mattson, M.P. (1997) Amyloid beta-peptide induces cell monolayer albumin permeability, impairs glucose transport, and induces apoptosis in vascular endothelial cells. *Journal of Neurochemistry* 68, 1870–1881.

Braak, H. and Braak, E. (1996) Evolution of the neuropathology of Alzheimer's disease. *Acta Neurologica Scandinavica* 165 (Suppl.), 3–12.

Brodaty, H. and Sachdev, P.S. (1997) Drugs for the prevention and treatment of Alzheimer's disease. *Medical Journal of Australia* 167, 447–452.

Bruce, A.J., Malfroy, B. and Baudry, M. (1996) β-Amyloid toxicity in organotypic hippocampal cultures: protection by EUK-8, a synthetic catalytic free radical scavenger. *Proceedings of the National Academy of Sciences, USA* 93, 2312–2316.

Butterfield, D.A. (1996) Alzheimer's disease: a disorder of oxidative stress. *Alzheimer's Disease Review* 1, 68–70.

Butterfield, D.A. (1997) β-Amyloid-associated free radical oxidative stress and neurotoxicity: implications for Alzheimer's disease. *Chemical Research in Toxicology* 10, 495–506.

Butterfield, D.A., Hensley, K., Harris, M., Mattson, M. and Carney J. (1994) β-Amyloid peptide free radical fragments initiate synaptosomal lipoperoxidation in a sequence-specific fashion: implications to Alzheimer's disease. *Biochemical and Biophysical Research Communications* 200, 710–715.

Buttke, T.M. and Sandstrom, P.A. (1994) Oxidative stress as a mediator of apoptosis (Review). *Immunology Today* 15, 7–10.

Café, C., Torri, C., Bertorelli, L., Angeretti, N., Lucca, E., Forloni, G. and Marzatico, F. (1996) Oxidative stress after acute and chronic application of beta-amyloid fragment 25–35 in cortical cultures. *Neuroscience Letters* 203, 61–65.

Cahill, A., Wang, X. and Hoek, J.B. (1997) Increased oxidative damage to mitochondrial DNA following chronic ethanol consumption. *Biochemical and Biophysical Research Communications* 235, 286–290.

Cai, S.D., Golde, T.E. and Younkin, S.G. (1993) Release of excess amyloid beta protein from a mutant amyloid beta protein precursor. *Science* 259, 514–516.

Cheeseman, K.H. and Slater, T.F. (1993) An introduction to free radical biochemistry. *British Medical Journal* 49, 481–493.

Citron, M., Oltersdorf, T., Haass, C., McConlogue, L., Hung, A.Y., Seubert, P., Vigo-Pelfrey, C., Lieberburg, I. and Selkoe, D.J. (1992) Mutation of the beta-amyloid precursor protein in familial Alzheimer's disease increases beta protein production. *Nature* 360, 672–674.

Citron, M., Vigo-Pelfrey, C., Teplow, D.B., Miller, C., Schenk, D., Johnston, J., Winblad, B., Venizelos, N., Lannfelt, L. and Selkoe, D.J. (1994) Excessive production of amyloid β protein by peripheral cells of symptomatic and presymptomatic patients carrying the Swedish familial Alzheimer's disease mutation. *Proceedings of the National Academy of Sciences, USA* 91, 11993–11997.

Citron, M., Teplow, D.B. and Selkoe, D.J. (1995) Generation of amyloid β protein from its precursor is sequence specific. *Neuron* 14, 661–670.

Colton, C.A., Snell, J., Chernyshev, O. and Gilbert, D.L. (1994) Induction of superoxide anion and nitric oxide production in cultured microglia. *Annals of the New York Academy of Sciences* 17, 54–63.

Cotman, C.W. and Anderson, A.J. (1995) A potential role for apoptosis in neuro-degeneration and Alzheimer's disease. *Molecular Neurobiology* 10, 19–45.

Craft, S., Zallen, G. and Baker, L. (1992) Glucose and memory in senile dementia of the Alzheimer type. *Journal of Clinical Experimental Neuropsychology* 141, 253–267.

Craft, S., Newcomber, J., Kanne, S., Dagogo-Jack, S., Cryer, P., Sheline, Y., Luby, J., Dagogo-Jack, A. and Alderson, A. (1996) Memory improvement following induced hyperinsulinemia in Alzheimer's disease. *Neurobiology of Aging* 17, 123–130.

Das, D. and Banerjee R.K. (1993) Effect of stress on the antioxidant enzymes and gastric ulceration. *Molecular and Cellular Biochemistry* 125, 115–125.

Davis, R.E., Miller, S., Herrnstadt, C., Ghosh, S.S., Fahy, E., Shinobu, L.A., Galasko, D., Thal, L.J., Beal, M.F., Howell, N. and Parker, W.D. Jr. (1997) Mutations in mitochondrial cytochrome c oxidase genes segregate with late-onset Alzheimer disease. *Proceedings of the National Academy of Sciences, USA* 94, 4526–4531.

Esch, F.S., Keim, P.S., Battie, E.C., Blacher, R.W., Culwell, A.R., Oltersdorf, T., McClure, D. and Ward, P.J. (1990) Cleavage of amyloid β peptide during constitutive processing of its precursor. *Science* 248, 1122–1124.

Estevez, A.G., Radi, R., Barbeito, L., Shin, J.T., Thompson, J.A. and Beckman, J.S. (1995) Peroxynitrite-induced cytotoxicity in PC12 cells: evidence for an apoptotic mechanism differentially modulated by neurotrophic factors. *Journal of Neurochemistry* 65, 1543–1550.

Evans, D.A., Funkenstein, H. and Albert, M.S. (1989) Prevalence of Alzheimer's disease in a community population of older persons. *Journal of the American Medical Association* 262, 2551–2556.

Fraser, P.E., Nguyen, J.T., Surewicz, W.K. and Kirschner, D.A. (1991) pH dependent structural transition of Alzheimer amyloid peptides. *Biophysics Journal* 60, 1190–1201.

Gaido, M.L. and Cidlowski, J.A. (1991) Identification, purification, and characterization of a calcium-dependent endonuclease (NUC-18) from apoptotic rat thymocytes. *Journal of Biological Chemistry* 266, 18580–18585.

Games, D., Adams, D., Allesandrini, R., Barbour, R., Berthelette, P., Blackwell, C., Carr, T., Clemens, J., Donaldson, T., Gillespie, F., Guido, T., Hagoplan, S., Johnson-Wood, K., Khan, K., Leem, M., Leibowitz, P., Lieburburg, I., Littles, S., Masliah, E., McConlogue, L., Montoya-Zavala, M., Muckk, L., Paganini, L., Penniman, E., Power, M., Schenk, D., Seubert, P., Snyder, B., Soriano, F., Tan, F., Vital, J., Wadsworth, S., Wolozin, B. and Zhao, J. (1995) Alzheimer type neuropathology in transgenic mice overexpressing V717F β amyloid precursor protein. *Nature* 373, 523–527.

Giannakis, C., Forbes, I.J. and Zalewski, P.D. (1991) Ca^{2+}/Mg^{2+} dependent endonuclease: tissue distribution, relationship to internucleosomal DNA fragmentation and inhibition by Zn^{2+}. *Biochemical and Biophysical Research Communications* 181, 915–920.

Glenner, G.G. and Wong, C.W. (1984) Alzheimer's disease: initial report of the purification and characterization of a novel cerebrovascular amyloid protein. *Biochemical and Biophysical Research Communications* 120, 885–890.

Goldgaber, D., Lerman, M.I., McBride, W.O., Saffiotti, U. and Gajdusek, D.C. (1987) Isolation, characterization, and chromosomal localization of human brain cDNA clones coding for the precursor of the amyloid of brain in Alzheimer's disease, Down's syndrome and aging. *Journal of Neural Transmission* 24 (Suppl.), 23–28.

Goodman, Y., Bruce, A.J., Chang, B. and Mattson, M.P. (1996) Estrogens attenuate and corticosterone exacerbates excitotoxicity, oxidative injury and amyloid B-peptide toxicity in hippocampal neurons. *Journal of Neurochemistry* 66, 1836–1844.

Grant, W.B. (1997) Dietary links to Alzheimer's disease. *Alzheimer's Disease Review* 2, 42–55.

Haass, C. and Selkoe D.J. (1993) Cellular processing of β-amyloid precursor protein and the genesis of amyloid β peptide. *Cell* 75, 1035–1042.

Haass, C., Hung, A.Y., Selkoe D.J. and Teplow, D.B. (1994) Mutations associated with a locus for familial Alzheimer's disease result in alternative processing of amyloid β protein precursor. *Journal of Biological Chemistry* 269, 17741–17748.

Halliwell, B. (1984) Oxygen radicals: a common sense look at their nature and medical importance. *Medical Biology* 62, 71–77.

Halliwell, B. (1991) Drug antioxidant effects. A basis for drug selection? *Drugs* 4, 569–605.

Halliwell, B. (1994) Free radicals, antioxidants and human disease: curiosity, cause of consequence? *Lancet* 344, 721–724.

Halliwell, B. and Gutteridge, J.M.C. (1985) The importance of free radicals and catalytic metal ions in human diseases. *Molecular Aspects in Medicine* 8, 189–193.

Halliwell, B. and Gutteridge, J.M.C. (1989) *Free Radicals in Biology and Medicine,* 2nd edn. Clarendon Press, Oxford.

Halliwell, B., Gutteridge, J.M. and Cross, C.E. (1992) Free radicals, antioxidants, and human disease: where are we now? *Journal of Laboratory and Clinical Medicine* 119, 598–620.

Hardy, J. (1996) New insights into the genetics of Alzheimer's disease. *Annals of Medicine* 28, 255–258.

Hardy, J. and Allsop, D. (1991) Amyloid deposition as the central event in the aetiology of Alzheimer's disease (Review). *Trends in Pharmacological Science* 12, 383–388.

Hardy, J.A. and Higgins, G.A. (1992) Alzheimer's disease: the amyloid cascade hypothesis. *Science* 256, 184–185.

Harman, D. (1956) Aging: a theory based on free radical and radation chemistry. *Journal of Gerontology* 11, 298–300.

Harman, D. (1988) Free radicals in aging. *Molecular and Cellular Biochemistry* 84, 155–161.

Harris, M.E., Hensley, K., Butterfield, D.A., Leedle, R.A. and Carney, J.M. (1995) Direct evidence of oxidative injury produced by the Alzheimer's β-amyloid peptide (1–40) in cultured hippocampal neurons. *Experimental Neurology* 131, 193–200.

Hendrie, H.C. (1997) Epidemiology of Alzheimer's disease. *Geriatrics* 52 (Suppl. 2), S4–S8.

Hertz, L. and Schousboe, A. (1986) Uptake of GABA and nipecotic acid in astrocytes and neurons in primary cultures: changes in the sodium coupling ratio during differentiation. *Journal of Neuroscience Research* 16, 699–708.

Higgins, L.S. and Cordell, B. (1995) Striving for useful phenotypes in beta-APP transgenic mice. *Neurobiology of Aging* 16, 707–709.

Hippeli, S. and Elstner, E.F. (1995) Biological and biochemical effects of air pollutants: synergistic effects of sulphite. *Biochemical Society Symposia* 61, 153–161.

Holsie, E., Schousboe, A. and Holsie, L. (1986) Amino acid uptake. In: Federoff, S. and Vernadakis, A. (eds) *Astrocytes.* Academic Press, Orlando, Florida, pp. 133–153.

Horwood, N. and Davies, D.C. (1994) Immunolabelling of hippocampal microvessel glucose transporter protein is reduced in Alzheimer's disease. *Virchows Archiv* 425, 69–71.

Hsiao, K.K., Borchelt, D.R., Olson, K., Johannsdottir, R., Kitt, C., Yunis, W., Xu, S., Eckman, C., Younkin, S. and Price, D. (1995) Age-related CNS disorder and early death in transgenic FVB/N mice overexpressing Alzheimer amyloid precursor proteins. *Neuron* 15, 1203–1218.

Jarret, J.T. and Lansbury, P.T. (1993) Seeding 'one dimensional crystallization' of amyloid: a pathogenic mechanism in Alzheimer's disease and scrapie. *Cell* 763, 1055–1058.

Joseph, R. and Han, E. (1992) Amyloid β protein fragment 25–35 causes activation of cytoplasmic calcium in neurons. *Biochemical and Biophysical Research Communications* 184, 1441–1447.

Kang, J., Lemaire, H.G., Unterbeck, A., Salbaum, J.M., Masters, C.L., Giaeshick, K.H., Multhaup, G., Beyreuther, K. and Muller-Hill, B. (1987) The precursor of Alzheimer's disease amyloid βA4 protein resembles a cell surface receptor. *Nature* 325, 733–736.

Kappus, H. (1987) A survey of chemicals inducing lipid peroxidation in biological systems. *Chemistry and Physics of Lipids* 45, 105–115.

Katzman, R. (1986) Alzheimer's disease. *New England Journal of Medicine* 314, 964–973.

Keller, J.M., Germeyer, A., Begley, J.G. and Mattson, M.P. (1997) 17-Beta-estradiol attenuates oxidative impairment of synaptic Na+/K+-ATPase activity, glucose transport, and glutamate transport induced by amyloid beta-peptide and iron. *Journal of Neuroscience Research* 50, 522–530.

Koh, J.Y., Yang, L.L. and Cotman, C.W. (1990) Beta-amyloid protein increases the vulnerability of cultured cortical neurons to excitotoxic damage. *Brain Research* 533, 315–320.

Kontos, H.A. (1989) Oxygen radicals in CNS damage. *Chemico-Biological Interactions* 72, 229–255.

LaFerla, F.M., Tinkle, B.T., Bieberich, C.J., Haudenschild, C.C. and Jay, G. (1995) The Alzheimer's A beta peptide induces neurodegeneration and apoptotic cell death in transgenic mice. *Nature Genetics* 9, 21–30.

Lassman, H., Bancher, C., Breitschopf, H., Weigel, J., Bobinski, M., Jellinger, K. and Wisniewski, H.M. (1995) Cell death in Alzheimer's disease evaluated by DNA fragmentation *in situ*. *Acta Neuropathologica* 89, 35–41.

Lawson, J.A. and Maxey, K.M. (1996) Isoprostanes: prostanoids that arise spontaneously in membrane phospholipids. *Cayman Currents* 2, 1–5.

Lennon, S.V., Martin, S.J. and Cotter, T.G. (1991) Dose dependent induction of apoptosis in human tumour cell lines by widely diverging stimuli. *Cell Proliferation*. 24, 203–214.

Levy-Lahad, E., Wijsman, E.M., Nemens, E., Anderson, L., Goddard, K.A., Weber, J.L., Bird, T.D. and Schellenberg, G.D. (1995) A familial Alzheimer's disease locus on chromosome 1. *Science* 269, 970–973.

Loo, D.T., Agata, C., Pike, C.J., Whittemore, E.R., Wulencewicz, A.J. and Cotman, C.W. (1993) Apoptosis is induced by β-amyloid in cultured central nervous system neurons. *Proceedings of the National Academy of Sciences, USA* 90, 7951–7955.

Mark, R.J., Pang, Z., Geedes, J.W., Uchida, K. and Mattson M.P. (1997) Amyloid beta-peptide impairs glucose transport in hippocampal and cortical neurons: involvement of membrane lipid peroxidation. *Journal of Neuroscience* 17, 1046–1054.

Markesberry, G., Sclicksupp, A., Hesse, L., Beher, D., Ruppert, T., Masters, C.L. and Beyreuther, K. (1996) The amyloid precursor protein of Alzheimer's disease in the reduction of copper (2) to copper (1). *Science* 271, 1406–1409.

Martins, R.N., Harper, C.G., Stokes, G.B. and Masters, C.L. (1986) Increased cerebral glucose-6-phosphate dehydrogenase activity in Alzheimer's disease may reflect oxidative stress. *Journal of Neurochemistry* 46, 1042–1045.

Martins, R.N., Clarnette, R., Fisher, C., Broe, G.A, Brooks, W.S., Montgomery, P. and Gandy, S.E. (1995) APOE genotypes in Australia: roles in early and late-onset Alzheimer's disease and Down Syndrome. *Neuroreport* 6, 1513–1516.

Masters, C.L., Simms, G., Weinman, N.A., Multhaup, G., McDonald, B.L. and Beyreuther, K. (1985) Amyloid plaque core protein in Alzheimer disease and Down syndrome. *Proceedings of the National Academy of Sciences, USA* 82(12), 4245–4249.

Matsuo, M. (1993) Age related alterations in antioxidant defences. In: Yu, B.P. (ed.) *Free Radicals in Aging*. CRC Press, London, pp. 143–181.

Mattson, M.P. (1995) Untangling the pathophysiology of β amyloid. *Nature Structural Biology* 926–928.

Mattson, M.P. (1997) Central role of oxyradicals in the mechanism of amyloid β-peptide cytotoxicity. *Alzheimer's Disease Review* 2, 1–14.

Mattson, M.P. (1998) Experimental models of Alzheimer's disease. *Science and Medicine,* March/April, 16–25.

Mattson, M.P., Cheng, B., Davis, D., Bryant, K., Lieberburg, I. and Rydel, R.E. (1992) β-Amyloid peptides destabilizes calcium homeostasis and render human cortical neurons more vulnerable to excitotoxicity. *Journal of Neuroscience* 12, 376–389.

Mattson, M.P., Barger, S.W., Cheng, B., Lieberburg, I., Smith-Swintosky, V.L. and Rydel, R.E. (1993) β-Amyloid precursor protein metabolites and loss of neuronal Ca^{2+} homeostasis in Alzheimer's disease. *Trends in Neuroscience* 16, 409–414.

McLennan, H. (1976) The autoradiographic localization of L-[^{3}H]glutamate in rat brain tissue. *Brain Research* 115, 139–144.

Mirzabekov, T., Lin, M., Yuan, W., Marshall, P.J., Carman, M., Tomaselli, K., Lieberburg, I. and Kagan, B.L. (1994) Channel formation in planar lipid bilayers by a neurotoxic fragment of the beta amyloid peptide. *Biochemical and Biophysical Research Communications* 202, 1142–1148.

Montine, K.S., Olson, S.J., Amarnath, V., Whetsell, W.O. Jr, Graham, D.G. and Montine, T.J. (1997) Immunohistochemical detection of 4-hydroxy-2-nonenal adducts in Alzheimer's disease is associated with inheritance of APOE4. *American Journal of Pathology* 150, 437–443.

Multhaup, G., Schlicksupp, A., Hesse, L., Beher, D., Ruppert, T., Masters, C.L. and Beyreuther, K. (1996) The amyloid prescursor protein of Alzheimer's disease in the reduction of copper(II) to copper. *Science* 271, 1406–1409.

Nagy, Z.S. and Esiri, M.M. (1997) Apoptosis related protein expression in the hippocampus in Alzheimer's disease. *Neurobiology of Aging* 18, 565–571.

Ott, A., Breteler, M.M.B., van Harskamp, F., Claus, J.J., van der Cammen, T.J., Grobbee, D.E. and Hoffman, A. (1995) Prevalence of Alzheimer's disease and vascular dementia: association with education. The Rotterdam Study. *British Medical Journal* 310, 970–973.

Pappolla, M.A., Sos, M., Omar, R.A., Bick, R.J., Hickson-Bick, D.L., Reiter, R.J., Efthimiopoulos, S. and Robakis, N.K. (1997) Melatonin prevents death of neuroblastoma cells exposed to Alzheimer amyloid peptide. *Journal of Neuroscience* 17, 1683–1690.

Parker, W.D. Jr, Parks, J., Filley, C.M. and Kleinschmidt-Demasters, B.K. (1994) Electron transport chain defects in Alzheimer's disease brain. *Neurology* 44, 1090–1096.

Patrono, C. and FitzGerald, G.A. (1997) Isoprostanes: potential markers of oxidant stress in atherothrombotic disease. *Arteriosclerosis, Thrombosis and Vascular Biology* 17, 2309–2315.

Pike, C.J., Walencewicz, A.J., Glabe, C.G. and Cotman, C.W. (1991) *In vitro* aging of beta-amyloid protein causes peptide aggregation and neurotoxicity. *Brain Research* 563, 311–314.

Pillot, T., Goethals, M., Vanloo, B., Talussot, C., Brasseur, R., Vandekerckhove, J., Rosseneu, M. and Lins, L. (1996) Fusogenic properties of the C-terminal domain of the Alzheimer β-amyloid peptide. *Journal of Biological Chemistry* 271, 28757–28765.

Pryor, W.A. (1986) Oxy-radicals and related species: their formation, lifetimes, and reactions. *Annual Reviews in Physiology* 48, 657–667.

Querfurt, H.W., Wisjsman, E.M., St George-Hyslop, P. and Selkoe, D.J. (1995) βAPP mRNA transcription is increased in cultured fibroblasts from the familial Alzheimer's disease 1 family. *Molecular Brain Research* 28, 319–337.

Rice-Evans, C.A. and Burdon, R.H. (1994) *Free Radical Damage and its Control.* Elsevier Science, New York.

Rice-Evans, C.A., Miller, N.J. and Paganga, G. (1996) Structure–antioxidant activity relationships of flavonoids and phenolic acids. *Free Radical Biology and Medicine* 20, 933–956.

Robakis, N.K., Ramakrishna, N., Wolfe, G. and Wisniewski, H.M. (1987) Molecular cloning and characterization of a cDNA encoding the cerebrovascular and the neuritic plaque amyloid peptides. *Proceedings of the National Academy of Sciences, USA* 84, 4190–4194.

Roher, A.E., Lowenson, J.D., Clarke, S., Woods, A.S., Cotter, R.J., Gowing, E. and Ball, M.J. (1993) beta-Amyloid 1–42 is a major component of cerebrovascular amyloid deposits: implications for the pathology of Alzheimer disease. *Proceedings of the National Academy of Sciences, USA* 90, 10836–10840.

Rong, Y., Li, L., Shah, V. and Lau, B.H.S. (1994) Pycnogenol protects vascular endothelial cells from *t*-butyl hydroperoxide induced oxidant injury. *Biotechnology Therapeutics* 5, 117–126.

Sandbrink, R., Masters, C.L. and Beyreuther, K. (1994) Amyloid protein precursor mRNA isoforms without exon 15 (L-APP mRNAs) are ubiquitously expressed in rat tissues including brains but not in neurons. *Journal of Biological Chemistry* 269, 1510–1517.

Schmidt, M.L., DiDario, A.G., Lee, V.M.-Y. and Trojanowski, J.Q. (1994) An extensive network of PHFτ-rich dystrophic neurites permeates neocortex and nearly all neuritic and diffuse plaques in Alzheimer's disease. *FEBS Letters* 344, 69–73.

Schubert, W., Prior, R., Weidemann, A., Dircksen, H., Multhaup, G., Masters, C.L. and Beyreuther, K. (1991) Localization of Alzheimer βA4 amyloid precursor protein at central and peripheral synaptic sites. *Brain Research* 563, 184–194.

Selkoe, D.J. (1996) Amyloid β protein and the genetics of Alzheimer's disease. *Journal of Biological Chemistry* 271, 18295–18298.

Seubert, P., Olsterdorf, T., Lee, M.G., Barbour, R., Blomqurst, C., Davis, D.L., Bryant, K., Fritz, L.C., Galasko, D. and Thal, L.J. (1993) Secretion of β-amyloid precursor protein cleaved at the amino terminus of the β-amyloid peptide. *Nature* 361, 260–263.

Sherrington, R., Rogaev, E.I., Liang, Y., Rogaeva, E.A., Levesque, G., Ikeda, M., Chi, H., Lin, C., Li, G., Holman, K., Tsuda, T., Mar, L., Foncin, J.F., Bruni, A.C., Montesi, M.P., Sorbi, S., Rainero, I., Pinessi, L., Nee, L., Chumakov, I., Pollen, D., Brookes, A., Sanseau, P., Polinsky, R.J., Wasco, W., Da Silva, H.A.R., Haines, J.L., Pericak-Vance, M.A., Tanzi, R.E., Roses, A.D., Fraser, P.E., Rommens, J.M. and St George-Hyslop, P.H. (1995) Cloning of a gene bearing missense mutations in early onset familial Alzheimers disease. *Nature* 375, 754–760.

Sheuner, D., Eckman, C., Jensen, M., Song, X., Citron, M., Suzuki, N., Bird, T., Hardy, J., Hutton, M., Kukull, W., Larson, E., Levy-Lahad, E., Vitannen, M., Peskind, E., Poorkaj, P., Scellenberg, G., Tanzi, R., Wasco, W., Lannfelt, L., Selkoe, D. and Younkin, S. (1996) Secreted amyloid β-protein similar to that in senile plaques of Alzheimer's disease is increased *in vivo* by the presenilin 1 and 2 and APP mutations linked to familial Alzheimer's disease. *Nature Medicine* 2, 864–870.

Shinobu, L.A. and Beal, M.F. (1997) The role of oxidative processes and metal ions in aging and Alzheimer's disease. In: Connor, J.R. (ed.) *Metals and Oxidative Damage in Neurological Disorders*. Plenum Press, New York, pp. 237–275.

Simons M., Ikonene E., Tienari P.J., Cid-Arregui, A., Monning, U., Beyreuther, K. and Dotti, C.G. (1995) Intracellular routing of human amyloid precursor protein: axonal delivery followed by transport to the dendrites. *Journal of Neuroscience Research* 41, 121–128.

Simpson, I.A., Koteswara, R.C., Davies-Hill, T., Hone, W.G. and Davies, P. (1994) Decreased concentrations of GLUT1 and GLUT3 glucose transporters in the brains of patients with AD. *Annals of Neurology* 35, 546.

Smith, C.D., Carney, J.M., Starke-Reed, P.E., Oliver, C.N., Stadtman, E.R., Floyd, R.A. and Markesbery, W.R. (1991) Excess brain protein oxidation and enzyme dysfunction in normal aging and in Alzheimer disease. *Proceedings of the National Academy of Sciences, USA* 88, 10540–10543.

Smith, M.A. and Perry, G. (1995) Free radical damage, iron and Alzheimer's disease. *Journal of the Neurological Sciences* 134 (Suppl.), 92–94.

Smith, M.A., Taneda, S., Richey, P.L., Mikyata, S., Yan, S., Stern, D., Sayer, L., Monnier, V.M. and Perry, G. (1994) Advanced Maillard reaction end products are associated with Alzheimer disease pathology. *Proceedings of the National Academy of Sciences, USA* 91, 5710–5714.

Sokoloff, L. (1960) The metabolism of the central nervous system *in vivo*. In: Field J., Magokin, H.W. and Hall, V.E. (eds) *Handbook of Physiology-Neurophysiology*, Vol. 3. American Physiological Society, Washington, DC, pp. 1843–1864.

Strittmatter, W.J., Saunders, A.M., Schmechel, D., Pericak-Vance, M., Enghild, J., Salvesen, G.S. and Roses, A.D. (1993a) Apolipoprotein E: high-affinity binding to beta amyloid; increased frequency of type 4 allele in late-onset familial Alzheimer's disease. *Proceedings of the National Academy of Sciences, USA* 90, 1977–1989.

Strittmatter, W.J., Weisgraber, K.H., Huang D.Y., Dong, L.M., Salvesen, G.S., Pericak-Vance, M., Scmechel, D., Saunders, A.M., Goldgaber, D. and Roses, A.D. (1993b) Binding of human apolipoprotein E to beta/A4 peptide: isoform specific effects and implications for late onset Alzheimer's disease. *Proceedings of the National Academy of Sciences, USA* 90, 8098–8102.

Subbaro, D.V., Richardson, J.S. and Ang, L.C. (1990) Autopsy samples of Alzheimer's cortex show increased peroxidation *in vitro*. *Journal of Neurochemistry* 55, 342–345.

Suzuki, N., Cheung, T.T., Xai, X.D., Odeika, A., Otvos, L., Eckman, C., Golde, T.E. and Younkin, S.G. (1994) An increased percentage of long amyloid beta-protein secreted by familial amyloid beta protein precursor APP 717 mutants. *Science* 264, 1336–1340.

Tang, M.-X., Jacobs, D., Stern, Y., Marder, K., Schofield, P., Gurland, B., Andrews, H. and Mayeux, R. (1996) Effect of oestrogen during menopause on risk and age at onset of Alzheimer's disease. *Lancet* 348, 429–432.

Tanzi, R.E., Gusella, J.F., Watkins, P.C., Bruns, G.A., St George-Hyslop, P., Van Keuren, M.L., Patterson, D., Pagan, S., Kurnit, D.M. and Neve, R.L. (1987) Amyloid beta protein gene: cDNA, mRNA distribution, and genetic linkage near the Alzheimer locus. *Science* 235, 880–884.

Teller, J.K., Russo, C., DeBusk, L.M., Angelini, G., Zaccheo, D., Dagna-Bricarelli, F., Scartezzini, P., Bertolini, S., Mann, D.M., Tabaton, M. and Gambetti, P. (1996) Presence of soluble amyloid beta-peptide precedes amyloid plaque formation in Down's syndrome. *Nature Medicine* 2, 93–95.

Tilly, J.L. and Hsueh, A.J.W. (1993) Microscale autoradiographic method for the qualitative and quantitative analysis of apoptotic DNA fragmentation. *Journal of Cellular Physiology* 154, 519–526.

Trojanowski, J.Q., Schmidt, M.L., Shin, R.W., Bramblett, G.T., Rao, D. and Lee, V.M.-Y. (1993) Altered tau and neurofilament proteins in neurodegenerative diseases: diagnostic implications for Alzheimer's disease and lewy body dementia. *Brain Pathology* 3, 45–54.

Uchida, S., Edamatsu, R., Hiramatsu, M., Mori, A., Nonaka, G., Nishioka, I., Niwa, M. and Ozaki, M. (1987) Condensed tannins scavenge active oxygen free radicals. *Medical Science Research* 15, 831–832.

Wisniewski, K.E., Dalton, A.J., McLachlan, C., Wen, G.Y. and Wisniewski, H.M. (1985) Alzheimer's disease in Down's syndrome: clinicpathologic studies. *Neurology* 35, 957–961.

Wisniewski, H.M., Bancher, C., Barcikowska, M., Wen, G.Y. and Curries, J. (1989) Spectrum of morphological appearance of amyloid deposits in Alzheimer's disease. *Acta Neuropathology* 78, 337–347.

Wyllie, A.H. (1980) Glucocorticoid-induced thymocyte apoptosis is associated with endogenous endonuclease activation. *Nature* 284, 555–556.

Yamaguchi, H., Hirai, S., Morimatsu, M., Shoji, M. and Ihara, Y. (1988) A variety of cerebral amyloid deposits in the brains of Alzheimer type dementia demonstrated by beta protein immunostaining. *Acta Neuropathology* 76, 541–549.

Yan, S.D., Chen, X., Schmidt, A.M., Brett, J., Goodman, G., Zou, Y.S., Scott, C.W., Caputo, C., Frappier, T., Smith, M.A., Perry, G., Yen, S.H. and Stern, D. (1994) Glycated tau protein in Alzheimer disease: a mechanism for induction of oxidant stress. *Proceedings of the National Academy of Sciences, USA* 91, 7787–7791.

Yoshikai, S., Sasaki, H., Doh-Via, K., Furuyu, H. and Sakaki, Y. (1990) Genomic organisation of the human amyloid beta-protein precursor gene. *Gene* 87, 257–263.

Younkin, S.G. (1995) Evidence that A beta 42 is the real culprit in Alzheimer's disease. *Annals of Neurology* 37, 287–288.

Zeleznick, A.J., Ihrig, L.L. and Basset, S.G. (1989) Developmental expression of Ca^{2+}/Mg^{2+}-dependent endonuclease activity in rat granulosa and luteal cells. *Endocrinology* 125, 2218–2220.

Zhou, Y., Gopalakrishnan, V. and Richardson, S.J. (1996) Actions of the neurotoxic β amyloid on calcium homeostasis and viability of PC12 cells are blocked by antioxidants but not by calcium channel antagonists. *Journal of Neurochemistry* 67, 1419–1425.

Isoprostanes: Indicators of Oxidative Stress *in Vivo* and Their Biological Activity

29

P. QUAGGIOTTO AND MANOHAR L. GARG

Discipline of Nutrition and Dietetics,
Faculty of Medicine and Health Sciences,
University of Newcastle, Callaghan, Australia

Introduction

The oxidation of macronutrients by metabolic pathways such as the citric acid cycle, β-oxidation and glycolysis is essential for the derivation of energy and the maintenance of bodily functions. However, free radical-catalysed oxidation is non-essential and has been associated with a number of degenerative diseases such as cancer, cardiovascular disease, rheumatoid arthritis, lupus and the acceleration of the ageing process. Detrimental oxidative process in the body can be initiated by pro-oxidants present in foods and the environment. Normal functions such as activation of the immune system due to infection can also contribute to the oxidative stress experienced by the body. Neutrophils which have migrated to the site of infection generate free radicals which attack the invading pathogen, however they can also damage the host's cells. Smoking and drug toxicities can also increase oxidation in the body.

The research on the relationship between oxidative damage and the pathogenesis of degenerative diseases and their prevention by dietary antioxidants has been hampered by the lack of a single, reliable marker of oxidative stress *in vivo*. Determination of malondialdehyde levels by the thiobarbituric acid reactive substances (TBARS) test, breath alkane levels, hydroperoxides, conjugated dienes, etc., while satisfactory in many circumstances, has met criticism by a number of investigators particularly when examining oxidative stress *in vivo*. Recently, the discovery of a group of prostaglandin-like compounds, formed via the free radical-catalysed oxidation of polyunsaturated fatty acids, has provided a new and dependable method of quantifying oxidative stress. This review will examine the recent knowledge about isoprostanes and their biological function, means of analysis and relationship to disease.

Structure and Biosynthesis

In 1990, Morrow and his associates discovered the presence of prostaglandin-like compounds formed via the cyclooxygenase-independent, free radical-catalysed oxidation of the polyunsaturated fatty acid (PUFA), arachidonic acid (20:4n-6). Free radicals have one or more unpaired electrons which makes them highly reactive and toxic to tissues (Stein *et al.*, 1996). The superoxide ion (O_2^-) and hydroperoxide (H_2O_2) are two prominent free radicals which can catalyse the conversion of arachidonic acid to isoprostanes (Fig. 29.1). The process begins with the abstraction of an allylic hydrogen atom of arachidonic acid to produce an arachidonyl radical, which is subsequently converted to a peroxyl radical by the insertion of oxygen. Four different peroxyl isomers can be thus created depending on the location of abstraction and insertion. The radical undergoes endocyclization, then another incorporation of oxygen. This produces four bicycloendoperoxide regioisomers that are subsequently reduced to F_2 isoprostanes. These regioisomers can theoretically be comprised of eight racemic diastereomers. As a result, this mechanism has the potential to form 64 isomeric structures. As they are isomeric with the enzymatically synthesized prostaglandin $F_{2\alpha}$, they are collectively referred to as the F_2 isoprostanes. Of these, 8-iso-prostaglandin $F_{2\alpha}$ (8-iso-PGF$_{2\alpha}$), also referred to in the literature as 8-epi-prostaglandin $F_{2\alpha}$, is the most abundant of the F_2 isoprostanes found in human tissues and fluids (Morrow and Roberts, 1997).

The non-enzymatic free radical-catalysed lipid peroxidation mechanism can also result in the formation of D_2 and E_2 isoprostanes, structurally isomeric with PGD$_2$ and PGE$_2$ respectively. The *in vivo* levels of D_2 and E_2 isoprostane were found to be only slightly less than that of the F_2 isoprostanes (Morrow *et al.*, 1994).

Arachidonic acid is not the only PUFA that can act as a substrate for the free radical-catalysed formation of isoprostanes. *In vitro* oxidation of the n-3 counterpart of arachidonic acid, eicosapentaenoic acid (EPA) (20:5n-3) yielded F_3 isoprostanes (Nourooz-Zadeh *et al.*, 1997). This study found that while EPA produced a range of F_3 isoprostanes, 8-iso-PGF$_{3\alpha}$ was a minor product. F_4 isoprostanes, produced from docosahexaenoic acid (DHA, 22:6n-3), have also been detected (Nourooz-Zadeh *et al.*, 1998). The production of F_3 isoprostanes correlated with other indices of lipid oxidation such as measurement of lipid hydroperoxides and TBARS. It remains to be seen whether F_3 isoprostanes can occur *in vivo* and which

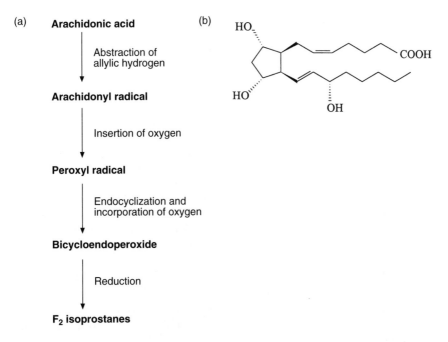

(a)

Arachidonic acid

↓ Abstraction of allylic hydrogen

Arachidonyl radical

↓ Insertion of oxygen

Peroxyl radical

↓ Endocyclization and incorporation of oxygen

Bicycloendoperoxide

↓ Reduction

F₂ isoprostanes

Fig. 29.1. (a) Biosynthetic pathway of isoprostane from arachidonic acid. (b) Structure of 8-epi-PGF$_{2\alpha}$ which is the predominant isoprostane in human fluids and tissues.

isoprostanes are the major F$_3$ isoprostane formed from the free radical-catalysed peroxidation of *n*-3 fatty acids.

F$_2$ isoprostanes have also been observed to be synthesized via enzyme-dependent mechanisms. Monocytes and platelets have shown the ability to synthesize 8-iso-PGF$_{2\alpha}$ via both cyclooxygenase-catalysed and free radical-catalysed mechanisms. They are one of the first examples of cells which can synthesize isoprostanes by both mechanisms (Pratico and FitzGerald, 1996). While the conditions under which such biosynthesis occurs have not been fully categorized, some authors suggest that enzymatically produced isoprostanes contribute only trivially to overall 8-iso-PGF$_{2\alpha}$ synthesis, even in conditions such as smoking and vascular reperfusion which are associated with increased oxidant stress. Cyclooxygenase-derived 8-iso-PGF$_{2\alpha}$ is produced in far less quantities in human platelets compared to thromboxane (Pratico *et al.*, 1995).

Biological Activity of Isoprostanes

8-iso-PGF$_{2\alpha}$ has been shown to be a potent vasoconstrictor in a variety of organs and tissues. Such activity has been reported in rat kidney (Takahashi *et al.*, 1992) and rabbit lung tissue (Banerjee *et al.*, 1992) as well as in cultured aortic smooth muscle cells (Fukunaga *et al.*, 1993a) and porcine and bovine, but not ovine, coronary arteries, with a potency twice that of $PGF_{2\alpha}$ (Kromer and Tippins, 1996). $8\text{-iso-PGF}_{2\alpha}$ has also been shown to stimulate constriction of non-pregnant pre-menopausal human myometrial tissue *in vitro* (Crankshaw, 1995). $8\text{-iso-PGF}_{2\alpha}$ reduced coronary blood flow by 50% when administered to isolated, perfused guinea pig hearts (Möbert *et al.*, 1997), and induced platelet shape change but not platelet aggregation (Pratico *et al.*, 1995).

The majority of isoprostane research has involved $8\text{-iso-PGF}_{2\alpha}$, however work has been performed on other isoprostanes. 8-iso-PGE_2 was also found to be a potent renal vasoconstrictor (Morrow *et al.*, 1994), reducing coronary flow as with $8\text{-iso-PGF}_{2\alpha}$, although to a lesser extent (Möbert *et al.*, 1997). 8-iso-PGE_2 also promoted the constriction of human and guinea pig airway smooth muscle *in vitro*, as well as stimulating airway obstruction and plasma exudation *in vivo* (Okazawa *et al.*, 1997). In cultured rat aortic smooth muscle cells, 8-iso-PGE_2 was found to be constrictive but with a potency less than that of $8\text{-iso-PGF}_{2\alpha}$ (Fukunaga *et al.*, 1993a). In rat aortic smooth muscle cells $8\text{-iso-PGF}_{2\alpha}$ stimulated both 1,4,5-inositol triphosphate generation and DNA synthesis (Fukunaga *et al.*, 1993b). In general, it seems that 8-iso-PGE_2 produces similar physiological responses to $8\text{-iso-PGF}_{2\alpha}$ but at a reduced potency.

Of the PUFA in a typical Western diet, those of the *n*-6 family such as arachidonic acid and linoleic acid (which can be endogenously elongated and desaturated to arachidonate) predominate. The last two decades have seen a substantial amount of work carried out on the health benefits of a diet containing fatty acids of the *n*-3 family such as eicosapentaenoic and docosahexanenoic acid (which are present in low amounts in a Western diet). The impact of this on isoprotane biology has received little attention, however it has been observed that $8\text{-iso-PGF}_{3\alpha}$ has a comparatively negligible effect on the constriction of human placental arteries compared to $8\text{-iso-PGF}_{2\alpha}$ (Read *et al.*, unpublished observations). It is likely that a diet containing *n*-3 fatty acids may improve blood flow following a heart attack simply by shifting isoprostane production from the vasoconstrictory F_2 family to the biologically inactive F_3 isoprostanes.

Putative Isoprostane Receptor

The prostanoids, which include the prostaglandins, thromboxanes and prostacyclins, elicit a wide variety of biological actions on a number of cells types. This is partly because each prostanoid can act through a range of receptors rather than a single receptor. Five distinct classes of prostanoid receptors have been recognized; DP, EP, FP, IP and TP, where each is specific for its corresponding substrate; PGD_2, PGE_2, PGF_2, PGI_2 and TXA_2, respectively. Each prostanoid can still bind to and exert an effect through receptors other than its specific counterpart, but at a potency lower by an order of magnitude. To further add to the complexity of prostanoid–receptor interactions, recent evidence also supports the existence of subtypes of at least some of these receptors (Coleman *et al.*, 1994).

Considering the structural similarities between prostanoids and isoprostanes, it seems reasonable to hypothesize that 8-iso-PGF$_{2\alpha}$ may also exert its physiological effects through more than one receptor. According to many reports, 8-iso-PGF$_{2\alpha}$ acts, in part, through the vascular thromboxane A$_2$/prostaglandin H$_2$ (TP) receptor (Takahashi *et al.*, 1992). Data also exist to support the contention that it may also act through a structurally similar yet clearly distinct 8-iso-PGF$_{2\alpha}$ specific receptor (Fukunaga *et al.*, 1997).

8-iso-PGF$_{2\alpha}$ has been shown to be a partial agonist to the TP receptor (Crankshaw, 1995). TP receptor antagonists were found to be effective in inhibiting the action of 8-iso-PGF$_{2\alpha}$ in isolated guinea-pig and human tracheal tissue (Kawikova *et al.*, 1996; Pratico and FitzGerald, 1996). Additionally, there is growing evidence to indicate that 8-iso-PGF$_{2\alpha}$ also acts through a novel receptor closely related to, but distinct from the TP receptor. Competitive binding assays on cultured bovine aortic endothelial cells showed that two distinct binding sites (one high- and one low-affinity) for 8-iso-PGF$_{2\alpha}$ were present (Fukunaga *et al.*, 1995). Most likely, the low-affinity site represents the TP receptor and the high-affinity site is indicative of a 8-iso-PGF$_{2\alpha}$ specific receptor.

A study examined the ability of 8-iso-PGF$_{2\alpha}$ to functionally couple to G proteins through direct action on the TP receptor as measured by mobilization of intracellular calcium. cDNA for the human placental TPα isoform and Gq or G11 were coexpressed in human embryonic kidney (HEK) 293 cells. They found that stimulation of these cells with 8-iso-PGF$_{2\alpha}$ and also the prostaglandin endoperoxide/thromboxane A$_2$ analogue U46619 resulted in a rise in intracellular calcium. Similar results were also observed with platelets (Kinsella *et al.*, 1997).

The data suggest that 8-iso-PGF$_{2\alpha}$ acts through a thromboxane receptor and another similar yet 8-iso-PGF$_{2\alpha}$-specific receptor. The crucial question remains as to whether, and in which tissues, 8-iso-PGF$_{2\alpha}$ acts through either receptor or a combination of the two.

Comparison of Isoprostanes and Prostanoids

Despite their structural resemblance, isoprostanes and prostanoids have several important differences in terms of their biological activity. Firstly, prostanoids are formed via enzyme-catalysed reactions, while isoprostanes are produced via an enzyme-independent free radical-catalysed process (Morrow and Roberts, 1996). Secondly, prostanoid formation requires the fatty acid substrate to be cleaved from the parent phospholipid by phospholipase A$_2$ before it can be acted upon by cyclooxygenase, while isoprostanes are formed while arachidonic acid is still esterified to its parent phospholipid, after which it is presumably cleaved by phospholipases (Morrow *et al.*, 1992). Whether the phospholipase is specific for isoprostanes is not known. Thirdly, isoprostanes are found in human fluids at concentrations an order of magnitude higher than prostanoids (Awad *et al.*, 1996a). Fourth, isoprostanes are chemically stable, whereas, for example, thromboxane A_2 has a half-life of approximately 30 s after which it rearranges to the biologically inactive thromboxane B_2 (Samuelsson, 1976). Finally, 8-iso-PGF$_{2\alpha}$ stimulates constriction of vascular smooth muscle as does thromboxane A_2, but unlike thromboxane A_2, it does not induce platelet shape-change (Pratico *et al.*, 1995).

$F_{2\alpha}$ Isoprostanes as an Index of Oxidative Stress

Several established methods exist to quantify lipid peroxidation (Table 29.1). Measurement of: conjugated dienes, lipid hydroperoxides, exhaled pentane (Cailleux and Allain, 1993), depletion of PUFA and/or vitamin E, and determination of malondialdehyde via the TBARS test. TBARS has been the most popular because of its simplicity, however it has received considerable criticism due to its lack of specificity (Halliwell and Grootveld, 1987; Gopaul *et al.*, 1994). Research into free radical-mediated injury has been hampered by the suitability of these techniques to *in vitro* applications only, and one cannot eliminate the potential for positive results to be merely artefactual (Roberts and Morrow, 1995).

Isoprostanes are becoming accepted as the most accurate indicator of oxidative stress and lipid peroxidation as: established methods exist for their quantification, they are generated *in vivo* and they are structurally stable, unlike lipid peroxides. As an indication, 8-iso-PGF$_{2\alpha}$ determination of carbon tetrachloride (CCl_4)-induced lipid peroxidation is believed to be 30 times more sensitive than measurement of TBARS (Awad *et al.*, 1996b).

The ability of several known stimulants of oxidation have been reported to induce *in vivo* increases in isoprostane levels. These include CCl_4 (Morrow *et al.*, 1994), the anaesthetic halothane (Awad *et al.*, 1996b) and ozone (O_3^-) (Hazbun *et al.*, 1993). Increased free radical production is one of the main causes of tissue damage during coronary reperfusion (Bhatnagar *et al.*, 1990). It was found that coronary reperfusion was associated with increased urinary levels of 8-iso-PGF$_{2\alpha}$ in canines as well as in human patients with acute myocardial infarction given lytic therapy (Delanty *et al.*, 1997). Significantly elevated levels of 8-iso-PGF$_{2\alpha}$ have also been reported in smokers. Morrow and co-workers (1995) discovered a significant correlation between urinary and circulatory F_2 isoprostanes in both smokers and non-smokers. Urinary analysis of isoprostanes is useful, as it can provide an indication of oxidative stress over specified periods of time. The major urinary metabolite of 8-iso-PGF$_{2\alpha}$ is 2,3-dinor-5,6-dihydro-8-iso-prostaglandin F$_{2\alpha}$ (Roberts *et al.*, 1996).

Table 29.1. Parameters affected by oxidation as measured in a variety of disorders and experimental models.

Condition	Reference	TBARS	8-iso-PGF2α	SOD	GP	Catalase	Conjugated dienes
Human CHD	Buczynski *et al.*, 1993	↑	–	↓	↓	↓	–
Human smoking	Bachi *et al.*, 1996	–	↑	–	–	–	–
Human smoking	Morrow *et al.*, 1995	–	↑	–	–	–	↑
Human hypertension	Parik *et al.*, 1996	↑	–	–	–	–	–
Human scleroderma	Stein *et al.*, 1996	–	↑	–	–	–	↑
Rat alcoholic liver disease	Nanji *et al.*, 1994	–	↑	–	–	–	↑
Cirrhotic rats	Marley *et al.*, 1997	–	↑	–	–	–	–

As stated, isoprostanes exist in a non-esterified (free) or esterified form. This can be useful in determining the site of oxidation or if some tissues or organs are more susceptible to oxidation, as esterified isoprostanes remain largely in the tissues where they were created whereas the non-esterified circulatory isoprostanes are indicative of general systemic oxidation (Burk *et al.*, 1995b). This is an advantage of isoprostane assessment compared with exhaled alkanes, for example, where localization of the site of oxidation is not possible (Awad *et al.*, 1994).

Some experiments have reported the detection of cyclooxygenase-catalysed production of 8-iso-PGF$_{2\alpha}$ (Pratico *et al.*, 1995; Pratico and FitzGerald, 1996). This may serve to confound its usefulness as an indication of free radical-mediated lipid oxidation. Since cyclooxygenase requires cleavage of arachidonic acid prior to catalysis, perhaps a more accurate assessment of lipid oxidation would be to restrict measurement of isoprostanes to only the esterified form, as the cyclooxygenase enzyme can only metabolize the free form of arachidonic acid.

Analysis and Quantification of Isoprostanes

Two major means of quantifying isoprostanes exist; gas chromatography–mass spectrometry (GC–MS) and enzyme immunoassay. Gas chromatography/negative-ion chemical ionization mass spectrometry (GC-NICIMS) has the advantage of being able to detect the multiple isomeric forms of isoprostanes. However, it is costly in terms of equipment and requires time and labour-intensive sample preparation protocols. The alternative is enzyme immuno-assay, available in a commercial kit form. This method is not as laborious and time consuming as a GC-MS protocol. However, its main disadvantage is that, at present, kits are available with antibodies specific for only the 8-iso-PGF$_{2\alpha}$ isoprostane isomer.

Isoprostanes as Oxidative Markers in Degenerative Diseases

Free radical-mediated tissue damage has been implicated in a wide variety of degenerative diseases. The exposed double bonds of the PUFA of cell membrane phospholipids are particularly susceptible to attack by free radicals. Increased isoprostane levels have been reported in a wide variety of disorders, from scleroderma (Stein *et al.*, 1996) to cystic fibrosis (Collins *et al.*, unpublished observations) and hepatorenal syndrome (Morrow *et al.*, 1993). High levels of free radicals found at a site of inflammation have been reported to reduce cell proliferation and increase the rate of apoptosis. Excessive DNA replication and damage can also occur upon reaching an inflamed area. Superoxide and hydroperoxide radicals are produced by the plasma membrane-bound NADPH oxidase of neutrophils, a process known as 'respiratory burst'. Recently it has been observed that non-inflammatory cells such as fibroblasts and endothelial cells are similarly capable when stimulated by pro-inflammatory cytokines such as tumour necrosis factor-α (TNF-α) and interleukin 1 (IL-1) (Burdon, 1997).

Lung and airway tissue, as the interface between the atmosphere and the body, are particularly susceptible to oxidative attack and damage. Using isolated guinea-pig and human tracheal tissue from respiratory failure patients, it has been demonstrated that 8-iso-PGF$_{2\alpha}$ constricted airway smooth muscle, and was more effective in the human tissue (Kawikova *et al.*, 1996). Administration of oxygen at levels higher than normal is in frequent clinical use. Such excessive oxygen exposure can cause pulmonary oedema in humans and animals. After acute and chronic hyperoxia, increased oxygen radical formation can occur, leading to toxic injury. Levels of 8-iso-PGF$_{2\alpha}$ were found to be significantly increased in lavage fluid obtained from rats exposed to 90% O_2 for 48 h compared with ambient atmosphere-exposed animals (Vacchiano and Tempel, 1994).

Cyclooxygenase and thromboxane synthetase inhibitors provide no beneficial effect for asthma sufferers (O'Byrne and Fuller, 1989) yet the TP receptor antagonist AA-2414 decreases bronchial hyperresponsiveness to methacholine (Fujimura *et al.*, 1991). The lungs of asthmatic patients have an imbalance of the oxidative/antioxidative system in their lungs (Smith *et al.*, 1994). Perhaps the discrepancy can be explained by considering possible isoprostane–receptor interactions. While thromboxane does not seem to have a role in asthma, TP receptors are involved. Increased oxidative stress associated with asthma increases lipid peroxidation and consequently isoprostane production, which stimulates the TP receptors. Dietary supplementation with antioxidants such as vitamin E may improve endogenous antioxidant levels, thereby reducing isoprostane production and ultimately alleviating the symptoms of asthma.

Cystic fibrosis, a common genetic disease, is characterized by chronic lung infection and inflammation. The 8-iso-PGF$_{2\alpha}$ in erythrocyte membranes of cystic fibrosis patients were found to be elevated compared to normal controls (Collins *et al.*, unpublished observations). These elevated levels correlated with a reduction in plasma β-carotene concentration despite antioxidant supplementation. Since diseases as cystic fibrosis and asthma have elevated isoprostanes levels, this marker can be used to test whether antioxidant supplements would be useful, and what type or types of antioxidant would be beneficial.

Atherosclerosis begins with the uptake of oxidized low-density lipoprotein (LDL) by macrophages, which become embedded in vascular smooth muscle and transform into foam cells. This forms the basis of an atherosclerotic lesion (Morrow *et al.*, 1995). Both free and total (free plus esterified) F_2 isoprostanes were found to increase with time in LDL incubated with cultured aortic endothelial cells over a 24 h period. This assessment of oxidation agreed with more established indexes of oxidation such as TBARS, conjugated dienes and lipid hydroperoxides (Gopaul *et al.*, 1994).

In experimentally induced alcoholic liver injury, researchers explored the relationship between eicosanoids, vitamin E and 8-iso-PGF$_{2\alpha}$ plasma levels in a rat model (Nanji *et al.*, 1994a). They discovered that the ratio of thromboxane B$_2$:6-ketoprostaglandin F$_{1\alpha}$ correlated inversely with vitamin E and positively with 8-iso-PGF$_{2\alpha}$. This study demonstrated two, possibly related, means by which experimental alcoholic liver disease can induce injury; enhancing oxidation and therefore lipid peroxidation (evidenced by increased isoprostane levels) by depletion of vitamin E antioxidant; and altering the thromboxane/prostacyclin balance in favour of the pro-aggregatory thromboxane.

A study was conducted to examine the relationship between pathological severity and lipid peroxidation, using intragastric fed rats as a model for alcoholic liver disease (Nanji *et al.*, 1994b). Oxidative stress was assessed by measurement of 8-iso-PGF$_{2\alpha}$ and microsome-conjugated dienes, as well as histological liver examination. It was found that animals fed a diet supplemented with ethanol and polyunsaturated fish oil had the highest amount of isoprostanes, and the most pathological damage, compared with a saturated fat and ethanol diet.

Liver cirrhosis is associated with increased free radical production and decreased levels of antioxidants such as vitamin E, glutathione and selenium. Livers from normal and bile duct-ligated cirrhotic rats were perfused with 8-iso-PGF$_{2\alpha}$ resulting in increased portal pressure in both experimental groups. There was a significantly greater change in portal pressure in response to 8-iso-PGF$_{2\alpha}$ perfusion in the cirrhotic animals. This action was completely blocked, in cirrhotic rats, by the addition of SQ29548, a thromboxane receptor antagonist, to the perfusate (Marley *et al.*, 1997).

The potential for free radicals to induce cancer has received increased scrutiny in recent times. High levels of free radicals induce excessive DNA replication (Burdon, 1997). 8-iso-PGF$_{2\alpha}$ has also been shown to increase DNA synthesis in rat aortic smooth muscle cells (Fukunaga *et al.*, 1993b). Smoking has been implicated in the pathogenesis of cancer due to oxidative damage of DNA. Cigarette smoke is known to contain large quantities of oxidants. It is not surprising that plasma levels of non-esterified and esterified F$_2$ isoprostanes are elevated in smokers (Morrow *et al.*, 1995).

Antioxidants and Their Use in Disease Prophylaxis

Antioxidants are essentially free radical scavengers. Enzymes such as superoxide dismutase, glutathione peroxidase and catalase are part of the endogenous mechanisms that the body possesses to combat oxidation. Superoxide dismutase metabolizes the superoxide ion (O$_2^-$) to hydroperoxide (H$_2$O$_2$) which is them acted upon by glutathione peroxidase (Burk *et al.*, 1995a). Vitamin E (α-tocopherol) and β-carotene are antioxidants that can be obtained from the diet (Awad *et al.*, 1994). Both *in vivo* and dietary antioxidants have a role in the prevention of lipid peroxidation, and isoprostanes provide a more accurate means of assessing their effectiveness.

Recently it was observed that reactive oxygen species can act as signalling molecules in the regulation of gene expression. Extracellular radicals can initiate cell signalling, and intracellular radicals can act as second messengers. Therefore the intake of dietary antioxidants enables alteration of radical-affected signalling pathways. Antioxidants may achieve this by several different mechanisms: by affecting the binding ability of transcription factors to DNA, by modifying redox-sensitive sites on signalling molecules, or by alteration of phosphorylation reactions (Palmer and Paulson, 1997).

Crosby and co-workers (1996) demonstrated that the type of fatty acids can affect antioxidant enzyme activity. Incubation of human vascular endothelial cells with the *n*-3 PUFA eicosapentaenoic acid (EPA) and docosahexaenoic acid (DHA) was associated with an increase in glutathione peroxidase activity. This may, in part, explain the anti-atherosclerotic effect of consuming a diet high in *n*-3 PUFA-rich marine foods (Charnock, 1994) and the pathogenesis of atherosclerosis is initiated by the oxidation of LDL (Klatt and Esterbauer, 1996). This study assessed lipid peroxidation as a function of conjugated diene formation.

The role of antioxidants in the prevention of apoptosis has also received attention (Patel and Gores, 1997). Apoptosis is programmed cell death which, although it is a feature of normal cells, can occur excessively as a result of oxidation and has been shown to be induced in hepatocytes following oxidative challenge. Using the antioxidant lazaroid U83836E, a 21-aminosteroid having an antioxidant potency 100-fold greater than vitamin E, researchers found that incubation of U83836E with cultured rat hepatocytes significantly reduced both lipid peroxidation, as measured by F_2 isoprostane assay, and glycochenodeoxycholate (GCDC)-induced apoptosis.

Iron can catalyse the generation of reactive oxygen radicals and excess iron has been shown to induce cellular oxidant injury. Dietary iron overload has been reported to increase hepatic F_2 isoprostane levels and reduce levels of the antioxidants α-tocopherol, β-carotene and ascorbic acid (Dabbagh *et al.*, 1994).

Selenium acts as an antioxidant by being an essential component of active glutathione peroxidase. A study involving selenium-deficient rats found that circulatory F_2 isoprostanes were elevated after dosing with diquat (Burk *et al.*, 1995a). Diquat, a bipyridyl compound, induces oxidation by transferring electrons from NADPH cytochrome P-4540 reductase to other receptor molecules, resulting in free radical production. Hepatic vein plasma contained higher F_2 isoprostane levels than the portal vein plasma, suggesting that the liver was producing isoprostanes. Subsequent administration of selenium prevented diquat-induced lipid peroxidation, as indicated by isoprostane quantification. The diquat-induced hepatic lipid peroxidation preceded hepatic necrosis, indicating that isoprostanes may have a role in the pathogenesis of liver disease.

The role of dietary selenium and vitamin E in the prevention of lipid peroxidation has also been examined. The first stage of the dietary intervention consisted of feeding rats a selenium- and vitamin E-deficient diet for a period of 12 weeks; afterwards they were divided into five secondary-stage groups fed diets deficient in: both selenium and vitamin E, selenium only, vitamin E only, a non-deficient control group, and also a control group that was immediately euthanased (Awad *et al.*, 1994). Analysis of tissue esterified F_2 isoprostanes showed that the group fed selenium- and vitamin E-deficient diets exhibited the most severe lipid peroxidation. The longer the period of time for which they were maintained on the diet, the greater the increase in tissue isoprostanes. The selenium-only and vitamin E-only rats exhibited lower isoprostane levels compared with the doubly deficient. The study showed that combined selenium and vitamin E deficiency was dramatically damaging compared with controls and that selenium or vitamin E supplementation was effective in reducing the oxidative stress.

Further studies examined the role of glutathione in liver and kidney necrosis by administering a glutathione-depleting agent, phorone, to selenium-deficient and control rats (Burk *et al.*, 1995b). Glutathione acts as a substrate for glutathione peroxidase. Plasma levels of free F_2 isoprostanes increased 13-fold after phorone treatment in selenium-deficient animals. Esterified liver F_2 isoprostanes were present at two orders of magnitude higher than circulatory levels. They were elevated in both experimental groups after phorone treatment. Kidney isoprostanes were unchanged in control organs, after phorone treatment, but increased 20-fold in selenium-deficient rats. Investigators demonstrated that glutathione depletion predisposes the liver and kidney to oxidative necrosis in the selenium-deficient but not the control rats.

Cystic fibrosis patients were shown to have elevated red blood cell 8-iso-PGF$_{2\alpha}$, and depressed β-carotene levels (Collins, unpublished observations). This study leads to the possibility of dietary supplementation with antioxidants as a means to reduce the oxidative damage sustained by tissues, and their efficacy can be assessed by isoprostane quantification. The question remains as to whether there is an ideal antioxidant or whether a combined treatment would be the most beneficial.

Hypertension affects 30% of adults and has been associated with diabetes mellitus (Cerielo *et al.*, 1997) and increased risk of atherosclerosis. The low, endogenous antioxidant status characteristic of hypertensive patients (Tse *et al.*, 1994) suggest that a possible treatment of hypertension could involve administration of antioxidants to supplement the body's internal stores. A randomized, double-blind, cross-over designed placebo control study, involving hypertensive and normotensive volunteers, was conducted to examine the effect of short-term (8 weeks), high-dose antioxidants on blood pressure. Daily administration of a combination of zinc sulphate, ascorbic acid (vitamin C), α-tocopherol (vitamin E) and β-carotene, resulted in a reduction in systolic blood pressure in both patient types (Galley *et al.*, 1997). Another study demonstrated that low-dose aspirin therapy was effective in inhibiting thromboxane (and, surprisingly, lipid peroxides) in placental cells taken from pre-eclamptic women. (Pre-eclampsia is a hypertensive disorder of human pregnancy that is a leading cause of premature delivery and fetal growth retardation (Wang and Walsh, 1995).) Such data raise the possibility of designing improved treatments by combining dietary antioxidants and non-steroidal anti-inflammatory drugs (NSAIDS) such as aspirin (Fig. 29.2).

Conclusions and Future Directions

Oxidation is a prominent feature of a considerable range of degenerative diseases; however, research into this area has been problematic due to the lack of a dependable indicator of oxidation. Isoprostanes provide researchers with such an indicator: dependable, stable and readily quantified. Its usefulness is especially apparent when applied to *in vivo* testing, a feature not part of previous techniques. A growing body of evidence demonstrates the occurence of higher levels of F_2 isoprostanes in

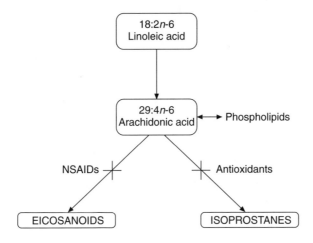

Fig. 29.2. Model for improved treatment of disorders with an inflammatory/oxidative injury component whereby both enzymatically and free radical-derived metabolites of polyunsaturated fatty acids are targeted for inhibition. NSAIDs, non-steriodal anti-inflammatory drugs.

a variety of diseases. The next step must be to determine whether isoprostanes have an active participation in disease pathogenesis and not simply exist as an artefact of oxidative injury. If the hypothetical role of isoprostanes in disease proves to be true, then the next step should be the determination of suitable antioxidants to prevent or ameliorate the symptoms of oxidative disorders. Specific analysis of 8-iso-PGF$_{2\alpha}$ provides the opportunity to evaluate the effects of antioxidant interventions in human disease characterized by excessive lipid peroxidation *in vivo*.

References

Awad, J.A., Morrow, J.D., Hill, K.H., Roberts, L.J. II and Burk, R.F. (1994) Detection and localisation of lipid peroxidation in selenium- and vitamin E-deficient rats using F$_2$-isoprostanes. *Journal of Nutrition* 124, 810–816.

Awad, J.A., Roberts, L.J. II, Burk, R.F. and Morrow, J.D. (1996a) Isoprostanes – prostaglandin-like compounds formed independently of cyclooxygenase. Use as clinical indicators of oxidant damage. *Gastroenterology Clinics of North America* 25, 409–427.

Awad, J.A., Horn, J.L., Roberts, L.J. II and Franks, J.J. (1996b) Demonstration of halothane-induced hepatic lipid peroxidation in rats by quantification of F$_2$-isoprostanes. *Anesthesiology* 84, 910–916.

Bachi, A., Zuccato, E., Baraldi, M., Fanelli, R. and Chiabrando, C. (1996) Measurement of urinary 8-epi-prostaglandin F$_{2\alpha}$, a novel index of lipid peroxidation *in vivo*. By immunoaffinity extraction/gas chromatography-mass spectrometry. Basal levels in smokers and nonsmokers. *Free Radical Biology and Medicine* 20, 619–624.

Banerjee, M., Kang, K.H., Morrow, J.D., Roberts, L.J. II and Newman, J.H. (1992) Effects of novel prostaglandin, 8-epi-PGF$_{2\alpha}$, in rabbit lung *in situ*. *American Journal of Physiology* 263, H660–H663.

Bhatnagar, A., Srivastava, S.K. and Szabo, G. (1990) Oxidative stress alters specific membrane currents in isolated cardiac myocytes. *Circulation Research* 67, 535–549.

Buczynski, A., Wachowicz, B., Kedziora-Kornatowska, K., Tkaczewski, W. and Kedziora, J. (1993) Changes in antioxidant enzymes activities, aggregability and malonyldialdehyde concentration in blood platelets from patients with coronary heart disease. *Atherosclerosis* 100, 223–228.

Burdon, R.H. (1997) Control of cell proliferation by reactive oxygen species. *Biochemical Society Transactions* 24, 1028–1032.

Burk, R.F., Hill, K.E., Awad, J.A., Morrow, J.D., Kato, T., Cockell, K.A. and Lyons, P.R. (1995a) Pathogenesis of diquat-induced liver necrosis in selenium-deficient rats: assessment of the roles of lipid peroxidation and selenoprotein P. *Hepatology* 21, 561–569.

Burk, R.F., Hill, K.E., Awad, J.A., Morrow, J.D. and Lyons, P.R. (1995b) Liver and kidney necrosis in selenium-deficient rats depleted of glutathione. *Laboratory Investigation* 72, 723–730.

Cailleux, A. and Allain, P. (1993) Is pentane a normal constituent of human breath? *Free Radical Research Communications* 18, 323–327.

Cerielo, A., Motz, E., Cavarape, A., Lizzio, S., Russo, A., Quatraro, A. and Giugliano, D. (1997) Hyperglycemia counterbalances the antihypertensive effect of glutathione in diabetic patients: evidence linking hypertension and glycemia through the oxidative stress in diabetes mellitus. *Journal of Diabetes and its Complications* 11, 250–255.

Charnock, J.S. (1994) Dietary fats and cardiac arrhythmia in primates. *Nutrition* 10, 161–169.

Coleman, R.A., Smith, W. and Narumiya, S. (1994) VIII. International Union of Pharmacology classification of prostanoid receptors: properties, distribution, and structure of the receptor and their subtypes. *Pharmacological Review* 46, 205–229.

Crankshaw, D. (1995) Effects of the isoprostane, 8-epi-prostaglandin F_{2a}, on the contractility of the human myometrium *in vitro*. *European Journal of Pharmacology* 285, 151–158.

Crosby, A.J., Wahle, K.W.J. and Duthie, G.G. (1996) Modulation of glutathione peroxidase activity in human vascular endothelial cells by fatty acids and the cytokine interleukin-1 β. *Biochimica et Biophysica Acta* 1303, 187–192.

Dabbagh, A.J., Mannion, T., Lynch, S.M. and Frei, B. (1994) The effect of iron overload on rat plasma and liver oxidant status *in vivo*. *Biochemical Journal* 300, 799–803.

Delanty, N., Reilly, M.P., Pratico, D., Lawson, J.A., McCarthy, J.F., Wood, A.E., Ohnishi, S.T., Fitzgerald, D.J. and FitzGerald, G.A. (1997) 8-epi PGF_{2a} generation during coronary reperfusion. A potential quantitative marker of oxidant stress *in vivo*. *Circulation* 95, 2492–2499.

Fujimura, M.S., Sakamoto, S., Saito, M., Mikaye, Y. and Matsuda, T. (1991) Effect of a thromboxane A2 receptor antagonist (AA-2414) on bronchial hyper-responsiveness to methacholine in subjects with asthma. *Journal of Allergy and Clinical Immunology* 87, 23–27.

Fukunaga, M., Takahashi, K. and Badr, K.F. (1993a) Vascular smooth muscle actions and receptor interactions of 8-iso-prostaglandin E_2, an E_2-isoprostane. *Biochemical and Biophysical Research Communications* 195, 507–515.

Fukunaga, M., Makita, N., Roberts, L.J. II, Morrow, J.D., Takahashi, K. and Badr, K.F. (1993b) Evidence for the existence of F_2-isoprostane receptors on rat vascular smooth muscle cells. *American Journal of Physiology* 264, C1619–C1624.

Fukunaga, M., Yura, T. and Badr, K.F. (1995) Stimulatory effect of 8-epi-PGF_{2a}, an isoprostane, on endothelin-1 release. *Journal of Cardiovascular Pharmacology* 26, S51–S52.

Fukunaga, M., Yura, T., Grygorczyk, R. and Badr, K.F. (1997) Evidence for the distinct nature of F_2-isoprostane receptors from those of thromboxane A_2. *American Journal of Physiology* 272 (*Renal Physiology* 41), F477–F483.

Galley, H.F., Thornton, J., Howdle, P.D., Walker, B.E. and Webster, N.R. (1997) Combination oral antioxidant supplementation reduces blood pressure. *Clinical Science* 92, 361–365.

Gopaul, N.K., Nourooz-Zadeh, J., Mallet, A.I. and Anggard, E.E. (1994) Formation of F_2-isoprostanes during aortic endothelial cell-mediated oxidation of low density lipoprotein. *FEBS Letters* 348, 297–300.

Halliwell, B. and Grootveld, M. (1987) The measurement of free radical reactions in humans. *FEBS Letters* 213, 9–14.

Hazbun, M.E., Hamilton, R., Holian, A. and Eschenbauer, W.L. (1993) Ozone-induced increases in substance P and 8-epi-prostaglandin $F_{2\alpha}$ in the airways of human subjects. *American Journal of Respiratory and Cell Molecular Biology* 9, 568–572.

Kawikova, I., Barnes, P.J., Takahashi, T., Tadjkarimi, S., Yacoub, M.H. and Belvisi, M.G. (1996) 8-epi-PGF$_{2\alpha}$, a novel noncyclooxygenase-derived prostaglandin, constricts airways *in vitro*. *American Journal of Respiratory and Critical Care Medicine* 135, 590–596.

Kinsella, B.T., O'Mahoney, D.J. and FitzGerald, G.A. (1997) The human thromboxane A2 receptor a isoform (TP$_\alpha$) functionally couples to the G proteins G$_q$ and G$_{11}$ *in vivo* and is activated by the isoprostane 8-epi-prostaglandin F$_{2\alpha}$. *The Journal of Pharmacology and Experimental Therapeutics* 281, 957–964.

Klatt, P. and Esterbauer, H. (1996) Oxidative hypothesis of atherogenesis. *Journal of Cardiovascular Risk* 3, 346–351.

Kromer, B.M. and Tippins, J.R. (1996) Coronary artery constriction by the isoprostane 8-epi-prostaglandin F$_{2\alpha}$. *British Journal of Pharmacology* 119, 1276–1280.

Marley, R., Harry, D., Anand, R., Fernando, B., Davies, S. and Moore, K. (1997) 8-iso-prostaglandin F$_{2\alpha}$, a product of lipid peroxidation, increases portal pressure in normal and cirrhotic rats. *Gastroenterology* 112, 208–213.

Môbert, J., Becker, B.F., Zahler, S. and Gerlach, E. (1997) Hemodynamic effects of isoprostanes (8-iso-prostaglandin F$_{2a}$ and E$_2$) in isolated guinea pig hearts. *Journal of Cardiovascular Pharmacology* 29, 789–794.

Morrow, J.D. and Roberts, L.J. II (1996) The isoprostanes. Current knowledge and directions for future research. *Biochemical Pharmacology* 51, 1–9.

Morrow, J.D. and Roberts, L.J. II (1997) The isoprostanes: unique bioactive products of lipid peroxidation. *Progress in Lipid Research* 36, 1–21.

Morrow, J.D., Hill, K.E., Burk, R.F., Nammour, T.M., Badr, K.F. and Roberts, L.J. II (1990) A series of prostaglandin F$_2$-like compounds are produced *in vivo* in humans by a non-cyclooxygenase, free radical-catalysed mechanism. *Proceedings of the National Academy of Sciences, USA* 87, 9383–9387.

Morrow, J.D., Awad, J.A., Boss, H.J., Blair, I.A. and Roberts, L.J. II (1992) Non-cyclooxygenase-derived prostanoids (F$_2$-isoprostanes) are formed *in situ* on phospholipids. *Proceedings of the National Academy of Sciences, USA* 89, 10721–10725.

Morrow, J.D., Moore, K.P., Awad, J.A., Ravenscraft, M.D., Marini, G., Badr, K.F., Williams, R. and Roberts, L.J. II (1993) Marked overproduction of non-cyclooxygenase derived prostanoids (F2-isoprostanes) in the hepatorenal syndrome. *Journal of Lipid Mediators* 6, 417–420.

Morrow, J.D., Minton, T.A., Mukundan, C.R., Campbell, M.D., Zackert, W.E., Daniel, V.C., Badr, K.F., Blair, I.A. and Roberts, L.J. II (1994) Free radical-induced generation of isoprostanes *in vivo*. Evidence for the formation of D-ring and E-ring isoprostanes. *Journal of Biological Chemistry* 269, 4317–4326.

Morrow, J.D., Frei, B., Longmire, A.W., Gaziano, J.M., Lynch, S.M., Shyr, Y., Strauss, W.E., Oates, J.A. and Roberts, L.J. II (1995) Increase in circulating products of lipid peroxidation (F$_2$-isoprostanes) in smokers. Smoking as a cause of oxidative damage. *New England Journal of Medicine* 332, 1198–1203.

Nanji, A.A., Khwaja, S. and Sadrzadeh, S.M.H. (1994a) Eicosanoid production in experimental alcoholic liver disease is related to vitamin E levels and lipid peroxidation. *Molecular and Cellular Biochemistry* 140, 85–89.

Nanji, A.A., Khwaja, S., Tahan, S.R. and Sadrzadeh, S.M.H. (1994b) Plasma levels of a novel noncyclooxygenase-derived prostanoid (8-isoprostane) correlate with severity of liver injury in experimental alcoholic liver disease. *The Journal of Pharmacology and Experimental Therapeutics* 269, 1280–1285.

Nourooz-Zadeh, J., Gopaul, N.K., Barrow, S., Mallet, A.I. and Anggard, E.E. (1995) Analysis of F_2-isoprostanes as indicators of non-enzymatic lipid peroxidation *in vivo* by gas chromatography-mass spectrometry: development of a solid-phase extraction procedure. *Journal of Chromatography B: Biomedical Applications* 667, 199–208.

Nourooz-Zadeh, J., Halliwell, B. and Anggard, E.E. (1997) Evidence for the formation of F_3-isoprostanes during peroxidation of eicosapentaenoic acid. *Biochemical and Biophysical Research Communications* 236, 467–472.

Nourooz-Zadeh, J., Liu, E.H., Anggard, E. and Halliwell, B. (1998) F_4-isoprostanes: a novel class of prostanoids formed during peroxidation of docosahexaenoic acid (DHA). *Biochemical and Biophysical Research Communications* 242, 338–344.

O'Byrne, P.M. and Fuller, R.W. (1989) The role of thromboxane A_2 in the pathogenesis of airway hyperresponsiveness. *European Respiratory Journal* 2, 782–786.

Okazawa, A., Kawikova, I., Cui, Z., Skoogh, B. and Lotvall, J. (1997) 8-epi-PGF$_{2\alpha}$ induces airflow obstruction and airway plasma exudation *in vivo*. *American Journal of Respiratory and Critical Care Medicine* 155, 436–441.

Palmer, H.J. and Paulson, K.E. (1997) Reactive oxygen species and antioxidants in signal transduction and gene expression. *Nutrition Reviews* 55, 353–361.

Parik, T., Allikmets, K., Teesalu, R. and Zilmer, M. (1996) Evidence for oxidative stress in essential hypertension: perspective for antioxidant therapy. *Journal of Cardiovascular Risk* 3, 49–54.

Patel, T. and Gores, G.J. (1997) Inhibition of bile-salt-induced hepatocyte apoptosis by the antioxidant Lazaroid U83836E. *Toxicology and Applied Pharmacology* 142, 116–122.

Pratico, D. and FitzGerald, G.A. (1996) Generation of 8-epiprostaglandin F_{2a} by human monocytes. Discriminate production by reactive oxygen species and prostaglandin endoperoxide synthase-2. *Journal of Biological Chemistry* 271, 8919–8924.

Pratico, D., Lawson, J.A. and FitzGerald, G.A. (1995) Cyclooxygenase-dependent formation of the isoprostane, 8-epi prostaglandin F_{2a}. *Journal of Biological Chemistry* 270, 9800–9808.

Roberts, L.J. II and Morrow, J.D. (1995) The isoprostanes: novel markers of lipid peroxidation and potential mediators of oxidant injury. *Advances in Prostaglandin, Thromboxane and Leukotriene Research* 23, 219–224.

Roberts, L.J. II, Moore, K.P., Zackert, W.E., Oates, J.A. and Morrow, J.D. (1996) Identification of the major urinary metabolite of the F_2-isoprostane 8-iso-prostaglandin F_{2a} in humans. *Journal of Biological Chemistry* 271, 20617–20620.

Samuelsson, B. (1976) Introduction: new trends in prostaglandin research. *Advances in Prostaglandin and Thromboxane Research* 1, 1–6.

Smith, L.J., Shamsudin, M. and Anderson, J. (1994) Oxidant–antioxidant balance in lungs of patients with asthma (abstract). *American Review of Respiratory and Critical Care Medicine* 149, A965.

Stein, C.M., Tanner, S.B., Awad, J.A., Roberts, L.J. II and Morrow, J.D. (1996) Evidence of free radical-mediated injury (isoprostane overproduction) in scleroderma. *Arthritis and Rheumatism* 39, 1146–1150.

Takahashi, K., Nammour, T.M., Fukunaga, M., Ebert, J.D., Morrow, J.D., Roberts, L.J. II, Hoover, R.L. and Badr, K.F. (1992) Glomerular actions of a free radical-generated novel prostaglandin, 8-epi-PGF$_{2a}$, in the rat. Evidence for interactions with thromboxane A_2 receptors. *Journal of Clinical Investigation* 90, 136–141.

Tse, W.Y., Maxwell, S.R., Thomason, H., Blann, A., Thorpe, G.H., Waite, M. and Holder, R. (1994) Antioxidant status in controlled and uncontrolled hypertension and its relationship to endothelial damage. *Journal of Human Hypertension* 8, 843–849.

Vacchiano, C. and Tempel, G.E. (1994) Role of nonenzymatically generated prostanoid, 8-iso-PGF$_{2\alpha}$, in pulmonary oxygen toxicity. *Journal of Applied Physiology* 77, 2912–2917.

Wang, Y. and Walsh, S.W. (1995) Aspirin inhibits both lipid peroxides and thromboxane in preeclamptic placentas. *Free Radical Biology & Medicine* 18, 585–591.

Indicators of Oxidative Stress, Antioxidants and Human Health

30

MÁRIA DUŠINSKÁ[1], JÁN LIETAVA[2], BEGOÑA OLMEDILLA[3], KATARÍNA RAŠLOVÁ[1], SUSAN SOUTHON[4] AND ANDREW R. COLLINS[5]

[1]*Institute of Preventive and Clinical Medicine, Bratislava, Slovakia;* [2]*2nd Department of Internal Medicine, Comenius University, Bratislava, Slovakia;* [3]*Servicio de Nutrición, Clínica Puerta de Hierro, Madrid, Spain;* [4]*Institute of Food Research, Norwich, UK;* [5]*Rowett Research Institute, Aberdeen, UK*

Introduction

It is generally accepted that oxidative stress is an inevitable feature of life, induced by reactive forms of oxygen released during normal respiration, by the oxidative burst of the macrophages in response to infection, and by a variety of exogenous agents including cigarette smoke and ionizing radiation. It is also agreed that excessive oxidative stress is something to be avoided, as it may be a contributing cause in a variety of human degenerative diseases. The presence of powerful antioxidant defences such as catalase, glutathione and associated enzymes within the cell points to the potential importance to the organism of protecting biomolecules against damage. Oxidation of DNA may lead to mutation (and hence to carcinogenesis); the most common altered base, 8-oxo-guanine, can pair with adenine (A) rather than cytosine (C) (Shibutani *et al.*, 1991), and so if it is present during replication, C→A transversions may result. In heart disease, too, oxidative stress is thought to be a causative factor; peroxidation of lipids occurs during the development of atherosclerotic plaques.

Reflecting this, the 'antioxidant hypothesis' has arisen – and has been accepted virtually without question – as an explanation for the epidemiological link between consumption of fruit and vegetables and decreased risk of both cardiovascular disease and cancer. The hypothesis proposes that it is the natural antioxidants in fruit and vegetables (vitamins C and E, carotenoids, flavonoids, etc.) that are protective, and that they act by scavenging reactive oxygen-derived free radicals before they can cause damage. To test the hypothesis, we need a biomarker for *in vivo* oxidative stress that can be correlated with antioxidant levels on the one hand and with disease on the other.

Here we describe studies of oxidative damage to DNA in white blood cells, measured by two distinct methods: the comet assay and high performance liquid chromatography (HPLC). This biomarker has been used to investigate protective effects of antioxidants *in vivo*, and to estimate levels of oxidative damage in various disease states. First, we provide some information about the two assays.

The Comet Assay (Single-cell Gel Electrophoresis)

Cells are embedded in agarose on microscope slides and lysed with Triton X-100 and 2.5 mol l^{-1} NaCl, which leaves the DNA, stripped of most protein, as nucleoids. The slides are placed in alkaline solution prior to electrophoresis. The still supercoiled loops of DNA resist electrophoresis; however, breaks in the DNA relax supercoils, and loops are then free to migrate. They form a 'tail' to the nucleoid 'head' (hence the designation of 'comet'), and the percentage of DNA that moves into the tail reflects quantitatively the frequency of DNA breaks, over a range from a few hundred per cell up to several thousand (Collins *et al.*, 1996). An assay for DNA breaks is of limited use in looking for endogenous oxidative damage to DNA since breaks can arise in a variety of ways unrelated to oxidation and, furthermore, breaks are quite rapidly repaired by cells. We have therefore modified the assay by incorporating a step, between lysis and electrophoresis, at which the DNA is digested with a bacterial repair endonuclease specific for certain kinds of DNA lesion (Collins *et al.*, 1996). Endonuclease III nicks DNA at sites of oxidized pyrimidines (Doetsch *et al.*, 1987); formamidopyrimidine glycosylase (FPG) recognizes damaged, ring-opened purines (formamidopyrimidines) as well as 8-oxo-guanine, removes them, and nicks the DNA at the resulting base-less sugar (Boiteux *et al.*, 1992). 8-Oxo-guanine is probably the principal substrate for FPG *in vivo* (Boiteux *et al.*, 1992). By measuring the increase in tail DNA in the presence of one of these enzymes, we can estimate the amount of oxidative base damage in a sample of cells. After staining with DAPI (4′,6-diamidine-2-phenylindole dihydrochloride, a fluorescent dye which binds to DNA), relative tail intensity is assessed either visually, by sorting 100 comets into classes from 0 (no detectable tail) to 4 (large tail, minimal head), giving an overall damage score of 0–400; or by computer image analysis, which gives the mean percentage of DNA in the tail. The scoring methods are equally reliable (Collins *et al.*, 1997a), and with each, results can be expressed in terms of actual DNA break frequency by use of a calibration curve established with ionizing radiation to introduce known numbers of DNA breaks (Collins *et al.*, 1996).

We have been able to estimate the normal amount of oxidized pyrimidines and altered purines in leukocytes from 36 healthy male volunteers in Scotland at around 1000 of each per cell (Collins *et al.*, 1997b). It should be appreciated that this measured damage is a steady state level, representing the balance between input and repair, both of which are presumably taking place continuously.

8-Oxo-deoxyguanosine Measured by HPLC

A more conventional method of measuring oxidative damage to DNA is to assay directly for 8-oxo-deoxyguanosine (8-oxo-dG) in hydrolysed DNA, using HPLC with electrochemical detection, or to analyse for 8-oxo-guanine with GC-MS. Reported values for endogenous damage in white blood cell DNA vary enormously – over at least two orders of magnitude (Collins *et al.*, 1997c). Oxidation during isolation and preparation of the DNA hydrolysate for analysis can account for some of the discrepancies, and recently developed methods aimed at eliminating this artefact produce lower values for endogenous damage (Ravanat *et al.*, 1995; Nakajima *et al.*, 1996; Helbock *et al.*, 1998). Taking leukocyte samples from the same 36 individuals sampled with the comet assay, and using an approach which minimizes oxidation during preparation, we found with HPLC a concentration of 8-oxo-dG equivalent to over 10,000 per cell (Collins *et al.*, 1997b). There is clearly an unresolved problem. Either the enzymic methods (the comet assay and other methods where damaged bases are converted to DNA breaks) underestimate damage, or spurious oxidation of dG is still affecting analysis by HPLC. The results to be presented here show that, in spite of this puzzling state of affairs, both approaches – the comet assay with oxidation-specific endonucleases, and HPLC – are apparently valid indicators of oxidative stress.

Oxidative DNA Damage is Linked to Dietary Antioxidant Levels

We have recently used the comet assay to measure DNA damage (strand breaks, oxidized pyrimidines and altered purines) in lymphocytes from Spanish participants in a carotenoid supplementation trial. The volunteers, divided into four matched groups, received daily for 12 weeks 15 mg of either α/β-carotene, lutein, lycopene or a placebo. Blood concentrations of these and other dietary antioxidants were measured by HPLC before and after supplementation. We found no significant effect of the supplements on DNA damage; however, levels of oxidized bases (especially endonuclease III-sensitive sites), measured only at the end of supplementation, showed a significant negative correlation with several of the carotenoids measured at the same time. Surprisingly, this correlation tended to be at least as strong with *pre*-supplementation carotenoid concentrations (Collins *et al.*, 1998a). Figure 30.1 shows, as an example, the negative correlation between endonuclease III sites measured after supplementation and β-carotene concentrations before and after supplementation. This supports the idea that carotenoids (or some other associated phytochemicals) taken up as part of the normal diet modulate the amount of endogenous oxidation occurring in the DNA and, presumably, in other biomolecules. Other antioxidants, such as vitamin C or E, did not show correlations with oxidative damage, but this should not be taken as definitive; it was noticeable that, in this population, baseline (unsupplemented) levels of carotenoids covered a much wider range of values than was seen for vitamin C or E, and so correlations with the latter blood constituents are less likely to emerge. In an earlier study, involving British volunteers, only weakly negative correlations were seen between oxidized pyrimidines and baseline plasma concentrations of carotenoids and antioxidant vitamins (Duthie *et al.*, 1996) – perhaps, again, reflecting limited variability in blood antioxidant levels in this population group.

Supplementation with Antioxidants Can Protect DNA Against Oxidation

In the study mentioned above (Duthie *et al.*, 1996), the main purpose was to investigate the effects of daily supplementation with a mixture of 100 mg of vitamin C, 25 mg of β-carotene and 280 mg of α-tocopherol (vitamin E). After 20 weeks, there was indeed a significant decrease in the levels of oxidized pyrimidines in lymphocytes from smokers and non-smokers (Fig. 30.2), indicating protection against endogenous oxidative damage, and this was reflected in an increased resistance of the lympho-cytes to oxidation incurred on incubation with H_2O_2 (Fig. 30.3). A similar increase in resistance of lymphocytes is seen immediately following a single very large dose of any of these three antioxidants (Fig. 30.4; Panayiotidis and Collins, 1997), and this provides a useful assay for putative antioxidant effects of other dietary constituents that can be administered in a purified form.

The fact that a dietary constituent has a demonstrable antioxidant activity in these assays is no guarantee that it will be beneficial for health,

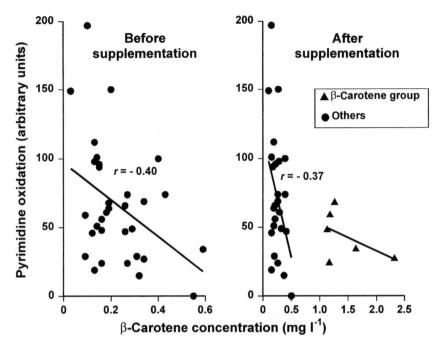

Fig. 30.1. Correlations between serum concentration of β-carotene and level of DNA damage (oxidized pyrimidines) in lymphocytes. Carotenoids were measured before and after the 12-week period during which one group received a supplement of β-carotene; the samples from this group are shown separately in the right-hand panel. DNA damage was measured only at the end of supplementation.

as has been demonstrated by the long-term β-carotene supplementation trials that have shown no effect, or even an increased cancer incidence, in groups receiving β-carotene (The Alpha-Tocopherol Beta-Carotene Cancer Prevention Study Group, 1994; Hennekens *et al.*, 1996; Omenn *et al.*, 1996). However, investigations of this kind are essential for establishing the mechanism of action of antioxidants *in vivo*.

Oxidative Damage is Elevated in Disease

Many human diseases have been associated with oxidative stress, as either cause or effect, and oxidative DNA damage may prove to be a useful biomarker in diagnosis, monitoring of treatment and aetiological investigations. Dandona *et al.* (1996) reported elevated levels of 8-oxo-dG in lymphocytes of diabetics (see also Chapter 20). We have measured DNA strand breaks, endonuclease III- and FPG-sensitive sites in lymphocytes from 10 patients with insulin-dependent diabetes mellitus (IDDM).

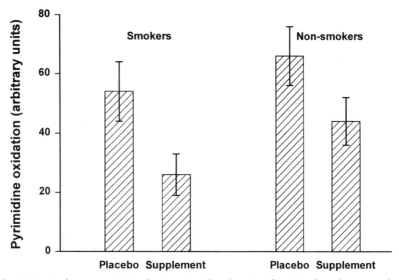

Fig. 30.2. Endogenous DNA damage (oxidized pyrimidines) in lymphocytes after 20 weeks of supplementation with vitamins C and E and β-carotene, or with a placebo. Bars indicate SE of means. Data redrawn from Duthie *et al.* (1996).

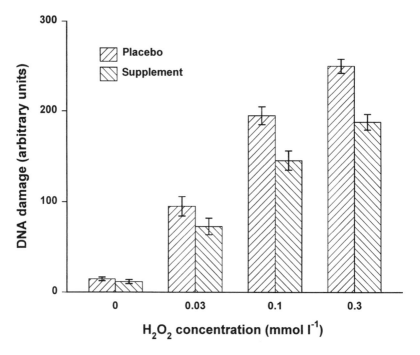

Fig. 30.3. Susceptibility of lymphocytes to *in vitro* DNA damage (strand breaks) on treatment with H_2O_2, after supplementation with antioxidants or placebo, as described in legend to Fig. 30.2. Data redrawn from Duthie *et al.* (1996).

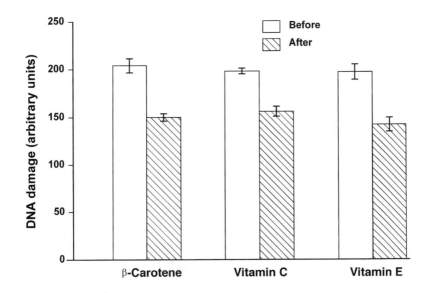

Fig. 30.4. Susceptibility of lymphocytes to *in vitro* DNA damage (strand breaks) on treatment with 0.24 mmol l^{-1} H$_2$O$_2$. Blood samples were taken before a single dose of 45 mg β-carotene, 1 g of vitamin C or 1 g of vitamin E, and 2 h later (vitamin C) or 24 h later (β-carotene and vitamin E). Data redrawn from Panayiotidis and Collins (1997).

Compared with an age- and sex-matched control group, the mean levels of strand breaks and of endonuclease III sites (oxidized pyrimidines) were significantly elevated (Fig. 30.5). In addition, we found a strong correlation between fasting blood glucose level in the IDDM patients and FPG-sensitive sites (Fig. 30.6). Three of the patients had normal blood glucose levels, and if these are excluded from the comparison of mean damage levels, FPG sites, as well as endonuclease III sites, show a significant difference from normal (Collins *et al.*, 1998b). These data are consistent with the idea that elevated blood sugar may play a causative role in oxidative damage in diabetics (Taniguchi *et al.*, 1996).

Rheumatoid conditions are characterized by severe inflammation, associated with the release of reactive oxygen species by macrophages. The resulting free radical damage is thought to exacerbate the condition (Halliwell, 1995). We recently studied eight male patients with ankylosing spondylitis, in which chronic interstitial inflammation, especially of connective tissue, is followed by ossification of the joints of the spine. Lymphocytes were examined with the comet assay; strand breaks and FPG sites were very significantly increased over the levels seen in normal controls (Fig. 30.5), consistent with the elevated oxidative stress.

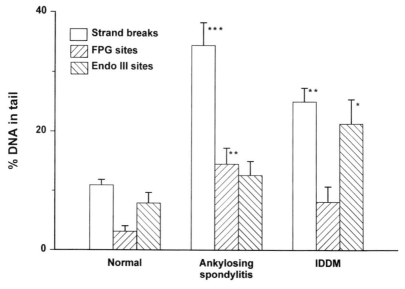

Fig. 30.5. DNA damage measured in lymphocytes of ten normal subjects, eight patients with ankylosing spondylitis, and ten with IDDM (all male; age range approximately 35–55). Mean values are shown, with SE, for DNA strand breaks, altered purines (FPG sites) and oxidized pyrimidines (endo III sites). $^*P < 0.05$; $^{**}P < 0.005$; $^{***}P < 0.0005$.

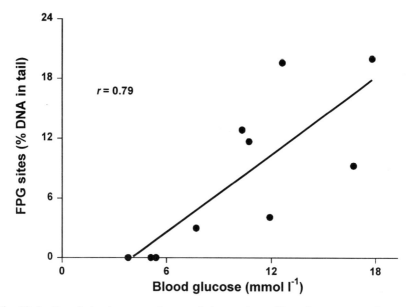

Fig. 30.6. Correlation between degree of glycaemia and lymphocyte DNA damage (FPG-sensitive sites) in a group of 10 IDDM patients. From Collins *et al.* (1998b) with permission from Elsevier Science Inc.

Correlations of Oxidative DNA Damage with Epidemiological Observations

We have measured 8-oxo-dG by HPLC in samples of lymphocytes from healthy, age-matched individuals from five European countries (Spain, France, the Netherlands, Ireland and the UK) (Collins *et al.*, 1998c). Individual samples were pooled to obtain sufficient material for analysis, and so only mean values (for men and women separately in each country) are available. Blood levels of antioxidants were measured in the same individuals (Table 30.1). We expected mean antioxidant levels to vary between countries, with higher levels in southern European groups, but in fact carotenoid and antioxidant vitamin levels were rather similar between countries. However, there was a striking difference in the pattern of oxidative DNA damage between sexes and countries. Levels of 8-oxo-dG in lymphocytes from women were not significantly different in the five countries. Men in the southern European countries (i.e. Spain and France) had similar levels of damage to the women. But in northern Europe, particularly in Ireland, men had up to five times more oxidative base damage than women. Since oxidative DNA damage is considered a likely participant in the process of carcinogenesis, we looked for correlations with cancer mortality at the national level and found a positive association with colorectal cancer in men, a negative association with gastric cancer in women, and no correlation with deaths from all cancers. The most impressive correlation, in fact, is with premature deaths (under the age of 65) from coronary heart disease (Fig. 30.7). This correlation is seen only for men. The geographical pattern of heart disease deaths for women is similar to that for men (though actual rates in each country are much lower), but other factors such as smoking patterns and protection by oestrogens probably obscure any link with oxidative stress.

Table 30.1. Concentration of antioxidants in different centres.

	France		Ireland		Spain	
	M	F	M	F	M	F
Vitamin C (μmol l^{-1})	58.5	65.6	50.5[a]	67.7	61.4[a]	70.0
In plasma	(4.4)	(6.8)	(3.9)	(6.5)	(2.9)	(5.4)
Carotenoids (mg l^{-1})	1.27	1.46	1.06	1.12	1.01	1.14
In serum	(0.07)	(0.15)	(0.08)	(0.11)	(0.12)	(0.10)

Data are means (SEM in parentheses) at week 0. From Collins *et al.* (1998c).
M, Men; F, Women. Within each sex, only samples with the same superscript letter are significantly different (*P*<0.05).

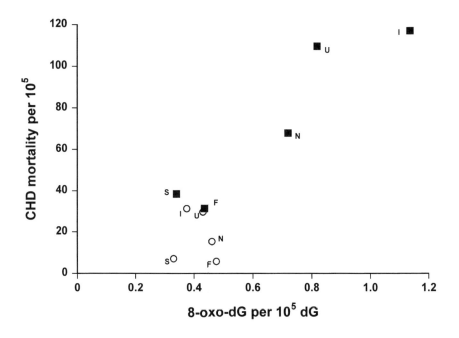

Fig. 30.7. Correlation between concentration of 8-oxo-dG in lymphocyte DNA (measured by HPLC) and national rates of premature death from heart disease. ■, male; ○, female; countries identified by initials (Spain, France, the Netherlands, the UK, Ireland). From Collins *et al.* (1998c) with permission of *FASEB Journal.*

Conclusions

Markers of oxidative damage to lymphocyte DNA are valid indicators of oxidative stress. The comet assay (modified by the use of lesion-specific enzymes) is particularly suitable for use as a biomonitoring tool; it requires extremely small quantities of blood and is simple, rapid and economical. Oxidative stress is clearly demonstrated in conditions such as diabetes, ankylosing spondylitis and hyperlipidaemia. DNA base oxidation is decreased in inverse relation to the presence of antioxidants in the blood. However, the significance of oxidative DNA damage in terms of carcinogenesis remains unproven; there are too many inconsistencies, such as the lack of an elevated cancer risk in diabetics (apart from pancreatic cancer, which might be expected from the nature of the disease), and the lack of correlation between DNA oxidation and cancer mortality at the national level. As with all biomarkers, it is one thing to establish that a correlation exists with other markers, or that a change is seen in particular disease states, and quite another to demonstrate a predictive power of the marker at the level of individual risk of disease.

Acknowledgements

We gratefully acknowledge the expert assistance of Martina Somorovská and Helena Petrovská. The work was funded by the Slovak Ministry of Health, EC contract CIPA-CT94–0129, the Scottish Office Agriculture, Environment and Fisheries Department, and the Ministry of Agriculture, Fisheries and Food.

References

The Alpha-Tocopherol Beta-Carotene Cancer Prevention Study Group (1994) The effect of vitamin E and beta carotene on the incidence of lung cancer and other cancers in male smokers. *New England Journal of Medicine* 330, 1029–1035.

Boiteux, S., Gajewski, E., Laval, J. and Dizdaroglu, M. (1992) Substrate specificity of the *Escherichia coli* Fpg protein (formamidopyrimidine-DNA glycosylase): Excision of purine lesions in DNA produced by ionizing radiation or photosensitization. *Biochemistry* 31, 106–110.

Collins, A.R., Dušinská, M., Gedik, C.M. and Štetina, R. (1996) Oxidative damage to DNA: do we have a reliable biomarker? *Environmental Health Perspectives* 104 (suppl. 3), 465–469.

Collins, A., Dušinská, M., Franklin, M., Somorovská, M., Petrovská, H., Duthie, S., Fillion, L., Panayiotidis, M., Rašlová, K. and Vaughan, N. (1997a) Comet assay in human biomonitoring studies: reliability, validation, and applications. *Environmental and Molecular Mutagenesis* 30, 139–146.

Collins, A.R., Duthie, S.J., Fillion, L., Gedik, C.M., Vaughan, N. and Wood, S.G. (1997b) Oxidative DNA damage in human cells: the influence of antioxidants and DNA repair. *Biochemical Society Transactions* 25, 326–331.

Collins, A., Cadet, J., Epe, B. and Gedik, C. (1997c) Problems in the measurement of 8-oxoguanine in human DNA. Report of a workshop, DNA Oxidation, held in Aberdeen, UK, 19–21 January, 1997. *Carcinogenesis* 18, 1833–1836.

Collins, A., Olmedilla, B., Southon, S., Granado, F. and Duthie, S. (1998a) Serum carotenoids and oxidative DNA damage in human lymphocytes. *Carcinogenesis* 19, 2159–2162.

Collins, A.R., Rašlová, K., Somorovská, M., Petrovská, H., Ondrušová, A., Vohnout, B., Fábry, R. and Dušinská, M. (1998b) DNA damage in diabetes; correlation with a clinical marker. *Free Radical Biology and Medicine* 25, 373–377.

Collins, A.R., Gedik, C.M., Olmedilla, B., Southon, S. and Bellizzi, M. (1998c) Oxidative DNA damage measured in human lymphocytes; large differences between sexes and between countries, and correlations with heart disease mortality rates. *FASEB Journal* 12, 1397–1400.

Dandona, P., Thusu, K., Cook, S., Snyder, B., Makowski, J., Armstrong, D. and Nicotera, T. (1996) Oxidative damage to DNA in diabetes mellitus. *Lancet* 347, 444–445.

Doetsch, P.W., Henner, W.D., Cunningham, R.P., Toney, J.H. and Helland, D.E. (1987) A highly conserved endonuclease activity present in *Escherichia coli*, bovine, and human cells recognizes oxidative DNA damage at sites of pyrimidines. *Molecular and Cellular Biology* 7, 26–32.

Duthie, S.J., Ma, A., Ross, M.A. and Collins, A.R. (1996) Antioxidant supplementation decreases oxidative DNA damage in human lymphocytes. *Cancer Research* 56, 1291–1295.

Halliwell, B. (1995) Oxygen radicals, nitric oxide and human inflammatory joint disease. *Annals of Rheumatoid Disease* 54, 505–510.

Helbock, H.J., Beckman, K.B., Shigenaga, M.K., Walter, P.B., Woodall, A.A., Yeo, H.C. and Ames, B.N. (1998) DNA oxidation matters: the HPLC-electrochemical detection assay of 8-oxo-deoxyguanosine and 8-oxo-guanine. *Proceedings of the National Academy of Sciences, USA* 95, 288–293.

Hennekens, C.H., Buring, J.E., Manson, J.E., Stampfer, M., Rosner, B., Cook, N.R., Belanger, C., LaMotte, F., Gaziano, J.M., Ridker, P.M., Willet, W. and Peto, R. (1996) Lack of effect of long-term supplementation with beta-carotene on the incidence of malignant neoplasms and cardiovascular disease. *New England Journal of Medicine* 334, 1145–1149.

Nakajima, M., Takeuchi, T., Takeshita, T. and Morimoto, K. (1996) 8-Hydroxydeoxyguanosine in human leukocyte DNA and daily health practice factors: effects of individual alcohol sensitivity. *Environmental Health Perspectives* 104, 1336–1338.

Omenn, G.S., Goodman, G., Thornquist, M.D., Balmes, J., Cullen, M.R., Glass, A., Keogh, J.P., Meyskens, F.L. Jr, Valanis, B., Williams, J.H. Jr, Barnhart, S., Chernaick, M.G., Brodkin, C.A. and Hammar, S. (1996) Effects of a combination of beta carotene and vitamin A on lung cancer and cardiovascular disease. *New England Journal of Medicine* 334, 1150–1155.

Panayiotidis, M. and Collins, A.R. (1997) *Ex vivo* assessment of lymphocyte antioxidant status using the comet assay. *Free Radical Research* 27, 533–537.

Ravanat, J.L., Turesky, R.J., Gremaud, E., Trudel, L.J. and Stadler, R.H. (1995) Determination of 8-oxoguanine in DNA by gas chromatography–mass spectrometry and HPLC-electrochemical detection: overestimation of the background level of the oxidized base by the gas chromatography mass spectrometry assay. *Chemical Research in Toxicology* 8, 1039–1045.

Shibutani, S., Takeshita, M. and Grollman, A.P. (1991) Insertion of specific bases during DNA synthesis past the oxidation-damaged base 8-oxodG. *Nature* 349, 431–434.

Taniguchi, N., Kaneto, H., Asahi, M., Takahashi, M., Wenyi, C., Higashiwama, S., Fujii, J., Keiichiro, S. and Kayanoki, Y. (1996) Involvement of glycation and oxidative stress in diabetic macroangiopathy. *Diabetes* 45 (suppl. 3), S81–S83.

Consumer Issues in Relation to Antioxidants

31

EFI FARMAKALIDIS

Austral Health, Killara, Australia

Introduction

The word 'antioxidants' conjures up definite images in the scientists' minds. There are no questions raised as to what these compounds do, what they are and how they might be beneficial to health and our bodies. However, for the average consumer 'antioxidants' are mysterious and unknown. Consumers recognize the word, which has virtually become part of the normal vocabulary. Most people identify a number of foods as being full of antioxidants and therefore good for you. This is especially true for those products that have received significant media coverage. The purpose of this concluding chapter of the book is to discuss how the consumer interacts with nutrition and the reasons why scientific communities need to be aware of their expectations when research is publicized in the 'name of providing them with information' so they can make better dietary choices.

Seeking Long-term Health

Research conducted in the USA shows that virtually everyone (94% of consumers) believes that food and nutrition have a strong/moderate impact on personal health (ADA, 1995, 1997). In fact, the number of consumers who claim they have changed their eating habits to select a healthier diet jumped by 5% to 97% from May 1995 to May 1996. The importance of nutrition is at an all-time high of 78% compared with the gold standard (88% taste; FMI, 1996). Today, seven out of ten consumers (73%) see a need to improve their own diet and recognize that they are not doing all they can to ensure proper nutrition. Overall, the number of health-conscious food shoppers remains stable at 58% (FMI, 1996). Consumer research conducted in Australia shows similar trends. A significant number of people think that a good diet and exercise together make up a 75% contribution to maintaining long-term health. Over 90% of the population believe that a 'good diet' plays an essential role in avoiding heart disease and cancer (L. Dangar, personal communication).

Research in Australia and the USA shows that while in the early 1990s the majority of consumers 'believed that health was due to luck and factors beyond their control in 1997 the majority of consumers disagree that their health is due to external factors or chance' (Sloan, 1997). Consumers believe that they can prevent chronic disease. Research from the Food Marketing Institute in the USA shows that food shoppers' understanding of the diet–disease link is at an all-time high (Table 31.1).

Consumer trends worldwide show that consumers have a far longer-term outlook on health than used to be the case. We know that the elasticity of age is well entrenched, i.e. the notion of being older/elderly stretches further out. Consumers are looking at prolonging personal vitality to maximize 'life options'. They are also interested in minimizing the risks of modern diseases and are adopting a preventative stance towards health.

Interest in vitamins and minerals has significantly increased, showing that there has been a fundamental shift in people's approach to nutrition. People are no longer passive; they are proactive with respect to nutrition and their health. They are re-orienting their health strategies from one of avoidance of macro ingredients such as cholesterol, fat and sodium to inclusion of health-promoting ingredients such as vitamins, minerals, botanicals and phytochemicals (Sloan, 1996).

Table 31.1. Research results from the Food Marketing Institute in the USA (FMI, 1996) showing the percentage of people who are aware of the diet/disease links.

Disease	Awareness (%)
High cholesterol	96
Heart disease	93
High blood pressure	92
Stroke	81
Diabetes	74
Colon cancer	64
Osteoporosis	60
Prostate cancer	46
Breast cancer	37

Increased Knowledge and the Role of the Media

People are interested in the relationship of specific foods or nutrients to diseases such as heart disease and cancer. The functionality of many familiar and new food components is being established by clinical and epidemiological research, and much of this research is often widely publicized. There is typically a 2-year lag before medical and nutrition reports published in the scientific literature begin to surface with any major impact in the consumer media (Applied Biometrics, 1996). Consumers perceive themselves to be far better informed about diet and health and its physical effects than their parents. However, we do know that actual nutrition knowledge is often superficial and misconceptions are widespread.

Surveys (ADA, 1997; L. Dangar, personal communication) show that the media play a vital role in educating people about food, nutrition and health. The major sources of information include television, magazines, newspapers, friends/relatives and books. Although television news is the largest source of information, only 24% of people judge it to be 'very valuable'. Dietitians and doctors are viewed as the most valued source (both at 52%), followed by specialty health/nutrition magazines (39%), nurses (38%) and women's magazines (36%). Newspaper sources of nutrition information are rated as 'very valuable' by 21%, followed by news magazines (17%), radio news (12%) and men's magazines (8%) (ADA, 1997).

The media play a major role in communicating nutrition information to the public by providing more 'user-friendly' information on health, diet and nutrition. A growing number of people (51%) like to hear about new nutrition studies, up from 43% 2 years ago (ADA, 1997). However, in brief news stories, where the media reporters are looking for the '10 second grab', news stories cannot put the new research findings in context. The Center for Media and Public Affairs in Washington, DC, analysed 3 months of news coverage (May–July 1995) from 37 local and national news outlets. The Center found that although the media frequently featured stories about research findings, the stories often omitted details that would allow readers to determine the relevance of the study results to their own lives. Few reports, for example, described the study's design, study conditions or the statistical significance of the results. These omissions do a grave injustice to the studies, because study design is critical to the interpretation of the results (Goldberg and Shuman, 1997).

It is common knowledge, from the scientists' point of view, that each study should be considered in the light of existing knowledge on the subject. However, even preliminary findings are reported as *faits accomplis* in the media. One recent example of this type of story is the media coverage of the study linking lycopene to cancer prevention. The media reports read as 'Tomatoes fight cancer!'.

The public responds to such headlines as they are looking for 'magic bullets' to all their nutrition issues. According to ADA (1997), the biggest perceived hurdles to eating well include the fear of giving up foods (40%), confusion or frustration over nutrition studies and reports (23%), and the belief that a healthful eating style takes too much time (21%). Although the number has declined since ADA's first trends survey in 1991, seven in ten Americans (72%) still believe that foods are either 'good' or 'bad' – one of the biggest food myths and a prime source of consumer confusion.

The four headlines 'Beta carotene; a nugget of nutritional gold', 'All that glitters is not beta-carotene', 'New benefit from beta-carotene', 'Beta no more' appeared in prominent magazines, newspapers, and journals between 1992 and 1996, prompting consumer confusion and frustration. Given the contradictions in the headlines, it is easy to understand why consumers are confused and frustrated (Goldberg and Shuman, 1997).

Consumers are Taking Control of Their Health

People identify with the concept of 'wellness/being healthy and want to choose health solutions for themselves' (L. Dangar, personal communication). Over 80% of non-prescription medicines sold are through self-selection; approximately three-quarters of consumers worldwide opt to self medicate. Consumers want greater autonomy/increased control and a healthier lifestyle. They want relevant, current, user-friendly information, which contributes to a quality self and addresses their needs and expectations.

Research shows that North Americans are shying away from the medical establishment and are taking responsibility for their own health (ADA, 1997). Single-vitamin usage is skyrocketing, as they believe that to achieve health benefits there is a need to take high doses of one vitamin rather than taking multivitamin supplements. The trend for people to take control of their own health coincides with increased visits to alternative health practitioners. Consumers' understanding and beliefs regarding vitamins and minerals have improved dramatically. The reasons for taking vitamins are now disease-prevention driven (Table 31.2).

Table 31.2. Consumers' nutrition knowledge regarding vitamins and minerals. From Sloan (1997).

1992	1995
Health/feel better, 83%	Prevent disease, 62%
Better job, 74%	Increase energy, 54%
Years to live, 55%	Improve fitness, 40%
Sex life, 30%	Increase alertness, 31%
Hair loss, 27%	Reduce stress, 27%
Intelligence quotient, 23%	Treat medical problems, 25%
Eat anything I want, 15%	Fight depression, 21%

Consumer research shows that almost 50% of Australians have used (non-prescribed) alternative medicine at least once in the past year, while 18% have used it two or more times. Twenty per cent of people have visited at least one alternative practitioner in the past 12 months and 30% are likely to do so in the near future. The attitude held by 49% of respondents is that conventional and alternative medicines are complementary. There is a strong belief (65%) in the validity of alternative medicine. Thirty-one per cent of people intend to visit a naturopath, 26% intend to use acupuncture and 19% intend to visit a homeopath for health care (L. Dangar, personal communication).

Estimate of the Self-medication Market: Natural Remedies/Vitamins

In 1993 a representative population survey of 3004 individuals 15 years or older living in South Australia assessed the rates of use and types of alternative medicine and therapists used by this population (Victoria, NSW and Queensland Departments of Health, 1997). The findings of this study were similar to those found in the USA. From that survey we know that Aus$621 million was spent on alternative medicines in Australia in 1993. A sum of Aus$309 million was spent on alternative therapists. The percentage share and dollar value of those (non-prescribed) is shown in Table 31.3.

In the USA traditional vitamins and minerals – now a US$4.6 billion business for nutritional supplements – lead the list of the most desired health-promoting substances. Vitamins E and C are by far the most popular, followed by calcium, the B vitamins, β-carotene and iron (Sloan, 1996). Perhaps the most noteworthy nutrition trend in the last couple of years is

Table 31.3. The percentage market shares and value of alternative medicines (non-prescribed) in Australia. From Victoria, NSW and Queensland Departments of Health (1997).

Treatment	Share of market (%)	Value (Aus $)
Vitamins (non-prescribed)	38	248 million
Herbal medicines	10	62 million
Mineral supplements	9	56 million
Evening primrose oil	8	49 million
Homeopathic medicines	4	24 million
Aromatherapy oils	4	24 million
Ginseng	3	18 million
Chinese medicines	2	12 million
Premenstrual treatments	1.5	9 million

the growing acceptance of botanicals by mainstream consumers. Sales of herbal remedies are growing by 15% annually, with 1995 year-end sales at about US$2.0 billion (Sloan, 1996). More than one-third of consumers surveyed by HealthFocus want to learn more about herbal remedies and how they relate to disease, while 29% want information about how to use or act on what they learn about them (Gilbert, 1995).

Sales of herbal teas are one indication of the growing interest in herbal food products. The sales of ready-to-drink teas grew 60.6% from 1994 to 1995, with total annual sales from all outlets approaching US$2 billion (Sloan, 1996). Sales of functional teas, designed to offer consumers specific health benefits are expected to increase from $60 million in 1995 to $100 million by 2000 (MIS, 1995). In Australia, it is estimated that the herbal market could easily reach Aus$550 million by the end of 1998. Based on herbal manufacturers' estimates that their products represent around 20/25% of the supplement market we can say that the market for herbals is worth Aus$100–120 million, while vitamins and minerals are worth Aus$386–396 million. The growth rate in the herbal/vitamin and mineral market is estimated at 30–35% per annum.

Consumer Trends for the New Millennium

Because of the recently accumulating scientific data demonstrating the relationship between food consumption and disease incidence, consumers are beginning to accept that, to a significant part, 'health is a controllable gift' (Goldberg, 1994). Preventative health measures are really coming of age. The maxim 'you are what you eat' does not just refer to how people feel today but relates also to their future quality of life. In terms of food, this puts a new emphasis not only on how various nutrients affect weight, energy, the general condition of body tone, skin, hair, eyes and so forth but also on their prophylactic effect, how they nourish the essential balance and strength of the body's systems (or 'inner' health).

Advances in science, technology and understanding of human health and disease, along with the blurring of the distinction between food and medicine, indicates that foods will be developed to meet strategic health and well-being objectives. Science will continue to unravel the health-promoting and curative powers of food components and natural substances. Americans' belief in food as medicine will continue to grow. Already 52% of Americans believe that foods can replace the use of drugs and 33% regularly use foods for treatment (Sloan, 1998). Nearly three-quarters (70%) have 'heard of naturally occurring food substances that help prevent disease, even cancer' (FMI, 1996). The contribution of food to health in the preventative sense is liable to become increasingly important. Building up immunities to, or otherwise counteracting, particular health problems (the province of so-called 'function foods') is a key new trend. In a recent food industry research and development (R&D)

survey, functional foods were identified as the single most important consumer trend impacting current new product development (Kevin, 1997).

Twenty years from now, marketing food products for disease prevention and treatment will be commonplace. Already marketing and R&D executives are predicting that the most important health claims 5 years from now will be 'reduce risk of heart disease' and 'reduce the risk of cancer'. Marketers will be directing food products to new generations of young adults who have grown up with existing health problems and risk factors for coronary heart disease and cancer. The incidence of heart disease has been rising since 1993 (Sloan, 1998).

There is no doubt that health will remain on the front burner way beyond the year 2020. Today, the number one health-related interest among food shoppers is 'boosting the immune system' followed by cancer-preventing chemicals in fruits, vegetables and grains, foods that 'reduce the risk of disease or enhance health' and then antioxidants. The ageing baby-boomers will dominate the market for the next 30 years (Sloan, 1998). As a result, health concerns will continue to be energy, immunity, ageing and disease prevention and treatment.

Brand Differentiation

Most food products represent mature categories where brand differentiation is a difficult challenge. Aggressive firms with strong technical development capability will use the interest in health and nutrition as an opportunistic way to differentiate and add value to their brand of product.

During the past few years we have seen the traditional vitamin supplement companies offer customized products for men, women, smokers, joggers, osteoporosis, menopause and children. Look for the food industry to follow suit. The nutraceutical/functional foods market will mature offering foods and beverages not only for improved lifestyle and performance, but also for those with risk factors for the major diseases and those afflicted with chronic conditions.

Over 100 companies are actively selling or developing products that could in due course fit into the category of functional foods. Over 70% of the products are estimated to be drinks; the remainder are foods. The distribution of ingredients in various potential functional foods is estimated to be dietary fibre (40%), calcium (20%), oligosaccharides (20%), lactic acid bacteria (10%) and other (10%) (R. Reid, personal communication).

Functional Foods

The concept of functional foods has broadened the scope of nutrition, health promotion and disease prevention beyond traditional definitions.

The search for a better understanding of why a high consumption of fruits and vegetables is associated with reduced incidence of several chronic diseases has led not only to a re-examination of the function of key vitamins, especially antioxidant vitamins, but also to an examination of the effects and metabolism of non-nutritive components, widely known as phytochemicals.

As a consequence of the attention given to functional foods, the West is giving renewed attention to the Eastern concept of food as medicine. A medical food in the US is defined as 'a food which is formulated to be consumed or administered enterally under the supervision of a physician and which is intended for the specific dietary management of a disease' (FDA, 1996). In Asia, the term 'medicinal food' simply means food used for medical purposes (Weng and Chen, 1996). In traditional Chinese medicine, food and medicine are of equal importance in preventing and treating disease. In the West, functional foods are distinctly not medical foods but are viewed loosely as having distinctly healthful properties beyond basic nutrition. The blurring of boundaries between Eastern and Western ideas about food and health is an indication of the need for more flexible approaches to diet and health, and it has the added benefit of focusing positively on well being.

Terms used to define functional foods

Confusion exists about how to describe this newly evolving area of food and food technology because numerous interchangeable or related terms have been suggested or published in the USA, Europe and Japan. These include terms such as pharmafoods, functional foods, chemopreventive agents and therapeutic foods (Goldberg, 1994). Other new terms, such as bioengineering, biotechnology and designer foods, relate to the technology available to develop phytochemical-rich foods (ADA, 1993).

Functional foods are defined in the US by the National Academy of Sciences as 'any modified food ingredient that may provide a health benefit beyond the traditional nutrients it contains' (Goldberg, 1994). In Japan, these foods are called 'foods for specified health use' and are foods where the components, which maintain body functions, have been processed and their efficacy and safety have been scientifically confirmed by clinical and animal trials (Okhuma, 1998). In Australia, they have been described as 'functional foods'. 'These foods are similar in appearance to conventional foods and are intended to be consumed as part of a usual diet, but have been modified to subserve physiological roles beyond the provision of simple nutrient requirements' (NFA, 1994). In Europe, the situation on 'functional foods' is still very much under discussion, without any concrete recommendations. Common to all of these terms is the assumption that these foods or components have a potential beneficial role in the prevention and treatment of disease.

World Trends in Functional Foods

Japan is currently the world leader in the development of functional foods. In Japan, functional foods (FOSHU) are considered as a major new product opportunity – a new dimension of a wide range of food and drink products.

The value of the Japanese market for functional foods, even without manufacturers being able to make explicit health claims, is of the order of $3 billion, but could well reach $7.5 billion, or approximately 5% of the processed food market in Japan (R. Reid, personal communication).

Less information is available for the European market. The total size of the health food market in Europe was $8.52 billion in 1987 (i.e. West Germany $4.82 billion, UK $2.28 billion and France $1.42 billion), which is about 44% of the US market (R. Reid, personal communication).

Health Claims

Food labels are recognized as important communication tools for dissemination of nutrition and health information.

> ... the enactment in 1990 of the US Nutrition, Labelling and Education Act (NLEA) was a formal recognition of the gains that could flow from moving the body of knowledge about diet and health into the marketplace and embracing the concept that the food label can be a way of communicating nutrition and disease related information to consumers to assist them in constructing healthier diets. (Taylor, 1995)

According to a national survey commissioned by the Australian New Zealand Food Authority (1996), consumers rated food labels as the third most important source of nutrition/health information to help them in their food choices at the point of purchase. The study also showed that labels were not the primary source of information for the consumer; but 'rather labels tended to be used as a tool whereby cumulative health and nutrition knowledge is put into practice to facilitate the purchase decision'. Research from the USA shows similar findings (ADA, 1997).

Food packages are unique as vehicles for information because of their ability to reach into every household. Messages on food packages have durability in that the consumer is able to review the message several times (unlike, for example the electronic broadcast media).

However, although health claims on labels are considered critical by the food industry for communicating the health benefits of a functional food, consumers do not share this view. For example, sales for Ocean Spray cranberry juice increased significantly in 1994 following the publication of a paper on the ability of this beverage to reduce urinary tract infections. Sales for St John's wort rose a staggering 11,449% in 1997 probably because this herb was featured on a prime television news programme. The critical factor in both cases was that the potential health benefits of these products were highly publicized in the media and it has been well documented that the major source of nutrition information for consumers is the media, not food labels (Hasler, 1998).

Diet Versus Supplement

While most Americans do not believe that it is necessary to take a nutrition supplement to ensure proper health, a growing number (35%) do believe so, up from 28% 2 years ago. Women (40%) increasingly believe that they need supplements to ensure proper health, up from 35% (1995) and 27% (1993). They are more likely to believe this than men (30%). Americans with fewer years of education (high school or less, 44%) are more likely than college graduates (29%) to believe that supplements are necessary (ADA, 1997).

Well-designed clinical trials, several of which have been completed (Blot *et al.*, 1993; Li *et al.*, 1993; The Alpha-Tocopherol, Beta-Carotene Cancer Prevention Study Group, 1994), indicate that the beneficial effects associated with a diet high in fruits and vegetables may not be demonstrated when individual nutrients, such as vitamins E and C or β-carotene, are consumed in supplement form. For example, in 1994, Greenberg and colleagues published the results of a 4-year, randomized, controlled clinical trial in which 864 patients were given supplemental vitamins E and C and β-carotene to prevent colorectal adenoma. They concluded that antioxidant supplements were not beneficial in reducing colorectal cancer risk and that 'additional dietary factors' (such as phytochemicals) may play a more important role (Greenberg, 1994).

Phytochemicals will clearly be the next growth opportunity and are quickly emerging as an opportunity for promoting traditional products. More than 70% of consumers have heard that naturally occurring food components may prevent disease, even cancer; 86% think it likely or somewhat likely that fruits, vegetables and grains contain these substances, and only 9% were somewhat dubious (FMI, 1995). More than half (51%) of consumers want to know more about cancer-preventing chemicals in foods.

Pharmaceutical companies will be motivated to isolate components in foods into pill or supplement form and market the individual components for their health benefit. As mentioned previously, consumers are spending an enormous amount of money on vitamin/mineral supplements with the expectation that supplement consumption will ensure optimal health (Sloan, 1997; R. Reid, personal communication). As the evidence of the health benefits of functional foods and phytochemicals grows, consumers may abuse supplements.

Consumption of supplements will only provide selected components in a concentrated form, not the diversity of phytochemicals that occur naturally in foods. In addition to the hundreds or even thousands of components already identified, additional phytochemicals remain to be found. Elucidation of the health benefits of such foods promises to bring new meaning to the traditional dietary recommendations for variety and moderation, as well as new avenues to enhance health.

The public must be convinced that the more appropriate choice would be to increase fruit and vegetable consumption and to incorporate other foods (in addition to fruits and vegetables) containing beneficial health components as part of a varied diet based on the Dietary Guidelines (Dietary Guidelines for Australians, 1992; Human Nutrition Information Service, 1992).

Summary

Never before has the focus on the health benefits of commonly available foods been so strong. The philosophy that food can be health promoting beyond its nutritional value is gaining acceptance within the public arena and among the scientific community as mounting research links diet/food components to disease prevention and treatment. Increasing the availability of healthful foods, including functional foods, is critical to ensuring a healthier population.

Consumers are interested in nutrition and are actively looking for 'magic bullets' to solve all their nutrition problems. The media are the most important source of nutrition information; unfortunately they perpetuate the myth of good and bad foods. Consumers are taking control of their own health and are shying away from traditional advice. They are confused and frustrated with nutrition science and find it difficult to select a proper diet. Thus, they find it easier to self medicate and opt for supplements.

Science is constantly evolving. The optimal levels for antioxidants, phytochemicals and functional food intake have yet to be determined. Health professionals making recommendations relating to antioxidants, phytochemicals and functional foods must recognize that requirements will probably be altered as new research findings come to light. The consumer and the media are hungry for nutrition information. We as scientists are anxious to communicate exciting new research; however, we must be aware that the consumer is anxious to find 'magic bullets'. Therefore it is preferable that nutrition communication should emphasize the need to consume whole foods not supplements.

References

ADA. (1993) Position of the American Dietetic Association: biotechnology and the future of food. *Journal of the American Dietetic Association* 93, 189–191.

ADA. (1995) *ADA 1995 Nutrition Trends Survey* (underwritten by Kraft Foods). American Dietetic Association, Chicago, Illinois.

ADA. (1997) *ADA 1997 Nutrition Trends Survey* (supported in part by the National Cattlemen's Beef Association). American Dietetic Association, Chicago, Illinois.

AGPS (1992) *Dietary Guidelines for Australians.* AGPS, Canberra.

The Alpha-Tocopherol, Beta-Carotene Cancer Prevention Study Group (1994) The effect of vitamin E and beta-carotene on the incidence of lung cancer and other cancers in male smokers. *New England Journal of Medicine* 330, 1029.

ANZFA. (1996) *National Consumer Survey on Food Labelling.* AGPS, Canberra.

Applied Biometrics. (1996) *Health Enhancing Ingredients, a National Profile of Supplement Users.* Applied Biometrics, North Palm Beach, Florida.

Blot, W.J., Li, J.-Y, Taylor, P.R., Guo, W., Dawsey, S., Wang, G.Q., Yang, C.S., Zheng, J.F., Gail, M. and Li, G.Y. (1993) Nutrition intervention trials in Linxian, China: supplementation with specific vitamin/mineral combinations, cancer incidence and disease-specific mortality in the general population. *Journal of National Cancer Institute* 85, 1483–1488.

FDA. (1996) *Regulation of Medical Foods.* Federal Register no. 61, p. S6.

FMI. (1995) *Trends in the United States: Consumer Attitudes and the Supermarket.* Food Marketing Institute, Washington, DC.

FMI. (1996) *Trends in the United States: Consumer Attitudes and the Supermarket.* Food Marketing Institute, Washington, DC.

Gilbert, L. (1995) Consumers and functional foods. Presented at NutraCon, 1995, Las Vegas, Nevada.

Goldberg, I. (1994) *Functional Foods, Designer Foods, Pharmafoods, Nutraceuticals.* Chapman & Hall, New York.

Goldberg, J.P. and Shuman, J.M. (1997) *Making Sense of Scientific Research about Diet. The Food and Nutrition Alliance (FANSA) Statement.* IFT, Chicago, Illinois.

Greenberg, E.R., Baron, J.A., Tosteson, T.D., Freeman, D.H., Beck, G.J., Colacchio, T.A., Coller, J.A., Frankl, H.D. and Haile, R.W. (1994) A clinical trial of antioxidant vitamins to prevent colo-rectal adenoma. *New England Journal of Medicine* 331, 141.

Hasler, C.M. (1998) The US functional foods industry: opportunities and challenges. *Functional Foods* 1, 24.

Human Nutrition Information Service (1992) *Food Guide Pyramid: a Guide to Daily Food Choices.* Department of Agriculture, Washington, DC.

Kevin, K. (1997) The 1997 top 100 R&D Survey. *Food Processing* 58, 70.

Li, J.-Y, Taylor, P.R., Li, B., Dawsey, S., Liu, S.F., Yang, C.S. and Shan, Q. (1993) Nutrition intervention trials in Linxian, China: multiple vitamin/mineral supplementation, cancer incidence, and disease-specific mortality among adults with esophageal dysplagia. *Journal of the National Cancer Institute* 85, 1492.

NFA. (1994) *Functional Foods.* Policy Discussion Paper, NFA, Canberra.

Okhuma, K. (1998) FOSHU: functional foods in Japan. *Functional Foods* 1, 26.

Sloan, E.A. (1996) America's Appetite '96. The Top 10 Trends to watch and work on. *Food Technology* 50, 54.

Sloan, E.A. (1997) Feel Good Foods and Beverages – Nutraceuticals on the Consumer Horizon. 2nd Annual Food and Beverage Conference on Consumer Trends, April 1997.

Sloan, E.A. (1998) Food industry forecast: consumer trends to 2020 and beyond. *Food Technology* 52, 37–44.

Taylor, M. (1995) ILSI Conference on Substantiation of the Impact of Nutrient and Non-Nutrient Antioxidants on Health. Washington, DC.

Victoria, New South Wales and Canberra (1997) *Towards a Safer Choice. The Practice of Traditional Chinese Medicine in Victoria*. AGPS, Canberra.

Weng, W. and Chen, J. (1996) The Eastern perspective on functional foods based on traditional Chinese medicine. *Nutrition Review* 54, S11–S14.

Index

Figures in **bold** indicate major references.
Figures in *italic* refer to diagrams, photographs and tables.